Dangerous Behavior in Clinical and Forensic Psychology

Series Editors

Greg Bohall, CHE Behavioral Health Services, Los Angeles, CA, USA

Mary-Jo Bautista, Mary-Jo Bautista, DBA, Behavior Specialist,
Whittier, CA, USA

Sabrina Musson, Tonawanda, NY, USA

This new series will close the gap between forensic rehabilitation and prediction/ intervention approaches. Taking a broad view of what is sometimes termed deviant behavior, the series will provide individual volumes on key problems such as domestic violence, bullying, homicide, and terrorism. Each topic will be handled in a systematic way that will cover major psychological concepts as well as policy issues, and clinical practice. Useful to a range of professionals who desire a brief evidence-based overview of problems critical to the health and well-being of individuals and society in general. It is particularly relevant to mental health professionals and forensic professionals as well as those in law enforcement.

More information about this series at http://link.springer.com/series/16078

Jennifer E. Vitale
Editor

The Complexity of Psychopathy

Springer

Editor
Jennifer E. Vitale
Hampden–Sydney College
Farmville, VA, USA

ISSN 2524-4051 ISSN 2524-406X (electronic)
Dangerous Behavior in Clinical and Forensic Psychology
ISBN 978-3-030-83155-4 ISBN 978-3-030-83156-1 (eBook)
https://doi.org/10.1007/978-3-030-83156-1

This Springer imprint is published by the registered company Springer Nature Switzerland AG
The registered company address is: Gewerbestrasse 11, 6330 Cham, Switzerland

Biographies of the Series Editors

Greg Bohall, Psy.D., C.R.C., MAC, ICADC, CADC-III: Principal Series Editor
Dr. Bohall is the co-owner of Innovative Psychological Solutions, A Professional Corporation, and is the current principal series editor of the series titled Dangerous Behavior in Clinical and Forensic Psychology through Springer. He earned a doctorate in psychology (Psy.D.) in clinical forensic psychology and provides consultation for numerous organizations throughout the United States. Dr. Bohall is currently internationally and nationally recognized as a Certified Rehabilitation Counselor (C.R.C.), as a Master Addiction Counselor (MAC), and as an International Certified Alcohol and Drug Counselor (ICADC). In the State of California, he is recognized as a Certified Alcohol and Drug Counselor-III (CADC-III). Recently, Dr. Bohall was the principal author in the co-authored textbook *The Psychologist's Guide to Professional Development (2017)* as well as writing *Legal System and Gender, Posttraumatic Stress Disorder and Gender,* and *Gender Conformity* in *The SAGE Encyclopedia of Psychology and Gender (2017).* Furthermore, his academic work can be found in the *Journal of Family Violence* and *Aggression and Violent Behavior.* Dr. Bohall also serves on the editorial board of the *Journal of Aggression, Maltreatment, & Trauma,* the *Journal of Family Trauma, Child Custody, & Child Development,* the *Journal of Child Sexual Abuse*, and the *Journal of Child & Adolescent Trauma.* Lastly, Dr. Bohall's academic and research interests include forensic assessment and intervention; crisis intervention and negotiation techniques; evaluation of interviewing, investigation, and interrogation procedures; psychopathy; and offender profiles and victimology of individuals involved in intimate partner violence cases.

Mary-Jo Bautista-Bohall, Psy.D.: Associate Series Editor
Dr. Bautista-Bohall is the co-owner of Innovative Psychological Solutions, A Professional Corporation, and is an associate series editor of the series titled Dangerous Behavior in Clinical and Forensic Psychology. Dr. Bautista-Bohall is an early career psychologist; she earned a doctorate in psychology (Psy.D.) in applied clinical psychology in 2013. She is a licensed clinical psychologist in the State of

California and currently provides services for various state and government funded agencies. Dr. Bautista-Bohall is an advocate for underprivileged populations and presents her work at national and international conferences promoting the need for mental health services for minorities. Her current projects include decreasing the stigma of mental health with Filipino Americans through the development of culturally specific interventions. Dr. Bautista-Bohall is also dedicated to educating practitioners on promising and effective interventions for individuals diagnosed with a neurodevelopmental disability. More specifically, she has extensive experience providing a variety of interventions for individuals with intellectual disabilities. In the forensic realm, Dr. Bautista-Bohall helps determine various capacities of individuals with a neurodevelopmental disability; this information is then used to determine ability to participate in the judicial process and to address other psycholegal questions. Dr. Bautista-Bohall's research interests include the identification of diversity factors that are associated with different deviant behaviors. Academically, she has been published three times in peer-reviewed works as well as her recent co-authored textbook, *The Psychologist's Guide to Professional Development (2017);* this text was designed to help students and fellow early career professionals reach their personal and academic goals.

Sabrina Musson, Ph.D., LMHC, CASAC: Associate Series Editor
Dr. Musson is an associate editor of the series titled Dangerous Behavior in Clinical and Forensic Psychology. Dr. Musson is a Clinical Assistant Professor in the Graduate School of Education's Counseling School and Educational Psychology Mental Health Counseling Program at the State University of New York at Buffalo since September 2018. Dr. Musson was also working for the University of Buffalo's Research Institute on Addictions as a project director for various research studies funded by the National Institutes of Health from 2013 to 2018. She has been the vice president of the not-for-profit Bridges From Borders since January 2021, assisting in mental health advocacy, training, and research within immigrant and refugee populations of Western New York. Her previous teaching experience was at Medaille College in the Division of Applied and Social Sciences as a clinical assistance professor from August 2016 to 2018, after working as an adjunct professor with Medaille since 2011. Dr. Musson served as the coleader for the Western New York Chapter of the New York Mental Health Counseling Association from 2019 to 2021. She earned her master's degree in mental health counseling from Medaille College and her Ph.D. in counselor education from the State University of New York at Buffalo. She has over 20 years of experience working in the human services field. During this span, Dr. Musson gained over 10 years of clinical experience and over 10 years of experience in research; in both areas she has performed in supervisory and practice roles. Her fields of specialization include addictions, homelessness, intimate partner violence, crisis intervention, and clinical supervision. Dr. Musson also serves as a reviewer for the *Journal of Aggression, Maltreatment & Trauma* and the *Journal of Child and Adolescent Trauma.*

Biography of the Volume Editor

Jennifer E. Vitale, Ph.D.: Volume Editor
Dr. Vitale is a professor of psychology at Hampden-Sydney College. Dr. Vitale received her Ph.D. in clinical psychology in 2003 from the University of Wisconsin-Madison. Dr. Vitale has written for both academic and clinical audiences, and has contributed review chapters on psychopathy to several key texts, including Patrick's (2018) *Handbook of Psychopathy,* Gacono's (2016) *Clinical and Forensic Assessment of Psychopathy: A Practitioner's Guide,* and Craighead, Miklowitz, and Craighead's (2013) *Psychopath ology: History, Diagnosis, and Empirical Foundations*. In addition, her original research in the areas of attention processing in psychopathy and psychopathy in women can be found in journals including the *Journal of Psychopathology and Behavioral Assessment*, *Criminal Justice and Behavior*, *Journal of Abnormal Psychology*, and *Neuropsychology.*

Preface

When considering the rapid expansion of specialties in the field of psychology coupled with disciplines outside of the behavioral sciences seeing the value of psychology in their day-to-day activities, researchers and clinicians alike are seeing "their place" in areas where they have traditionally not been before. For example, developmental psychologists whose expertise is in development across the lifespan may be involved in providing expert testimony on developmental factors as it relates to addressing various psycholegal questions. Sport psychology has typically centered on athlete performance; however, sport psychologists are implementing more clinical interventions as "grit" and "determination" can only take an individual so far in their athletic performance. Clinical interventions to increase employee job satisfaction, improve employee motivation, and improve organizational communication have been sought from the clinical psychology specialty when it has not been as prominently involved historically (I/O psychology). Indeed, this expansion of ideas and researcher/clinician endorsement is exciting for the future of psychology.

Identifying and implementing various theories or clinical perspectives from these specialties to a central issue or population is an incredible benefit in psychology today. Moreover, many of these central issues or populations have not been explored for some of the various theories/perspectives or even within some specialties themselves; we believe the expansive nature of the volumes in this series provide an answer to that deficiency. As series editors, our goal was to identify these various clinical and forensic considerations in need of further exploration, identify the various components of each central issue or population, and help develop an expansive volume on the central issue or population where numerous perspectives are involved in order to improve understanding as well as how to effectively intervene.

The central issues and populations in this series were selected by the series editors; all have clinical and/or forensic aspects that make them important for publication at this time. Volume editors were selected for their specific expertise as it relates to the central issue or population. For this volume, Dr. Jennifer E. Vitale has been appointed based on her expertise and willingness to direct this expansive project through its completion. Chapter authors were selected in the same manner to ensure that each volume will serve as a valuable reference for academics and clinicians alike. Through ongoing collaboration with the series editorial team, Dr. Vitale has been able to strike a successful balance of authors that include those with a strong research background and/or a strong clinical background.

This volume synthesizes the important research and practice developments in the field of psychopathy. As the reader will review, psychopathy has undergone numerous conceptualizations over the past century and it continues to evolve in its understanding. The addition of various perspectives coupled with this unique approach to psychopathy makes this volume in the series titled *Dangerous Behavior in Clinical and Forensic Psychology* an essential resource for researchers and clinicians.

Los Angeles, CA, USA
Greg Bohall
Mary-Jo Bautista-Bohall

Buffalo, NY, USA
Sabrina Musson

Contents

Contributors

John R. Anderson Department of Psychology, Rosalind Franklin University of Medicine and Science, North Chicago, IL, USA

Arielle R. Baskin-Sommers Department of Psychology, Yale University, New Haven, CT, USA

Blair D. Batky Department of Psychology, The University of Alabama, Tuscaloosa, AL, USA

Julie Blais Department of Psychology and Neuroscience, Dalhousie University, Life Sciences Centre, Halifax, NS, Canada

Katherine W. Bogen Department of Psychology, University of Nebraska-Lincoln, Lincoln, Nebraska, USA

Greg Bohall Innovative Psychological Solutions, A Professional Corporation, Los Angeles, CA, USA

Andrew P. Bontemps Department of Psychology, The University of Alabama, Tuscaloosa, AL, USA

Nadia Bounoua Department of Psychological and Brain Sciences, University of Delaware, Newark, DE, USA

Andrew E. Brankley Kurt Freund Phallometric Lab & Sexual Behaviours Clinic, Toronto, ON, Canada

Grace M. Brennan Department of Psychology, Yale University, New Haven, CT, USA

Susan Cooper Consultant Forensic Psychologist, Durham Therapy Centre, Durham, UK

Cristina Crego Department of Psychology, Longwood University, Farmville, VA, USA

Mark R. Dadds School of Psychology, The University of Sydney, Camperdown/Darlington, NSW, Australia

Monika Dargis Department of Psychiatry, New York Presbyterian- Weill Cornell Medical Center, New York, NY, USA

Corine de Ruiter Faculty of Psychology & Neuroscience, Maastricht University, Maastricht, the Netherlands

Stephen Arthur Diamond Licensed Clinical and Forensic Psychologist, Marina del Rey, CA, USA

Lauren F. Fournier Department of Psychology, University of South Florida, Tampa, FL, USA

Gianni Francesetti IPsiG – International Institute for Gestalt Therapy and Psychopathology, Department of Psychology, University of Torino, Turin, Italy

Katy Drorit Gaines Neuro Health, Inc., Beverly Hills, CA, USA

David J. Hawes School of Psychology, The University of Sydney, Camperdown/Darlington, NSW, Australia

Martin Hildebrand Private Practice, Amsterdam, the Netherlands

Jerry L. Jennings Liberty Healthcare Corporation, Bala Cynwyd, PA, USA

Shan Jumper IDHS Treatment and Detention Facility, Rushville, IL, USA

Salpi Kevorkian Injury and Violence Prevention Research Lab, Virginia Commonwealth University Health, Richmond, VA, USA

David Kosson Department of Psychology, College of Health Professions, Rosalind Franklin University of Medicine and Science, North Chicago, IL, USA

Jennifer Lamb Teesside University, Durham, UK

Darren Lemon Applied Behavioral Alternatives, Inc, Arcadia, CA, USA

Natasha S. Maltais Department of Psychology, Carleton University, Ottawa, ON, Canada

Annette McKeown Kolvin Service, Cumbria, Northumberland Tyne and Wear NHS Foundation Trust, Newcastle University, Newcastle upon Tyne, UK

Beatriz Mendez Department of Psychology, The University of Alabama, Tuscaloosa, AL, USA

Rickie Miglin Department of Psychological and Brain Sciences, University of Delaware, Newark, DE, USA

Devon L. L. Polaschek Te Kura Whatu Oho Mauri School of Psychology, Te Puna Haumaru NZ Institute for Security and Crime Science, Te Whare Wānanga o Waikato The University of Waikato, Hamilton, New Zealand

Dennis E. Reidy School of Public Health & Center for Research on Interpersonal Violence, Georgia State University, Atlanta, GA, USA

Naomi Sadeh Department of Psychological and Brain Sciences, University of Delaware, Newark, DE, USA

Randall T. Salekin Department of Psychology, The University of Alabama, Tuscaloosa, AL, USA

Vilas Sawrikar School of Health and Social Sciences, The University of Edinburgh, Edinburgh, UK

Allison M. Stuppy-Sullivan Department of Psychology, Yale University, New Haven, CT, USA

Nicholas D. Thomson Department of Surgery, Virginia Commonwealth University Health, Richmond, VA, USA

Adelaide A. Verdugo-Thomson Injury and Violence Prevention Research Lab, Virginia Commonwealth University Health, Richmond, VA, USA

Edelyn Verona Department of Psychology, University of South Florida, Tampa, FL, USA

Jennifer E. Vitale Department of Psychology, Hampden-Sydney College, Hampden-Sydney, VA, USA

Jessica Yakeley British Psychoanalytical Society, Forensic Psychotherapy and Portman Clinic Tavistock and Portman NHS Foundation Trust, London, UK

Chapter 1
Introduction to Psychopathy

Jennifer E. Vitale

Abstract Lewis (Psychol Med 4:133–140, 1974) referred to psychopathy as "the elusive category", a terminology that remains relevant even after decades of research on the construct. The associated characteristics (e.g., shallow emotionality, callousness, lack of guilt, manipulativeness, impulsivity, and irresponsibility) delineate individuals who often exploit those around them and who engage in criminal and other antisocial behaviors. Although the PCL-R (Hare RD, Can Psychol 57:21–34, 2003) opened the door to decades of important psychopathy research, questions regarding the construct still proliferate. This volume captures that continued interest in chapters that address the field's conceptualizations of the construct, our understanding of the points at which psychopathy touches other clinical syndromes that are classified within DSM-V, and ongoing attempts to design and/or implement effective treatments. The chapters assembled in this volume highlight a diversity of developments and perspectives in both research and clinical arenas, and look ahead to future avenues of exploration.

Keywords Psychopathy · PCL-R · ASPD

Lewis (1974) referred to psychopathy as "the elusive category", a terminology that remains relevant even after decades of research on the construct. Certainly, psychopathy still stands somewhat separate from many other syndromes, with no direct representation in our primary diagnostic tools (e.g., DSM-5), and with a history of being conceptualized and applied as a forensic construct just as often as a clinical one. The associated characteristics (e.g., shallow emotionality, callousness, lack of guilt, manipulativeness, impulsivity, and irresponsibility) delineate individuals who often exploit those around them and who engage in criminal and other antisocial behaviors. In the absence of diagnostic criteria provided by the Diagnostic and Statistical Manuals (DSM through DSM 5) of the American Psychiatric Association, the introduction of the Psychopathy Checklist – Revised (PCL-R; Hare, 2003)

J. E. Vitale (✉)
Hampden-Sydney College, Hampden-Sydney, VA, USA
e-mail: jvitale@hsc.edu

J. E. Vitale (ed.), *The Complexity of Psychopathy*, Dangerous Behavior in Clinical and Forensic Psychology, https://doi.org/10.1007/978-3-030-83156-1_1

provided a both a means for assessing the syndrome consistently across samples as well as a common vocabulary for describing the psychopathic individual.

Although the PCL-R opened the door to decades of important psychopathy research, questions regarding the central components of psychopathy (e.g., Cooke et al., 2006; Hare, 1998; Lilienfeld, 1994), the generalizability of the construct across groups (e.g., Cooke & Michie, 1999; Sullivan et al., 2006; Verona & Vitale, 2018), and the relation between psychopathy and other clinical syndromes (especially Antisocial Personality Disorder) (e.g. Hare, 2016; Lykken, 1995; Verona et al., 2012) proliferated. Today, the psychopathy literature can appear even less cohesive than it did in the mid-1990's, as assessment tools representing alternative conceptualizations of the construct are developed and validated (e.g., the TriPM, Patrick, 2010; the CAPP, Kreis et al., 2012) and conceptualizations that place an emphasis on dimensional and personality-based approaches gain ground, not just within the psychopathy literature, but across psychology and psychiatry more broadly (e.g., Crego, Chap. 12, this volume). Given these myriad threads, it is not surprising that a simple "psychopathy" keyword search reveals the several thousand articles that have been published in just the past few decades, highlighting the significant interest that surrounds the syndrome.

The current volume captures that continued interest in chapters that address the field's conceptualizations of the construct (e.g., Bontemps et al., Chap. 10; Gaines, Chap. 20; McKeown et al., Chap. 4; Vitale, Chap. 2), as well as our understanding of the points at which psychopathy touches other clinical syndromes that are classified within DSM-V, including neurodevelopmental disorders (Bohall et al., Chap. 6), schizophrenia and psychotic disorders (Anderson & Kosson, Chap. 7), mood disorders (Dargis, Chap. 8), and substance use disorders (Brennan et al., Chap. 11). Other chapters address ongoing attempts by clinicians to design and/or implement effective treatments (e.g., Blais et al., Chap. 13; de Ruiter & Hildebrand, Chap. 14; Jennings & Jumper, Chap. 18; Sawrikar et al., Chap. 19). Additionally, a variety of empirical and clinical perspectives are represented, as authors draw on their own research or clinical work. While each chapter reviews and analyzes a different aspect of the syndrome, a comprehensive reading reveals important, overlapping threads across chapters that speak to current pivotal issues in the field.

First, throughout the volume, authors repeatedly confront the question of heterogeneity within the psychopathy construct. This has been a consistent issue within the literature, as Karpman (1941) distinguished between "primary" and "secondary" psychopaths, and—more recently—Lykken (1995) drew a distinction between psychopaths and sociopaths. Consistent with these distinctions, some chapters in the volume highlight the associations between individual components of psychopathy (e.g., factors/facets) and other key variables, whereas other chapters invoke the long-standing distinction between "primary" and "secondary" psychopathy types. In Chap. 3, Bounoua et al. address the multidimensional conceptualization of psychopathy in adolescents and highlight the particular importance of callous/unemotional traits in this population. Similarly, the components of psychopathy and their relations to other clinical syndromes are highlighted in chapters by Bontemps et al. (Chap. 10), Thomson et al. (Chap. 5), Dargis (Chap. 8), Fournier and Verona (Chap.

9), and Brennan et al. (Chap. 11). Finally, the heterogeneity of psychopathy is touched upon in the clinical chapters, where these distinctions are particularly noted in the context of rehabilitation models (Blais et al., Chap. 13) and family therapy contexts (Sawrikar et al., Chap. 19), as well as by existential (Diamond, Chap. 16) and psychodynamic approaches (Yakeley, Chap. 15).

Second, as authors unpack the components of psychopathy, they also identify points where the early experiences of psychopathic individuals become potentially necessary considerations in our discussion of the factors that contribute to the development of the syndrome. Despite the historical tendency to view psychopathic individuals as "born, not made", research makes clear that experience may matter. These connections become especially apparent in the chapters examining psychopathy's association with trauma (Fournier & Verona, Chap. 9), differences in the development and expression of psychopathy across gender (McKeown et al., Chap. 4), and development of psychopathy in youth (Bounoua et al., Chap. 3). The role these factors may play in the effectiveness of interventions are also addressed (e.g., Jennings & Jumper, Chap. 18).

Third, across multiple chapters, authors note that a traditional view of psychopathy as "untreatable" and the associated focus on psychopathy as a forensic, rather than a clinical, construct has potentially inhibited intervention research and implementation (e.g., de Ruiter, Chap. 14; Polaschek, Chap. 21). Well-validated models for the treatment of antisocial behavior exist, and such models could be fruitfully applied to psychopathy. Simultaneously, in other chapters, clinicians draw on their experiences of working with psychopathic individuals to explore and describe ways in which psychopathy can be addressed through the lenses of existential (Diamond, Chap. 16), psychoanalytic (Yakeley, Chap. 15) and gestalt (Francesetti, Chap. 17) perspectives.

Across these chapters, authors examine the experiences and backgrounds of the psychopathic individual and the ways in which these can contribute to psychopathic behavior. However, at no point is the significant harm that can be caused by these individuals forgotten. Throughout the volume, vivid reminders of the costs of psychopathy to individuals and to the broader community are presented. For example, Thomson et al. (Chap. 5) explore the associations between psychopathy and aggression/violence, while Reidy and Bogen (Chap. 22) present a public health perspective on the syndrome that illustrates its far-reaching negative effects.

The chapters assembled in this volume highlight a diversity of developments and perspectives in the field. New approaches to the assessment of the psychopathy syndrome reflect changes in our conceptualization of the construct. Explorations of the ways that psychopathy relates to other clinical syndromes increases interest in how both psychobiological and environmental factors can influence the expression of psychopathy. Further, changes regarding the treatability of psychopathy will lead to important changes in how psychopathy interventions are designed and implemented. Certainly, this shifting landscape makes clear that psychopathy, in many ways, remains an "elusive category". However, as the literature reviewed in this volume makes clear, it is one in which a number of researchers and clinicians remain engaged in active and lively pursuit.

References

Cooke, D. J., & Michie, C. (1999). Psychopathy across cultures: North America and Scotland compared. *Journal of Abnormal Psychology, 108*, 58–68.

Cooke, D. J., Michie, C., & Hart, S. D. (2006). Facets of clinical psychopathy: Towards clearer measurement. In C. Patrick (Ed.), *Handbook of psychopathy* (pp. 91–106). Guilford Press.

Hare, R. D. (1998). Psychopaths and their nature: Implications for the mental health and criminal justice systems. In T. Millon & E. Sorenson (Eds.), *Psychopathy: Antisocial, criminal, and violent behavior* (pp. 188–212). Guilford Press.

Hare, R. D. (2003). *Manual for the Hare psychopathy checklist–revised* (2nd ed.). Multi-Health Systems.

Hare, R. D. (2016). Psychopathy, the PCL-R, and criminal justice: Some new findings and current issues. *Canadian Psychology, 57*, 21–34.

Karpman, B. (1941). On the need of separating psychopathy into two distinct clinical types: The symptomatic and the idiopathic. *Journal of Criminal Psychopathology, 3*, 112–137.

Kreis, M. K. F., Cooke, D. J., Michie, C., Hoff, H. A., & Logan, C. (2012). The Comprehensive Assessment of Psychopathic Personality (CAPP): Content validation using prototypical analysis. *Journal of Personality Disorders, 26*, 402–413.

Lewis, A. (1974). Psychopathic personality: A most elusive category. *Psychological Medicine, 4*, 133–140.

Lilienfeld, S. O. (1994). Conceptual problems in the assessment of psychopathy. *Clinical Psychology Review, 14*, 17–38.

Lykken, D. T. (1995). *The antisocial personalities*. Erlbaum.

Patrick, C. J. (2010). *Operationalizing the triarchic conceptualization of psychopathy: Preliminary description of brief scales for assessment of boldness, meanness, and disinhibition*. Unpublished manual, Department of Psychology, Florida State University.

Sullivan, E. A., Abramowitz, C. S., Lopez, M., & Kosson, D. S. (2006). Reliability and construct validity of the psychopathy checklist-revised for Latino, European American, and African American male inmates. *Psychological Assessment, 18*, 382–392.

Verona, E., & Vitale, J. E. (2018). Psychopathy in women: Assessment, manifestations, and etiology. In C. Patrick (Ed.), *Handbook of psychopathy* (2nd ed., pp. 509–528). Guilford Press.

Verona, E., Sprague, J., & Sadeh, N. (2012). Inhibitory control and negative emotion processing psychopathy and antisocial personality disorder. *Journal of Abnormal Psychology, 121*, 498–510.

Chapter 2
Profile and Assessment of Psychopathy

Jennifer E. Vitale

Abstract Clinicians and legal professionals are often familiar with psychopathic individuals, who account for a sizable portion of most incarcerated or forensic populations, and whose characteristic interpersonal, affective, and behavioral features distinguish them from other antisocial individuals. Psychopathy represents as a construct distinct from other antisocial syndromes, associated with different causal models and treatment responses (Hare RD, Can Psychol 57:21–54, 2016; Lykken DT, The antisocial personalities. Erlbaum, Hillsdale, 1995; Verona E, Sprague J, Sadeh N, J Abnormal Psychol 121:498–510, 2012). This chapter will provide an overview of the clinical features of psychopathy, with a primary emphasis on those characteristics highlighted by Cleckley (*The Mask of Sanity*. Mosby, St. Louis, 1941/1988) in his seminal work *The Mask of Sanity*. It will then review the most commonly used diagnostic instruments, including the PCL-R and its progeny, as well as several well-validated, alternate measures of the construct. Throughout, the chapter will consider some of the key points of contention or controversy relevant to assessment of the syndrome, including the underlying structure and potential heterogeneity of psychopathy.

Keywords Psychopathy · Assessment · PCL-R · Self-report psychopathy · Cleckley

2.1 Introduction and Clinical Description

Clinicians and legal professionals are often familiar with psychopathic individuals, who account for a sizable portion of most incarcerated or forensic populations, and whose characteristic interpersonal, affective, and behavioral features distinguish them from other antisocial individuals. Individuals exhibiting those features now associated consistently with the construct of psychopathy are found throughout psychiatric history, although not always under the "psychopathy" label. For example,

J. E. Vitale (✉)
Hampden-Sydney College, Hampden-Sydney, VA, USA
e-mail: jvitale@hsc.edu

J. E. Vitale (ed.), *The Complexity of Psychopathy*, Dangerous Behavior in Clinical and Forensic Psychology, https://doi.org/10.1007/978-3-030-83156-1_2

texts will often trace the concept to Pinel's (1806) "manie sans delire", which was characterized by a tendency towards engaging in impulsive and destructive behavior despite otherwise intact reasoning. Similarly, those same impulsive and antisocial features would have been captured by Kraepelin's "morbid personalities", Schneider's "affectionless" personalities, or Millon's "aggressive personalities". The recurrence of callous, impulsive, and antisocial behavior as core features of these conceptualizations would also lay the groundwork for the sometimes-controversial association between what we now consider "psychopathy" and criminality and violence. Such associations would be presaged by Rush's "innate, preternatural moral depravity" (1812, p.112), or Prichard's (1835) "moral insanity". Even the later editions of the Diagnostic and Statistical Manual (DSM) of the American Psychiatric Association (i.e., DSM III, III-R, IV, and 5) folded features typical of the psychopathic individual into their diagnosis for Antisocial Personality Disorder (ASPD), the classification most strongly associated with criminal behavior.

Many key features of psychopathy overlap with the characteristics of ASPD. Nevertheless, researchers have consistently argued that, as a result of distinct patterns in prevalence, etiology, and efficacy of intervention, the two constructs can and should be differentiated (e.g., Crego & Widiger, 2015; Verona et al., 2012). Importantly, although the DSM has historically included criteria for ASPD that are also characteristic of the prototypical psychopath (e.g., guiltlessness, impulsivity), these criteria were not meant to identify this subgroup of antisocial individuals, specifically. As a result, the prevalence of ASPD is higher (roughly 2–3 times greater than psychopathy), suggesting there will be many individuals who meet DSM criteria for ASPD who are not psychopathic (Hare & Neumann, 2008; Ogloff, 2006). Further, as the criteria for ASPD grew more behavioral in nature across DSM editions (e.g., conduct disorder present before age 15, repeatedly performing acts that are grounds for arrest), there was an associated increase in the likelihood of excluding some individuals who would be considered psychopathic.

Psychopathy represents as a construct distinct from other antisocial syndromes, associated with different causal models and treatment responses (Hare, 2016; Lykken, 1995; Verona et al., 2012). This chapter will provide an overview of the clinical features of psychopathy, with a primary emphasis on those characteristics highlighted by Cleckley (1941/1988) in his seminal work *The Mask of Sanity*. It will then review the most commonly used diagnostic instruments, including the PCL-R and its progeny, as well as several well-validated, alternate measures of the construct. Throughout, the chapter will consider some of the key points of contention or controversy relevant to assessment of the syndrome, including the underlying structure and potential heterogeneity of psychopathy.

2.1.1 The Mask of Sanity

Several comprehensive clinical descriptions of the psychopathic individual have been presented throughout history. For example, McCord and McCord (1964) emphasized the characteristics of impulsivity, excitement-seeking, guiltlessness, and "warped capacity for love" in their conceptualization of the psychopath, and referenced historical figures such as "Billy the Kid" as early examples of the prototype. Despite these other presentations, Cleckley's (1941/1988) work, *The Mask of Sanity* is considered by most to be the first comprehensive clinical description of the psychopathy syndrome and has often served as the standard against which other conceptualizations are measured. Cleckley's (1941/1988) intention was to facilitate a more clear understanding of a group of patients who "constitute a most grave and constant problem to the hospital and to the community" (p. xi). To that end, he paid considerable attention not only to describing the key aspects of the psychopathic personality, but also to differentiating the syndrome from other psychopathology. While acknowledging that too little is understood regarding psychopathy, Cleckley (1941/1988) was clear that the syndrome can and should be differentiated from other conditions, including psychosis, psychoneurosis, and "ordinary" criminality. In his book, Cleckley presented a set of detailed case histories from which he derived 16 criteria. Among the 16 criteria (see Table 2.1.), six have consistently and particularly influenced current conceptualizations of the psychopathy syndrome.

Superficial charm and good intelligence. This feature of psychopathy highlights how the often self-defeating behavior exhibited by the psychopathic individual stems neither from a lack of intelligence nor from an inability to interact effectively with others. As Cleckley noted, "The typical psychopath will seem particularly agreeable and make a distinctly positive impression when he is first encountered... signs of affectation or excessive affability are not characteristic. He looks like the real thing." (p. 338) This feature may be especially important for modern conceptualizations of the "successful psychopath", who is more likely to be found in the higher reaches of the boardroom than in a prison (e.g., Boddy et al., 2010).

Lack of remorse or shame. It is notable that the psychopathic individual does not express genuine contrition for the antisocial acts he or she commits. When

Table 2.1 Cleckley (1941/1988) criteria for psychopathy

Superficial charm and good "intelligence."
Absence of delusions and other signs of irrational thinking.
Absence of "nervousness" or psychoneurotic manifestations.
Unreliability.
Untruthfulness and insincerity.
Lack of remorse or shame.
Inadequately motivated antisocial behavior.
Poor judgment and failure to learn by experience.
Pathological egocentricity and incapacity for love.
General poverty in major affective reactions.
Specific loss of insight.
Unresponsiveness in general interpersonal relations.
Fantastic and uninviting behavior with drink and sometimes without.
Suicide rarely carried out.
Sex life impersonal, trivial, and poorly integrated.
Failure to follow any life plan.

confronted, the psychopathic individual may be unable to articulate the purpose in feeling such remorse. Cleckley wrote: "Usually he denies emphatically all responsibility and directly accuses others as responsible, but often he will go through an idle ritual of saying that much of his trouble is his own fault.... More detailed questioning about just what he blames himself for and why may show that a serious attitude is not only absent but altogether inconceivable to him" (p. 343). Because "lack of remorse" is a criterion for ASPD, this feature is one that can contribute to the difficulty in differentiating psychopathy from ASPD; although, this becomes less challenging when the presence of other features is considered.

Inadequately motivated antisocial *behavior.* Although there is some debate regarding the centrality of criminal behavior to the conceptualization of psychopathy (see Sect. 2.3.1.3), most assessments of the syndrome will include some measure of antisocial behavior. Importantly, Cleckley allowed for a wide range of behaviors in this category, ranging from minor infractions such as lying and cheating, to more serious, aggressive offenses. For Cleckley, what was important was not the type or severity of the acts, but the psychopath's tendency to "commit such deeds in the absence of any apparent goal at all" (p. 343). Thus, the "inadequately motivated" was the key piece of this criterion; one that distinguished the behavior of the psychopath from the behavior of other criminals.

Poor judgment and failure to learn by experience. Although characterized by "good intelligence", the psychopathic individual continues to make self-defeating choices. Further, even when the psychopathic individual can explain "what went wrong" in a particular situation (i.e., what he did that may have resulted in the poor outcome), this understanding does not translate to future situations. Cleckley saw this as a key feature, noting: "One important point that distinguishes the psychopath is his failure to learn and adopt a better and more fulfilling pattern of life" (p. 78).

Incapacity for love. Cleckley noted that, although the psychopathic individual may be "capable of fondness, of likes, of dislikes ... these affective reactions are, however, always strictly limited in degree" (p. 348). He wrote of one case example, "As his feelings...were discussed, it remained impossible to detect any sort of affective content to which those words might refer. The more one investigated...the more strictly verbal his statements appeared" (p. 86). Psychopathic individuals, as Maslow (1951) would write "have no love identifications with other human beings and can therefore hurt them or even kill them casually, without hate, and without pleasure" (p. 173).

General poverty in major affective reactions. Consistent with their apparent "incapacity for love", psychopathic individuals generally do not demonstrate those behaviors or attitudes that would be demonstrative of deep, long-lasting emotional experience. Although the psychopathic individual may express himself in ways that suggest that he is experiencing affective reactions (e.g., a short temper, a declaration of affection), there is no "mature, wholehearted anger, true or consistent indignation, honest, solid grief, sustaining pride, deep joy, and genuine despair" (p. 348). This apparent inability to experience deep emotion or to connect emotionally with others is one of the most central features of the disorder, and an important criterion for distinguishing the psychopath from other antisocial individuals (e.g., Cleckley, 1941/1988; Cooke et al., 2006; Lykken, 1995).

In summary, the psychopathic individual can be identified based on certain interpersonal, affective, and behavioral features that have been depicted and well-described in a number of case studies. These features reflect an individual who does not appear to appreciate the negative impact of their behavior on themselves or others. They also describe an individual who fails to form deep, emotional connections, and who engages in self-defeating, reckless behavior despite normal intelligence. As a result, although psychopathic individuals may never voluntarily seek treatment or assistance, they will often come before clinicians as a consequence of their illegal or harmful behaviors.

2.2 Epidemiology

Although the number and types of psychopathy assessment tools has been growing in the past decades, the Psychopathy Checklist-Revised (PCL-R; Hare, 2003) is generally considered to remain among the most influential tools for the assessment of the syndrome, particularly in forensic settings. The PCL-R is composed of 20 items, which are rated as 0 "not applicable to the individual", 1 "applicable only to a certain extent", or 2 "applicable to the individual" on the basis of information collected from both interview and file review (Hare, 2003). Although the PCL-R can be conceptualized as a dimensional instrument (e.g., Walters et al., 2007, 2015), a cut score is often used to classify individuals as psychopathic (Hare, 2003). Historically, a cut score of 30 is recommended (Hare, 2003), although researchers- particularly in Europe- have also employed other cut scores (e.g, 25). Overall, the rate of PCL-R assessed psychopathy in offender populations has been reported between 10% and 15% in forensic psychiatric settings, and 15–50% in non-psychiatric prison populations (Hare, 1991, 2003; Herve et al., 2004; Salekin et al., 1998). Rates appear to differ, however, across gender, racial, and cultural groups.

2.2.1 North American Samples Versus European Samples

Evidence for differences in psychopathy prevalence across regions is difficult to interpret. For example, research does suggest that there is a significant difference between the mean PCL-R scores of incarcerated North American offenders ($M = 22.1$; $SD = 7.9$) and those of incarcerated European offenders ($M = 17.5$; $SD = 7.3$; Sullivan & Kosson, 2006). However, other studies show that the difference in mean scores between psychiatric samples (i.e., patients or inmates in psychiatric or secure hospitals) across North America and Europe are considerably smaller (i.e., a mean of 21.5 (6.9) in North American samples and 22.5(8.0) in European samples). As a result, it has been suggested that the larger differences observed in incarcerated samples may not reflect differences in levels of the syndrome across nations, but instead result from differences in incarceration base rates

(Rasmussen et al., 1999) as well as differences in how mentally disordered offenders are classified and placed within different nations' legal systems (Hobson & Shine, 1998).

2.2.2 *Male Samples Versus Female Samples*

There are well-documented differences in the mean scores and rates of psychopathy between male and female offender populations (see Verona & Vitale, 2018, for a review). The majority of studies using PCL-based measures (i.e., PCL-R, PCL-YV, PCL-SV) have found lower rates of psychopathy among female offenders compared to males, with reported prevalence rates for female offender samples as low as 6% (Jackson et al., 2002), and several falling between 11% and 17% (e.g., O'Connor, 2001; Warren et al., 2003). These differences also maintain when other measures of the syndrome are used. For example, in a self-report study examining psychopathy in community samples across nations, Neumann et al. (2012) found that levels of psychopathy assessed using the Self Report Psychopathy Scale (SRP) were generally lower for females than for males across world regions. This finding is consistent with differences in the mean scores for males and females that have been reported in institutionalized, undergraduate, noninstitutionalized, and adolescent samples (see Verona & Vitale, 2018).

2.2.3 *African American Samples Versus European American Samples*

Early reviews based on a relatively limited number of samples suggested differences in mean PCL-R scores across racial groups. Because African American offenders attained higher scores than European American offenders in these studies (e.g., Cooke et al., 2001; Kosson et al., 1990), these data lead some to conclude that psychopathy rates were elevated in this group (Lynn, 2002). However, this conclusion has been strongly challenged, as there has been an important shift in the interpretation of mean scores and rates of psychopathy among African American offender populations. Most notably, in a meta-analysis of 21 studies (n = 8890), only a small (i.e., an average of less than 1 point)—albeit statistically significant—difference in PCL-R total scores across race was found (Skeem et al., 2004), disputing the argument that levels of psychopathy differ in any clinically meaningful way between African American and European American samples.

In summary, rates of psychopathy tend to be higher in offender populations than in community samples. Further, there is good evidence for differences in the rates of psychopathy across region and gender, although the source of these differences is much less clear. These differences may represent differences in the true base rate of the syndrome. However, there is also evidence to suggest that these rates may instead reflect differences in how individuals are moved through the criminal justice system (i.e., whether individuals are incarcerated or hospitalized) and what features of the psychopathy syndrome may be most apparent in these populations (i.e., the likelihood of aggressive behavior).

2.3 Assessment of Psychopathy

Although Cleckley's criteria and case descriptions provided some guidance on how to identify the psychopathic individual, they did not represent a systematic, reliable assessment tool. Following the development of the "Cleckley criteria", clinicians relied primarily on either case-based "psychopathy prototype" assessments (e.g., Hare et al., 1978) or the use of self-report measures believed to capture the personality traits associated with the syndrome, such as the Socialization (So) subscale of the California Personality Inventory and the Psychopathic Deviate (Pd) scale of the MMPI. However, these methods were limited in diagnostic reliability. In addition, a lack of diagnostic uniformity made it difficult to generalize findings across studies. There was clearly a need for a reliable, widely accepted assessment of psychopathy. That need led to the development of the Psychopathy Checklist and its progeny (i.e., the PCL-R, the Psychopathy Checklist: Screening Version, and the Psychopathy Checklist: Youth Version), which eventually emerged as the most influential diagnostic tool and the standard against which other psychopathy assessment instruments were typically measured (DeMatteo et al., 2014; Fulero, 1995; Hare, 2016).

2.3.1 The PCL and Related Measures

Using Cleckley's criteria as a standard, Hare first developed the Research Scale for the Assessment of Psychopathy in 1980 (Psychopathy Checklist; Hare, 1980). This early version of the PCL was a 22-item measure that was scored on the basis of a semi-structured interview and review of institutional files. A revised version of the checklist (i.e., PCL-R) that removed two of the original scale items was released in 1991 and the scale has remained unchanged since then (Hare, 1991, 2003). As described in Sect. 2.2, each item on the 20-item checklist is scored using interview and file review as 0, 1, or 2. Items tap the interpersonal (e.g., "superficial charm"), affective (e.g., "lack of remorse or guilt"), and impulsive/antisocial lifestyle (e.g., "irresponsibility, "juvenile delinquency") features of the syndrome. Scores range from 0 to 40 and although there is taxonometric evidence suggesting the scale indexes a continuous construct (e.g., Walters et al., 2007, 2015), a diagnostic cut-off of 30 is often used in North American, male samples.

The PCL-R rose quickly to prominence, giving researchers both a reliable diagnostic tool, as well as a common vocabulary for describing psychopathy and for comparing results across studies. Not surprisingly, given its wide influence, criticisms have emerged that have challenged the outsized influence of the PCL-R in the field. Questions have arisen surrounding the factor structure of the PCL-R and the components of psychopathy (e.g., Bishopp & Hare, 2008; Cooke et al., 2006), the utility of an assessment tool that requires considerable collateral evidence to rate and score (e.g., Skeem et al., 2011), and the generalizability of the PCL-R across populations (e.g., Cooke & Michie, 1999; Kosson et al., 1990; Verona & Vitale, 2018).

2.3.1.1 The Structure of the PCL-R

On the basis of initial Exploratory Factor Analysis of the PCL-R, early studies seemed to support a correlated, two-factor structure (Harpur et al., 1988) of the instrument. Factor 1 was labeled the "affective/interpersonal factor", and included items representing many of the deficient emotional and interpersonally manipulative characteristics of the syndrome (e.g., glib/superficial charm, manipulative, callous, shallow affect). Factor 2 included items capturing the psychopathic individual's antisocial and criminal behavior (e.g., poor behavioral controls, impulsivity, early behavior problems), and became known as the social deviance or "impulsive/antisocial lifestyle" factor. Hare and colleagues (e.g., Hare, 2003, 2016; Neumann et al., 2007) have proposed that psychopathy is best conceptualized as a unidimensional construct. However, research has revealed that there are unique correlates of Factors 1 and 2 (Dolan & Anderson, 2003; Salekin et al., 2004), suggesting that the true relationship between psychopathy and other variables may be obscured if these differential associations are not taken into account.

In one of the first challenges to the two-factor conceptualization of psychopathy, Cooke et al. (2006) argued for a three-factor model that included an "Interpersonal" Factor 1, an "Affective" Factor 2, and a "Lifestyle" Factor 3. The first two factors essentially divided the original Factor 1 into two component parts (i.e., interpersonal and affective). However, this three-factor solution, although a significantly better fit to existing data than the traditional two-factor model (Cooke et al., 2004) also excluded 7 PCL-R items, limiting its relevance to the full PCL-R.

Both the original two-factor model and Cooke's proposed three-factor structure have since been superseded by a widely-accepted four-facet structure that can be used to model the higher-order two-factor structure (Hare, 2016; Hare & Neumann, 2008; Neumann et al., 2007). These facets are the "interpersonal" facet (including the items glib/superficial charm, grandiose sense of self-worth, pathological deception, conning/manipulative), the "affective" facet (including the items lack of remorse or guilt, shallow affect, callous/lack of empathy, failure to accept responsibility), the "lifestyle" facet (including the items need for stimulation/proneness to boredom, parasitic lifestyle, lack of realistic long-term goals, impulsivity, irresponsibility), and the "antisocial" facet (including the items poor behavioral controls, early behavior problems, juvenile delinquency, revocation of conditional release, criminal versatility).

It is important to note that the debate surrounding the factor structure of the PCL-R is not just relevant for researchers particularly interested in measurement theory.

Rather, the debate has important implications for the field's conceptualization of the psychopathy construct. One implication is the potential heterogeneity of psychopathy, which may be important for understanding differences in psychopathic individuals' behaviors and responses to treatment. The second is the question of the centrality of criminal and/or violent behavior to our understanding of psychopathy and our prototype of the psychopathic individual.

2.3.1.2 Factors, Facets, and Psychopathy "Subtypes"

As already noted, research reveals differential relationships between the Factors/Facets of the PCL-R and important variables. For example, in their study of sexual offender treatment outcomes, Sewall and Olver (2019) found that the affective facet, specifically, was associated with lower levels of therapeutic progress, whereas the affective and lifestyle facets together predicted treatment noncompletion. In another study, an examination of abuse history showed that whereas sexual abuse history was associated with the interpersonal and lifestyle facets, a history of physical abuse was related to the lifestyle and antisocial facets (Krstic et al., 2016). Factor and facet differences have also been observed in event-related potential (ERP) studies (Anderson et al., 2015; Steele et al., 2016; Venables et al., 2015; Veit et al., 2013), as well as in executive functioning as assessed by performance on the Wisconsin Card Sort (Pera-Guardiola et al., 2016).

Given findings such as these, researchers have noted the utility of considering subtypes of psychopathy (see Hicks & Drislane, 2018; Poythress & Skeem, 2006, for reviews). Most prominent among these has historically been the distinction between "primary" and "secondary" psychopathy. Typically, the primary psychopathy type is characterized by deficits in affective responses, whereas the secondary psychopath will evidence anxiety, depression, and negative emotionality (Dargis & Koenigs, 2018; Karpman, 1948; Lykken, 1995; Newman et al., 2005). Consistent with this distinction, studies using the PCL-R, as well as other psychopathy measures, have identified important differences between these types. For example, compared to the primary psychopathy subgroup, the secondary psychopathy type has been associated with the presence of fewer adaptive traits (i.e., leadership, focus; Bronchain et al., 2020), more self-injury behaviors and thoughts (Fadoir et al., 2019), higher rates of childhood maltreatment (e.g., Dargis & Koenigs, 2018), and lower rates of treatment non-completion (Klein Haneveld et al., 2018).

Despite this evidence for the existence of unique correlates of the Factors/Facets, as well as the increasing interest in distinguishing subgroups of psychopathic individuals, some researchers caution against perceiving any one component of the syndrome to be held superior over the others (e.g., Hare, 2003; Neumann et al., 2007). Rather, these individuals argue that PCL-R psychopathy is best conceptualized as a whole and that this "'whole' may be greater than the sum of the 'parts'" (Neumann et al., 2007). Nevertheless, there does appear to be increasing evidence that a failure to examine associations at the factor/facet level or to consider the heterogeneity of the construct may lead to incomplete understanding of psychopathy's relation to other variables.

2.3.1.3 Criminal Behavior and the PCL-R

The PCL-R was designed for use within institutionalized populations, as evidenced by its inclusion of items directly assessing criminality (e.g., "revocation of conditional release", "criminal versatility") as well as the reliance on extensive collateral information. Not surprisingly, scores on the measure are consistently associated with criminal behavior and predict general, violent, and sexual reoffending (Hare, 1996; Hemphill et al., 1998). As a result, the instrument is commonly used for risk assessment, management, and monitoring, particularly in North America. Although these associations have led to an increased use of PCL-R within forensic contexts (Fulero, 1995; Hare, 1998; Hurducas et al., 2014; Neal & Grisso, 2014), they have also been a source of criticism from those who challenge the importance of criminal behavior—and especially violent criminal behavior—as a core feature of psychopathy (e.g., Cooke et al., 2006; Lilienfeld, 1994; Skeem & Cooke, 2010; Skeem et al., 2011).

Although Cleckley (1941/1988) included "inadequately motivated antisocial behavior" among his original criteria, he did not present violent criminal behavior as a necessary component of the syndrome. Rather, he argued that "many persons showing the characteristics of those described here do commit major crimes and sometimes crimes of maximal violence. There are so many, however, who do not, that such tendencies should be regarded as the exception rather than as the rule" (Cleckley, 1941/1988, p. 262). Consistent with Cleckley's conceptualization, it is noteworthy that among the 7 PCL-R items that were omitted from Cooke et al.'s (2006) three-factor model of the PCL-R were those items specific to criminal or violent behavior.

While the ascendance of the PCL-R and the subsequent factor debates brought this issue to the forefront, the tension between conceptualizations of psychopathy and the role of violence precedes the development of the measure. For example, Lewis (1974) criticized what he called "a preoccupation with the nosological status of the concept … its forensic implications, its subdivisions, limits, [and] the propriety of identifying psychopathic personality with antisocial behavior…" (pp. 137–138). Similarly, Millon (1981) noted: "50 years ago the same issues were in the forefront, notably whether the psychopathic personality was or was not synonymous with overt antisocial behavior" (p. 184).

Researchers have turned to a variety of methods to address their concerns regarding the role of criminality in PCL-R psychopathy. As noted earlier, one solution has been to examine separately the contributions of the interpersonal and affective factor/facets and the antisocial/lifestyle factor/facets when studying the syndrome (e.g., Hansen et al., 2007; Patrick et al., 1993; Vaidyanathan et al., 2011). Another approach has been for researchers to develop alternative measures of psychopathy that are not as reliant as the PCL-R on either criminal behavior or corroborating evidence for the rating and scoring of individuals (e.g., Brislin et al., 2015; Lilienfeld & Andrews, 1996). Determining what features are considered "core" to psychopathy is necessary not only for guiding the refinement or development of assessment measures, but also for informing our examinations of these measures across populations. As a result, this debate is directly relevant to the next criticism of the PCL-R, which involves the generalizability of PCL-R psychopathy assessment across groups.

2.3.1.4 Generalizability Across Groups

Given the PCL-R's use in applied clinical and forensic settings, the generalizability of the measure across samples is a highly relevant consideration (e.g., Cooke & Michie, 1999; Kosson et al., 1990; Sullivan et al., 2006; Verona & Vitale, 2018). Much of the early research using the PCL-R was limited to samples of incarcerated, European American males in the US and Canada. Although differences in the expression of psychopathy across gender, cultural, and racial groups would have important implications for the use of the PCL-R in applied settings, there was for many years only limited research on the generalizability of the construct across populations. Fortunately, there was a marked increase in research in these areas in at the turn of the century, with numerous studies focused on the expression and correlates of psychopathy in other groups, particularly female offenders and African-American offenders (see Beryl et al., 2014; Sullivan & Kosson, 2006; Verona & Vitale, 2018 for reviews). However, the results of this research have not always been clear-cut. For example, although evidence supports the reliability of psychopathy assessments among female populations (e.g., Miller et al., 2011a, b; Salekin et al., 1997; Vitale et al., 2002) and across racial and cultural groups (e.g., Vachon et al., 2012), the evidence for the generalizability of behavioral and etiological-relevant correlates of psychopathy is less consistent.

Several key deficits in emotion-related responding have not been demonstrated among African American offenders (e.g., Baskin-Sommers et al., 2011; Lorenz & Newman, 2002; Newman et al., 1997) nor among female offenders (e.g., Anton et al., 2012; Vitale et al., 2011). Similarly, abnormalities in response perseveration and passive avoidance learning that have been reliably demonstrated among psychopathic males have not been reported among psychopathic females (e.g., Vitale et al., 2011). Differences across gender have also been found in laboratory-based assessments of adolescents with high levels of psychopathy traits (e.g., Isen et al., 2010; Vitale et al., 2005; Wang et al., 2012).

Even the well-established associations between PCL-R psychopathy and criminal behavior may be limited across samples. For example, Walsh (2013) showed that in a sample of 424 adult male jail inmates, PCL-R scores were a better predictor of violence among European American offenders than among either African American or Latino offenders. Similarly, Edens et al. (2007) reported meta-analytic results suggesting that within ethnically diverse juvenile samples, psychopathy was a weaker correlate of violent recidivism than within primarily European American samples. Finally, some research provides evidence that psychopathy may be a less powerful predictor of recidivism in incarcerated female samples (Weizmann-Henelius et al., 2015). Notably, other research identifying gender differences when using other alternative measures of psychopathy (e.g., Eichenbaum et al., 2019) suggest that these concerns might not be specific to PCL-R psychopathy, but may reflect more general limitations in how the psychopathy construct is conceptualized and assessed across groups.

Ideally, these inconsistencies would raise questions about the source of these differences. Is the PCL-R identifying a slightly different syndrome across different groups? Are certain items/facets disproportionately affecting total scores across groups? Some researchers have investigated these differences. For example, Neumann et al. (2012) conducted a large-scale (n = 33,016; 58% female/42% male) self-report psychopathy study across gender and world regions, and found that, in their female sample, Gross Domestic Product per capita (GDPpc) was negatively correlated with the expression of the interpersonal/affective psychopathy traits, suggesting an association between GDPpc and the expression of core psychopathy features. In a different study, Walsh and Kosson (2007) found that Socioeconomic Status (SES) moderated the relationship between psychopathy and crime differently across race, with a significant SES x psychopathy interaction on recidivism emerging among European American but not African American participants. Taken together, these findings highlight the possibility that the expression of psychopathy may be influenced by macro-level environmental factors such as SES and GDP.

In summary, it is clear that PCL-R assessed psychopathy is an influential construct in the field and particularly within institutional and forensic settings. In the past decades, the assessment landscape has changed, however. Although still at the forefront of psychopathy assessment, there are some debates surrounding the PCL-R's dominance. These debates include the role of criminal behavior and violence in the conceptualization of the syndrome and limitations of the generalizability of the construct across populations.

The desire of the field to generalize psychopathy findings to alternate samples leads directly to the final challenge to the PCL-R, which is the inability to use the measure to assess psychopathy in noninstitutionalized populations. As a result of this limitation, as well as the concerns surrounding the instrument's reliance on overt criminal behavior, there is a strong emphasis in the field on the continued development and validation of alternate or self-report measures that focus on psychopathy specifically (as opposed to more general personality traits) and that can be used with noninstitutionalized populations. In the next section, an overview of several of these measures is provided.

2.3.2 *Other Measures of Psychopathy*

Alternative measures of psychopathy have primarily been developed along two paths. The first path includes measures meant to be used with noninstitutionalized adults. These measures are designed to circumvent the necessity of a lengthy clinical interview and/or the use of extensive, corroborating file information. The second path includes measures that have been developed for use among adolescent populations. These measures are meant to capture the syndrome as it might appear prior to adulthood and place less emphasis on characteristics unlikely to be seen in adolescent samples (e.g., engaging in short-term marital relationships).

2.3.2.1 Self-Report and Other Alternative Measures

Along the first path, two measures that were developed as alternatives to the PCL-R are direct descendants of the original measure. These are the PCL: Screening Version (PCL:SV; Forth et al., 1996), designed to be less reliant on long interviews and extensive files review, and the Self-Report Psychopathy scale (SRP-II, -III; Williams & Paulhus, 2004), designed to provide a pen-and-pencil self-report assessment of the syndrome. The PCL: SV (Forth et al., 1996) was an early variation of the PCL-R, created to assess psychopathy using less information and without formal criminal records. Generally, research suggests that the PCL: SV captures a syndrome similar to the PCL-R. The two measures are highly correlated (with an average correlation of .8) (Cooke et al., 1999) and the PCL: SV exhibits a factor structure and item functioning similar to the PCL-R (Hill et al., 2004). Consistent with its close association to the original PCL-R, the PCL: SV is a good predictor of violent behavior (e.g., Douglas et al., 1999; Skeem & Mulvey, 2001). The Self-Report Psychopathy scale (SRP, SRP-II, SRP-III) was developed by Hare and colleagues (e.g., Hare et al., 1989; Williams et al., 2007) as a self-report measure of the syndrome in adult samples. The SRP-II and SRP-III are reliable (Neal & Sellbom, 2012) and relate in expected ways with correlates of the psychopathy syndrome, including scores on the PCL-R as well as measures of alcohol abuse, narcissism, empathy, Machiavellianism, agreeableness, and conscientiousness (e.g., Paulhus & Williams, 2002; Tew et al., 2015; Zagon & Jackson, 1994; Watt & Brooks, 2012).

Other researchers, wanting to emphasize theoretical conceptualizations of psychopathy distinct from the PCL-R have developed other, independent, measures of the syndrome. These measures were developed on the basis of those traits believed to be central to psychopathy, with less emphasis on the numbers or types of disinhibited behaviors or criminal acts committed by the individual. These have included the Primary and Secondary Psychopathy Scales (SRPS; Levenson et al., 1995), the Psychopathic Personality Inventory (PPI; Lilienfeld & Andrews, 1996), the Triarchic Psychopathy Measure (TriPM; Patrick, 2010), and the Comprehensive Assessment of Psychopathic Personality (CAPP; Kreis et al., 2012).

The SRPS is a 26-item self-report measure developed by Levenson et al. (1995) that has two components: the "primary scale" and the "secondary" scale. Scores on the primary scale are positively correlated with disinhibition and boredom susceptibility and negatively correlated with harm avoidance. Scores on the secondary scale are associated with stress reactions. Scores on the SRPS are correlated with PCL-R scores, substance use, criminal versatility, self-reported delinquency, low-agreeableness, and passive avoidance task performance (Brinkley et al., 2001; Lynam et al., 1999; Sellbom, 2011). More recently, scores on the SRPS have been related to abnormalities in ERP responses in a startle paradigm (De Pacalis et al., 2019) consistent with theories of psychopathy,

The PPI (Lilienfeld & Andrews, 1996) is a 187-item self-report measure with 8 subscales, including Machiavellian Egocentricity, Coldheartedness, Social Potency, Carefree Nonplanfulness, Fearlessness, Impulsive Nonconformity, Blame Externalization, and Stress Immunity. Research shows that the PPI correlates with PCL-R total scores (Poythress et al., 1998), and also with adult and childhood antisocial behavior and institutional misconduct (Edens et al., 2008a, b), measures of emotional empathy (Sandoval et al., 2000), and self-report aggression and dominance (Edens et al., 2001). The PPI has also been associated with abnormalities in affective startle responses (Anderson et al., 2011), in behavioral and neurological responses to incentives (Bjork et al., 2012), and in visual-spatial attention processes (Carolan et al., 2020).

The TriPM is based on the Triarchic Personality Model of Psychopathy (Patrick et al., 2009; Brislin et al., 2015), which places the three traits of meanness, disinhibition, and boldness at the core of the syndrome. Research has consistently shown expected associations with psychopathy-relevant variables. For example, research utilizing the triarchic conceptualization of psychopathy has shown expected correlations with other measures of psychopathy, antisocial behavior, and self-reported empathy (Sellbom et al., 2015a, b), structural differences in the amygdala (Vieira et al., 2015), deficits in emotion responses (Somma et al., 2015), and behavioral dysregulation (Ribes-Guardiola et al., 2020). However, there is some debate regarding the factor structure of the instrument (e.g., Collison et al., 2016; Roy et al., 2020), as well as the relative importance of all three factors (e.g., Hanniball et al., 2019; Sleep et al., 2019; Shou et al., 2018).

Just as the TriPM was developed to reflect a theoretical model of psychopathy centered around three neurobiologically-based traits, the Comprehensive Assessment of Psychopathic Personality (CAPP; Cooke et al., 2004; Hoff et al., 2012) is a conceptual model of the syndrome built through reference to the clinical and empirical literature. The CAPP includes 33 symptoms that are collected under six domains: Attachment (e.g., detached, unempathic), Behavioral (e.g., reckless, aggressive), Cognitive (e.g., suspicious, intolerant), Dominance (e.g., manipulative, garrulous), Self (e.g., self-justifying, self-aggrandizing), and Emotional (e.g., lacks remorse, lacks emotional depth). A growing body of research supports the utility of the CAPP model, which has been shown to translate across languages (Hoff et al., 2014), to intercorrelate with the PCL-R (Sandvik et al., 2012), and to relate in expected ways to criminal recidivism (Pedersen et al., 2010).

Early tests of the model utilized the CAPP- Institutional Rating Scale (CAPP-IRS; Cooke et al., 2004, 2012). However, the CAPP-IRS was developed for use in institutionalized settings, and its reliance on clinical interviews and extensive file reviews made it both time-intensive and impractical for application to noninstitutionalized populations. As a result, both the CAPP-Self Report (CAPP-SR; Sellbom et al., 2019) and the CAPP Lexical Rating Scale (LRS; Sellbom et al., 2015a, b; Kavish et al., 2020) have been more recently developed. Early results from research with both instruments provide evidence that these measures are reliable and valid assessments of the CAPP model and lay the groundwork for future research in this area.

Consistent with both the TriPM and CAPP models' emphasis on psychopathic traits, other researchers have developed alternative psychopathy conceptualizations rooted strongly in personality theory. For example, Lynam and colleagues (e.g., Lynam & Derefinko, 2006; Miller & Lynam, 2015) have argued that psychopathy is best conceptualized according to the traditional Five-Factor Model (FFM) of personality, and that psychopathy is easily captured by the traits and facets of personality measures like the NEO-PI-R. Proponents of this approach note that conceptualizing psychopathy in accordance with existing personality traits places the syndrome within the context of well-validated personality theory that is already strongly connected to research in diverse areas, including genetics, development, and neurobiology (Lynam & Derefinko, 2006; Widiger et al., 2012; Widiger & Trull, 2007).

In regards to measurement, Widiger and Lynam (1998) suggested that each item of the PCL-R could be represented by facets within the FFM. Miller et al. (2001) tested this proposal by asking psychopathy experts to generate an FFM profile of the prototypical psychopath on the basis of their understanding and knowledge of the syndrome. Importantly, the profile generated by these experts was similar to that generated by the theorists, which held, for example, that "glibness/superficial charm" would represented by low self-consciousness, and "shallow affect" by low warmth, low positive emotionality, low altruism, and low tender-mindedness.

On the basis of this early work, Lynam and colleagues (Lynam & Widiger, 2001; Miller & Lynam, 2003) went on to calculate the Psychopathy Resemblance Index (PRI), which was a measure of the extent to which an individual resembles the FFM prototype. Research showed that these scores were associated with an earlier age of onset of delinquency, greater criminal versatility, earlier drug use, higher rates of substance abuse, risky sexual behavior, and low internalizing problems (Miller et al., 2001; Miller & Lynam, 2003). Scores were also predictive of performance on psychopathy-related laboratory tasks (i.e., the use of aggressive responses on a social-information task, and less willingness to delay gratification on a time-discounting task) (Miller & Lynam, 2003).

To provide a measure based on the FFM but specific to psychopathy, Lynam et al. (2011) have developed the Elemental Psychopathy Assessment (EPA), which has both short and long forms. The long-form of the scale assesses the 18 traits that have been consistently associated with psychopathy, and which comprise four factors: Antagonism, Emotional Stability, Disinhibition, and Narcissism. In forensic, undergraduate, and community samples, scores on the EPA have correlated with existing psychopathy measures (i.e., SRP-III, PPI-R), as well as with aggressive social cognitions, antisocial personality features, romantic infidelity, alcohol use, and antisocial behavior (Collison et al., 2016; Lynam et al., 2011; Miller et al., 2011a, b; Miller et al., 2014; Wilson et al., 2011).

2.3.2.2 Measures for Use with Juvenile Samples

Developing separately from those measures meant to assess psychopathy in noninstitutionalized populations were measures designed to assess the construct among juvenile samples. Interest in reliable and valid assessments of the syndrome in these samples has only heightened in light of evidence for stability in psychopathic traits across childhood and adolescence (Hawes et al., 2018; Hemphälä et al., 2015; Lopez-Romero et al., 2014). A measure derived from the PCL is among those that have been established for use with adolescents. However, as in adult samples, other measures developed separately from the PCL have also grown in prominence.

The PCL: YV (Forth et al., 2003) is a modified version of the PCL-R that can be used with adolescents ages 12–18 (Forth et al., 2003). Research has demonstrated reliability of the measure in both male and female samples (e.g., Bauer et al., 2011), although there is some evidence for differential item functioning across gender (Tsang et al., 2015) and ethnicity (Tsang et al., 2014). Importantly, the measure also relates to criterion variables in ways that are consistent with PCL-R research with adults. For example, relative to adolescents with low scores, adolescents with high scores on the instrument commit more and more violent crimes and show lower levels of familial attachment (Kosson et al., 2002).

The PCL: YV, like the PCL-R, requires a lengthy interview procedure and is best utilized in institutional settings. As a result, more easily administered measures of psychopathy for juveniles have been developed. Primary among these has been the Antisocial Process Screening Device (APSD; Frick & Hare, 2001), a 20-item rating scale that can be used as a self-report measure or as a teacher and parent report measure. The ASPD has been widely utilized, and research has shown that scores on the measure are reliably associated with many of the personality traits and laboratory deficits exhibited by psychopathic adults. For example, high scores on the APSD delineate a group of individuals who exhibit higher rates of conduct problems and police contacts, and stronger family histories of antisocial behavior than groups characterized by lower scores (Christian et al., 1997; Fung et al., 2010; Munoz & Frick, 2007; Pechorro et al., 2014). Higher scores on the APSD are also associated with decreased empathy, perspective taking, and fearfulness (Blair et al., 2001).

The ASPD captures the interpersonal (e.g., superficial charm, lack of empathy), emotional (e.g., shallow affect), and behavioral (e.g., reckless antisocial behaviors, impulsivity) characteristics of psychopathy. Over time, particular interest has emerged in the callous/unemotional (CU) traits assessed by the measure, which may serve to distinguish those adolescents who are most closely similar to our conceptualization of an adult psychopathic individual. For example, laboratory studies have demonstrated that adolescents characterized by high scores on the CU traits exhibit abnormal neural responses (e.g., Sebastian et al., 2012), performance deficits on a task requiring them to modify an initial reward-oriented response strategy in light of increasing rates of punishment (e.g., O'Brien & Frick, 1996), reduced interference on a Picture-Word Stroop, and deficits in passive avoidance on a go-no-go task (Vitale et al., 2005)—all deficits associated with psychopathy in adults.

The Youth Psychopathic Traits Inventory (YPI and YPI-Short Form; Andershed et al., 2002) and YPI–Child Version (YPI-CV) are alternatives to the ASPD. The YPI has been shown to be moderately correlated with factors of the PCL: YV (Andershed et al., 2007), and other self-report measures of psychopathy (Cambell et al., 2009; Gillen et al., 2019). Further, the measure has been associated with key correlates of psychopathy, including conduct problems and proactive aggression (Leenarts et al., 2017; Rucevic, 2010; van Baardewijk et al., 2011), as well as self-reported antisocial attitudes and impulsivity (Campbell et al., 2009; Eisenbarth & Centifanti, 2020). However, results are mixed. Some studies have not found expected associations with criminal behavior or substance use (Colins et al., 2015; Shepherd & Strand, 2015) and others have provided only weak evidence that the measure captures key personality features of psychopathy (i.e., callous-unemotional traits) (Oshukova et al., 2015).

In summary, there is evidence that measures such as the PCL: YV, the ASPD, and—potentially—the YPI, capture a syndrome among adolescents that is similar to adult psychopathy. Further, assessments of juvenile psychopathy appear to be relatively stable across adolescence (e.g., Lynam et al., 2009; Neumann et al., 2011). That does not mean that the field is without controversy, however. For example, it is not apparent that psychopathy assessments in adolescents have the same utility in forensic contexts as assessments made for adults (Cauffman et al., 2009), suggesting that caution is required when these assessments are made in certain applied settings. Consistent with this caution, given the historic association between psychopathy and increased dangerousness and poor treatment response (e.g., Edens, 2006; Lykken, 1995), some critics have also argued that the psychopathy label may result in decreased attention to intervention and treatment for youth with this classification.

2.4 Conclusions and Recommendations

Psychopathy is a recognizable syndrome that is associated with significant negative effects for both the psychopathic individual, whose callous, irresponsible, manipulative, and sometimes aggressive behavior often results in punitive consequences, as well as for those persons who become their unwitting victims. The need to understand psychopathy derives from the desire to control better the behavior of these individuals in order to lessen the occurrence of harmful behaviors and their consequences. Despite a rich clinical history, psychopathy remains a somewhat controversial classification. Distinct from those disorders included in the various editions of the Diagnostic and Statistical Manual of the American Psychiatric Association (e.g., DSM-5; APA, 2013), psychopathy has been captured via numerous methodologies, from relatively subjective diagnoses based on clinical impressions to highly structured diagnostic rating scales. The emergence of the PCL-R in the early 1990's brought a new focus to psychopathy assessment, as the field rapidly adopted the instrument for use in both research and clinical/forensic contexts.

However, dissatisfaction with the limits of the PCL-R include concerns about its generalizability across diverse samples, the inability to apply it easily to noninstitutionalized populations, and more fundamental disputes over the nature of the psychopathy construct as assessed by the measure. These issues have resulted in a more varied assessment landscape in recent years. Measures built on theoretical models such as the TriPM and the CAPP-SR, instruments geared towards assessing the construct in adolescents including the APSD and YPI, and approaches rooted in general personality theory especially as reflected in the EPA, are all increasingly represented in the literature. This growing diversity in assessment tools brings its own challenges, however.

As researchers continue to pursue alternative methods of psychopathy assessment, it will be important to determine the extent to which these different instruments capture a similar construct. When the measures do diverge, it is important to clarify which components or characteristics of psychopathy are represented, and which aspects of the syndrome are not. In the absence of this clarity, the shared vocabulary the field has benefited from in recent decades will be diminished. Research should also continue to focus on the generalizability of results using these different measures across populations, and to try to determine, when differences do arise, whether they represent differences in the application or performance of the measure, differences in the composition of the samples, or fundamental differences in the expression of the psychopathy syndrome. Ideally, researchers would employ more than one psychopathy assessment measure in their studies, which would better enable direct comparisons across instruments. The importance of and interest in the psychopathy construct is unlikely to diminish in the near future. Developing, validating, and clarifying the limitations of measures of the construct will continue to be a necessary undertaking, as these tools will serve as the foundation on which all studies of the causes, consequences, and treatments for psychopathy will be built.

References

American Psychiatric Association. (2013). *Diagnostic and statistical manual of mental disorders* (5th ed.). Author.

Andershed, H., Kerr, M., Stattin, H., & Levander, S. (2002). Psychopathic traits in non-referred youths: A new assessment tool. In E. Blaauw & L. Sheridan (Eds.), *Psychopaths: Current international perspectives* (pp. 131–158). Elsevier.

Andershed, H., Hodgins, S., & Tengstrom, A. (2007). Convergent validity of the Youth Psychopathic Traits Inventory (YPI): Association with the Psychopathy Checklist: Youth Version (PCL:YV). *Assessment, 14*, 144–154.

Anderson, N. E., Stanford, M. S., Wan, L., & Young, K. A. (2011). High psychopathic trait females exhibit reduced startle potentiation and increased P3 amplitude. *Behavioral Sciences & the Law, 29*, 649–666.

Anderson, N. E., Steele, V. R., Maurer, J. M., Bernat, E. M., & Kiehl, K. A. (2015). Psychopathy, attention, and oddball target detection: New insights from PCL-R facet scores. *Psychophysiology, 52*, 1194–1204.

Anton, M., Baskin-Sommers, A. R., Vitale, J., Curtin, J. J., & Newman, J. P. (2012). Differential effects of psychopathy and antisocial personality disorder symptoms on cognitive and fear processing in female offenders. *Cognitive, Affective, & Behavioral Neuroscience, 12*, 761–776.

Baskin-Sommers, A. R., Newman, J. P., Sathasivam, N., & Curtin, J. J. (2011). Evaluating the generalizability of a fear deficit in psychopathic African American offenders. *Journal of Abnormal Psychology, 120*, 71–78.

Bauer, D. L., Whitman, L. A., & Kosson, D. S. (2011). Reliability and construct validity of Psychopathy Checklist: Youth Version scores among incarcerated adolescent girls. *Criminal Justice and Behavior, 38*, 965–987.

Beryl, R., Chou, S., & Völlm, B. (2014). A systematic review of psychopathy in women within secure settings. *Personality and Individual Differences, 71*, 185–195.

Bishopp, D., & Hare, R. D. (2008). A multidimensional scaling analysis of the PCL-R: Unfolding the structure of psychopathy. *Psychology, Crime & Law, 14*, 117–132.

Bjork, J. M., Chen, G., & Hommer, D. W. (2012). Psychopathic tendencies and mesolimbic recruitment by cues for instrumental and passively obtained rewards. *Biological Psychology, 89*, 408–415.

Blair, R. J. R., Monson, J., & Frederickson, N. (2001). Moral reasoning and conduct problems in children with emotional and behavioural difficulties. *Personality and Individual Differences, 5*, 799–811.

Boddy, C. R. P., Ladyshewsky, R., & Galvin, P. (2010). Leaders without ethics in global business: Corporate psychopaths. *Journal of Public Affairs, 10*, 121–138.

Brinkley, C. A., Schmitt, W. A., Smith, S. S., & Newman, J. P. (2001). Construct-validation of a self report psychopathy scale: Does Levenson's SRPS measure the same construct as Hare's PCL-R? *Personality and Individual Differences, 31*, 1021–1038.

Brislin, S. J., Drislane, L. E., Smith, S. T., Edens, J. F., & Patrick, C. J. (2015). Development and validation of triarchic psychopathy scales from the Multidimensional Personality Questionnaire. *Psychological Assessment, 27*, 838–851.

Bronchain, J., Raynal, P., & Chabrol, H. (2020). Heterogeneity of adaptive features among psychopathy variants. *Personality Disorders, Theory, Research, and Treatment, 11*, 63–68.

Campbell, M. A., Doucette, N. L., & French, S. (2009). Validity and stability of the Youth Psychopathic Traits Inventory in a nonforensic sample of young adults. *Journal of Personality Assessment, 91*, 584–592.

Carolan, P. L., Gaspar, J. M., Kleffner, K., & Liotti, M. (2020). Electrophysiological evidence that psychopathic personality traits are associated with atypical response to salient distractors. *Cognitive, Affective, & Behavioral Neuroscience, 20*, 195–213.

Cauffman, E., Kimonis, E. R., Dmitrieva, J., & Monahan, K. C. (2009). A multimethod assessment of juvenile psychopathy: Comparing the predictive utility of the PCL:YV, YPI, and the NEO PRI. *Psychological Assessment, 21*, 528–542.

Christian, R. E., Frick, P. J., Hill, N. L., Tyler, A. L., & Frazer, D. (1997). Psychopathy and conduct problems in children: II. Implications for subtyping children with conduct problems. *Journal of the American Academy of Child & Adolescent Psychiatry, 36*, 233–241.

Cleckley, H. (1941/1988). *The Mask of Sanity*. Mosby.

Colins, O. F., Andershed, H., & Pardini, D. A. (2015). Psychopathic traits as predictors of future criminality, intimate partner aggression, and substance use in young adult men. *Law and Human Behavior, 39*, 547–558.

Collison, K. L., Miller, J. D., Gaughan, E. T., Widiger, T. A., & Lynam, D. R. (2016). Development and validation of the super-short form of the Elemental Psychopathy Assessment. *Journal of Criminal Justice, 47*, 143–150.

Cooke, D. J., & Michie, C. (1999). Psychopathy across cultures: North America and Scotland compared. *Journal of Abnormal Psychology, 108*, 58–68.

Cooke, D. J., Michie, C., Hart, S. D., & Hare, R. D. (1999). Evaluating the Screening Version of the Hare Psychopathy Checklist–Revised: An item response theory analysis. *Psychological Assessment, 11*, 3–13.

Cooke, D. J., Kosson, D. S., & Michie, C. (2001). Psychopathy and ethnicity: Structural, item, and test generalizability of the Psychopathy Checklist—Revised (PCL-R) in Caucasian and African American participants. *Psychological Assessment, 13*, 531–542.

Cooke, D. J., Michie, C., Hart, S. D., & Clark, D. (2004). Reconstructing psychopathy: Clarifying the significance of antisocial and socially deviant behavior in the diagnosis of psychopathic personality disorder. *Journal of Personality Disorder, 18*, 337–357.

Cooke, D. J., Michie, C., & Hart, S. D. (2006). Facets of clinical psychopathy: Towards clearer measurement. In C. Patrick (Ed.), *Handbook of psychopathy* (pp. 91–106). Guilford Press.

Cooke, D. J., Hart, S. D., Logan, C., & Michie, C. (2012). Explicating the construct of psychopathy: Development and validation of a conceptual model, the Comprehensive Assessment of Psychopathic Personality (CAPP). *The International Journal of Forensic Mental Health, 11*, 242–252.

Crego, C., & Widiger, T. A. (2015). Psychopathy, DSM-5, and a caution. *Personality Disorders, Theory, Research, and Treatment, 5*, 335–347.

Dargis, M., & Koenigs, M. (2018). Two substypes of psychopathic criminals differ in negative affect and history of childhood abuse. *Psychological Trauma Theory Research Practice and Policy, 10*, 444–451.

De Pascalis, V., Scacchia, P., Sommer, K., & Checcucci, C. (2019). Psychopathy traits and reinforcement sensitivity theory: Prepulse inhibition and ERP responses. *Biological Psychology, 148*, Article 107771.

DeMatteo, D., Edens, J. F., Galloway, M., Cox, J., Smith, S. T., Koller, J. P., & Bersoff, B. (2014). Investigating the role of the Psychopathy Checklist-Revised in United States case law. *Psychology, Public Policy, and Law, 20*, 96–107.

Dolan, M. C., & Anderson, I. M. (2003). The relationship between seratonergic function and the Psychopathy Checklist: Screening Version. *Journal of Psychopharmacology, 17*, 216–222.

Douglas, K. S., Ogloff, J. R. P., Nicholls, T. L., & Grant, I. (1999). Assessing risk for violence among psychiatric patients: The HCR-20 violence risk assessment scheme and the Psychopathy Checklist: Screening Version. *Journal of Consulting and Clinical Psychology, 67*, 917–930.

Edens, J. F. (2006). Unresolved controversies concerning Psychopathy: Implications for clinical and forensic decision making. *Professional Psychology: Research and Practice, 37*, 59–65.

Edens, J. F., Poythress, N. G., & Watkins, M. M. (2001). Further validation of the Psychopathic Personality Inventory among offenders: Personality and behavioral correlates. *Journal of Personality Disorders, 15*, 403–415.

Edens, J. F., Campbell, J. S., & Weir, J. M. (2007). Youth psychopathy and criminal recidivism: A meta-analysis of the psychopathy checklist measures. *Law and Human Behavior, 31*, 53–75.

Edens, J. F., Poythress, N. G., Lilienfeld, S. O., & Patrick, C. J. (2008a). A prospective comparison of two measures of psychopathy in the prediction of institutional misconduct. *Behavioral Sciences & the Law, 26*, 529–541.

Edens, J. F., Poythress, N. G., Lilienfeld, S. O., Patrick, C. J., & Test, A. (2008b). Further evidence of the divergent correlates of the Psychopathic Personality Inventory factors: Prediction of institutional misconduct among male prisoners. *Psychological Assessment, 20*, 86–91.

Eichenbaum, A. E., Marcus, D. K., & French, B. F. (2019). Item response theory analysis of the Psychopathic Personality Inventory- Revised. *Assessment, 26*, 1046–1058.

Eisenbarth, H., & Centifanti, C. M. (2020). Dimensions of psychopathic traits in a community sample: Implications from different measures for impulsivity and delinquency. *European Journal of Psychological Assessment, 36*, 1–11.

Fadoir, N. A., Lutz-Zois, C. J., & Goodnight, J. A. (2019). Psychopathy and suicide: The mediating effects of emotional and behavioral dysregulation. *Personality and Individual Differences, 142*, 1–6.

Forth, A. E., Brown, S. L., Hart, S. D., & Hare, R. D. (1996). The assessment of psychopathy in male and female noncriminals: Reliability and validity. *Personality and Individual Differences, 20*, 531–543.

Forth, A. E., Kosson, D. S., & Hare, R. D. (2003). *The Psychopathy Checklist: Youth Version*. Multi-Health Systems.

Frick, P. J., & Hare, R. D. (2001). *The antisocial process screening device*. Multi-Health Systems.

Fulero, S. M. (1995). Review of the Hare Psychopathy Checklist–Revised. In J. C. Conoley & J. C. Impara (Eds.), *Twelfth mental measurements yearbook* (pp. 453–454). Buros Institute.

Fung, A. L., Gao, Y., & Raine, A. (2010). The utility of the child and adolescent psychopathy construct in Hong Kong, China. *Journal of Clinical Child and Adolescent Psychology, 39*, 134–140.

Gillen, C. T. A., MacDougall, E. A. M., Forth, A. E., Barry, C. T., & Salekin, R. T. (2019). Validity of the Youth Psychopathic Traits Inventory- Short Version in justice-involved and at-risk adolescents. *Assessment, 26*, 479–491.

Hanniball, K. B., Gatner, D. T., Douglas, K. S., Viljoen, J. L., & Aknin, L. B. (2019). Examining the triarchic psychopathy measure and comprehensive assessment of psychopathic personality in self-identified offender populations. *Personality Disorders, Theory, Research, and Treatment, 10*, 340–353.

Hansen, A. L., Johnsen, B. H., Thornton, D., Waage, L., & Thayer, J. F. (2007). Facets of psychopathy, heart rate variability and cognitive function. *Journal of Personality Disorders, 21*, 568–582.

Hare, R. D. (1980). A research scale for the assessment of psychopathy in criminal populations. *Personality and Individual Differences, 1*, 111–119.

Hare, R. D. (1991). *Manual for the Hare Psychopathy Checklist–Revised* (1st ed.). Multi-Health Systems.

Hare, R. D. (1996). Psychopathy: A clinical construct whose time has come. *Criminal Justice and Behavior, 23*, 25–54.

Hare, R. D. (1998). Psychopaths and their nature: Implications for the mental health and criminal justice systems. In T. Millon & E. Sorenson (Eds.), *Psychopathy: Antisocial, criminal, and violent behavior* (pp. 188–212). Guilford Press.

Hare, R. D. (2003). *Manual for the Hare Psychopathy Checklist–Revised* (2nd ed.). Multi-Health Systems.

Hare, R. D. (2016). Psychopathy, the PCL-R, and criminal justice: Some new findings and current issues. *Canadian Psychology, 57*, 21–34.

Hare, R. D., & Neumann, C. S. (2008). Psychopathy as a clinical and empirical construct. *Annual Review of Clinical Psychology, 4*, 217–246.

Hare, R. D., Frazelle, J., & Cox, D. N. (1978). Psychopathy and physiological responses to threat of an aversive stimulus. *Psychophysiology, 15*, 165–172.

Hare, R. D., Harpur, T. J., & Hemphill, J. D. (1989). *Scoring pamphlet for the Self-Report Psychopathy scale: SRP-II*. Unpublished manuscript, Simon Fraser University, Vancouver, British Columbia, Canada.

Harpur, T. J., Hakstian, A. R., & Hare, R. D. (1988). Factor structure of the Psychopathy Checklist. *Journal of Consulting and Clinical Psychology, 56*, 741–747.

Hawes, S. W., Byrd, A. L., Gonzalez, R., Cavanagh, C., Bechtold, J., Lynam, D. R., & Pardini, D. A. (2018). The developmental course of psychopathic features: Investigating stability, change, and long-term outcomes. *Journal of Research in Personality, 77*, 83–89.

Hemphälä, M., Kosson, D., Westerman, J., & Hodgins, S. (2015). Stability and predictors of psychopathic traits from mid-adolescence through early adulthood. *Scandinavian Journal of Psychology, 56*, 649–658.

Hemphill, J. F., Templeman, R., Wong, S., & Hare, R. D. (1998). Psychopathy and crime: Recidivism and criminal careers. In D. J. Cooke, R. D. Hare, & A. Forth (Eds.), *Psychopathy: Theory, research and implications for society* (pp. 375–399). Kluwer Academic Publishers.

Herve, H., Mitchell, D., & Cooper, B. S. (2004). Psychopathy and unlawful confinement: An examination of perpetrator and event characteristics. *Canadian Journal of Behavioural Science, 36*, 137–145.

Hicks, B. M., & Drislane, L. E. (2018). Variants ("subtypes") of psychopathy. In C. Patrick (Ed.), *Handbook of psychopathy* (2nd ed., pp. 297–334). Guilford Press.

Hill, C. D., Neumann, C. S., & Rogers, R. (2004). Confirmatory factor analysis of the Psychopathy Checklist: Screening Version in offenders with Axis I disorders. *Psychological Assessment, 16*, 90–95.

Hobson, J., & Shine, J. (1998). Measurement of psychopathy in a UK prison population referred for long-term psychotherapy. *British Journal of Criminology, 38*, 504–515.

Hoff, H. A., Rypdal, K., Mykletun, A., & Cooke, D. J. (2012). A prototypicality validation of the Comprehensive Assessment of Psychopathic Personality (CAPP). *Journal of Personality Disorders, 26*, 414–427.

Hoff, H. A., Rypdal, K., Hystad, S. W., Hart, S. D., Mykletun, A., Kreis, M. K. F., & Cooke, D. J. (2014). Cross-language consistency of the Comprehensive Assessment of Psychopathic Personality (CAPP) model. *Personality Disorders: Theory, Research, and Treatment, 5(4)*, 356–368. https://doi.org/10.1037/per0000069

Hurducas, C. C., Singh, J. P., de Ruiter, C., & Petrila, J. (2014). Violence risk assessment tools: A systematic review of surveys. *The International Journal of Forensic Mental Health, 13*, 181–192.

Isen, J., Raine, A., Baker, L., Dawson, M., Bezdjian, S., & Lozano, D. I. (2010). Sex-specific association between psychopathic traits and electrodermal reactivity in children. *Journal of Abnormal Psychology, 119*, 216–225.

Jackson R.L., Rogers R., Neumann C.S., & Lambert, P.L. (2002). Psychopathy in female offenders: An investigation of its underlying dimensions. *Criminal Justice and Behavior, 29*, 692–704. https://doi.org/10.1177/009385402237922

Karpman, B. (1948). The myth of the psychopathic personality. *The American Journal of Psychiatry, 104*, 523–534.

Kavish, N., Schiafo, M., Sellbom, M., & Anderson, J. L. (2020). Construct validity of the Comprehensive Assessment of Psychopathic Personality (CAPP) Lexical Rating Scale. *Personality Disorders, Theory, Research, and Treatment, 11*, 418–430.

Klein Haneveld, E., Neumann, C. S., Smid, W., Wever, E., & Kamphuis, J. H. (2018). Treatment responsiveness of replicated psychopathy profiles. *Law and Human Behavior, 42*, 484–495.

Kosson, D. S., Smith, S. S., & Newman, J. P. (1990). Evaluating the construct validity of psychopathy in Black and White male inmates: Three preliminary studies. *Journal of Abnormal Psychology, 99*, 250–259.

Kosson, D. S., Cyterski, T. D., Steuerwald, B. L., Neumann, C. S., & Walker-Matthews, S. (2002). The reliability and validity of the Psychopathy Checklist: Youth Version (PCL: YV) in nonincarcerated adolescent males. *Psychological Assessment, 14*, 97–109.

Kreis, M. K. F., Cooke, D. J., Michie, C., Hoff, H. A., & Logan, C. (2012). The Comprehensive Assessment of Psychopathic Personality (CAPP): Content validation using prototypical analysis. *Journal of Personality Disorders, 26*, 402–413.

Krstic, S., Knight, R. A., & Robertson, C. A. (2016). Developmental antecedents of the facets of psychopathy: The role of multiple abuse experiences. *Journal of Personality Disorders, 30*, 677–693.

Leenarts, L. E. W., Dölitzsch, C., Pérez, T., Schmeck, K., Fegert, J. M., & Schmid, M. (2017). The relationships between gender, psychopathic traits and self-reported delinquency: A comparison between a general population sample and a high-risk sample for juvenile delinquency. *Child and Adolescent Psychiatry and Mental Health, 11*, Article 64.

Levenson, M. R., Kiehl, K. A., & Fitzpatrick, C. M. (1995). Assessing psychopathic attributes in a noninstitutionalized population. *Journal of Personality and Social Psychology, 68*, 151–158.

Lewis, A. (1974). Psychopathic Personality: A most elusive category. *Psychological Medicine, 4*, 133–140.

Lilienfeld, S. O. (1994). Conceptual problems in the assessment of psychopathy. *Clinical Psychology Review, 14*, 17–38.

Lilienfeld, S. O., & Andrews, B. P. (1996). Development and preliminary validation of a self-report measure of psychopathic personality traits in noncriminal populations. *Journal of Personality Assessment, 66*, 488–524.
Lopez-Romero, L., Romero, E., & Villar, P. (2014). Assessing the stability of psychopathic traits: Adolescent outcomes in a six-year follow-up. *Spanish Journal of Psychology, 17*, 1–11.
Lorenz, A. R., & Newman, J. P. (2002). Do emotion and information processing deficiencies found in Caucasian psychopaths generalize to African-American psychopaths? *Personality and Individual Differences, 32*, 1077–1086.
Lykken, D. T. (1995). *The antisocial personalities*. Erlbaum.
Lynam, D. R., & Derefinko, K. J. (2006). Psychopathy and personality. In C. Patrick (Ed.), *Handbook of psychopathy* (pp. 133–155). Guilford Press.
Lynam, D. R., & Widiger, T. A. (2001). Using the Five Factor Model to represent the DSM-IV personality disorders: An expert consensus approach. *Journal of Abnormal Psychology, 110*, 401–412.
Lynam, D. R., Whiteside, S., & Jones, S. (1999). Self-reported psychopathy: A validation study. *Journal of Personality Assessment, 73*, 110–132.
Lynam, D. R., Charnigo, R., Moffitt, T. E., Raine, A., Loeber, R., & Stouthamer-Loeber, M. (2009). The stability of psychopathy across adolescence. *Development and Psychopathology, 21*, 1133–1153.
Lynam, D. R., Gaughan, E. R., Miller, J. D., Miller, D. J., Mullins-Sweatt, S., & Widiger, T. A. (2011). Assessing the basic traits associated with psychopathy: Development and validation of the Elemental Psychopathy Assessment. *Psychological Assessment, 23*, 108–124.
Lynn, R. (2002). Racial and ethnic differences in psychopathic personality. *Personality and Individual Differences, 32*, 273–316.
Maslow, A. H. (1951). *Principles of abnormal psychology: The dynamics of psychic illness*. Harper.
McCord, W., & McCord, J. (1964). *The psychopath: An essay on the criminal mind*. Van Nostrand.
Miller, J. D., & Lynam, D. R. (2003). Psychopathy and the Five Factor Model of personality: A replication and extension. *Journal of Personality Assessment, 81*, 168–178.
Miller, J. D., & Lynam, D. R. (2015). Understanding psychopathy using the basic elements of personality. *Social and Personality Psychology Compass, 9*, 223–237.
Miller, J. D., Lynam, D. R., Widiger, T. A., & Leukefeld, C. (2001). Personality disorders as extreme variants of common personality dimensions: Can the Five Factor Model adequately represent psychopathy? *Journal of Personality, 69*, 253–276.
Miller, J. D., Gaughan, E. T., Maples, J., Gentile, B., Lynam, D. R., & Widiger, T. A. (2011a). Examining the construct validity of the Elemental Psychopathy Assessment. *Assessment, 18*, 106–114.
Miller, J. D., Watts, A., & Jones, S. E. (2011b). Does psychopathy manifest divergent relations with components of its nomological network depending on gender? *Personality and Individual Differences, 50*, 564–569.
Miller, J. D., Hyatt, C. S., Rausher, S., Maples, J. L., & Zeichner, A. (2014). A test of the construct validity of the Elemental Psychopathy Assessment scores in a community sample of adults. *Psychological Assessment, 26*, 555–562.
Millon, T. (1981). *Disorders of personality: DSM-III: Axis II*. Wiley.
Munoz, L. C., & Frick, P. J. (2007). The reliability, stability, and predictive validity of the self-report version of the Antisocial Process Screening Device. *Scandinavian Journal of Psychology, 48*, 299–312.
Neal, T. M. S., & Grisso, T. (2014). Assessment practices and expert judgment methods in forensic psychology and psychiatry: An international snapshot. *Criminal Justice and Behavior, 41*, 1406–1421.
Neal, T. M. S., & Sellbom, M. (2012). Examining the factor structure of the Hare Self-Report Psychopathy Scale. *Journal of Personality Assessment, 94*, 244–253.
Neumann, C. S., Hare, R. D., & Newman, J. P. (2007). The super-ordinate nature of psychopathy. *Journal of Personality Disorders, 21*, 102–117.

Neumann, C. S., Wampler, M., Taylor, J., Blonigen, D. M., & Iacono, W. G. (2011). Stability and invariance of psychopathic traits from late adolescence to young adulthood. *Journal of Research in Personality, 45*, 145–152.

Neumann, C. S., Schmitt, D. S., Carter, R., Embley, I., & Hare, R. D. (2012). Psychopathic traits in females and males across the globe. *Behavioral Sciences & the Law, 30*, 557–574.

Newman, J. P., Schmitt, W. A., & Voss, W. (1997). Processing of contextual cues in psychopathic and nonpsychopathic offenders. *Journal of Abnormal Psychology, 106*, 563–575.

Newman, J. P., MacCoon, D. G., Vaughn, L. J., & Sadeh, N. (2005). Validating a distinction between primary and secondary psychopathy with measures of Gray's BIS and BAS constructs. *Journal of Abnormal Psychology, 114*, 319–323.

O'Connor, D. A. (2001). *The female psychopath: Validity and factor structure of the revised Psychopathy Checklist (PCL-R) in women inmates*. Unpublished doctoral dissertation, Florida State University, Tallahassee.

O'Brien, B. S., & Frick, P. J. (1996). Reward dominance: Associations with anxiety, conduct problems, and psychopathy in children. *Journal of Abnormal Child Psychology, 24*, 223–240.

Ogloff, J. R. (2006). Psychopathy/antisocial personality disorder conundrum. *Australian and New Zealand Journal of Psychiatry, 40*, 519–528.

Oshukova, S., Kaltiala-Heino, R., Miettunen, K., Marttila, R., Tani, P., Aronen, E. T., Marttunen, M., Kaivosoja, M., & Lindberg, N. (2015). Self-reported psychopathic traits among non-referred Finnish adolescents: Psychometric properties of the Youth Psychopathic Traits Inventory and the Antisocial Process Screening Device. *Child and Adolescent Psychiatry and Mental Health, 9*, 15.

Patrick, C. J. (2010). *Operationalizing the triarchic conceptualization of psychopathy: Preliminary description of brief scales for assessment of boldness, meanness, and disinhibition*. Unpublished manual, Department of Psychology, Florida State University.

Patrick, C. J., Bradley, M. M., & Lang, P. J. (1993). Emotion in the criminal psychopath: Startle reflex modulation. *Journal of Abnormal Psychology, 102*, 82–92.

Patrick, C. J., Fowles, D. C., & Krueger, R. F. (2009). Triarchic conceptualization of psychopathy: Developmental origins of disinhibition, boldness, and meanness. *Development and Psychopathology, 21*, 913–938.

Paulhus, D. L., & Williams, K. M. (2002). The Dark Triad of personality: Narcissism, Machiavellianism and psychopathy. *Journal of Research in Personality, 36*, 556–563.

Pechorro, P. S., Poiares, C. A., Vieira, R. X., Maroco, J., Nunes, C., & de Jesus, S. N. (2014). Psychological and behavioral adjustment in female youths with high or low psychopathic traits. *International Journal of Law and Psychiatry, 37*, 619–627.

Pedersen, L., Kunz, C., Rasmussen, K., & Elsass, P. (2010). Psychopathy as a risk factor for violent recidivism: Investigating the Psychopathy Checklist Screening Version (PCL: SV) and the Comprehensive Assessment of Psychopathic Personality (CAPP) in a forensic psychiatric setting. *International Journal of Mental Health, 9*, 308–315.

Pera-Guardiola, V., Batalla, I., Bosque, J., Kosson, D., Pifarré, J., Hernández-Ribas, R., Goldberg, X., Contreras-Rodríguez, O., Menchón, J. M., Soriano-Mas, C., & Cardoner, N. (2016). Modulatory effects of psychopathy on Wisconsin Card Sorting Test performance in male offenders with Antisocial Personality Disorder. *Psychiatry Research, 235*, 43–48.

Pinel, P. (1806). *A treatise on insanity* (Translated by D. Davis). Hafner.

Poythress, N. G., & Skeem, J. L. (2006). Disaggregating psychopathy: Where and how to look for subtypes. In C. Patrick (Ed.), *Handbook of psychopathy* (pp. 172–192). Guilford Press.

Poythress, N. G., Edens, J. F., & Lilienfeld, S. O. (1998). Criterion-related validity of the Psychopathic Personality Inventory in a prison sample. *Psychological Assessment, 10*, 426–430.

Prichard, J. C. (1835). *A treatise on insanity and other disorders affecting the mind*. Sherwood, Gilbert, & Piper.

Rasmussen, K., Storsæter, O., & Levander, S. (1999). Personality disorders, psychopathy, and crime in a Norwegian prison population. *International Journal of Law and Psychiatry, 22*, 91–97.

Ribes-Guardiola, P., Poy, R., Segarra, P., Brandchadell, V., & Moltó, J. (2020). Response perseveration and the triarchic model of psychopathy in an undergraduate sample. *Personality Disorders, Theory, Research, and Treatment, 11*, 54–62.

Roy, S., Vize, C., Uzieblo, K., can Dongen, J. D. M., Miller, J., Lynam, D., Brazil, I., Yoon, D., Mokros, A., Gray, N. S., Snowden, R., & Neumann, C. S. (2020). Triarchic or septarchic?—Uncovering the Triarchic Psychopathy Measure's (TriPM) structure. *Personality Disorders, Theory, Research, and Treatment, 12*, 1–15.

Ručević, S. (2010). Psychopathic personality traits and delinquent and risky sexual behaviors in Croatian sample of non-referred boys and girls. *Law and Human Behavior, 34*, 379–391.

Rush, B. (1812). *Medical inquiries and observations, upon the diseases of the mind*. Kimber and Richardson.

Salekin, R. T., Rogers, R., & Sewell, K. W. (1997). Construct validity of psychopathy in a female offender sample: A multitrait-multimethod evaluation. *Journal of Abnormal Psychology, 106*, 576–585.

Salekin, R. T., Rogers, R., Ustad, K. L., & Sewell, K. W. (1998). Psychopathy and recidivism among female inmates. *Law and Human Behavior, 22*, 109–128.

Salekin, R. T., Neumann, C. S., Leistico, A.-M. R., & Zalot, A. A. (2004). Psychopathy in youth and intelligence: An investigation of Cleckley's hypothesis. *Journal of Clinical Child and Adolescent Psychology, 33*, 731–742.

Sandoval, A. R., Hancock, D., Poythress, N., Edens, J., & Lilienfeld, S. (2000). Construct validity of the Psychopathic Personality Inventory in a correctional sample. *Journal of Personality Assessment, 74*, 262–281.

Sandvik, A. M., Hansen, A. L., Kristensen, M. V., Johnsen, B. H., Logan, C., & Thornton, D. (2012). Assessment of psychopathy: Inter-correlations between Psychopathy Checklist Revised, Comprehensive Assessment of Psychopathic Personality—Institutional Rating Scale, and Self-Report of Psychopathy Scale—III. *The International Journal of Forensic Mental Health, 11*, 280–288.

Sebastian, C. L., McCrory, E. J. P., Cecil, C. A. M., Lockwood, P. L., De Brito, S. A., Fontaine, N. M. G., & Viding, E. (2012). Neural responses to affective and cognitive theory of mind in children with conduct problems and varying levels of callous-unemotional traits. *JAMA Psychiatry, 69*, 814–822.

Sellbom, M. (2011). Elaborating on the construct validity of the Levenson Self-Report Psychopathy Scale in incarcerated and non-incarcerated samples. *Law and Human Behavior, 35*, 440–451.

Sellbom, M., Cooke, D. J., & Hart, S. D. (2015a). Construct validity of the Comprehensive Assessment of Psychopathic Personality (CAPP) concept map: Getting closer to the core of psychopathy. *The International Journal of Forensic Mental Health, 14*, 172–180.

Sellbom, M., Wygant, D. B., & Drislane, L. E. (2015b). Elucidating the construct validity of the psychopathic personality inventory triarchic scales. *Journal of Personality Assessment, 97*, 374–381.

Sellbom, M., Cooke, D. J., & Shou, Y. (2019). Development and initial validation of the Comprehensive Assessment of Psychopathic Personality—Self-Report (CAPP-SR). *Psychological Assessment, 31*, 878–894.

Sewall, L. A., & Olver, M. E. (2019). Psychopathy and treatment outcome: Results from a sexual violence reduction program. *Personality Disorders, Theory, Research, and Treatment, 10*, 59–69.

Shepherd, S. M., & Strand, S. (2015). The utility of the Psychopathy Checklist: Youth Version (PCL: YV) and the youth psychopathic trait inventory (YPI)- Is it meaningful to measure psychopathy in young offenders? *Psychological Assessment, 28*, 405–415.

Shou, Y., Sellbom, M., & Xu, J. (2018). Psychometric properties of the Triarchic Psychopathy Measure: An item response theory approach. *Personality Disorders, Theory, Research, and Treatment, 9*, 217–227.

Skeem, J. L., & Cooke, D. J. (2010). Is criminal behavior a central component of psychopathy? Conceptual directions for resolving the debate. *Psychological Assessment, 22*, 433–445.

Skeem, J. L., & Mulvey, E. P. (2001). Psychopathy and community violence among civil psychiatric patients: Results from the MacArthur Violence Risk Assessment Study. *Journal of Consulting and Clinical Psychology, 69*, 358–374.

Skeem, J. L., Edens, J. F., Camp, J., & Colwell, L. H. (2004). Are there ethnic differences in levels of psychopathy? A meta-analysis. *Law and Human Behavior, 28*, 505–527.

Skeem, J. L., Polaschek, D. L. L., Patrick, C. J., & Lilienfeld, S. O. (2011). Psychopathic personality: Bridging the gap between scientific evidence and public policy. *Psychological Science in the Public Interest, 12*, 95–162.

Sleep, C. E., Weiss, B., Lynam, D. R., & Miller, J. D. (2019). An examination of the Triarchic Model of psychopathy's nomological network: A meta-analytic review. *Clinical Psychology Review, 71*, 1–26. https://doi.org/10.1016/j.cpr.2019.04.005

Somma, A., Borroni, S., Drislane, L. E., & Fossatti, A. (2015). Assessing the Triarchic Model of Psychopathy in adolescence: Reliability and validity of the Triarchic Psychopathy Measure (TriPM) in three samples of Italian community-dwelling adolescents. *Psychological Assessment, 28*, 36–48.

Steele, V. R., Maurer, J. M., Bernat, E. M., Calhoun, V. D., & Kiehl, K. A. (2016). Error-related rocessing in adult males with elevated psychopathic traits. *Personality Disorders, Theory, Research, and Treatment, 7*, 80–90.

Sullivan, E. A., & Kosson, D. S. (2006). Ethnic and cultural variations in psychopathy. In C. Patrick (Ed.), *Handbook of psychopathy* (pp. 437–458). Guilford Press.

Sullivan, E. A., Abramowitz, C. S., Lopez, M., & Kosson, D. S. (2006). Reliability and construct validity of the psychopathy checklist-revised for Latino, European American, and African American male inmates. *Psychological Assessment, 18*, 382–392.

Tew, J., Harkins, L., & Dixon, L. (2015). Assessing the reliability and validity of the Self-Report Psychopathy Scales in a UK offender population. *Journal of Forensic Psychiatry and Psychology, 26*, 166–184.

Tsang, S., Piquero, A. R., & Cauffman, E. (2014). An examination of the Psychopathy Checklist: Youth Version (PCL:YV) among male adolescent offenders: An item response theory analysis. *Psychological Assessment, 26*, 1333–1346.

Tsang, S., Schmidt, K. M., Vincent, G. M., Salekin, R. T., Moretti, M. M., & Odgers, C. L. (2015). Assessing psychopathy among justice involved adolescents with the PCL: YV: An item response theory examination across gender. *Personality Disorders, Theory, Research, and Treatment, 6*, 22–31.

Vachon, D. D., Lynam, D. R., Loeber, R., & Stouthamer-Loeber, M. (2012). Generalizing the nomological network of psychopathy across populations differing on race and conviction status. *Journal of Abnormal Psychology, 121*, 263–269.

Vaidyanathan, U., Hall, J. R., Patrick, C. J., & Bernat, E. M. (2011). Clarifying the role of defensive reactivity deficits in psychopathy and antisocial personality using startle reflect methodology. *Journal of Abnormal Psychology, 120*, 253–258.

van Baardewijk, Y., Vermeiren, R., Stegge, H., & Doreleijers, T. (2011). Self-reported psychopathic traits in children: Their stability and concurrent and prospective association with conduct problems and aggression. *Journal of Psychopathology and Behavioral Assessment, 33*, 235–245.

Veit, R., Konicar, L., Klinzing, J. G., Barth, B., Yilmaz, O., & Birbaumer, N. (2013). Deficient fear conditioning in psychopathy as a function of interpersonal and affective disturbances. *Frontiers in Human Neuroscience, 25*, 706.

Venables, N. C., Hall, J. R., Yancey, J. R., & Patrick, C. J. (2015). Factors of psychopathy and electrocortical response to emotional pictures: Further evidence for a two-process theory. *Journal of Abnormal Psychology, 124*, 319–328.

Verona, E., & Vitale, J. E. (2018). Psychopathy in women: Assessment, manifestations, and etiology. In C. Patrick (Ed.), *Handbook of psychopathy* (2nd ed., pp. 509–528). Guilford Press.

Verona, E., Sprague, J., & Sadeh, N. (2012). Inhibitory control and negative emotion processing psychopathy and antisocial personality disorder. *Journal of Abnormal Psychology, 121*, 498–510.

Vieira, J. B., Ferreira-Santos, F., Almeida, P. R., Barbosa, F., Marques-Teixeira, J., & Marsh, A. A. (2015). Psychopathic traits are associated with cortical and subcortical volume alterations in healthy individuals. *Social Cognitive and Affective Neuroscience, 10*, 1693–1704.

Vitale, J. E., Smith, S. S., Brinkley, C. A., & Newman, J. P. (2002). The reliability and validity of the Psychopathy Checklist-Revised in a sample of female offenders. *Criminal Justice and Behavior, 29*, 202–231.

Vitale, J. E., Newman, J. P., Bates, J. E., Goodnight, J., Dodge, K. A., & Petit, G. S. (2005). Deficient behavioral inhibition and anomalous selective attention in a community sample of adolescents with psychopathic and low-anxiety traits. *Journal of Abnormal Child Psychology, 33*, 461–470.

Vitale, J. E., MacCoon, G. D., & Newman, J. P. (2011). Emotion facilitation and passive avoidance learning in psychopathic female offenders. *Criminal Justice and Behavior, 38*, 641–658.

Walsh, Z. (2013). Psychopathy and criminal violence: The moderating effect of ethnicity. *Law and Human Behavior, 37*, 303–311.

Walsh, Z., & Kosson, D. S. (2007). Psychopathy and violent crime: A prospective study of the influence of socioeconomic status and ethnicity. *Law and Human Behavior, 31*, 209–229.

Walters, G. D., Duncan, S. A., & Mitchell-Perez, K. (2007). The latent structure of psychopathy: A taxonometric investigation of the Psychopathy Checklist–Revised in a heterogeneous sample of male inmates. *Assessment, 14*, 270–278.

Walters, G. D., Ermer, E., Knight, R. A., & Kiehl, K. A. (2015). Paralimbic biomarkers in taxometric analyses of psychopathy: Does changing the indicators change the conclusion? *Personality Disorders, Theory, Research, and Treatment, 6*, 41–52.

Wang, P., Baker, L. A., Gao, Y., Raine, A., & Lozano, D. I. (2012). Psychopathic traits and physiological responses to aversive stimuli in children aged 9–11 years. *Journal of Abnormal Child Psychology, 40*, 759–769.

Warren, J. I., Burnette, M. L., South, S. C., Preeti, C., Bale, R., Friend, R., & Van Patten, I. (2003). Psychopathy in women: Structural modeling and comorbidity. *International Journal of Law and Psychiatry, 26*, 223–242.

Watt, B. D., & Brooks, N. S. (2012). Self-report psychopathy in an Australian community sample. *Psychiatry, Psychology and Law, 19*, 389–401.

Weizmann-Henelius, G., Virkkunen, M., Gammelgard, M., Eronen, M., & Putkonen, H. (2015). The PCL-R and violent recidivism in a prospective follow-up of a nationwide sample of female offenders. *Journal of Forensic Psychiatry and Psychology, 26*, 667–685.

Widiger, T. A., & Lynam, D. (1998). Psychopathy and the five-factor model of personality. In T. Millon, E. Simonsen, M. Birket-Smith, & R. Davis (Eds.), *Psychopathy: Antisocial, criminal, and violent behavior* (pp. 171–187). Guilford Press.

Widiger, T. A., & Trull, T. J. (2007). Plate tectonics in the classification of personality disorder: Shifting to a dimensional model. *American Psychologist, 62*, 71–83.

Widiger, T. A., Samuel, D. B., Mullins-Sweatt, S., Gore, W. L., & Crego, C. (2012). An integration of normal and abnormal personality structure: The Five-Factor Model. In T. A. Widiger (Ed.), *Oxford library of psychology. The Oxford handbook of personality disorders* (pp. 82–107). Oxford University Press.

Williams, K. M., & Paulhus, D. L. (2004). Factor structure of the Self-Report Psychopathy scale (SRP-II) in non-forensic samples. *Personality and Individual Differences, 37*, 765–778.

Williams, K. M., Paulhus, D. L., & Hare, R. D. (2007). Capturing the four-factor structure of psychopathy in college students via self-report. *Journal of Personality Assessment, 88*, 205–219.

Wilson, L., Miller, J. D., Zeichner, A., Lynam, D. R., & Widiger, T. A. (2011). An examination of the validity of the elemental psychopathy assessment: Relations with other psychopathy measures, aggression, and externalizing behaviors. *Journal of Psychopathology and Behavioral Assessment, 33*, 315–322.

Zagon, I., & Jackson, H. (1994). Construct validity of a psychopathy measure. *Personality and Individual Differences, 17*, 125–135.

Chapter 3
Developmental Considerations in Psychopathy

Nadia Bounoua, Rickie Miglin, and Naomi Sadeh

Abstract Psychopathy is a personality disorder that was originally conceptualized based on abnormal affective, interpersonal, and behavioral tendencies observed in adults, many of whom displayed chronic antisocial behavior (Cleckley H, *The Mask of Sanity*. Mosby, 1941). Given that adults with psychopathic traits typically begin to display symptoms early in life (Frick et al., J Abnorm Child Psychol 31(4):457–470, 2003a; Frick et al., Behav Sci Law 21(6):713–736, 2003b), efforts to understand the developmental trajectory of this disorder have resulted in mounting research on risk factors for, and symptoms of, psychopathy that manifest in childhood and adolescence. This chapter will provide an overview of developmental considerations in the study of psychopathy. The topics covered include methods for assessing psychopathic traits in youth, prominent etiological models of the disorder, and emerging issues in the field with regard to intervention and treatment.

Keywords Psychopathic youth · Callous-unemotional traits · Downward translations · Etiological models · Youth interventions

3.1 Introduction

Psychopathy is a personality disorder that was originally conceptualized based on abnormal affective, interpersonal, and behavioral tendencies observed in adults, many of whom displayed chronic antisocial behavior (Cleckley, 1941). Given that adults with psychopathic traits typically begin to display symptoms early in life (Frick et al., 2003a, b), efforts to understand the developmental trajectory of this disorder have resulted in mounting research on risk factors for, and symptoms of, psychopathy that manifest in childhood and adolescence. This chapter will provide an overview of developmental considerations in the study of psychopathy. The topics covered include methods for assessing psychopathic traits in youth, prominent

N. Bounoua · R. Miglin · N. Sadeh (✉)
University of Delaware, Newark, DE, USA
e-mail: nsadeh@psych.udel.edu

J. E. Vitale (ed.), *The Complexity of Psychopathy*, Dangerous Behavior in Clinical and Forensic Psychology, https://doi.org/10.1007/978-3-030-83156-1_3

etiological models of the disorder, and emerging issues in the field with regard to intervention and treatment.

Psychopathic traits in youth are typically marked by a constellation of symptoms that span affective (e.g., callousness, shallow emotions), interpersonal (e.g., grandiosity, deceitfulness), and behavioral (e.g., impulsivity, aggressiveness) domains. Paralleling the adult literature, the affective-interpersonal characteristics are conceptualized as central to the construct in youth and differentiate psychopathic traits from other externalizing and antisocial behavior problems in childhood (Barry et al., 2000). That is, children with psychopathic traits present with callous attitudes and blunted emotional reactivity, traits that set them apart from youth with other disruptive behavior problems (Haas et al., 2015). Further, many studies have shown that youth who present with another disruptive behavior and callous-unemotional (CU) traits have poorer outcomes compared to their counterparts with no CU traits, including more behavior problems and greater social impairment (Kimonis et al., 2004; Waschbusch & Willoughby, 2008). High levels of such traits are associated with increased risk of engaging in severe antisocial behaviors and the development of psychopathic traits in adulthood (Blonigen et al., 2006; Lynam et al., 2007). Thus, although children and adolescents cannot be diagnosed with psychopathy, many of the features of the disorder are evident in youth, including emotional deficits, elevated impulsivity and a tendency to violate social norms (Pardini & Loeber, 2007). However, caution must be taken when labeling youth as "psychopathic", as certain behaviors that seem psychopathic may in fact be a normal and transitory part of development during childhood and adolescence (Steinberg, 2002).

3.2 Measurement of Psychopathic Traits

One of the first methodological hurdles the field had to overcome was developing measures to reliably assess psychopathic traits in youth. Overwhelmingly, researchers have adopted a downward translation approach to solve this problem. This approach involves revising adult psychopathy assessments to make them developmentally-appropriate for children and adolescents by removing items that are irrelevant (e.g., engaging in multiple short-term marital relationships) or altering them to reflect behaviors that are more characteristic of youth and/or do not pathologize normative behavior in kids (e.g., changing the parasitic lifestyle item to parasitic orientation). To date, several reliable measures have been developed to assess psychopathic traits in children and adolescents using a downward translation approach.

The most widely-used interview-based assessment of psychopathic symptoms among youth is the Hare Psychopathy Checklist: Youth Version (PCL:YV; Forth et al., 2003). The PCL:YV was developed through downward translation of the Psychopathy Checklist -Revised (PCL-R, Hare, 2003), the gold standard method of assessing psychopathic traits in adults. Items on the PCL:YV are typically scored by trained coders, based on a child's interview responses, available court documentation, and, at times, an interview with a parent or guardian.

A wealth of research has demonstrated concurrent validity between PCL:YV scores and externalizing problems (Schmidt et al., 2006). Among youth offenders, scores on the PCL:YV have been shown to predict a range of important outcomes, including recidivism (Corrado et al., 2004; Hempel et al., 2013), and adult violence and antisocial behavior (Gretton et al., 2004). It is important to note that the predictive validity of the PCL:YV has been shown to vary across samples. For example, weaker associations between scores on the PCL:YV and recidivism have been reported among female than male adolescents (Schmidt et al., 2006). Further, work by Shepherd and Strand (2016) calls into question the utility of the PCL:YV in high-risk, justice-involved youth. This study examined the predictive validity of the PCL:YV after a 6 month follow-up period and found that, while the PCL:YV identified youth high in psychopathic traits, it did not show much utility as a predictor of future antisocial behavior. Although the antisocial facet modestly predicted violent recidivism, none of the PCL:YV scores predicted general recidivism during the follow-up period, and age was a superior predictor of both violent and general recidivism to the PCL:YV total score (Shepherd & Strand, 2016). These findings suggest that the usefulness of the PCL:YV for predicting recidivistic outcomes may be diminished in high-risk, offender samples. Still, this interview-based tool is widely considered a valid and developmentally appropriate measure of psychopathic traits in youth.

There are several multi-informant scales, many of which were initially derived from the PCL-R and PCL-YV, that have been introduced with the goal of providing a more efficient means of screening for psychopathic traits than interview-based measurement. Research has demonstrated that self-report questionnaires are reliable and valid methods for assessing psychopathic traits in youth (Vahl et al., 2014). However, some limitations that arise with self-report measures in youth, particularly in relation to undesirable behaviors or traits, include lack of insight/awareness or tendencies to underreport. To address these concerns, parent/caregiver and teacher reports are often combined with youth self-reports of psychopathic traits, which has been shown to offer some advantages in terms of accurately predicting recidivism and other outcomes compared to self-report measures alone (Colins et al., 2012).

The Antisocial Process Screening Device (APSD; Frick & Hare, 2001), formerly known as the Psychopathy Screening Device, is the most widely researched questionnaire-based assessment of psychopathic traits in youth. It was modeled as a downward extension of the adult PCL-R. The APSD is short, easy to administer, and can be used and combined across multiple informants. It has also demonstrated reliability (Sharp & Kine, 2008) and predictive validity in terms of recidivism, program non-compliance, and severe patterns of violence in incarcerated populations (Falkenbach et al., 2003; Kruh et al., 2005). However, others have found that the APSD fails to distinguish children that go on to develop psychopathic traits in adulthood from those who do not (Lynam, 1997) and have criticized the development of the instrument based on the PCL-R, given this tool was not developed for self-report purposes (Andershed et al., 2002).

The CU traits subscale of the APSD is limited in that it is only comprised of six items, has a restricted number of response options (3-point Likert scale), and has only shown moderate internal consistency in many samples (Loney et al., 2003). To address the psychometric limitations of the original CU subscale on the APSD, Frick (2004) developed the Inventory of Callous-Unemotional Traits (ICU). To create the ICU, the four items of the APSD that loaded consistently on the CU factor were expanded with six new items for each original item, and the resulting 24 items were put on a 4-point rating scale. The ICU loads on a general CU factor as well as on three distinct factors: callousness, uncaring, and unemotional. It can be used with multiple informants (self, parent, teacher) and has demonstrated good convergent validity with other measures of antisocial behavior in youth (Kimonis et al., 2008; Roose et al., 2010).

In summary, there have been great advancements in the development of tools to measure psychopathic traits in youth using a downward translation approach. Although this type of research has yielded a great deal of information about the extension of psychopathy to youth, it is important to note the limitations of this approach. Conceptualizing psychopathic traits in youth based on adult psychopathy means that the validity of the construct in youth depends on the accuracy of our conceptualization and measurement of psychopathy in adulthood. Further, there is growing evidence that personality traits change over development and interact with the environment (Caspi et al., 2005; Newton-Howes et al., 2015). For example, the stability of psychopathic traits has been found to be substantially less over a 2 year period in adolescence (r = .33) than in adulthood ($r = .71$), potentially as a result of the psychosocial maturation that occurs during the former period (Cauffman et al., 2016). Therefore, more research is needed to establish that youth who exhibit psychopathic traits manifest similar symptoms in adulthood and to ensure that the existing measures adequately capture the construct in youth. Despite these limitations, much has been learned from research on the assessment of psychopathic traits in youth.

3.2.1 Evidence of a Multidimensional Construct

As a means of evaluating the construct validity of youth psychopathy measures, researchers have examined structural models of psychopathic traits in children and adolescents and compared them to those found with adult measures. Substantial research indicates that adult psychopathy is a multidimensional construct comprised of at least two primary dimensions: Factor 1 represents the affective and interpersonal symptoms of psychopathy (e.g., lack of remorse, shallow affect, superficial charm, deceitfulness) and Factor 2 captures the chronic engagement in impulsive and antisocial acts (e.g., need for stimulation, irresponsibility, criminal behavior). More recently, additional factor structures have been proposed that parse the two factors into more specific facets. For example, a recent review of studies using exploratory factor analyses (EFAs) to examine the structure of adult psychopathy reported empirical support for models of two to five latent factors (Neumann et al., 2006).

Similar findings have emerged for youth psychopathy; Neumann et al. (2006) report that several models, including two, three and four factors, provided good fit among adolescents. These findings suggest that psychopathic traits in youth consist of separable affective, interpersonal, impulsive, and antisocial facets (Frick et al., 2000; Gorin et al., 2019; Salekin, 2017). There is also evidence that the factor structure of psychopathic traits changes in different settings, with the two-factor model appearing to better characterize clinical inpatient populations (Fite et al., 2009) and the three-factor model working well with non-referred community children (Dadds et al., 2005) and incarcerated adolescents (Vitacco et al., 2003).

Research on the multidimensional nature of psychopathic traits in youth has focused on scales developed as downward extensions of adult measures, such as the PCL: YV and APSD. As an alternative to youth-adapted versions of adult psychopathy measures, Patrick et al. (2009) proposed a triarchic model meant to reconcile competing conceptualizations and to summarize commonly observed features of psychopathy. In particular, Patrick and colleagues have argued that the boldness dimension of psychopathy is not well represented in existing youth measures and a more developmentally-informed approach needs to be taken to index the core neurobiological processes that lead to the development of psychopathy in adulthood. The Triarchic model of psychopathy addresses these limitations and it is composed of three distinguishable yet related phenotypic components: boldness, meanness, and disinhibition. Unlike other factor oriented models of psychopathy (Hare & Neumann, 2006; Frick & Marsee, 2006), the Triarchic model was not designed based on any one adult assessment instrument, though the Triarchic Psychopathy Measure (TriPM; Patrick, 2010) has been used to operationalize the phenotypic constructs of the model. The boldness facet reflects the temperamental fearlessness, lack of anxiety, resilience to psychopathological distress, and interpersonal dominance that is characteristic of psychopathy. The meanness facet relates to the callous and unemotional features of psychopathy (e.g. lack of empathy, callous-aggression), and the disinhibition facet reflects the lack of inhibitory control that is core to psychopathy as well as impulsive conduct problems and externalizing disorders (Patrick et al., 2009). Compared to downward translation conceptualizations of psychopathy and their associated measures, research on the Triarchic model is still in its infancy and more research is needed to establish its construct validity. For example, although in its early stages, a recent meta-analytic study by Sleep et al. (2019) suggests that the boldness dimension is not central to prototypical psychopathy, but rather represents a positive, socially-dominant interpersonal style that is associated with adaptive outcomes rather than maladaptive behavior. Thus, the usefulness of the Triarchic model for understanding and measuring developmental risk for psychopathy remains an empirical question.

Although there is still disagreement among researchers in terms of the dimensions that most accurately capture the construct of psychopathic traits in youth, CU traits (e.g. lack of guilt, lack of empathy, callous use of others) make up an important component in most conceptualizations and measurements of psychopathy (Barry et al., 2000). CU Traits have been shown to distinguish an important subgroup of youth on an etiological trajectory associated with chronic, severe, and premeditated types of violent behavior (Frick et al., 2003a; Frick & Dickens, 2006). As a consequence, research on CU traits has dominated the study of psychopathy in youth. CU traits remain relatively stable across childhood and adolescence compared to other measures of personality (Frick et al., 2003b, 2005; Lynam et al., 2007), and are predictive of both juvenile and adult arrests as well as early adult personality disorder symptoms and diagnosis (Lynam et al., 2007; McMahon et al., 2010).

3.3 The Etiology of Psychopathic Traits

The causes of psychopathic traits in youth still remain largely unknown. However, research on risk factors and causal mechanisms is expanding rapidly. The next section provides an overview of key areas of research on contributors to the development of psychopathic traits in youth. Three levels of analysis are reviewed: environmental, genetic, and neurobiological factors.

3.3.1 Environmental Factors

Environmental factors have historically not been emphasized in research on psychopathy, given that seminal theorists postulated psychopaths are "free from social or emotional impediments" (Cleckley, 1941) and are difficult to socialize using traditional environmental reinforcements, like punishment (Lykken, 1995). However, as research on psychopathy grew, it became apparent that not all individuals who manifest psychopathic traits show low levels of social and emotional reactivity. Accordingly, scientists interested in the etiology of psychopathy often differentiate "primary" or innate psychopathy from "secondary" or acquired psychopathy (Skeem et al., 2003) using measures of trait anxiety, internalizing psychopathology, or emotional reactivity (Craig & Moretti, 2018; Eisenbarth et al., 2019; Kimonis et al., 2012). In primary psychopathy, a constitutional deficit in fear reactivity is theorized to increase risk-taking behavior, social dominance, and a failure to internalize punishment (expressed as guiltlessness) (Berg et al., 2013; Lilienfeld & Hess, 2001; Lykken, 1995). By contrast, secondary psychopathy is thought to result from early exposure to environmental adversity that leads to the appearance of an "acquired callousness" that masks high levels of emotional turmoil (Kerig et al., 2010). Thus, primary and secondary psychopathic individuals appear similarly callous, impulsive, and antisocial in their behavior, but they differ in their causal pathways (i.e., heritable liability towards low fear reactivity vs. environmental exposure to adversity) and their experience of distress (Karpman, 1948; Lykken, 1995; Porter, 1996).

Primary and secondary psychopathy subtypes have consistently been found in adult incarcerated populations (Hicks et al., 2004, 2010; Newman et al., 2005), but research has only recently explored these variants in youth. Although research on psychopathic subtypes in youth is less well developed than in adult samples, a number of studies have found that youth who score high on psychopathic or CU traits can be parsed into primary and secondary subtypes based on measures of anxiety, depression, or exposure to trauma (Kimonis et al., 2011, 2012; Tatar et al., 2012; Vaughn et al., 2009). Thus, the primary-secondary distinction appears to be useful for considering etiological models of psychopathy in youth, and potentially for identifying environmentally-mediated trajectories of risk.

Several theoretical models posit that environmental factors play an integral role in the etiology of youth psychopathy (Karpman, 1941; Kerig et al., 2010; Porter, 1996). These theories suggest that exposure to various forms of environmental risk factors may lead to an array of delinquent and antisocial behaviors and the development of youth psychopathy, particularly "secondary" psychopathic traits (Karpman, 1941; Lee et al., 2010).

While research has implicated a multitude of environmental risk factors related to youth psychopathic traits, a thorough review of these factors is outside the scope of this chapter (for a review of sociocultural factors and youth psychopathy, see Rubio et al., 2014). Instead, here we highlight empirical support for three key environmental factors that have been implicated in etiological models of youth psychopathy—trauma exposure, parenting practices, and peer influences.

Trauma exposure is a key environmental factor represented in etiological models of youth psychopathy. In samples of boys and girls, research has pointed to high rates of exposure to traumatic events and victimization among youth with psychopathic traits (Kahn et al., 2013; Krischer & Sevecke, 2008; Maikovich et al., 2008; O'Neill et al., 2003; Schraft et al., 2013; Sharf et al., 2014; Tatar et al., 2012; Vaughn et al., 2009). Theoretical models have posited that youth who experience trauma may acquire strategies to cope with these traumatic experiences, including detachment from others or a "mask" of callousness. These acquired mechanisms are posited to then lead to the presentation of callousness and reduced emotionality, consistent with the secondary subtype of psychopathy (Ford et al., 2006; Porter, 1996).

Several mechanisms underlying the relationship between trauma and secondary psychopathic traits have been examined. One robust finding is that alterations in various emotional processing strategies may serve as the link between trauma exposure and psychopathic traits among youth. For example, Bennett and Kerig (2014) found that traumatized detained youth with CU traits had greater difficulty with a range of emotion regulation strategies than their non-traumatized counterparts. Similarly, other research has shown that psychopathic youth who have experienced chronic trauma are more likely to engage in emotional numbing, or the avoidance of distressing emotions (Kalisch et al., 2005). Further, studies have demonstrated that emotional numbing mediates the relationship between exposure to trauma and youth psychopathic traits (Allwood et al., 2011; Kerig et al., 2010).

This body of research points to robust associations between exposure to stressful and traumatic events and psychopathic traits, with the most support for this association among youth with secondary or acquired CU traits. Although these associations have been well-documented, more work is needed to better understand the mechanisms through which exposure to traumatic events confers risk for later psychopathic and delinquent behaviors. Promising mechanisms include emotional processing strategies (discussed above), which may represent adaptive *immediate* responses to trauma, but subsequently lead to the development of CU traits and engagement in delinquent behaviors.

Family characteristics are also believed to play a pivotal role in the etiology of youth psychopathy. Dimensions of negative parenting practices, in particular, have emerged as robust predictors of a range of psychopathic traits, including CU features and antisocial behavior in youth (Craig et al., 2013; Farrington et al., 2010; Fisher & Brown, 2018; Larsson et al., 2008; Mills-Koonce et al., 2016; Waller et al., 2018a). In addition to concurrent associations, prospective studies have reported causal links between the development of CU traits and negative parenting practices, such as harsh parenting (Barker et al., 2011; Frick et al., 2003b; Waller et al., 2012, 2015) and corporal punishment (Childs et al., 2014; Pardini et al., 2007). These relationships are thought to emerge through various mechanisms, including disrupted parent-child attachment (Kosson et al., 2002; Pasalich et al., 2012; Willoughby et al., 2014). Interestingly, recent longitudinal work has shown that the association with parenting and psychopathic traits may continue into adulthood, with negative parenting in childhood predicting an array of adult antisocial behaviors through increased CU traits (Goulter et al., 2020). This research points to negative parenting practices as a key risk factor for the development of youth psychopathic traits that may persist into adulthood.

In addition to negative parenting, other parental practices such as the monitoring of children's behaviors and level of supervision have also been implicated in psychopathic traits among youth (Crum et al., 2015; Fisher & Brown, 2018; Hawes et al., 2011; Waller et al., 2018a). It is worth mentioning that, while the relationship between low parental monitoring and the development of CU traits seems to be causal, studies have also shown that this relationship may be bidirectional. That is, longitudinal research indicates CU traits influence monitoring and supervision efforts in parents, with parents of children high in CU traits reducing their surveillance behaviors over time (Muñoz et al., 2011; Salihovic et al., 2012; Tuvblad et al., 2013). These findings suggest that, in addition to a causal mechanism, decreased parental monitoring may be a reaction to the expression of CU traits in youth. More research is needed to distinguish between "child-driven" effects on parenting practices and vice versa to clarify how parenting practices impact the development of psychopathic traits (Hawes et al., 2011; Larsson et al., 2008).

While extant research has focused on risk factors for the development of CU traits in youth, a line of research has also sought to identify protective factors that reduce the manifestation of these traits. Positive parenting practices, such as parental warmth and responsivity, have been shown to be inversely related to youth psychopathic traits (Clark & Frick, 2018; Muratori et al., 2016; Pasalich et al., 2011). Further, studies have shown that positive parenting can lead to decreases in youth CU traits and conduct problems over time (Dishion et al., 2008; Waller et al., 2014; Wright et al., 2018).

In sum, a consistent and robust relationship has emerged between parenting practices and the development of psychopathic traits early in life. In addition to establishing associations between negative parenting and the presence of CU traits, research has also demonstrated that parenting can predict the future development of psychopathic traits. Further, research has shown that positive parenting styles, such as positive-reinforcement of prosocial behaviors and parental warmth, have a positive impact on youth who are at risk for developing CU traits as well as those who already evidence them. Additional research is needed to clarify how other individual difference factors may moderate the impact of parenting practices. For example, studies have shown that the association between parenting and psychopathic traits may vary by sex and the age of youth (Hawes et al., 2011). However, other studies point to consistency across sexes in relation to the role of parenting and psychopathic traits (Hicks et al., 2012; Salihovic et al., 2012). Thus, the specific pathways through which family characteristics impact psychopathic traits in youth requires further study and other individual difference factors should be considered to accurately model the impact of family environment on psychopathy trajectories.

Peer influences represent another key environmental risk factor that may be particularly salient in relation to youth psychopathic traits. Indeed, research studies have reported concurrent links between peer influences, CU traits, and delinquency among adolescents (Burnette et al., 2012; Kerr et al., 2012; Kimonis et al., 2004; Mobarake et al., 2014; Muñoz et al., 2008; Slattery & Meyers, 2014). These peer influences appear to be especially relevant for youth during middle adolescence (Monahan et al., 2009). However, to date, mixed results regarding the strength and directionality of effects in this association have been reported. Some research suggests that youth with psychopathic traits are more likely to be rejected by peers, which then increases the likelihood that these youth will engage in a range of delinquent behaviors (Hicks et al., 2012). On the other hand, research has also demonstrated that affiliation with deviant peers increases the opportunity for youth to participate in antisocial behaviors and may provide positive reinforcement for these behaviors (Dishion et al., 1995). Further, longitudinal work has found that social relationships may moderate the stability of youth psychopathic traits, such that youth with positive social interactions may show decreases in traits like aggression over time (Barry et al., 2008). Given the mixed findings in the literature to date, more research is needed to further clarify what role, if any, peer relationships play in the etiology of psychopathic traits among children and adolescents. Longitudinal studies would be particularly informative, as they could help parse out whether youth with psychopathic traits are more likely to seek out deviant peers (vs. the peers impacting the manifestation of psychopathic traits) and how youth with CU traits impact their peers' delinquent behavior.

3.3.2 Genetic Factors

There is strong evidence that genetic factors play a significant role in the development of psychopathic traits, especially for individuals who manifest high levels of these traits early in development and those that demonstrate "primary" CU traits

(Moore et al., 2019). The majority of empirical support for genetic contributors to psychopathic traits in youth comes from behavioral genetics research, with twin studies consistently showing moderate to strong heritability of CU traits (36–67%, Moore et al., 2019) and environmental contributors typically accounting for much less of the phenotypic variability (Viding & McCrory, 2012a, b). The limited evidence that exists from longitudinal investigations suggests that genetic influences account for a substantial portion of the stability in CU traits over time in late childhood (estimated at 89% for stability between ages 7 and 12; Henry et al., 2018a, b) and adolescence (estimated at 58% for stability between ages 17 and 24; Blonigen et al., 2006). These findings are consistent with theoretical models that postulate CU traits are temperamental and largely attributable to biological causes that make youth who inherit these traits less reactive to environmental influences and, consequently, more difficult to socialize (e.g., the Low Fear Hypothesis; Lykken, 1995).

However, emerging research calls into question the long-held assumption that youth with psychopathic traits are relatively unaffected by environmental factors. Although the majority of twin studies have found minimal effects of shared environmental factors (i.e., experiences that increase the similarity of twins) on the development of CU traits (e.g., Bezdjian et al., 2011), there are exceptions. In a mixed-sex sample of over five-thousand twin pairs, Henry et al. (2016) reported that 26% of the variation in CU traits was accounted for by shared environmental influences, which is a higher proportion than has been found in most previous work. Similarly, a few studies implicate a greater, though still modest, effect of shared environmental influences on psychopathic traits in girls than boys, especially for girls with elevated and stable CU traits (Fontaine et al., 2010; Viding et al., 2007), suggesting social forces may shape CU expressions in girls more so than boys. A recent longitudinal investigation of 227 twin pairs revealed that small differences in the manner in which parents treat identical twins influenced levels of CU traits, such that those siblings who experienced harsher parenting demonstrated higher levels of callousness and unemotionality (Waller et al., 2018a, b). An related finding from a sample of 662 twin pairs suggested that the heritability of CU traits was diminished in the presence of high vs. low warm/ rewarding parenting (Henry et al., 2018a, b). The relatively novel influence of environmental forces detected in these studies may be due to improvements in the experimental design of behavioral genetic research, such as the use of more reliable measures of psychopathic traits and prospective designs. Notably, these findings challenge the assumption that psychopathic trajectories are determinate and immune to what is happening in a child's environment, although the degree of environmental influence does appear to be diminished relative to genetic factors in youth with CU traits.

The substantial empirical support for the heritability of psychopathic traits suggests that there may be a specific set or class of genes that confer risk for low emotionality and, in turn, CU traits. There have only been a few genetic studies to date that have examined candidate gene associations with CU traits in youth, and the majority of research has been conducted on genes involved in the oxytocin and serotonin systems (Beichtman et al., 2012; Fowler et al., 2009; Malik et al., 2012; Moore et al., 2019; Moul & Dadds, 2013). The oxytocin receptor gene (OXTR) has been of interest to psychopathy researchers given that genetic variations in OXTR have been associated with prosocial behaviors, such as affiliation and attachment (Lee et al., 2009), as well as antisocial behavior, such as aggression and criminality (LoParo et al., 2016), including in adolescents (Hovey et al., 2016; Smearman et al., 2015). A study by Dadds et al., (2014) reported a novel association between the rs1042778 SNP of OXTR and the co-occurrence of CU traits and conduct problems in two samples of children ages 4–16. Gene-environment interactions have also emerged in genetic association studies on psychopathic traits. For example, Sadeh et al. (2010) found that youth who carried the long allele of the serotonin transporter gene (5HTTLPR) evidenced higher levels of CU traits than carriers of the short allele if they also lived in socioeconomically disadvantaged environments. Studies such as these provide preliminary evidence that oxytocin and serotonin may be involved in the development of psychopathic traits, though more research is needed to determine the replicability of the findings.

Like research on other complex psychiatric phenotypes, candidate gene studies on psychopathic traits has suffered from failures to replicate. Methodological considerations, such as underpowered studies and inconsistencies in the measurement of psychopathic traits across studies, may have contributed to replication inconsistencies. The complexity of the psychopathy construct may also have hampered the search for specific genes, as it is unlikely that a single common genetic variant will be able to account for the complex behaviors associated with psychopathy. Further, the search for candidate genes has relied on the ability of scientists to predict in advance which genetic variants will confer risk for psychopathic traits, potentially limiting the discovery of relevant genes and causal pathways (Dick et al., 2015). To move the field forward, it will be necessary to take a more exploratory and comprehensive approach to examining genetic influences, especially methodologies that evaluate the entire genome (e.g., genome-wide association studies, development of polygenic risk scores, consideration of nonadditive genetic effects), those that examine epigenetic mechanisms, and studies linking genetic factors with intermediate mechanisms (e.g., neurocognitive factors, emotional processes).

These types of studies have started to emerge, though data are limited. Only one genome wide association study has been conducted to date and it did not reveal any significant genetic associations with CU traits in youth (Viding et al., 2010). Epigenetic studies have begun to examine methylation of psychopathy-linked genes, specifically the OXTR, and found higher levels of CU traits were associated with greater methylation of this gene (Cecil et al., 2014; Dadds et al., 2014). Research evaluating the mechanisms by which genetic risk translates into psychopathic phenotypes has also gained momentum in recent years, shedding light on how risk is conferred across levels of analysis. For example, an interesting study by Ezpeleta et al. (2019) examined the contributions of stressful life events and the OXTR gene to the developmental trajectories of CU traits in a sample of children assessed annually from ages three to nine. Latent growth models revealed three distinct developmental trajectories that differed in reports of stressful life events and fluctuations of CU traits. The first class was the largest and characterized by low levels of stress exposure and low CU traits that were relatively stable over time. The second class was marked by high and ascending CU traits, but low levels of stress exposure, whereas the third class was characterized by persistently high CU traits and high stress exposure. Notably, carriers of the OXTR A allele were more likely to belong to the third class, but not the other two developmental trajectories. Studies such as these highlight the interplay of genetic and environmental risk on the course of psychopathic traits in youth and show promise for untangling developmental pathways in future research.

Although the majority of research has examined genetic risk for CU traits, studies have also examined how genes influence the co-occurrence of these traits and conduct problems. Twin studies suggest that the heritability of antisocial and disruptive behavior is stronger in youth with CU traits (Viding et al., 2009) and that genetic factors are important for explaining the covariation in these behavior problems (Fontaine et al., 2018). It is important to note that genetic risk factors likely differ between youth who display disruptive behaviors with and without CU traits (e.g., Sadeh et al., 2010), and there is evidence to suggest environmental influences have a greater impact on the trajectories of the latter children (Viding et al., 2005). Moving forward, genetically-informed research that differentiates children high and low in CU traits will be important for parsing developmental pathways to antisocial and psychopathic behavior.

The need to consider genetic factors in developmental models of psychopathy is no longer in question. However, it is necessary to recognize that a genetic predisposition to develop CU traits does not determine whether or not an individual will manifest psychopathic behaviors. Rather, it influences the probability that these phenotypes will be expressed. Growing evidence that environmental factors influence the manifestation of CU phenotypes underscores the point that even highly heritable traits are potentially amenable to treatment intervention. Research on the genetic underpinnings of complex behavioral patterns, including disruptive behavior disorders, unequivocally implicates the interplay of a multitude of risk and protective factors, with genetic liability representing only one facet. Thus, genetic contributions need to be considered in the context of other risk processes, such as social, cognitive, affective and neurobiological factors.

3.3.3 Neurobiological Factors

For youth who demonstrate CU or psychopathic traits, biological predispositions for aberrant brain activity in regions that support emotion, cognition, and decision-making. These biological factors may influence these youths towards a trajectory that engenders engagement in more severe acts of violence and chronic antisocial behavior. Neural abnormalities have been linked to both the CU dimension and impulsive-antisocial dimension of psychopathic traits in youth. However, the types of neural abnormalities that are observed have been found to differ across these symptom dimensions.

Given that lack of empathy is a core component of CU behavior, it is not surprising that numerous investigations have sought to identify this construct's neural underpinnings. During conditions meant to elicit empathy, such as the viewing of fearful faces, CU traits in youth have been consistently linked with hypoactive functioning of the amygdala, a brain region involved in perceiving and processing emotion, compared to typically developing youth (Marsh et al., 2008; Jones et al., 2009; Viding et al., 2012). This finding is consistent with etiological models that emphasize blunted fear processing in the development of psychopathy (e.g., Lykken, 1995), which could contribute to impaired empathy in terms of detecting expressions of fear in others. Indeed, studies consistently show impaired recognition of fearful, sad, and happy facial expressions in youth with psychopathic traits (Dawel et al., 2012). Thus, hypoactivation in amygdala to fearful faces may reflect the amygdala's role in the processing and recognition of emotional expression and indicate youth with psychopathic traits have deficits in the recognition of emotion that extend beyond fearful faces.

The anterior cingulate cortex and putamen (Marsh et al., 2013) have also been identified as abnormal in youth with CU traits in conditions meant to elicit empathy, such as fearful facial expressions, as well as during affective theory of mind tasks (Sebastian et al., 2012). The anterior cingulate and putamen regions are implicated in affective processing and reinforcement-based learning, respectively, suggesting youth high on CU traits have deficits in these cognitive functions, which are important for engendering empathy. Notably, the clinical significance of functional neural abnormalities in youth psychopathy has also been investigated. For example, among youth with high CU traits, hypoactive amygdala functioning in response to fearful faces has been shown to mediate the relationship between CU traits and proactive aggressive behavior (Lozier et al., 2014). Thus, abnormal neurocognitive functioning in response to empathy-eliciting stimuli appear to at least partially explain aggressive behavior related to CU traits.

It should also be noted that, in addition to the emotional empathy deficits reviewed above, youth with psychopathic traits may have diminished cognitive empathy (Dadds et al., 2009), though findings are mixed (Jones et al., 2010) and seem to differ by gender (Dadds et al., 2009). That is, girls with psychopathic traits are less likely to display cognitive empathy deficits, which has been attributed to socialization factors that encourage taking others' perspectives more so in girls than boys (Brouns et al., 2013). Cognitive empathy refers to the ability to know or accurately label what another person is feeling, but it does not require an individual to have affective response to (or "feel") the other person's emotional state. Unlike the findings for emotional empathy tasks, some fMRI studies have demonstrated that youth high in psychopathic traits show normal recruitment of key brain regions during cognitive empathy tasks, such as the medial frontal cortex, temporal parietal junction, temporal pole, and posterior cingulate cortex (Sebastian et al., 2012). This finding is consistent with etiological models that posit psychopathic individuals' ability to recognize another person's emotional state is intact, but their ability to subjectively feel another person's emotions is impaired (Cleckley, 1941).

In addition to functional impairments, CU traits have been associated with cortical and subcortical neuroanatomical abnormalities. Youth who display high levels of CU traits, for instance, have been found to also exhibit reduced gray matter, lower total cortical surface area, and reduced gyrification in several temporal and prefrontal regions thought to be related to behavioral inhibition, social cognition, and emotional regulation (Bolhuis et al., 2019a).

Additionally, many studies have found reduced amygdala (Fairchild et al., 2013; Wallace et al., 2014), and ventromedial prefrontal cortex (vmPFC) volumes and thickness (Huebner et al., 2008; Ermer et al., 2013) among youth with conduct disorder, though there is conflicting evidence regarding the latter (De Brito et al., 2009). Researchers have interpreted these findings as support for the conceptualization of pediatric callous traits as a neurodevelopmental condition (Bolhuis et al., 2019b). Longitudinal research on the neuroanatomical correlates of CU traits should be given priority in future efforts in order to ascertain whether these structural abnormalities are evident in early childhood or whether they develop over time.

Another neurocognitive abnormality linked with psychopathic traits in youth is impaired reinforcement learning, or in other words, deficits in the ability to link outcomes (rewards or punishments) with stimuli or responses. Much neuroimaging work has shown that youths with psychopathic traits demonstrate abnormal patterns of functioning in reward and punishment processing regions, such as the vmPFC and the striatum (Cohn et al., 2015; White et al., 2013), in response to receiving or attempting to predict the value of rewards. For example, Finger et al. (2008) demonstrated that children with psychopathic traits (compared to healthy controls and children with ADHD) displayed lower vmPFC activity during a task that probed the ability to adjust and update learning in response to the reversal of previously rewarding stimuli to punishments. This line of research suggests that youth with psychopathic traits demonstrate impairments in both stimulus-response learning and aversive conditioning, and such impairments in childhood may constitute risk factors that predispose individuals to adult antisocial behavior in longitudinal studies (Gao et al., 2009).

Blair (2013) integrated a theoretical neurocognitive model to argue that dysfunction of emotion processing regions, such as the amygdala, as well as reward processing (e.g., striatum, caudate, nucleus accumbens, vmPFC) regions can lead to problems creating reinforcement contingencies between stimuli and conditioned responses. In other words, youth with psychopathic traits may be difficult to socialize, because they fail to encode the negative consequences associated with their problematic behaviors. This disruption in reinforcement learning could, in turn, influence the development and maintenance of maladaptive behavioral choices, such as aggressive and violent behavior. Future efforts ought to investigate how neurocognitive systems interact with genetic and environmental contributions, with the goal of understanding how such deficits can be modified to improve reinforcement-based decision making (Blair, 2015).

In addition to empathic responding and reinforcement-learning, another line of research has revealed that CU traits in youth are associated with attentional deficits that impact emotional processing. For example, researchers have investigated whether youth with psychopathic traits attend to the eye region of other people's faces to the same extent as non-psychopathic youth. Attention to the eye region is known to be especially important for social information processing, including non-verbal communication of emotional experiences, such as fear perception (Adolphs, 2008). Monitoring of other people's eye gaze has also been linked to the functioning of the amygdala, which appears to play an important role in directing attention to the eye region (Kawashima et al., 1999).

Based on this literature, researchers hypothesized and found that youth with CU traits displayed reduced attention to the eye region of other's faces, a finding not observed with other childhood maladjustment problems (e.g. anxiety, hyperactivity, other emotional difficulties) (Dadds et al., 2008). This deficit in attention to the eye region appears to partially explain why these youth have difficulty recognizing fear in others (Dadds et al., 2006), though it is not clear why this effect is observed or its implications for understanding the etiology of psychopathy. It is possible that youth high on CU traits attend less to the eye region as a function of reduced amygdala activation, which would make them more difficult for caregivers to socialize using eye contact and non-verbal emotional communication. It is also possible, however, that the parents of youth high on CU are less likely to make eye contact with their offspring (as a function of their own CU traits) and, thus, these children are less likely to learn that eye contact is a useful tool for communicating emotion, which in turn could impact amygdala reactivity to these stimuli. Longitudinal neuroimaging studies are needed to parse the directionality of these effects. Interestingly, this body of research has also shown that a simple manipulation of asking youth with CU traits to look at the eye region increases their recognition of fearful faces, though whether or not this manipulation could lead to true functional changes has not been determined (Dadds et al., 2012). Further research is needed to determine if attempting to modify these attentional deficits could lead to an increased ability to respond to emotionally salient aspects of the environment.

A relatively new line of study in this literature involves examination of neurodevelopmental biomarkers that may confer risk for psychopathic traits in youth. Certain prenatal risk factors can influence the development of neural abnormalities that contribute to the expression of psychopathic traits. For example, prenatal alcohol exposure (Swayze et al., 1997) and genetic factors (May et al., 2004) are thought to contribute to cavum septum pellucidum, a marker of fetal limbic system maldevelopment that has been hypothesized to predispose individuals towards antisocial behavior (Raine et al., 2010). Since limbic and paralimbic structures (e.g., amygdala, hippocampus, thalamus) play a crucial role in emotional processing, it follows that such abnormalities could be of etiological significance in regards to psychopathic behavior. Further investigation into such biomarkers is important to inform clinical and educational prevention efforts to improve prenatal health in at-risk mothers. Comparatively, relatively little research has been conducted on neurodevelopmental risk markers, but awareness of the importance of the prenatal environment on developmental outcomes is growing.

3.4 Emergent Issues in Treatment & Interventions

Like most forms of psychopathology, psychopathic traits are assumed to be more malleable in youth than adults, because the symptoms and behaviors are less ingrained (Hawes & Dadds, 2007). Consequently, there has been a push in the field to consider and develop novel prevention and intervention strategies to reduce the long-term negative outcomes associated with the manifestation of psychopathic traits in youth. In this section, we provide an overview of emerging issues and recent advances in this research literature.

Empirical studies on the treatment of psychopathic traits is relatively limited compared to other disruptive behavior disorders and results from the studies that have been conducted to date have been inconsistent (for a recent review, see Wilkinson et al., 2016), though the majority of studies have reported poorer outcomes for youth with CU traits (Frick et al., 2014). Much of this work has examined whether interventions previously found to be effective at reducing conduct problems could be used to treat callousness in children and adolescents. For example, Hawes and Dadds (2005) investigated the benefits conferred by family-based interventions like parent training for youth (ages 4–8) with CU traits and conduct problems. In a modest sample of boys referred for disruptive behavior problems (N = 56), high levels of CU traits were associated with worse pre-treatment functioning and less responsiveness to the parent training intervention. This is consistent with a number of studies showing that youth with psychopathic traits represent a particularly challenging group to treat (Falkenbach et al., 2003; Spain et al., 2004). For example, evidence suggests that these children and adolescents tend to be less engaged in treatment (O'Neil et al., 2003), more likely to demonstrate poor outcomes in psychiatric settings (Hicks et al., 2010; Stellwagen & Kerig, 2010), and show higher recidivism after completing treatment programs (Gretton et al., 2001).

Given the difficulties associated with treatment for youth with CU traits, recent interventions have been developed that specifically target this at-risk and treatment-resistant group of youth. One such treatment is an adapted Parent–Child Interaction Therapy for youth with CU traits (PCIT-CU; Kimonis et al., 2013, 2019; Kimonis et al., 2012). In this treatment, components of traditional PCIT, such as Child-Directed Interaction (CDI) and Parent-Child Interactions (PDI), were slightly modified to address specific difficulties common among youth with CU traits. Specifically, parents are explicitly coached to increase expressions of warmth and to utilize a token economy system to motivate and reinforce positive child behaviors. In addition to these modifications, an additional module, termed Coaching and Rewarding Emotional Skills (CARES), is implemented to address the youth's insensitivity to distress (Datyner et al., 2016; Kimonis & Armstrong, 2012; Kimonis & Hunt, 2012). A recent open trial pilot study found that PCIT-CU successfully reduced conduct problems and CU traits and increased empathy among youth with co-occurring conduct problems and CU traits (Kimonis et al., 2019).

Very few studies to date have employed rigorous experimental methods to evaluate the efficacy of treatments, including large samples with adequate control conditions. One exception is a study by Somech and Elizure (2012) who conducted a longitudinal randomized controlled trial to examine the effects of an intensive co-parent training program on conduct problems in young children (ages 3–5). Results of this study suggested an early parenting intervention was beneficial in reducing CU traits at post-treatment, gains that were maintained over the year follow-up based on parent report. It is unclear why the intervention described in this study was more effective than some other behavioral treatments, but it may be that recruitment of a community (vs. clinical) sample resulted in a less severe sample in terms of conduct problems and CU traits. Another possibility is that the treatment elements (frequency of treatment; skills training techniques) more effectively targeted the needs of youth with CU traits and their families.

While these findings provide preliminary support of intervention effects on CU traits, this line of research is still in its early stages. More research is needed to identify: (a) what key therapeutic ingredients are necessary to elicit change, (b) which (if any) parent- (e.g., warmth, responsivity) and child-level (e.g. empathy, sensitivity) factors serve as mechanisms of change, and (c) whether individual differences, such as age, gender, quality of CU traits (e.g. secondary vs. primary) influence the efficacy of these treatments. Regardless, studies such as these provide hope that the trajectories of young children with CU traits can be improved by family systems and/or parenting interventions.

A relatively new line of research has emerged examining the potential utility of pharmacological treatments for addressing psychopathic traits in youth, with initial findings from these studies resulting in mixed evidence that limits generalizability. One review suggests that antipsychotic (e.g. risperidone) and stimulant (e.g., methylphenidate) medications may be effective in reducing aggression among children and adolescents with conduct disorder; however, few and inconsistent findings regarding the modulating role of CU traits on medication efficacy have been found (Balia et al., 2018). Further, another meta-analysis noted that, aside from strong evidence for the use of antipsychotic medication for youth with oppositional defiant disorder, conduct disorder, and aggression, less support is found for the use of other forms of psychotropic medications for these conditions (Pringsheim et al., 2015). Together, while some evidence points to the efficacy of psychotropic medication for dimensions of psychopathic traits, the majority of studies point to inconclusive findings, particularly as it relates to CU traits among youth. This will be an important area for future research, and future clinical trials comparing psychotropic medication and behavioral/family interventions will be needed to bolster the evidence of psychotropic interventions for these youth. Research on genetic contributors to psychopathic traits in youth may also lead to new advances in pharmacological research by identifying novel gene pathways that can be targeted with medication development.

Compared to other disruptive behavior disorders, the development and evaluation of treatments for psychopathic traits in youth has received little attention. This trend in the literature may reflect the assumption that psychopathic traits stem from an "evil" predisposition that is not amenable to psychological, systems-based, or psychotropic intervention. However, the responsivity of youth with psychopathic traits to treatment largely remains an unanswered question. Research showing that psychopathic traits are less stable in adolescence than adulthood (Cauffman et al., 2016) and CU traits are more affected by environmental influences than previously thought (e.g., Henry et al., 2018a, b; Waller et al., 2018b) underscores the importance of implementing prevention and intervention efforts early in development, before psychopathic traits solidify in adulthood. The major challenge faced by the scientific community will be creating evidence-based, innovative therapies and treatments that target the environmental, genetic, and neurocognitive characteristics of youth with psychopathic traits.

3.5 Conclusions

Empirical evidence on the assessment of psychopathic traits in youth and etiological mechanisms that confer risk for the disorder have grown substantially in the last two decades, and the field will only continue to grow as more information is collected on the developmental trajectories of these youth. Historically, research on developmental considerations in psychopathy has focused on creating tools to assess the construct of psychopathy in youth and investigated the usefulness of adult etiological models for understanding the manifestation of psychopathic traits in children and adolescents. With the development of novel technology and more sophisticated analytic methods, research on risk and protective factors has expanded to include new levels of analysis—from genetic liability to neurocognitive abnormalities.

The future of developmental research on psychopathy is unknown but building and testing increasingly complex and integrative etiological models that assess interactions across multiple levels of analysis over time are needed to move the field forward. Multilevel longitudinal models can help parse heterogeneity in the developmental trajectories of youth with psychopathic traits—moving beyond just "primary" and "secondary" subtypes to include more nuanced pathway models—and to identify risk factors and etiological mechanisms that are unique to specific trajectories. In addition, there is a need for more clinical intervention studies that specifically target psychopathic traits in youth. The growing evidence base on the etiology of this disorder holds promise for uncovering novel and more personalized prevention and treatment efforts. Continued research into the causes and consequences of psychopathic traits in youth as well as effective preventive and intervention strategies will be crucial for addressing the unique needs of this type of disruptive behavior in youth.

References

Adolphs, R. (2008). Fear, faces, and the human amygdala. *Current Opinion in Neurobiology, 18*(2), 166–172. https://doi.org/10.1016/j.conb.2008.06.006

Allwood, M. A., Bell, D. J., & Horan, J. (2011). Posttrauma numbing of fear, detachment, and arousal predict delinquent behaviors in early adolescence. *Journal of Clinical Child & Adolescent Psychology, 40*(5), 659–667. https://doi.org/10.1080/15374416.2011.597081

Andershed, H. A., Kerr, M., Stattin, H., & Levander, S. (2002). Psychopathic traits in nonreferred youths: A new assessment tool. In E. Blaauw & L. Sheridan (Eds.), *Psychopaths: Current international perspectives* (pp. 131–158). Elsevier.

Balia, C., Carucci, S., Coghill, D., & Zuddas, A. (2018). The pharmacological treatment of aggression in children and adolescents with conduct disorder. Do callous—Unemotional traits modulate the efficacy of medication? *Neuroscience & Biobehavioral Reviews, 91*, 218–238. https://doi.org/10.1016/j.neubiorev.2017.01.024

Barker, E. D., Oliver, B. R., Viding, E., Salekin, R. T., & Maughan, B. (2011). The impact of prenatal maternal risk, fearless temperament and early parenting on adolescent callous unemotional traits: A 14-year longitudinal investigation. *Journal of Child Psychology and Psychiatry, 52*(8), 878–888. https://doi.org/10.1111/j.1469-7610.2011.02397

Barry, C. T., Frick, P. J., DeShazo, T. M., McCoy, M., Ellis, M., & Loney, B. R. (2000). The importance of callous–unemotional traits for extending the concept of psychopathy to children. *Journal of Abnormal Psychology, 109*(2), 335. https://doi.org/10.1037/0021-843X.109.2.335

Barry, T. D., Barry, C. T., Deming, A. M., & Lochman, J. E. (2008). Stability of psychopathic characteristics in childhood: The influence of social relationships. *Criminal Justice and Behavior, 35*(2), 244–262. https://doi.org/10.1177/0093854807310508

Beitchman, J. H., Zai, C. C., Muir, K., Berall, L., Nowrouzi, B., Choi, E., & Kennedy, J. L. (2012). Childhood aggression, callous-unemotional traits and oxytocin genes. *European Child & Adolescent Psychiatry, 21*(3), 125–132. https://doi.org/10.1007/s00787-012-0240-6

Bennett, D. C., & Kerig, P. K. (2014). Investigating the construct of trauma-related acquired callousness among delinquent youth: Differences in emotion processing. *Journal of Traumatic Stress, 27*(4), 415–422. https://doi.org/10.1002/jts.21931

Berg, J. M., Smith, S. F., Watts, A. L., Ammirati, R., Green, S. E., & Lilienfeld, S. O. (2013). Misconceptions regarding psychopathic personality: Implications for clinical practice and research. *Neuropsychiatry, 3*(1), 63.

Bezdjian, S., Raine, A., Baker, L. A., & Lynam, D. R. (2011). Psychopathic personality in children: Genetic and environmental contributions. *Psychological Medicine, 41*(3), 589–600. https://doi.org/10.1017/S0033291710000966

Blair, R. J. R. (2013). The neurobiology of psychopathic traits in youths. *Nature Reviews Neuroscience, 14*(11), 786. https://doi.org/10.1038/nrn3577

Blair, R. J. (2015). Reward processing, functional connectivity, psychopathy, and research domain criteria. *Biological Psychiatry, 78*(9), 592–593. https://doi.org/10.1016/j.biopsych.2015.08.014

Blonigen, D. M., Hicks, B. M., Krueger, R. F., Patrick, C. J., & Iacono, W. G. (2006). Continuity and change in psychopathic traits as measured via normal-range personality: A longitudinal biometric study. *Journal of Abnormal Psychology, 115*(1), 85. https://doi.org/10.1037/0021843X.115.1.85

Bolhuis, K., Muetzel, R. L., Stringaris, A., Hudziak, J. J., Jaddoe, V. W., Hillegers, M. H., White, T., Kushner, S. A., & Tiemeier, H. (2019a). Structural brain connectivity in childhood disruptive behavior problems: A multidimensional approach. *Biological Psychiatry, 85*(4), 336–344. https://doi.org/10.1016/j.biopsych.2018.07.005

Bolhuis, K., Viding, E., Muetzel, R. L., El Marroun, H., Kocevska, D., White, T., Tiemeier, H., & Cecil, C. A. (2019b). Neural profile of callous traits in children: A population-based neuroimaging study. *Biological Psychiatry, 85*(5), 399–407. https://doi.org/10.1016/j.biopsych.2018.10.015

Brouns, B. H., de Wied, M. A., Keijsers, L., Branje, S., van Goozen, S. H., & Meeus, W. H. (2013). Concurrent and prospective effects of psychopathic traits on affective and cognitive empathy in a community sample of late adolescents. *Journal of Child Psychology and Psychiatry, 54*(9), 969–976. https://doi.org/10.1111/jcpp.12052

Burnette, M. L., Oshri, A., Lax, R., Richards, D., & Ragbeer, S. N. (2012). Pathways from harsh parenting to adolescent antisocial behavior: A multidomain test of gender moderation. *Development and Psychopathology, 24*(3), 857–870. https://doi.org/10.1017/S0954579412000417

Caspi, A., Roberts, B. W., & Shiner, R. L. (2005). Personality development: Stability and change. *Annual Review of Psychology, 56*, 453–484. https://doi.org/10.1146/annurev.psych.55.090902.141913

Cauffman, E., Skeem, J., Dmitrieva, J., & Cavanagh, C. (2016). Comparing the stability of psychopathy scores in adolescents versus adults: How often is "fledgling psychopathy" misdiagnosed? *Psychology, Public Policy, and Law, 22*(1), 77–91. https://doi.org/10.1037/law0000078

Cecil, C. A., Lysenko, L. J., Jaffee, S. R., Pingault, J. B., Smith, R. G., Relton, C. L., Woodward, G., McArdle, W., Mill, J., & Barker, E. D. (2014). Environmental risk, Oxytocin Receptor Gene (OXTR) methylation and youth callous-unemotional traits: A 13-year longitudinal study. *Molecular Psychiatry, 19*(10), 1071. https://doi.org/10.1038/mp.2014.95

Childs, A. W., Fite, P. J., Moore, T. M., Lochman, J. E., & Pardini, D. A. (2014). Bidirectional associations between parenting behavior and child callous-unemotional traits: Does parental depression moderate this link? *Journal of Abnormal Child Psychology, 42*(7), 1141–1151. https://doi.org/10.1007/s10802-014-9856-y

Clark, J. E., & Frick, P. J. (2018). Positive parenting and callous-unemotional traits: Their association with school behavior problems in young children. *Journal of Clinical Child & Adolescent Psychology, 47*(sup1), S242–S254. https://doi.org/10.1080/15374416.2016.1253016

Cleckley, H. (1941). *The Mask of Sanity*. Mosby.

Cohn, M. D., Pape, L. E., Schmaal, L., van den Brink, W., van Wingen, G., Vermeiren, R. R., Doreleijers, T. A. H., Veltman, D. J., & Popma, A. (2015). Differential relations between juvenile psychopathic traits and resting state network connectivity. *Human Brain Mapping, 36*(6), 2396–2405. https://doi.org/10.1002/hbm.22779

Colins, O. F., Noom, M., & Vanderplasschen, W. (2012). Youth Psychopathic Traits Inventory-Short Version: A further test of the internal consistency and criterion validity. *Journal of Psychopathology and Behavioral Assessment, 34*(4), 476–486. https://doi.org/10.1007/s10862012-9299-0

Corrado, R. R., Vincent, G. M., Hart, S. D., & Cohen, I. M. (2004). Predictive validity of the Psychopathy Checklist: Youth Version for general and violent recidivism. *Behavioral Sciences & the Law, 22*(1), 5–22. https://doi.org/10.1002/bsl.574

Craig, S. G., & Moretti, M. M. (2018). Profiles of primary and secondary callous-unemotional features in youth: The role of emotion regulation. *Development and Psychopathology, 31*(4), 1–12. https://doi.org/10.1017/S0954579418001062

Craig, R. L., Gray, N. S., & Snowden, R. J. (2013). Recalled parental bonding, current attachment, and the triarchic conceptualisation of psychopathy. *Personality and Individual Differences, 55*(4), 345–350. https://doi.org/10.1016/j.paid.2013.03.012

Crum, K. I., Waschbusch, D. A., Bagner, D. M., & Coxe, S. (2015). Effects of callous–unemotional traits on the association between parenting and child conduct problems. *Child Psychiatry & Human Development, 46*(6), 967–980. https://doi.org/10.1007/s10578-015-0535-1

Dadds, M. R., Fraser, J., Frost, A., & Hawes, D. J. (2005). Disentangling the underlying dimensions of psychopathy and conduct problems in childhood: A community study. *Journal of Consulting and Clinical Psychology, 73*(3), 400. https://doi.org/10.1037/0022-006X.73.3.400

Dadds, M. R., Perry, Y., Hawes, D. J., Merz, S., Riddell, A. C., Haines, D. J., Solak, E., & Abeygunawardane, A. I. (2006). Attention to the eyes and fear-recognition deficits in child psychopathy. *The British Journal of Psychiatry, 189*(3), 280–281. https://doi.org/10.1192/bjp.bp.105.018150

Dadds, M. R., El Masry, Y., Wimalaweera, S., & Guastella, A. J. (2008). Reduced eye gaze explains "fear blindness" in childhood psychopathic traits. *Journal of the American Academy of Child & Adolescent Psychiatry, 47*(4), 455–463. https://doi.org/10.1097/CHI.0b013e31816407f1

Dadds, M. R., Hawes, D. J., Frost, A. D., Vassallo, S., Bunn, P., Hunter, K., & Merz, S. (2009). Learning to 'talk the talk': The relationship of psychopathic traits to deficits in empathy across childhood. *Journal of Child Psychology and Psychiatry, 50*(5), 599–606. https://doi.org/10.1111/j.14697610.2008.02058.x

Dadds, M. R., Cauchi, A. J., Wimalaweera, S., Hawes, D. J., & Brennan, J. (2012). Outcomes, moderators, and mediators of empathic-emotion recognition training for complex conduct problems in childhood. *Psychiatry Research, 199*(3), 201–207. https://doi.org/10.1016/j.psychres.2012.04.033

Dadds, M. R., Moul, C., Cauchi, A., Dobson-Stone, C., Hawes, D. J., Brennan, J., & Ebstein, R. E. (2014). Methylation of the oxytocin receptor gene and oxytocin blood levels in the development of psychopathy. *Development and Psychopathology, 26*(1), 33–40. https://doi.org/10.1017/S0954579413000497

Datyner, A., Kimonis, E. R., Hunt, E., & Armstrong, K. (2016). Using a novel emotional skills module to enhance empathic responding for a child with conduct disorder with limited prosocial emotions. *Clinical Case Studies, 15*(1), 35–52. https://doi.org/10.1177/1534650115588978

Dawel, A., O'Kearney, R., McKone, E., & Palermo, R. (2012). Not just fear and sadness: Metaanalytic evidence of pervasive emotion recognition deficits for facial and vocal expressions in psychopathy. *Neuroscience & Biobehavioral Reviews, 36*(10), 2288–2304. https://doi.org/10.1016/j.neubiorev.2012.08.006

De Brito, S. A., Mechelli, A., Wilke, M., Laurens, K. R., Jones, A. P., Barker, G. J., Hodgins, S., & Viding, E. (2009). Size matters: Increased grey matter in boys with conduct problems and callous–unemotional traits. *Brain, 132*(4), 843–852. https://doi.org/10.1093/brain/awp011

Dick, D. M., Agrawal, A., Keller, M. C., Adkins, A., Aliev, F., Monroe, S., Hewitt, J. K., Kendler, K. S., & Sher, K. J. (2015). Candidate gene–environment interaction research: Reflections and recommendations. *Perspectives on Psychological Science, 10*(1), 37–59. https://doi.org/10.1177/1745691614556682

Dishion, T. J., Andrews, D. W., & Crosby, L. (1995). Antisocial boys and their friends in early adolescence: Relationship characteristics, quality, and interactional process. *Child Development, 66*(1), 139–151. https://doi.org/10.1111/j.1467-8624.1995.tb00861.x

Dishion, T. J., Shaw, D., Connell, A., Gardner, F., Weaver, C., & Wilson, M. (2008). The family check-up with high-risk indigent families: Preventing problem behavior by increasing parents' positive behavior support in early childhood. *Child Development, 79*(5), 1395–1414. https://doi.org/10.1111/j.1467-8624.2008.01195.x

Eisenbarth, H., Godinez, D., du Pont, A., Corley, R. P., Stallings, M. C., & Rhee, S. H. (2019). The influence of stressful life events, psychopathy, and their interaction on internalizing and externalizing psychopathology. *Psychiatry Research, 272*, 438–446. https://doi.org/10.1016/j.psychres.2018.12.145

Ermer, E., Cope, L. M., Nyalakanti, P. K., Calhoun, V. D., & Kiehl, K. A. (2013). Aberrant paralimbic gray matter in incarcerated male adolescents with psychopathic traits. *Journal of the American Academy of Child & Adolescent Psychiatry, 52*(1), 94–103. https://doi.org/10.1016/j.jaac.2012.10.013

Eva R., Kimonis Paul J., Frick Elizabeth, Cauffman Asha, Goldweber Jennifer, Skeem (2012) Primary and secondary variants of juvenile psychopathy differ in emotional processing. *Development and Psychopathology 24*(3), 1091–1103. https://doi.org/10.1017/S0954579412000557

Ezpeleta, L., Penelo, E., de la Osa, N., Navarro, J. B., Fañanás, L., & Fatjó-Vilas, M. (2019). Association of OXTR rs53576 with the developmental trajectories of callous- unemotional traits and stressful life events in 3-to 9-year-old community children. *Journal of Abnormal Child Psychology, 47*, 1651–1662. https://doi.org/10.1007/s10802-019-00548-z

Fairchild, G., Van Goozen, S. H., Calder, A. J., & Goodyer, I. M. (2013). Research review: Evaluating and reformulating the developmental taxonomic theory of antisocial behaviour. *Journal of Child Psychology and Psychiatry, 54*(9), 924–940. https://doi.org/10.1111/jcpp.12102

Falkenbach, D. M., Poythress, N. G., & Heide, K. M. (2003). Psychopathic features in a juvenile diversion population: Reliability and predictive validity of two self-report measures. *Behavioral Sciences & the Law, 21*(6), 787–805. https://doi.org/10.1002/bsl.562

Farrington, D. P., Ullrich, S., & Salekin, R. T. (2010). Environmental influences on child and adolescent psychopathy. In R. T. Salekin & D. R. Lynam (Eds.), *Handbook of child and adolescent psychopathy* (pp. 202–230). The Guilford Press.

Finger, E. C., Marsh, A. A., Mitchell, D. G., Reid, M. E., Sims, C., Budhani, S., Kosson, D. S., Chen, G., Towbin, K. E., Leibenluft, E., Pine, D. S., & Pine, D. S. (2008). Abnormal ventromedial prefrontal cortex function in children with psychopathic traits during reversal learning. *Archives of General Psychiatry, 65*(5), 586–594. https://doi.org/10.1001/archpsyc.65.5.586

Fisher, J. H., & Brown, J. L. (2018). A prospective, longitudinal examination of the influence of childhood home and school contexts on psychopathic characteristics in adolescence. *Journal of Youth and Adolescence, 47*(10), 2041–2059. https://doi.org/10.1007/s10964-018-0861-2

Fite, P. J., Greening, L., Stoppelbein, L., & Fabiano, G. A. (2009). Confirmatory factor analysis of the Antisocial Process Screening Device with a clinical inpatient population. *Assessment, 16*(1), 103–114. https://doi.org/10.1177/1073191108319893

Fontaine, N. M., Rijsdijk, F. V., McCrory, E. J., & Viding, E. (2010). Etiology of different developmental trajectories of callous-unemotional traits. *Journal of the American Academy of Child & Adolescent Psychiatry, 49*(7), 656–664. https://doi.org/10.1016/j.jaac.2010.03.014

Fontaine, N. M., McCrory, E. J., & Viding, E. (2018). Genetic contributions to the development of psychopathic traits and antisocial behavior in youths. In *The Wiley Blackwell handbook of forensic neuroscience* (Vol. 1, pp. 481–506). https://doi.org/10.1002/9781118650868.ch18

Ford, J. D., Chapman, J., MACK, J. M., & Pearson, G. (2006). Pathways from traumatic child victimization to delinquency: Implications for juvenile and permanency court proceedings and decisions. *Juvenile and Family Court Journal, 57*(1), 13–26. https://doi.org/10.1111/j.17556988.2006.tb00111

Forth, A. E., Kosson, D. S., & Hare, R. D. (2003). *Hare Psychopathy Checklist: Youth Version*. Multi-Health Systems.

Fowler, T., Langley, K., Rice, F., van den Bree, M. B., Ross, K., Wilkinson, L. S., Owen, M. J., O'Donovan, M. C., & Thapar, A. (2009). Psychopathy trait scores in adolescents with childhood ADHD: The contribution of genotypes affecting MAOA, 5HTT and COMT activity. *Psychiatric Genetics, 19*(6), 312–319. https://doi.org/10.1097/YPG.0b013e3283328df4

Frick, P. J. (2004). *The inventory of callous-unemotional traits*. Unpublished rating scale.

Frick, P. J., & Dickens, C. (2006). Current perspectives on conduct disorder. *Current Psychiatry Reports, 8*(1), 59–72.

Frick, P. J., & Hare, R. D. (2001). *Antisocial process screening device: APSD*. Multi-Health Systems.

Frick, P. J., & Marsee, M. A. (2006). Psychopathy and Developmental Pathways to Antisocial Behavior. In *Youth Handbook of psychopathy* (pp. 353–374).

Frick, P. J., Bodin, S. D., & Barry, C. T. (2000). Psychopathic traits and conduct problems in community and clinic-referred samples of children: Further development of the psychopathy screening device. *Psychological Assessment, 12*(4), 382. https://doi.org/10.1037/10403590.12.4.382

Frick, P. J., Cornell, A. H., Barry, C. T., Bodin, S. D., & Dane, H. E. (2003a). Callous unemotional traits and conduct problems in the prediction of conduct problem severity, aggression, and self-report of delinquency. *Journal of Abnormal Child Psychology, 31*(4), 457–470.

Frick, P. J., Kimonis, E. R., Dandreaux, D. M., & Farell, J. M. (2003b). The 4 year stability of psychopathic traits in non-referred youth. *Behavioral Sciences & the Law, 21*(6), 713–736.

Frick, P. J., Stickle, T. R., Dandreaux, D. M., Farrell, J. M., & Kimonis, E. R. (2005). Callous–unemotional traits in predicting the severity and stability of conduct problems and delinquency. *Journal of Abnormal Child Psychology, 33*(4), 471–487.

Frick, P. J., Marsee, M. A., & Patrick, C. (2006). Psychopathy and developmental pathways to antisocial behavior in youth. In C. Patrick (Ed.), *Handbook of psychopathy* (pp. 353–374). Guilford Press.

Frick, P. J., Ray, J. V., Thornton, L. C., & Kahn, R. E. (2014). Can callous-unemotional traits enhance the understanding, diagnosis, and treatment of serious conduct problems in children and adolescents? A comprehensive review. *Psychological Bulletin, 140*(1), 1–57. https://doi.org/10.1037/a0033076

Gao, Y., Raine, A., Venables, P. H., Dawson, M. E., & Mednick, S. A. (2009). Association of poor childhood fear conditioning and adult crime. *American Journal of Psychiatry, 167*(1), 5660. https://doi.org/10.1176/appi.ajp.2009.09040499

Gorin, H. M., Kosson, D. S., Miller, S. A., Fontaine, N. M., Vitaro, F., Séguin, J. R., Boivin, M., Cote, S., & Tremblay, R. E. (2019). Psychopathic traits in middle childhood: Evidence of a hierarchical three-factor structure. *Journal of Psychopathology and Behavioral Assessment, 41*(3), 341–352. https://doi.org/10.1007/s10862-019-09733-2

Goulter, N., McMahon, R. J., Pasalich, D. S., & Dodge, K. A. (2020). Indirect effects of early parenting on adult antisocial outcomes via adolescent conduct disorder symptoms and callous unemotional traits. *Journal of Clinical Child & Adolescent Psychology, 49*, 930–942. https://doi.org/10.1080/15374416.2019.1613999

Gretton, H. M., McBride, M., Hare, R. D., O'Shaughnessy, R., & Kumka, G. (2001). Psychopathy and recidivism in adolescent sex offenders. *Criminal Justice and Behavior, 28*(4), 427–449. https://doi.org/10.1177/009385480102800403

Gretton, H. M., Hare, R. D., & Catchpole, R. E. (2004). Psychopathy and offending from adolescence to adulthood: A 10-year follow-up. *Journal of Consulting and Clinical Psychology, 72*(4), 636–645. https://doi.org/10.1037/0022-006X.72.4.636

Haas, S. M., Waschbusch, D. A., King, S., & Walsh, T. M. (2015). Examining the role of callous-unemotional traits in the attributional styles and self-competence evaluations of children with conduct problems and ADHD. *Journal of Psychopathology and Behavioral Assessment, 37*(2), 196–206. https://doi.org/10.1037/0021-843X.109.2.335

Hare, R. D. (2003). *The Hare Psychopathy Checklist-Revised*. MultiHealth Systems.

Hare, R. D., & Neumann, C. S. (2006). The PCL-R assessment of psychopathy. In C. Patrick (Ed.), *Handbook of psychopathy* (pp. 58–88). Guilford Press.

Hawes, D. J., & Dadds, M. R. (2005). The treatment of conduct problems in children with callous-unemotional traits. *Journal of Consulting and Clinical Psychology, 73*(4), 737–741. https://doi.org/10.1037/0022-006X.73.4.737

Hawes, D. J., & Dadds, M. R. (2007). Stability and malleability of callous-unemotional traits during treatment for childhood conduct problems. *Journal of Clinical Child and Adolescent Psychology, 36*(3), 347–355. https://doi.org/10.1080/15374410701444298

Hawes, D. J., Dadds, M. R., Frost, A. D., & Hasking, P. A. (2011). Do childhood callous unemotional traits drive change in parenting practices? *Journal of Clinical Child & Adolescent Psychology, 40*(4), 507–518. https://doi.org/10.1080/15374416.2011.581624

Hempel, I., Buck, N., Cima, M., & Van Marle, H. (2013). Review of risk assessment instruments for juvenile sex offenders: What is next? *International Journal of Offender Therapy and Comparative Criminology, 57*(2), 208–228. https://doi.org/10.1177/0306624X11428315

Henry, J., Pingault, J. B., Boivin, M., Rijsdijk, F., & Viding, E. (2016). Genetic and environmental aetiology of the dimensions of Callous-Unemotional traits. *Psychological Medicine, 46*(2), 405–414. https://doi.org/10.1017/S0033291715001919

Henry, J., Dionne, G., Viding, E., Petitclerc, A., Feng, B., Vitaro, F., Brendgen, M., Tremblay, R. E., & Boivin, M. (2018a). A longitudinal twin study of callous-unemotional traits during childhood. *Journal of Abnormal Psychology, 127*(4), 374–384.

Henry, J., Dionne, G., Viding, E., Vitaro, F., Brendgen, M., Tremblay, R. E., & Boivin, M. (2018b). Early warm-rewarding parenting moderates the genetic contributions to callous–unemotional traits in childhood. *Journal of Child Psychology and Psychiatry, 59*(12), 1282–1288. https://doi.org/10.1111/jcpp.12918

Hicks, B. M., Markon, K. E., Patrick, C. J., Krueger, R. F., & Newman, J. P. (2004). Identifying psychopathy subtypes on the basis of personality structure. *Psychological Assessment, 16*(3), 276. https://doi.org/10.1037/1040-3590.16.3.276

Hicks, B. M., Vaidyanathan, U., & Patrick, C. J. (2010). Validating female psychopathy subtypes: Differences in personality, antisocial and violent behavior, substance abuse, trauma, and mental health. *Personality Disorders, Theory, Research, and Treatment, 1*(1), 38–57. https://doi.org/10.1037/a0018135

Hicks, B. M., Carlson, M. D., Blonigen, D. M., Patrick, C. J., Iacono, W. G., & MGue, M. (2012). Psychopathic personality traits and environmental contexts: Differential correlates, gender differences, and genetic mediation. *Personality Disorders, Theory, Research, and Treatment, 3*(3), 209. https://doi.org/10.1037/a0025084

Hovey, D., Lindstedt, M., Zettergren, A., Jonsson, L., Johansson, A., Melke, J., et al. (2016). Antisocial behavior and polymorphisms in the oxytocin receptor gene: Findings in two independent samples. *Molecular Psychiatry, 21*(7), 983–988. https://doi.org/10.1038/mp.2015.144

Huebner, T., Vloet, T. D., Marx, I. V. O., Konrad, K., Fink, G. R., Herpertz, S. C., & Herpertz Dahlmann, B. (2008). Morphometric brain abnormalities in boys with conduct disorder. *Journal of the American Academy of Child & Adolescent Psychiatry, 47*(5), 540–547. https://doi.org/10.1097/CHI.0b013e3181676545

Jones, A. P., Laurens, K. R., Herba, C. M., Barker, G. J., & Viding, E. (2009). Amygdala hypoactivity to fearful faces in boys with conduct problems and callous-unemotional traits. *American Journal of Psychiatry, 166*(1), 95–102. https://doi.org/10.1176/appi.ajp.2008.07071050

Jones, A. P., Happé, F. G., Gilbert, F., Burnett, S., & Viding, E. (2010). Feeling, caring, knowing: Different types of empathy deficit in boys with psychopathic tendencies and autism spectrum disorder. *Journal of Child Psychology and Psychiatry, 51*(11), 1188–1197. https://doi.org/10.1111/j.1469-7610.2010.02280.x

Kahn, R. E., Frick, P. J., Youngstrom, E. A., Kogos Youngstrom, J., Feeny, N. C., & Findling, R. L. (2013). Distinguishing primary and secondary variants of callous-unemotional traits among adolescents in a clinic-referred sample. *Psychological Assessment, 25*(3), 966–978. https://doi.org/10.1037/a0032880

Kalisch, R., Wiech, K., Critchley, H. D., Seymour, B., O'doherty, J. P., Oakley, D. A., Allen, P., & Dolan, R. J. (2005). Anxiety reduction through detachment: Subjective, physiological, and neural effects. *Journal of Cognitive Neuroscience, 17*(6), 874–883. https://doi.org/10.1162/0898929054021184

Karpman, B. (1941). On the need of separating psychopathy into two distinct clinical types: The symptomatic and the idiopathic. *Journal of Criminal Psychopathology, 3*, 112–137.

Karpman, B. (1948). Conscience in the psychopath: Another version. *American Journal of Orthopsychiatry, 18*(3), 455–491.

Kawashima, R., Sugiura, M., Kato, T., Nakamura, A., Hatano, K., Ito, K., Fukuda, H., Kojima, S., & Nakamura, K. (1999). The human amygdala plays an important role in gaze monitoring: A PET study. *Brain, 122*(4), 779–783. https://doi.org/10.1093/brain/122.4.779

Kerig, P. K., Becker, S. P., & Egan, S. (2010). From internalizing to externalizing: Theoretical models of the processes linking PTSD to juvenile delinquency. *Posttraumatic Stress Disorder (PTSD): Causes, Symptoms and Treatment, 33*, 78.

Kerig, P. K., Bennett, D. C., Thompson, M., & Becker, S. P. (2012). "Nothing really matters": Emotional numbing as a link between trauma exposure and callousness in delinquent youth. *Journal of Traumatic Stress, 25*(3), 272–279. https://doi.org/10.1002/jts.21700

Kerr, M., Van Zalk, M., & Stattin, H. (2012). Psychopathic traits moderate peer influence on adolescent delinquency. *Journal of Child Psychology and Psychiatry, 53*(8), 826–835. https://doi.org/10.1111/j.1469-7610.2011.02492.x

Kimonis, E. R., & Armstrong, K. (2012). Adapting parent–child interaction therapy to treat severe conduct problems with callous-unemotional traits: A case study. *Clinical Case Studies, 11*(3), 234–252. https://doi.org/10.1177/1534650112448835

Kimonis, E. R., & Hunt, E. (2012). *Coaching and rewarding emotional skills: Treatment manual* (CARES Module, Version 3.0). Unpublished manuscript.

Kimonis, E. R., Frick, P. J., & Barry, C. T. (2004). Callous-unemotional traits and delinquent peer affiliation. *Journal of Consulting and Clinical Psychology, 72*(6), 956. https://doi.org/10.1037/0022-006X.72.6.956

Kimonis, E. R., Frick, P. J., Skeem, J. L., Marsee, M. A., Cruise, K., Munoz, L. C., Aucoin, K. J., & Morris, A. S. (2008). Assessing callous–unemotional traits in adolescent offenders: Validation of the Inventory of Callous–Unemotional Traits. *International Journal of Law and Psychiatry, 31*(3), 241–252. https://doi.org/10.1016/j.ijlp.2008.04.002

Kimonis, E. R., Skeem, J. L., Cauffman, E., & Dmitrieva, J. (2011). Are secondary variants of juvenile psychopathy more reactively violent and less psychosocially mature than primary variants? *Law and Human Behavior, 35*(5), 381–391. https://doi.org/10.1007/s10979-010-92433

Kimonis, E. R., Frick, P. J., Cauffman, E., Goldweber, A., & Skeem, J. (2012). Primary and secondary variants of juvenile psychopathy differ in emotional processing. *Development and Psychopathology, 24*(3), 1091–1103. https://doi.org/10.1017/S0954579412000557

Kimonis, E. R., Hunt, E., Bagner, D., & Byrd, A. (2013, June). Adapting Parent-Child Interaction Therapy to treat young children with callous-unemotional conduct problems. In A. Byrd (Chair), *A multi-faceted examination of callous-unemotional traits: Construct validity, predictive utility, and treatment implications. Paper symposium presented at the Society for the Scientific Study of Psychopathy biennial conference, Washington, DC.*

Kimonis, E. R., Fleming, G., Briggs, N., Brouwer-French, L., Frick, P. J., Hawes, D. J., Bagner, D. M., Thomas, R., & Dadds, M. (2019). Parent-Child Interaction Therapy adapted for preschoolers with callous unemotional traits: An open trial pilot study. *Journal of Clinical Child & Adolescent Psychology, 48*(sup1), S347–S361. https://doi.org/10.1080/15374416.2018.1479966

Kosson, D. S., Cyterski, T. D., Steuerwald, B. L., Neumann, C. S., & Walker-Matthews, S. (2002). The reliability and validity of the Psychopathy Checklist: Youth Version (PCL: YV) in nonincarcerated adolescent males. *Psychological Assessment, 14*(1), 97. https://doi.org/10.1037/1040-3590.14.1.97

Krischer, M. K., & Sevecke, K. (2008). Early traumatization and psychopathy in female and male juvenile offenders. *International Journal of Law and Psychiatry, 31*(3), 253–262. https://doi.org/10.1016/j.ijlp.2008.04.008

Kruh, I. P., Frick, P. J., & Clements, C. B. (2005). Historical and personality correlates to the violence patterns of juveniles tried as adults. *Criminal Justice and Behavior, 32*(1), 69–96. https://doi.org/10.1177/0093854804270629

Larsson, H., Viding, E., & Plomin, R. (2008). Callous—Unemotional traits and antisocial behavior: Genetic, environmental, and early parenting characteristics. *Criminal Justice and Behavior, 35*(2), 197–211. https://doi.org/10.1007/s10802-007-9151-2

Lee, H.-J., Macbeth, A. H., Pagani, J. H., & Young, W. S. (2009). Oxytocin: The great facilitator of life. *Progress in Neurobiology, 88*(2), 127–151. https://doi.org/10.1016/j.pneurobio.2009.04.001

Lee, Z., Salekin, R. T., & Iselin, A. M. R. (2010). Psychopathic traits in youth: Is there evidence for primary and secondary subtypes? *Journal of Abnormal Child Psychology, 38*(3), 381–393. https://doi.org/10.1007/s10802-009-9372-7

Lilienfeld, S. O., & Hess, T. H. (2001). Psychopathic personality traits and somatization: Sex differences and the mediating role of negative emotionality. *Journal of Psychopathology and Behavioral Assessment, 23*(1), 11–24. https://doi.org/10.1023/A:1011035306061

Loney, B. R., Frick, P. J., Clements, C. B., Ellis, M. L., & Kerlin, K. (2003). Callous unemotional traits, impulsivity, and emotional processing in adolescents with antisocial behavior problems.

Journal of Clinical Child and Adolescent Psychology, 32(1), 66–80. https://doi.org/10.1207/S15374424JCCP3201_07
LoParo, D., Johansson, A., Walum, H., Westberg, L., Santtila, P., & Waldman, I. (2016). Rigorous tests of gene–environment interactions in a lab study of the oxytocin receptor gene (OXTR), alcohol exposure, and aggression. *American Journal of Medical Genetics Part B: Neuropsychiatric Genetics, 171*(5), 589–602. https://doi.org/10.1002/ajmg.b.32359
Lozier, L. M., Cardinale, E. M., Van Meter, J. W., & Marsh, A. A. (2014). Mediation of the relationship between callous-unemotional traits and proactive aggression by amygdala response to fear among children with conduct problems. *JAMA Psychiatry, 71*(6), 627–636. https://doi.org/10.1001/jamapsychiatry.2013.4540
Lykken, D. T. (1995). *The antisocial personalities*. Psychology Press.
Lynam, D. R. (1997). Pursuing the psychopath: Capturing the fledgling psychopath in a nomological net. *Journal of Abnormal Psychology, 106*(3), 425–438.
Lynam, D. R., Caspi, A., Moffitt, T. E., Loeber, R., & Stouthamer-Loeber, M. (2007). Longitudinal evidence that psychopathy scores in early adolescence predict adult psychopathy. *Journal of Abnormal Psychology, 116*(1), 155–165. https://doi.org/10.1037/0021-843X.116.1.155
Maikovich, A. K., Jaffee, S. R., Odgers, C. L., & Gallop, R. (2008). Effects of family violence on psychopathology symptoms in children previously exposed to maltreatment. *Child Development, 79*(5), 1498–1512. https://doi.org/10.1111/j.1467-8624.2008.01201
Malik, A. I., Zai, C. C., Abu, Z., Nowrouzi, B., & Beitchman, J. H. (2012). The role of oxytocin and oxytocin receptor gene variants in childhood-onset aggression. *Genes, Brain and Behavior, 11*(5), 545–551. https://doi.org/10.1111/j.1601-183X.2012.00776.x
Marsh, A. A., Finger, E. C., Mitchell, D. G., Reid, M. E., Sims, C., Kosson, D. S., Towbin, K. E., Leibenluft, E., Pine, D. S., & Blair, R. J. R. (2008). Reduced amygdala response to fearful expressions in children and adolescents with callous-unemotional traits and disruptive behavior disorders. *American Journal of Psychiatry, 165*(6), 712–720. https://doi.org/10.1176/appi.ajp.2007.07071145
Marsh, A. A., Finger, E. C., Fowler, K. A., Adalio, C. J., Jurkowitz, I. T., Schechter, J. C., Pine, D. S., Decety, J., & Blair, R. J. R. (2013). Empathic responsiveness in amygdala and anterior cingulate cortex in youths with psychopathic traits. *Journal of Child Psychology and Psychiatry, 54*(8), 900–910. https://doi.org/10.1111/jcpp.12063
May, F. S., Chen, Q. C., Gilbertson, M. W., Shenton, M. E., & Pitman, R. K. (2004). Cavum septum pellucidum in monozygotic twins discordant for combat exposure: Relationship to posttraumatic stress disorder. *Biological Psychiatry, 55*(6), 656–658. https://doi.org/10.1016/j.biopsych.2003.09.018
McMahon, R. J., Witkiewitz, K., & Kotler, J. S. (2010). Predictive validity of callous–unemotional traits measured in early adolescence with respect to multiple antisocial outcomes. *Journal of Abnormal Psychology, 119*(4), 752–763.
Mills-Koonce, W. R., Willoughby, M. T., Garrett-Peters, P., Wagner, N., Vernon-Feagans, L., & Family Life Project Key Investigators. (2016). The interplay among socioeconomic status, household chaos, and parenting in the prediction of child conduct problems and callous–unemotional behaviors. *Development and Psychopathology, 28*(3), 757–771. https://doi.org/10.1017/S0954579416000298
Mobarake, R. K., Juhari, R., Yaacob, S. N., & Esmaeili, N. S. (2014). The moderating role of self-control in the relationship between peer affiliation and adolescents antisocial behavior in Tehran, Iran. *Asian Social Science, 10*(9), 71–81. https://doi.org/10.5539/ass.v10n9p71
Monahan, K. C., Steinberg, L., & Cauffman, E. (2009). Affiliation with antisocial peers, susceptibility to peer influence, and antisocial behavior during the transition to adulthood. *Developmental Psychology, 45*(6), 1520–1530. https://doi.org/10.1037/a0017417
Moore, A. A., Blair, R. J., Hettema, J. M., & Roberson-Nay, R. (2019). The genetic underpinnings of callous-unemotional traits: A systematic research review. *Neuroscience & Biobehavioral Reviews, 60*(6), 638–645. https://doi.org/10.1016/j.neubiorev.2019.02.018

Moul, C., & Dadds, M. R. (2013). Learning-style bias and the development of psychopathy. *Journal of Personality Disorders, 27*(1), 85–98. https://doi.org/10.1521/pedi.2013.27.1.85

Muñoz, L. C., Kerr, M., & Besic, N. (2008). The peer relationships of youths with psychopathic personality traits: A matter of perspective. *Criminal Justice and Behavior, 35*(2), 212–227. https://doi.org/10.1177/0093854807310159

Muñoz, L. C., Pakalniskiene, V., & Frick, P. J. (2011). Parental monitoring and youth behavior problems: Moderation by callous-unemotional traits over time. *European Child & Adolescent Psychiatry, 20*(5), 261–269. https://doi.org/10.1007/s00787-011-0172-6

Muratori, P., Lochman, J. E., Manfredi, A., Milone, A., Nocentini, A., Pisano, S., & Masi, G. (2016). Callous unemotional traits in children with disruptive behavior disorder: Predictors of developmental trajectories and adolescent outcomes. *Psychiatry Research, 236*, 35–41. https://doi.org/10.1016/j.psychres.2016.01.003

Neumann, C. S., Kosson, D. S., Forth, A. E., & Hare, R. D. (2006). Factor structure of the Hare Psychopathy Checklist: Youth Version (PCL: YV) in incarcerated adolescents. *Psychological Assessment, 18*(2), 142–154. https://doi.org/10.1037/1040-3590.18.2.142

Newman, J. P., Mac Coon, D. G., Vaughn, L. J., & Sadeh, N. (2005). Validating a distinction between primary and secondary psychopathy with measures of Gray's BIS and BAS constructs. *Journal of Abnormal Psychology, 114*(2), 319–323. https://doi.org/10.1037/0021-843X.114.2.319

Newton-Howes, G., Clark, L. A., & Chanen, A. (2015). Personality disorder across the life course. *The Lancet, 385*(9969), 727–734. https://doi.org/10.1016/S0140-6736(14)61283-6

O'Neill, M. L., Lidz, V., & Heilbrun, K. (2003). Adolescents with psychopathic characteristics in a substance abusing cohort: Treatment process and outcomes. *Law and Human Behavior, 27*(3), 299–313. https://doi.org/10.1023/A:1023435924569

Pardini, D. A., & Loeber, R. (2007). Interpersonal and affective features of psychopathy in children and adolescents: Advancing a developmental perspective introduction to special section. *Journal of Clinical Child and Adolescent Psychology, 36*(3), 269–275. https://doi.org/10.1080/15374410701441575

Pardini, D. A., Lochman, J. E., & Powell, N. (2007). The development of callous-unemotional traits and antisocial behavior in children: Are there shared and/or unique predictors? *Journal of Clinical Child and Adolescent Psychology, 36*(3), 319–333. https://doi.org/10.1080/15374410701444215

Pasalich, D. S., Dadds, M. R., Hawes, D. J., & Brennan, J. (2011). Do callous-unemotional traits moderate the relative importance of parental coercion versus warmth in child conduct problems? An observational study. *Journal of Child Psychology and Psychiatry, 52*(12), 1308–1315. https://doi.org/10.1111/j.1469-7610.2011.02435

Pasalich, D. S., Dadds, M. R., Hawes, D. J., & Brennan, J. (2012). Attachment and callous unemotional traits in children with early-onset conduct problems. *Journal of Child Psychology and Psychiatry, 53*(8), 838–845. https://doi.org/10.1111/j.1469-7610.2012.02544

Patrick, C. J. (2010). *Operationalizing the triarchic conceptualization of psychopathy: Preliminary description of brief scales for assessment of boldness, meanness, and disinhibition*. Unpublished test manual, Florida State University, Tallahassee.

Patrick, C. J., Fowles, D. C., & Krueger, R. F. (2009). Triarchic conceptualization of psychopathy: Developmental origins of disinhibition, boldness, and meanness. *Development and Psychopathology, 21*(3), 913–938. https://doi.org/10.1017/S0954579409000492

Porter, S. (1996). Without conscience or without active conscience? The etiology of psychopathy revisited. *Aggression and Violent Behavior, 1*(2), 179–189. https://doi.org/10.1016/13591789(95)00010-0

Pringsheim, T., Hirsch, L., Gardner, D., & Gorman, D. A. (2015). The pharmacological management of oppositional behaviour, conduct problems, and aggression in children and adolescents with attention-deficit hyperactivity disorder, oppositional defiant disorder, and conduct disorder: A systematic review and meta-analysis. Part 1: Psychostimulants, alpha-2 agonists, and atomoxetine. *The Canadian Journal of Psychiatry, 60*(2), 42–51. https://doi.org/10.1177/070674371506000202

Raine, A., Lee, L., Yang, Y., & Colletti, P. (2010). Neurodevelopmental marker for limbic maldevelopment in antisocial personality disorder and psychopathy. *The British Journal of Psychiatry, 197*(3), 186–192. https://doi.org/10.1192/bjp.bp.110.078485

Roose, A., Bijttebier, P., Decoene, S., Claes, L., & Frick, P. J. (2010). Assessing the affective features of psychopathy in adolescence: A further validation of the inventory of callous and unemotional traits. *Assessment, 17*(1), 44–57. https://doi.org/10.1177/1073191109344153

Rubio, J. S., Krieger, M. A., Finney, E. J., & Coker, K. L. (2014). A review of the relationship between sociocultural factors and juvenile psychopathy. *Aggression and Violent Behavior, 19*(1), 23–31. https://doi.org/10.1016/j.avb.2013.11.001

Sadeh, N., Javdani, S., Jackson, J. J., Reynolds, E. K., Potenza, M. N., Gelernter, J., Lejuez, C. W., & Verona, E. (2010). Serotonin transporter gene associations with psychopathic traits in youth vary as a function of socioeconomic resources. *Journal of Abnormal Psychology, 119*(3), 604–609. https://doi.org/10.1037/a0019709

Salekin, R. T. (2017). Research review: What do we know about psychopathic traits in children? *Journal of Child Psychology and Psychiatry, 58*(11), 1180–1200. https://doi.org/10.1111/jcpp.12738

Salihovic, S., Kerr, M., Özdemir, M., & Pakalniskiene, V. (2012). Directions of effects between adolescent psychopathic traits and parental behavior. *Journal of Abnormal Child Psychology, 40*(6), 957–969. https://doi.org/10.1007/s10802-012-9623-x

Schmidt, F., McKinnon, L., Chattha, H. K., & Brownlee, K. (2006). Concurrent and predictive validity of the Psychopathy Checklist: Youth version across gender and ethnicity. *Psychological Assessment, 18*(4), 393. https://doi.org/10.1037/1040-3590.18.4.393

Schraft, C. V., Kosson, D. S., & McBride, C. K. (2013). Exposure to violence within home and community environments and psychopathic tendencies in detained adolescents. *Criminal Justice and Behavior, 40*(9), 1027–1043. https://doi.org/10.1177/0093854813486887

Sebastian, C. L., McCrory, E. J., Cecil, C. A., Lockwood, P. L., De Brito, S. A., Fontaine, N. M., & Viding, E. (2012). Neural responses to affective and cognitive theory of mind in children with conduct problems and varying levels of callous-unemotional traits. *Archives of General Psychiatry, 69*(8), 814–822. https://doi.org/10.1080/17470919.2015.1044672

Sharf, A., Kimonis, E. R., & Howard, A. (2014). Negative life events and posttraumatic stress disorder among incarcerated boys with callous-unemotional traits. *Journal of Psychopathology and Behavioral Assessment, 36*(3), 401–414. https://doi.org/10.1007/s10862-013-9404-z

Sharp, C., & Kine, S. (2008). The assessment of juvenile psychopathy: Strengths and weaknesses of currently used questionnaire measures. *Child and Adolescent Mental Health, 13*(2), 85–95. https://doi.org/10.1111/j.1475-3588.2008.00483.x

Shepherd, S. M., & Strand, S. (2016). The utility of the Psychopathy Checklist: Youth Version (PCL: YV) and the Youth Psychopathic Trait Inventory (YPI)—Is it meaningful to measure psychopathy in young offenders? *Psychological Assessment, 28*(4), 405–415. https://doi.org/10.1037/pas0000182

Skeem, J. L., Poythress, N., Edens, J. F., Lilienfeld, S. O., & Cale, E. M. (2003). Psychopathic personality or personalities? Exploring potential variants of psychopathy and their implications for risk assessment. *Aggression and Violent Behavior, 8*(5), 513–546. https://doi.org/10.1016/S1359-1789(02)00098-8

Slattery, T. L., & Meyers, S. A. (2014). Contextual predictors of adolescent antisocial behavior: The developmental influence of family, peer, and neighborhood factors. *Child and Adolescent Social Work Journal, 31*(1), 39–59. https://doi.org/10.1007/s10560-013-0309-1

Sleep, C. E., Weiss, B., Lynam, D. R., & Miller, J. D. (2019). An examination of the Triarchic Model of psychopathy's nomological network: A meta-analytic review. *Clinical Psychology Review, 71*, 1–26. https://doi.org/10.1016/j.cpr.2019.04.005

Smearman, E. L., Winiarski, D. A., Brennan, P. A., Najman, J., & Johnson, K. C. (2015). Social stress and the oxytocin receptor gene interact to predict antisocial behavior in an at-risk cohort. *Development and Psychopathology, 27*(1), 309–318. https://doi.org/10.1017/S0954579414000649

Somech, L. Y., & Elizur, Y. (2012). Promoting self-regulation and cooperation in prekindergarten children with conduct problems: A randomized controlled trial. *Journal of the American Academy of Child & Adolescent Psychiatry, 51*(4), 412–422. https://doi.org/10.1016/j.jaac.2012.01.019

Spain, S. E., Douglas, K. S., Poythress, N. G., & Epstein, M. (2004). The relationship between psychopathic features, violence and treatment outcome: The comparison of three youth measures of psychopathic features. *Behavioral Sciences & the Law, 22*(1), 85–102. https://doi.org/10.1002/bsl.576

Steinberg, L. (2002). Clinical adolescent psychology: What it is, and what it needs to be. *Journal of Consulting and Clinical Psychology, 70*(1), 124–128. https://doi.org/10.1037/0022006X.70.1.124

Stellwagen, K. K., & Kerig, P. K. (2010). Relation of callous-unemotional traits to length of stay among youth hospitalized at a state psychiatric inpatient facility. *Child Psychiatry & Human Development, 41*(3), 251–261. https://doi.org/10.1007/s10578-009-0164-7

Swayze, V. W., Johnson, V. P., Hanson, J. W., Piven, J., Sato, Y., Giedd, J. N., Mosnik, D., & Andreasen, N. C. (1997). Magnetic resonance imaging of brain anomalies in fetal alcohol syndrome. *Pediatrics, 99*(2), 232–240. https://doi.org/10.1542/peds.99.2.232

Tatar, J. R., Cauffman, E., Kimonis, E. R., & Skeem, J. L. (2012). Victimization history and post-traumatic stress: An analysis of psychopathy variants in male juvenile offenders. *Journal of Child & Adolescent Trauma, 5*(2), 102–113. https://doi.org/10.1080/19361521.2012.671794

Tuvblad, C., Bezdjian, S., Raine, A., & Baker, L. A. (2013). Psychopathic personality and negative parent-to-child affect: A longitudinal cross-lag twin study. *Journal of Criminal Justice, 41*(5), 331–341. https://doi.org/10.1016/j.jcrimjus.2013.07.001

Vahl, P., Colins, O. F., Lodewijks, H. P., Markus, M. T., Doreleijers, T. A., & Vermeiren, R. R. (2014). Psychopathic-like traits in detained adolescents: Clinical usefulness of self-report. *European Child & Adolescent Psychiatry, 23*(8), 691–699. https://doi.org/10.1007/s00787-0130497-4

Vaughn, M. G., Edens, J. F., Howard, M. O., & Smith, S. T. (2009). An investigation of primary and secondary psychopathy in a statewide sample of incarcerated youth. *Youth Violence and Juvenile Justice, 7*(3), 172–188. https://doi.org/10.1177/1541204009333792

Viding, E., & McCrory, E. J. (2012a). Genetic and neurocognitive contributions to the development of psychopathy. *Development and Psychopathology, 24*(3), 969–983. https://doi.org/10.1017/S095457941200048X

Viding, E., & McCrory, E. J. (2012b). Why should we care about measuring callous–unemotional traits in children? *The British Journal of Psychiatry, 200*(3), 177–178. https://doi.org/10.1192/bjp.bp.111.099770

Viding, E., Blair, R. J. R., Moffitt, T. E., & Plomin, R. (2005). Evidence for substantial genetic risk for psychopathy in 7-year-olds. *Journal of Child Psychology and Psychiatry, 46*(6), 592–597. https://doi.org/10.1111/j.1469-7610.2004.00393.x

Viding, E., Frick, P. J., & Plomin, R. (2007). Aetiology of the relationship between callous unemotional traits and conduct problems in childhood. *The British Journal of Psychiatry, 190*(S49), s33–s38. https://doi.org/10.1192/bjp.190.5.s33

Viding, E., Fontaine, N. M., Oliver, B. R., & Plomin, R. (2009). Negative parental discipline, conduct problems and callous–unemotional traits: Monozygotic twin differences study. *The British Journal of Psychiatry, 195*(5), 414–419. https://doi.org/10.1192/bjp.bp.108.061192

Viding, E., Hanscombe, K. B., Curtis, C. J., Davis, O. S., Meaburn, E. L., & Plomin, R. (2010). In search of genes associated with risk for psychopathic tendencies in children: A two- stage genome-wide association study of pooled DNA. *Journal of Child Psychology and Psychiatry, 51*(7), 780–788. https://doi.org/10.1111/j.1469-7610.2010.02236.x

Viding, E., Sebastian, C. L., Dadds, M. R., Lockwood, P. L., Cecil, C. A., De Brito, S. A., & McCrory, E. J. (2012). Amygdala response to preattentive masked fear in children with conduct problems: The role of callous-unemotional traits. *American Journal of Psychiatry, 169*(10), 1109–1116. https://doi.org/10.1176/appi.ajp.2012.12020191

Vitacco, M. J., Rogers, R., & Neumann, C. S. (2003). The Antisocial Process Screening Device: An examination of its construct and criterion-related validity. *Assessment, 10*(2), 143–150. https://doi.org/10.1177/1073191103010002005

Wallace, G. L., White, S. F., Robustelli, B., Sinclair, S., Hwang, S., Martin, A., & Blair, R. J. R. (2014). Cortical and subcortical abnormalities in youths with conduct disorder and elevated callous-unemotional traits. *Journal of the American Academy of Child & Adolescent Psychiatry, 53*(4), 456–465. https://doi.org/10.1016/j.jaac.2013.12.008

Waller, R., Gardner, F., Hyde, L. W., Shaw, D. S., Dishion, T. J., & Wilson, M. N. (2012). Do harsh and positive parenting predict parent reports of deceitful-callous behavior in early childhood? *Journal of Child Psychology and Psychiatry, 53*(9), 946–953. https://doi.org/10.1111/j.1469-7610.2012.02550

Waller, R., Gardner, F., Viding, E., Shaw, D. S., Dishion, T. J., Wilson, M. N., & Hyde, L. W. (2014). Bidirectional associations between parental warmth, callous unemotional behavior, and behavior problems in high-risk preschoolers. *Journal of Abnormal Child Psychology, 42*(8), 1275–1285. https://doi.org/10.1007/s10802-014-9871-z

Waller, R., Wright, A. G., Shaw, D. S., Gardner, F., Dishion, T. J., Wilson, M. N., & Hyde, L. W. (2015). Factor structure and construct validity of the parent-reported Inventory of Callous Unemotional Traits among high-risk 9-year-olds. *Assessment, 22*(5), 561–580. https://doi.org/10.1177/1073191114556101

Waller, R., Baskin-Sommers, A. R., & Hyde, L. W. (2018a). Examining predictors of callous unemotional traits trajectories across adolescence among high-risk males. *Journal of Clinical Child & Adolescent Psychology, 47*(3), 444–457. https://doi.org/10.1080/15374416.2015.1102070

Waller, R., Hyde, L. W., Klump, K. L., & Burt, S. A. (2018b). Parenting is an environmental predictor of callous-unemotional traits and aggression: A monozygotic twin differences study. *Journal of the American Academy of Child & Adolescent Psychiatry, 57*(12), 955–963. https://doi.org/10.1016/j.jaac.2018.07.882

Waschbusch, D. A., & Willoughby, M. T. (2008). Attention-deficit/hyperactivity disorder and callous-unemotional traits as moderators of conduct problems when examining impairment and aggression in elementary school children. *Aggressive Behavior, 34*(2), 139–153. https://doi.org/10.1002/ab.20224

White, S. F., Brislin, S., Sinclair, S., Fowler, K. A., Pope, K., & Blair, R. J. R. (2013). The relationship between large cavum septum pellucidum and antisocial behavior, callous- unemotional traits and psychopathy in adolescents. *Journal of Child Psychology and Psychiatry, 54*(5), 575–581. https://doi.org/10.1111/jcpp.12063

Wilkinson, S., Waller, R., & Viding, E. (2016). Practitioner review: Involving young people with callous unemotional traits in treatment–does it work? A systematic review. *Journal of Child Psychology and Psychiatry, 57*(5), 552–565. https://doi.org/10.1111/jcpp.12494

Willoughby, M. T., Mills-Koonce, W. R., Gottfredson, N. C., & Wagner, N. J. (2014). Measuring callous unemotional behaviors in early childhood: Factor structure and the prediction of stable aggression in middle childhood. *Journal of Psychopathology and Behavioral Assessment, 36*(1), 30–42. https://doi.org/10.1007/s10862-013-9379-9

Wright, N., Hill, J., Sharp, H., & Pickles, A. (2018). Maternal sensitivity to distress, attachment and the development of callous-unemotional traits in young children. *Journal of Child Psychology and Psychiatry, 59*(7), 790–800. https://doi.org/10.1111/jcpp.12867

Chapter 4
Psychopathy and Gender: How Relevant Is the Construct of Psychopathy in Females?

Annette McKeown, Susan Cooper, and Jennifer Lamb

Abstract This chapter will consider the relevance of the construct of psychopathy to adult women and adolescent girls. First, there will first be an outline of theoretical considerations in understanding psychopathy in females. This will be followed by consideration of the construct of psychopathy in adolescent girls and pathways to adult psychopathy in women. The role of trauma and survival strategies in understanding the development of personality traits will be considered. The chapter will then focus on whether there is a role for psychopathy in clinical assessment and treatment planning, and conclude with specific recommendations for the clinical application of psychopathy in females.

Keywords Psychopathy · Females · Gender · Trauma · Formulation · Assessment · Treatment

4.1 How Relevant Is the Construct of Psychopathy in Females?

This chapter will consider the relevance of the construct of psychopathy to adult women and adolescent girls. First, there will first be an outline of theoretical considerations in understanding psychopathy in females. This will be followed by consideration of the construct of psychopathy in adolescent girls and pathways to adult psychopathy in women. The role of trauma and survival strategies in understanding

A. McKeown (✉)
Kolvin Service, Cumbria, Northumberland Tyne and Wear NHS Foundation Trust & Newcastle University, Newcastle upon Tyne, UK
e-mail: Annette.McKeown@cntw.nhs.uk

S. Cooper
Durham Therapy Centre, Durham, UK

J. Lamb
Teesside University, Middlesbrough, UK

J. E. Vitale (ed.), *The Complexity of Psychopathy*, Dangerous Behavior in Clinical and Forensic Psychology, https://doi.org/10.1007/978-3-030-83156-1_4

the development of personality traits will be considered. The chapter will then focus on whether there is a role for psychopathy in clinical assessment and treatment planning, and conclude with specific recommendations for the clinical application of psychopathy in females.

4.1.1 Gender and Theoretical Considerations in Psychopathy

From the early stages of the twentieth century onwards, literature began to increasingly consider psychopathy in women. In 1916, the criminal case of Marion Smith was described by the lead psychiatrist at the first Psychopathic Department in Boston State Hospital (Southard, 1916). Ms. Smith's grandmother said she was attempting to control her property and described her as a "nymphomaniac" (as cited in Lunbeck, 2006, p. 49). In hospital, Ms. Smith was described as a "model patient," "well mannered" with no presenting psychotic symptoms (as cited in Lunbeck, 2006, p. 49). It contrast, she was also described as sexually promiscuous, impulsive and irresponsible in her decision-making. Ms. Smith was assessed as having a psychopathic personality (Southard, 1916). This was one of the early case studies highlighting psychopathy in women, and themes of impulsivity, conning behaviour and promiscuity predominated the case. In 1939, the Scottish psychiatrist, David Henderson, used terminology including "hypersexual" and emotional instability when he described his case studies of female psychopathy. These early commentaries on the characteristics of psychopathy in women started to grow over time.

It was Cleckley's (1941, 1988) pivotal work that informed modern day conceptualisations of psychopathy. In *The Mask of Sanity*, Cleckley (1941) presented 15 clinical case studies which provided rich clinical representations of his understanding of psychopathy. These 15 case studies informed 16 characteristics that Cleckley proposed underpinned psychopathy. Traits included superficial charm, absence of delusions, untruthfulness, poor insight, lack of shame and general lack of major affective reactions. Of Cleckley's 15 clinical case studies, only two – Roberta and Anna – were female. It is worth noting that both Anna and Roberta were characterised by relatively minor forensic histories (e.g., fraud and theft). Therefore, the views Cleckley presented on female psychopathy generally reflected women without a history of violence. With this caveat in mind, Cleckley identified some similarities in his conceptualisation of psychopathy in male and female psychopathic individuals. He identified that a lack of emotional depth tended to typify both male and female psychopathic individuals. For example, in the case of Cleckley's female case studies, when Roberta's mother was asked about her daughter's emotional functioning she commented:

> She has such sweet feelings ... but they don't amount to much. She's not hard or heartless, but she's all on the surface. I really believe she means to stop doing all those terrible things, but she doesn't mean it enough to matter (Cleckley, 1941, p. 49).

Other early case studies of psychopathy found a lack of empathy and depth of emotional understanding characterised both female and male psychopathy (Batchelor, 1954; Greenacre, 1945; Henderson, 1939). Gender differences in psychopathy were also identified in early research. Psychopathy in women was more often found to present with emotional instability (Ballard & Miller, 1945; Fremming, 1947; Henderson, 1939). For example, Fremming (1947) found in his psychopathic sample that female psychopaths were more mood labile in comparison to men. Promiscuity and "hypersexual behaviour" was found to be particularly characteristic of psychopathy in females (Batchelor, 1954; Greenacre, 1945; Henderson, 1939). Self-harm and attempted suicide was also suggested to be a notable feature of some psychopathic women (Barchelor, 1954; Greenacre, 1945). These findings were notably in conflict to Cleckley's (1988) view, which suggested that psychopathy presented relative immunity to suicide. Complicating the issue, for the first half of the twentieth century, although assessments of psychopathy were undertaken, there were no standardised psychopathy measures for either men or women.

4.1.2 Development of the Psychopathy Checklist (PCL): When the Construct Starts to Become Synonymous with the Measure

Over 30 years later, Hare (1980) developed the first version of the *Psychopathy Checklist* (PCL) assessment of psychopathy. The PCL was developed from psychometric analysis of Cleckley's (1941) criteria and validated on adult male prisoners in Canada. Over time, to some extent, this measure started to become synonymous with the construct of psychopathy. Anecdotally, it was noted that many clinicians began to view psychopathy as characterised by traits contained within the PCL. When Hare (1991) went on to develop the first version of the *Psychopathy Checklist – Revised* (PCL-R), he acknowledged further research with women with forensic histories would be beneficial. For example, he noted that some PCL-R items may need *"modification"* when applied to females, and that psychopathy may be *"expressed"* differently in females (p. 64). Generally, however, he took the view that the PCL-R was equally applicable to female offenders. The second version of the PCL-R (Hare, 2003) included minor revisions and provided extended descriptive data in relation to specific groups, including women.

The PCL-R consists of twenty items with each item scored using a three-point scale (0, 1 or 2) to identify the degree to which each item reflects the individual (Hare, 2003). It is currently the most commonly used assessment of psychopathy, and in many contexts is viewed as the *"gold standard"* assessment of the construct particularly in males (e.g., Lynam & Gudonis, 2005, p. 383) and one of the most reliable clinical constructs in the criminal justice system (Hemphill & Hare, 2004; Weizmann-Henelius et al., 2015). Scores range between 0 and 40 and a cut-off score of 30 has been applied in North American populations to define psychopathy (Boduszek & Debowska, 2016; Patrick, 2005). In the United Kingdom (UK), cut-off scores of 25 and above have been adopted as it appears lowered PCL-R cut-off scores may reflect increased levels of psychopathy in this population (Hare, 2008).

4.1.2.1 PCL-R Factor Structure

The most recent version of the PCL-R (Hare, 2003) includes two factors and each factor is inclusive of two facets. Factor 1 is characterised by grandiosity, superficiality and empathy deficits and encapsulates the (i) affective and (ii) interpersonal facets. The interpersonal facet includes the PCL-R items of glibness/superficial charm, grandiose sense of self-worth, pathological lying, and conning/manipulation. The affective facet includes the PCL-R items of lack of remorse, shallow affect, lack of empathy, and failure to accept responsibility. Factor 2 is characterised by traits associated with antisocial behaviour and criminality and encapsulates the (iii) criminal lifestyle and (iv) antisocial facets. The lifestyle facet includes the PCL-R items of need for stimulation, lack of realistic goals, parasitic lifestyle, impulsivity, and irresponsibility. The antisocial facet includes the PCL-R items of poor behavioural controls, early behavioural problems, juvenile delinquency, revocation of conditional release, and criminal versatility.

Various factor structures have been proposed including Hare's (1991) original two-factor model and subsequent four-factor model (affective, interpersonal, lifestyle, antisocial) (Hare, 2003). Cooke and Michie (2001) presented a three-factor hierarchical model of the PCL-R, which comprised three factors: Arrogant/Deceitful Interpersonal Style, Deficient Affective Experiences, and Impulsive/Irresponsible Behaviour Style. The three-factor model omits antisocial items as these can be viewed as a consequence, rather than a core feature of psychopathy (Boduszek & Debowska, 2016; deVogel & Lancel, 2016; Efferson & Glenn, 2018). As women have been found to score lower on antisocial items than men, there are some suggestions that the three-factor model can be particularly applicable to assessment of psychopathy in women (Beryl et al., 2014; Gray & Snowdon, 2016). There is also conflicting research suggesting the applicability of Hare's (2003) four-factor model with females. It is important to again note that the PCL-R was developed for men, predominantly used and normed with forensic males. This highlights valid questions about whether it adequately encapsulates the differing presentations of psychopathy presented by females (Eisenbarth et al., 2018; Hare & Neumann, 2005; Neumann et al., 2015). It is noteworthy, that existing research with women often refers to total, factor scores, and facet scores of the PCL-R (Coid et al., 2009; Hare & Neumann, 2005). It has also simultaneously been acknowledged that there is more limited research on use of the PCL-R in female samples in the UK (Kreis & Cooke, 2012). Overall, early clinical case studies and subsequent literature on the development of the PCL-R tentatively suggested the construct of psychopathy may present differently in women.

4.1.2.2 Prevalence and Gender Differences in PCL-R Scores

There are relatively consistent findings that female PCL-R scores tend to be lower than those of males (Grann, 2000; Guay et al., 2018; Jackson et al., 2002; Logan, 2009; Logan & Weizmann-Henelius, 2012; Nicholls et al., 2005; Salekin et al., 1997; Vitale et al., 2002; Warren et al., 2003). Given these findings, some researchers have proposed that PCL-R cut-off scores should be adjusted according to gender including some suggestion of 30 for men and 23 for women (Pauli et al., 2018). DeVogel and Lancel (2016) used these cut-off scores in their study and found prevalence rates for psychopathy were similar, 20.8% for men and 19.3% for women. However, they found gender differences in comorbid personality disorders with men more often diagnosed with Antisocial Personality Disorder (ASPD) and women more often Borderline Personality Disorder (BPD) (de Vogel & Lancel, 2016).

Differing PCL-R cut-off scores often adopted in different studies complicate measuring prevalence rates. Prevalence rates for women have varied between 1.05% (Logan & Blackburn, 2009) and 31% (Strachan, 1993) when the cut-off of 30 has been adopted (Beryl et al., 2014). It is noteworthy that lower prevalence rates tend to be identified in Europe, with higher prevalence rates identified in North America and Canada (Coid et al., 2009). In the general female forensic population in the US, the average PCL-R score has been found to be 19 (Hare, 2003). In contrast, in the general female population in the UK, the average PCL-R score has been found to be 8.3 (Coid et al., 2009). Some argue this discrepancy may be partially due to inclusion of more specifically selected high-risk violent females in North American samples (Coid et al., 2009). It is also suggested that differences may reflect the fact that the PCL-R was developed with a sample of Canadian male offenders, and is therefore perhaps less representative of European female samples (Beryl et al., 2014).

When using a cut-off score of 25, North American studies have found female psychopathy prevalence rates of 46.4% in forensic samples (Warren et al., 2003), whereas European studies found much lower rates of 21.6% (Weizmann-Henelius et al., 2010). Additional findings in Europe include De Vogel and de Ruiter's (2005) sample, where 10% of females versus 24% of men scored over 26 on the PCL-R. In the UK, Bell (2009) compared male and female high-risk offenders on psychopathy, Axis I mental disorder, Axis II personality disorder and index offence. Women scored lower on the PCL-R ($M = 16.4$) than men ($M = 17.8$) although this difference was not significant. Bell (2009) also found 16.2% women scored over 25 on the PCL-R in comparison to 21% of men. When a PCL-R score over 30 was applied, 2.9% of women and 5.6% of men scored over this cut-off (Bell, 2009). What seems clear is that women generally seem to score lower on the PCL-R than men. It is unclear whether this means that that psychopathy levels *per se* are lower in women, whether psychopathy is less common in women, or whether the PCL-R does not measure the construct as accurately in women (Guay et al., 2018; Klein Tuente et al., 2014). What is also clear, however, is that the cut-off scores for females are somewhat arbitrary and a dimensional approach to understanding this construct in women may be most appropriate (Guay et al., 2018).

4.1.3 The Role of Gender in Expressions of Psychopathy

Existing literature suggests that characteristics of psychopathy may be expressed differently in men and women (e.g., Efferson & Glenn, 2018; Fourozan & Cooke, 2005; Wiezmann-Henelius et al., 2015). In terms of interpersonal psychopathic traits, research has suggested strategies of meeting their own needs, sometimes referred to as "manipulation", *may be expressed differently in women (Vablais,* 2007; De Vogel et al., 2012). For example, it was suggested that women might be more likely to employ strategies such as flirtation as a means of meeting their own needs. In some cases, flirtation may also link to superficial charm. However, this may not always be the case, as for some women the primary function of flirtation may be to ensure their needs are met. Subsequent literature has also identified that superficial charm and grandiosity appear to be less characteristic of psychopathy in women to the same degree as men (Kreis & Cooke, 2011; Kruepke, 2015; Rogstad & Rogers, 2008; Wynn et al., 2012).

When assessing antisocial PCL-R items such as *early behavioural problems, juvenile delinquency, revocation of conditional release,* and *criminal versatility*, it is important to consider gender differences as statistics indicate that female offending tends to have a later onset and less chronic offending trajectory than observed in men (Verona & Vitale, 2006). In addition, behavioural manifestations of impulsivity and conduct disorder in females have been found to be more likely to include self-harm, running away, and being complicit in offending (Fourozan, 2003), whereas in males, behavioural manifestations were more likely to be characterised by overt aggression and violent behaviour. In adult male and females, differences have also been found in the behavioural expressions of aggression. The aggression of male psychopathic offenders has been found to be more instrumental and proactive in comparison to more frequent reactive expressions of violence in female psychopathic offenders (Hunt et al., 2015; Kruepke, 2015; Wynn et al., 2012). It is also noteworthy that females with higher levels of psychopathy have been found to present with higher levels of emotional instability and suicidal behaviour in comparison to male psychopathic offenders (de Vogel et al., 2019; Dolan & Völlm, 2009; Sprague et al., 2012; Verona et al., 2012).

Impulsivity and *poor behavioural controls* can also be characteristic of borderline personality disorder (BPD) as well as psychopathy, which can result in the same behaviours and characteristics being applied to infer presence of both borderline and psychopathic traits (deVogel et al., 2016; deVogel & Lancel, 2016; Kruepke, 2015; Logan & Weizmann-Henelius, 2012). This highlights the importance of considering the presence of BPD potentially inflating PCL-R scores to an extent that is perhaps not warranted. In women, *promiscuous sexual behaviour* may be linked to particular strategies of meeting their own needs (Kreis & Cooke, 2011). For example, in women, sexual behaviour may be used to improve access to potential partners, secure financial gains, and to manipulate social circles (Fourozan & Cooke, 2005; Thornton & Blud, 2007; Wynn et al., 2012). The possibility that sexually promiscuous behaviour may represent a symptom of trauma must also be considered (e.g.,

Covington & Bloom, 2007; Espinosa & Sorensen, 2015). For example, in some cases promiscuity may represent re-enactments of previous childhood traumatic experiences (Trippany et al., 2006). Therefore, careful examination of the function and characteristics of the presenting behaviour is incredibly important when employing a formulation. Societal understanding of gender can also influence what it is viewed to be *parasitic behaviour* (Fourozan & Cooke, 2005). For example, across many cultures financial dependence of women on men is not viewed as parasitic; although when men engage in the same behaviour it can be viewed as manipulative and parasitic behaviour (Logan & Weizmann-Henelius, 2012; Wynn et al., 2012). Overall, this highlights the importance of careful examination of the function of the presenting behaviour when examining psychopathic traits.

Rorschach (1942) assessments are psychodynamic measures of personality which examine the unconscious. Psychoanalytic Rorschach research comparing PCL-R scores of female and males have identified patterns of findings (e.g., Cunliffe et al., 2013). Cunliffe et al. (2013) found females with higher levels of psychopathy presented with lower levels of self-esteem and grandiosity than males. Preliminary findings indicated psychopathic women appeared to have greater capacity for relating with others, which initially suggested a greater female interest in reciprocal relationships. Upon further exploration, however, findings indicated the motivation underpinning apparent interest in relationships actually tended to be characterised by attempts to meet the woman's own needs (Cunliffe et al., 2013).

Cunliffe et al. (2013) did not find any gender differences in antisocial PCL-R items such as conning, manipulative behaviour, and pathological lying. Psychopathic women were twice as likely as men to perpetrate an offence towards an individual known to them. When administering the PCL-R with women, the authors highlighted the importance of awareness of impression management and need for praise; they postulate this is less present in male psychopathic offenders. Assessors were encouraged not to assume that depressive symptoms or low self-esteem are synonymous or necessarily indicative of guilt. Practitioners were also encouraged not to dismiss the possibility of women presenting with shallow emotions if they present with explicitly high levels of emotional instability. Attention was drawn to the importance of exploring this domain, particularly in women with BPD (Gacono et al., 2001). Overall, the findings highlight the importance of practitioners considering potential gender differences in psychopathy and manifestation of psychopathic traits. Adopting a psychological formulation approach to draw on theory and literature to understand and explain the function of presenting behaviours is also likely to be extremely useful (Johnstone & Dallos, 2013).

4.1.4 Primary and Secondary Psychopathy in Females

Cleckley (1941) and Karpman (1941, 1948) originally introduced the distinction between *"primary psychopaths"* and *"secondary psychopaths"*. Cleckley (1941) and Karpman (1941) viewed primary psychopathy as biologically and genetically driven, as opposed to secondary psychopathy which was more acquired and influenced by environmental and learning experiences. This distinction was also largely based on the difference between individuals' capacity for depth of emotion, anxiety, empathy, and desire for a meaningful relationship with others. Primary psychopaths were theorized to particularly struggle with the emotional functioning skills due to biologically driven affective deficits.

Hicks et al. (2010) applied this model to distinguish between primary psychopaths and secondary psychopaths in samples of female offenders. Hicks et al. (2010) found primary psychopathy tended to be characterised by features of generalised criminality with few presenting mental health problems, whereas those with secondary psychopathy characteristics were described as more impulsive in nature, with criminality occurring from a young age. Heightened levels of substance use, mental health difficulties, post-traumatic stress symptoms, suicidal behaviour and violent behaviour were also noted to characterise the secondary psychopath (Hicks et al., 2010). It was noted that secondary psychopathy appeared to be more consistent with emotional instability characteristics of personality disorder (e.g., Hicks et al., 2004, 2010). Falkenbach et al. (2017) also found the secondary group generated the most behavioural activation in that they were motivated towards reward through impulsivity.

4.1.5 Use of the PCL Youth Version with Adolescent Girls

Forth et al. (1990) propose that psychopathy is a chronic disorder, which first manifests at an early age and is relatively stable across the lifespan. It is important to note, however, that psychiatric guidelines (DSM-5 and ICD-10) indicate that personality disorders cannot be defined until an individual is aged 18 or over. Vincent and Hart (2002) note, 'presumably, the traits of a personality disorder do not have a sudden onset at the moment an individual turns 18 years of age' (p. 153). Developmental considerations, including the possibility of developmental trauma, must be considered when formulating and understanding these presentations (e.g., Van der Kolk, 2015).

Despite these important considerations, the PCL-R was modified for adolescents. It was formally developed and published as the Psychopathy Checklist-Youth Version in 2003 (PCL-YV; Forth et al., 2003) for adolescents aged 13–18. The PCL-YV measures essentially the same personality traits as the PCL-R. The PCL-YV has modifications to certain items to reflect the limited life span and experiences of adolescents and the greater influence of family, peers, and school on their lives as opposed to intimate or marital partners and work experience. For example, the item 'many short-term marital relationships' was changed to 'unstable interpersonal relationships'.

The issue of gender has been considered in adolescents using the PCL-YV. Forth et al. (2003) combined six samples and found males scored slightly higher on the PCL-YV than females. Cooper (2008) found no significant gender differences in total or factor PCL-YV scores. Sevecke et al. (2016), however, found that incarcerated male adolescents were significantly higher than incarcerated female adolescents on the PCL-YV total score as well as all four PCL-YV dimensions. Beyond total and factor scores, researchers have also examined the expression of psychopathic traits in adolescent females. Cooper (2008) found that higher PCL-YV scores were significantly associated with direct and indirect bullying in female adolescents in secure settings, but not males. This is consistent with the notion that there are gender differences in the expression of personality difficulties, with higher PCL-YV scores related to the perpetration of direct and indirect aggression in females.

In terms of the predictive validity in females, Odgers et al. (2005) found the affective traits of the PCL-YV were related to aggression in female adolescents. The PCL-YV did not predict future offending but victimisation significantly increased risk of reoffending, indicating victimisation may be a more important risk factor in females. Penny and Moretti (2007) examined the relationship between PCL-SV scores and aggressive and antisocial behavior in a sample of high-risk adolescent girls and boys. They found that the relationships between PCL-SV scores and outcomes were equivalent for boys and girls, and that deficits in affect were most consistently associated with aggression.

It is extremely important to note that the concept of psychopathy in adolescents has been challenged. Edens et al. (2001) and Seagrave and Grisso (2002) suggest that several features of psychopathy (such as impulsivity, lack of empathy, proneness to boredom, and irresponsibility) are normal and temporary traits in adolescence rather than indicative of a disturbed personality. In an early study of psychopathy in youth, Forth and Burke (1998) found adolescents score high on need for stimulation and impulsivity, which is consistent with this argument. This might suggest that these traits in young people reflect psychosocial immaturity rather than an underlying personality dysfunction. It is therefore important to consider whether using the PCL-YV in young people could result in pathologising adolescents who may be showing behavioural patterns consistent with developmental immaturity and may well in some cases reflect developmental trauma. Forth et al. (2003) suggest that when scoring items on the PCL-YV, raters should compare the individual to adolescents of his/her own age; adolescents would then only score higher if their traits are outside the normal range. However, making such within-age comparisons may still not be appropriate as adolescents mature at different rates. Several researchers also point out the ethical implications of extending the concept of psychopathy from adults to young people (Forth et al., 2003; Cruise et al., 2003). The main ethical issues relate to the potential impact of developmental trauma, labelling young people and misusing the PCL-YV.

4.2 Etiology: Is It Psychopathy or Is It Trauma?

Traumatic experiences are particularly characteristic of female pathways into the criminal justice system (Gottfried, Harrop, Anestis, Venables & Sellbom, 2018; McKeown, 2010; Salisbury & Van Voorhis, 2009; Gottfried et al., 2018). Maladaptive early experiences can influence development of both personality difficulties (Fonagy et al., 2003) and psychopathic traits (Buck, 2015). Understanding these factors alongside genetic factors, biological factors, and psychosocial factors can help us to understand developmental pathways into personality difficulties (Leichsenring et al., 2011; Linehan, 2014). Recent research indicated that women scoring highly on the PCL-R were more likely to have childhood experiences characterised by victimisation, behavioural difficulties, and attachment difficulties with parental figures (Forouzan & Nicholls, 2015). Early research also emphasised the links between early experiences of trauma (emotional, physical and sexual) and the development of psychopathic traits (de Vogel et al., 2016; Hicks et al., 2010). Interestingly, Forouzan and Nicholls (2015) found that experiencing maternal childhood neglect, and personality and mental health difficulties in the build-up to foster care placement were negatively associated with psychopathy. Conversely, paternal abuse and childhood impulsivity increased the likelihood of higher psychopathy scores. Recent research has found that physical trauma was the only form of trauma significantly related to psychopathy in both males and females (Gobin et al., 2015).

Additional research found that sexual abuse had a unique positive association with Factor 2 psychopathy scores (Verona et al., 2005). In contrast, neither physical nor sexual abuse were significantly associated with the interpersonal and affective characteristics associated with Factor 1 psychopathy scores (Verona et al., 2005). This research is consistent with findings that sexually abused females are more likely to develop conduct disorder, in comparison to females who have not experienced sexual abuse (Spataro et al., 2004). What appears clear is that early experiences and trauma pathways can contribute, to varying degrees, to emerging personality difficulties.

A lack of a gender-responsive theoretical framework in the literature has led to PCL defined psychopathy being viewed with some scepticism (Salekin et al., 1996). Furthermore, the literature on female offending more generally often focuses on pathways into offending and the unique needs of females. Recognizing the elevated rates of historical trauma amongst female offenders, gender-sensitive approaches to assessment and intervention have been developed (Covington, 2014; Grella, 2008) that consider the gendered context (or "pathways") of female offending (Salisbury & Van Voorhis, 2009; Simpson et al., 2008). Within these models of female offending, the behaviours that result in the woman's entry into the criminal justice system are viewed as survival strategies, rather than features of a psychopathic or other personality disorder.

4.2.1 Survival Strategies

If it is accepted that women with psychopathic personality traits have had adverse life experiences, then it is reasonable to suggest that these personality traits may well be developed over time as a way of surviving such adverse life experiences. Therapies for the treatment of trauma and complex trauma emphasise the importance of addressing the underlying trauma. Perhaps a woman with a history of abuse has learnt that dissociating from her emotions is a way of keeping herself safe. Likewise a woman who has been abused as a child might learn that to survive and ensure her needs are met and exploit others. If women can understand their personality in this context, then there are more opportunities for compassion for self and others.

This is consistent with the notion that there are gender differences in the manifestation of psychopathic traits. For example, drug use might be considered a feature of stimulation seeking in males, related to pleasure and peer pressure, but some research suggests that women's patterns of drug abuse are more socially embedded than men's and serve as a coping mechanism (Bloom et al., 2003; Inciardi et al., 1993). It is important to understand why such personality traits have developed for the individual woman. If women with psychopathic traits understand their personality traits as a way of adapting to an adverse environment, they might be motivated to explore their environment and how such strategies may no longer be helpful or necessary.

4.3 Assessment Considerations

As stated earlier, there appears to be differences in the expression of psychopathic traits between men and women, with women displaying more manipulation and emotional instability, and men more antisocial and criminal behaviours (de Vogel & Lancel, 2016). Given that the PCL-R was created and validated with adult males, results from these assessments may not adequately reflect the construct of psychopathy in females, and therefore such results should be interpreted with caution (Forouzan & Cooke, 2005). Further, the PCL-R adopts a personality-based view of psychopathy, with the inclusion of antisocial items more commonly associated with males. There have been divided opinions on the relevance of these items as core constructs of psychopathy (e.g., Skeem et al., 2007). Due to the differing symptomology and expression of psychopathy in males and females, and the lack of a clear consensus of the core constructs of psychopathy in general, alternative assessment instruments have been devised.

The Comprehensive Assessment of Psychopathic Personality (CAPP; Cooke et al., 2012) is a personality-based model which was created as a means to conceptualise psychopathy. Where the PCL-R has been criticised for being rigid in its focus on an individual's historic behaviours, the CAPP was developed to assess the fluctuating and remissive nature of psychopathic personality traits (Pauli et al., 2018). The CAPP uses a lexical approach which focuses on personality pathology, rather than antisocial behaviours or acts (Kreis & Cooke, 2011). The intention is that the assessment identifies personality deviance rather than cultural or social deviance (Pauli et al., 2018). Through the exclusion of these items, it is thought that the CAPP provides a more gender-neutral framework for assessing female psychopathy (Kreis & Cooke, 2011).

The model is comprised of 33 symptoms which were identified from relevant, scientific literature and conceptual frameworks concerning Psychopathic Personality Disorder (PPD) with each symptom defined by a selection of trait-descriptives. The symptoms and trait-descriptives are then subsequently divided into six domains: *attachment, behavioural, cognitive, dominance, emotional,* and *self*. The *attachment* domain includes attachment difficulties with others and difficulties developing and maintaining close relationships. The *behavioural* domain relates to behaviour regulation difficulties and difficulties with planning. The *cognitive* domain includes difficulties with concentration, cognitive flexibility and adaptability. The *dominance* domain reflects expressions of attempts to obtain power and control over others. The *emotional* domain encapsulates difficulties with emotional stability and emotional depth. The *self* domain relates to identity difficulties and individuality. There have been various translations of the CAPP with studies showing support for the validity of the model's descriptive symptoms and domains of psychopathy (Kreis et al., 2012).

Previous studies which focused on the gender prototypicality of the CAPP found that psychopathy symptoms were more indicative of males. However, the model reflected a similar personality profile in both males and females, providing support for its content validity across gender (Kreis & Cooke, 2011; Sellbom et al., 2015; Pauli et al., 2018). Whilst similarities were identified, it is of note that gender differences were recognised, with men scoring high in domains such as attachment, behavioural, and cognitive, and women in attachment, dominance, and self (Kreis & Cooke, 2011). Studies of the effectiveness of the CAPP show promising findings for its gender-neutral approach to psychopathy assessment, however, its clinical validation remains in infancy.

In studies that have examined gender-differences in psychopathy, higher prevalence rate of ASPD in men as opposed to higher prevalence of BPD in women have been found (Pauli et al., 2018). The reasons for this are uncertain but have led to the proposal that psychopathy and BPD could be variants of the same underlying phenotype (Viljoen et al., 2015; Pauli et al., 2018). Using a similar strategy to the CAPP model, the Comprehensive Assessment of Borderline Personality Disorder (CABP) was created by Cook et al. (2013) to assess this possible overlap, as well as BPD symptoms.

Similar to the CAPP model, limited research has been conducted to provide empirical support of the CAPB. Only two known studies have been conducted which include both the CAPP and CAPB models, with both producing conflicting findings. In one study conducted by Pauli et al. (2018), participants were found to be adept in distinguishing the symptoms of psychopathy and BPD, with a number of borderline symptoms being observed as typical of psychopathy, thus giving support to the theory of an overlap. Yet, there was no evidence between genders for BPD being more commonly associated with females. In contrast, Viljoen et al. (2015) found BPD symptoms to be more typical of psychopathy in females. A note of caution is that in both of these studies the participants were either correctional staff, trainees or mental health professionals, none of which identified as experienced within the field of personality disorder.

An assessment tool which acknowledged the gender differences in clinical and forensic settings was in the development of the Female Additional Manual (FAM; de Vogel et al., 2014). This was created for additional use with the Historical, Clinical, Risk Management-20 (HCR-20; Webster et al., 1997; Strand & Selenius, 2019) risk assessment tool to identify specific risk factors for women. The FAM consists of eight additional risk factors within the historical items of personality disorder and traumatic experiences of the HCR-20; pregnancy at a young age, parenting difficulties, prostitution, suicide attempt/self-harm, low self-esteem, manipulative behaviour, problematic childcare responsibilities, and problematic future intimate relationships (de Vogel et al., 2019). Three additional items are included: victimisation, self-destructive behaviour, and non-violent criminal behaviour.

A recent study of the FAM conducted by Strand and Selenius (2019) in a forensic psychiatric unit found that the HCR-20v2 showed significant reliability without the additional use of the FAM in assessing risks of physical violence in women. Yet, they proposed that using this additional tool as a means to identify specific risk factors more commonly manifesting in females was useful to guide formulation and treatment pathways (Strand & Selenius, 2019). This suggests the potential value of the addition of the FAM in the assessment of women who may present with psychopathic traits as a way to help develop understanding and a psychological formulation collaboratively with them (de Vogel & Lancel, 2016).

4.4 Psychological Formulation

Psychological formulation to understand the woman's early history and development of presenting problems is a collaborative process to inform treatment provision and risk management approaches (Logan, 2014, 2017; Johnstone & Dallos, 2013). Psychological formulation can also help the females themselves develop greater self-understanding. Identifying strengths is also a vital component of psychological formulation and key to collaboratively helping women working towards more prosocial strategies of meeting needs (de Vogel et al., 2011).

Formulation approaches can be underpinned by a variety of different theoretical approaches to help women and the teams working with them develop shared understanding of complex problems. The Power Threat Meaning (PTM) Framework is also a recent conceptual development encapsulating biological, social, and psychological factors as an alternative to diagnostic approaches (Johnstone et al., 2018). At its core is the conjecture that individuals make sense of their experiences in relation to their social, cultural, material, and spiritual environments (Grant & Gadsby, 2018). The PTM framework is a progressive approach to understanding complex problems and represents a paradigm shift away from *"what is wrong with you"* to exploration of *"what has happened to you"*. There are four key concepts of the framework which are interrelated, that mediate emotional and psychological distress and problematic behaviour (Johnstone et al., 2018).

- *Power:* Exploring the concept of power and how it is operating within their life in asking '*what has happened to you?*' Individuals can experience adversity and social inequalities as a consequence of various sources of power such as economical, legal, relational, and ideological contexts.
- *Threat:* Investigating the threats that are posed by the negative effects of power in asking '*how did this affect you?*' Threats can be perceived as potential or actual loss of a person's fundamental needs such as, personal safety and security, material needs, attachments to children, families and the community (Johnstone & Boyle, 2018). The threats manifest from power imbalances when there is a threat to the fulfilment of basic functional needs and result in in distress.
- *Meaning:* Enabling a person to express the meaning of the situation and experiences from their perspective by asking, '*What sense did you make of it?*' Meaning can be viewed as being comprised of feelings, beliefs, and bodily reactions. Through their personal narrative, they can describe their experience and perceptions of power, threat, and the mental distress that can ensue.
- Response: '*What did you do to survive?*' The correlation of the above concepts informs an individual response to perceived threat. Adversity, and its subsequent effects, can be viewed as cumulative, and as such increases the threat responses. An individual's responses to threat can be viewed as survival strategy (i.e. forming attachments, regulating emotions). Threat responses evolve from our earliest attachments and are thoughts, behaviours, reactions, and expressions that we can employ to ensure social, emotional, and physical survival when encountering the negative impact of power.
- Within therapeutic settings the following questions can also be added; '*What are your strengths?*', and in collating all the available information, '*What is your story*?' Through exploration of these areas, an individual can create a discursive narrative of their experiences of distress.

Behaviour and its resulting outcomes are shaped by multiple factors which can be complex, interactional, and shaped by personal meaning and agency. The focus within the PTM framework is on accessing the meaning of an individual's response to negative power imbalances, threat, and the resulting behavioural responses. It seeks to digress from a cause-effect relationship as seen within psychiatric diagnostic systems, thus shifting the focus from a biological perspective of symptoms and disorders in the hope of distinguishing nonmedical causal pathways.

The resulting behavioural and emotional difficulties expressed by the psychopathic female may be the result of these negative power imbalances experienced in their history- for example, poverty, victim of abuse, and/or sexual violence. Histories of complex developmental trauma and poor attachments can be predisposing factors which contribute to mental health illness and offending behaviour (Willmott & Evershed, 2018). The PTM framework is a useful tool for discovering links between psychosocial experiences, patterns of behavioural outcomes, and identifying the reasoned response of utilising problematic behavioural coping mechanisms. The aim being to restore the links between meaning-based threats and meaning-based responses (Johnstone & Boyle, 2018). In turn, this may inform treatment pathways.

Overall, the PTM framework may be a useful approach to assisting the development of narratives to help understand women presenting with personality patterns that can present problems for themselves and others. In turn, it may also help to inform treatment pathway approaches with this complex client group.

4.5 Treatment Considerations

Assessment and formulation guide the development of treatment pathways for women presenting with problematic personality patterns (Johnstone & Dallos, 2013). The interpersonal and affective deficits which are characteristic of psychopathy (i.e. grandiosity, superficiality, shallow emotional responses), can undeniably have an impact upon treatment adherence and outcomes. In forensic settings women may feel that they have little control over their lives. They may engage in treatment directed by criminal justice agencies to secure release or discharge rather than due to intrinsic motivation. The early experiences of women may result in enactments within the therapeutic relationship and this may have an impact upon building the strength of therapeutic alliance, engagement, and the therapeutic pathway (e.g., McKeown & Harvey, 2018; Motz, 2016). Boundaries, honesty, and empathy are just some of the characteristics needed to foster a therapeutic relationship. Experiencing these therapeutic qualities within a therapeutic context may be challenging for a woman in a forensic setting for a variety of reasons. For example, women may resist this alliance due to hypervigilance of potential threats presented by relationships or due to power dynamics, where they may perceive the therapist as more powerful, and may wish to regain feelings of control and power. The relational dynamics can be challenging within a therapeutic context, although also present a rich opportunity for the woman to collaboratively self-reflect upon some of these challenges.

The difficulties of treatment adherence and outcomes lay within the broadness and etiology each individual's journey into the therapeutic context. For those who attribute their behaviors and any adverse consequences to external situations, it may be challenging to promote acknowledgement of personal responsibility. Promoting safety, compassion, and understanding within the therapeutic context can create safer environments to explore some of these domains (e.g., Gilbert, 2005).

Treatment planning based on the principles of risk, need, and responsivity have been found to be effective in efforts to reduce violence and recidivism (Bonta & Andrews, 2007; Polaschek & Daley, 2013). Treatment intensity, which correlates to the level of risk posed by the woman (risk), targets dynamic risk factors such as substance misuse and criminal attitudes (need), and is delivered in a manner to foster positive engagement within the treatment approach (responsivity). Comprehensive understanding and formulation of the woman is key, as well as promoting openness, transparency, and safety (Motz, 2016, 2019). Compassion-focused approaches to considering the woman's journey into therapy and the survival strategies developed is also likely to be useful (Gilbert, 2005). Supervision and reflection for practitioners working with women with invariably complex histories is also a vital part of the scaffolding required to undertake such work.

4.6 Conclusion and Recommendations

Over time, the applicability of the construct of psychopathy to females has seen growing interest. The PCL-R has predominated many research studies, although more recently the CAPP has presented a welcome development to magnify gender considerations further. In recent times, emphasis has been increasingly placed on understanding the origin of presenting difficulties and shifting the paradigm from labelling and diagnostic approaches to trauma-informed, formulation-driven approaches of understanding. Psychological formulation is a vital component understanding women in forensic settings. The Power Threat Meaning (PTM) Framework also represents a recent non-diagnostic approach that warrants further exploration as we attempt to understand and develop treatment pathways for this complex client group. Although a woman may present with interpersonal and affective difficulties that may suggest personality difficulties, developing a meaningful collaborative narrative to understand and work on these areas represents the real development forward.

References

Ballard, S. I., & Miller, H. G. (1945). Psychiatric casualties in a women's service. *British Medical Journal, 1*(4391), 293–295.

Batchelor, I. R. C. (1954). Psychopathic states and attempted suicide. *British Medical Journal, 1*(4875), 1342.

Bell, L. E. (2009). *Psychopathology and neuropsychological functioning among male and female prisoners in England and Wales*. Doctoral dissertation. Retrieved from https://qmro.qmul.ac.uk/xmlui/bitstream/handle/123456789/396/BELLPsychopathology2009.pdf?sequence=1

Beryl, R., Chou, S., & Völlm, B. (2014). A systematic view of psychopathy in women in secure settings. *Personality and Individual Differences, 71*, 185–195.

Bloom, B. E., Owen, B., & Covington, S. S. (2003). *Gender-responsive strategies: Research, practice, and guiding principles for women offenders*. National Institute of Corrections.

Boduszek, D., & Debowska, A. (2016). Critical evaluation of psychopathy measurement (PSCL-R and SRP-III/SF) and recommendations for future research. *Journal of Criminal Justice, 44*, 1–12.

Bonta, J., & Andrews, D. A. (2007). Risk-Need-Responsivity: Model for offender assessment and rehabilitation. *Rehabilitation, 6*, 1–22.

Buck, K. A. (2015). Understanding adolescent psychopathic traits from early risk and protective factors: Relations among inhibitory control, maternal sensitivity, and attachment representation. *Journal of Adolescence, 44*, 97–105.

Cleckley, H. (1941). *The mask of sanity*. Mosby.

Cleckley, H. (1988). *The mask of sanity: An attempt to clarify some issues about the so-called psychopathic personality* (3rd ed.). Mosby Company.

Coid, J., Yang, M., Ullrich, S., Roberts, A., Moran, P., Bebbington, P., Brugha, T., Jenkins, R., Farrell, M., Lewis, G., Singleton, N., & Hare, R. (2009). Psychopathy among prisoners in England and Wales. *International Journal of Law and Psychiatry, 32*(3), 134–141.

Cook, A. N., Layden, B. K., Viljoen, S., Murray, A. A., McGinnis, C. R., & Hart, S. D. (2013). *The Comprehensive Assessment of Borderline Personality Disorder (CAPB).* Simon Fraser University.

Cooke, D. J., & Michie, C. (2001). Refining the construct of psychopathy: Towards a hierarchical model. *Psychological Assessment, 13*(2), 171.

Cooke, D. J., Hart, S. D., Logan, C., & Michie, C. (2012). Explicating the construct of psychopathy: Development and validation of a conceptual model, the Comprehensive Assessment of Psychopathic Personality (CAPP). *International Journal of Forensic Mental Health, 11*(4), 242–252.

Cooper, S. (2008). *Unpublished data comparing PCL: YV scores across gender.*

Covington, S. S., & Bloom, B. E. (2007). Gender responsive treatment and services in correctional settings. *Women & Therapy, 29*(3–4), 9–33.

Covington, S. S. (2014). Beyond Anger and Violence. A Program for Women Participant Workbook. John Wiley & Sons.

Cruise, K. R., Coiwell, L. H., Lyons, P. M., & Baker, M. D. (2003). Prototypical analysis of adolescent psychopathy: Investigating the juvenile justice perspective. *Behavioural Sciences and the Law, 21*(6), 829–846.

Cunliffe, T., Gacono, C. B., Meloy, J. R., & Taylor, E. (2013). Are male and female psychopaths equivalent? A Rorschach study. In J. B. Helfgott (Ed.), *Criminal psychology* (pp. 423–459). Praeger.

De Vogel, V., & de Ruiter, C. (2005). The HCR-20 in personality disordered female offenders: A comparison with a matched sample of males. *Clinical Psychology & Psychotherapy, 12*(3), 226–240.

De Vogel, V., & Lancel, M. (2016). Gender differences the assessment and manifestation of psychopathy: Results from a multicentre study in forensic psychiatric patients. *International Journal of Forensic Mental Health, 15*(1), 97–110.

De Vogel, V., de Vries Robbé, M., de Ruiter, C., & Bouman, Y. H. (2011). Assessing protective factors in forensic psychiatric practice: Introducing the SAPROF. *International Journal of Forensic Mental Health, 10*(3), 171–177.

De Vogel, V., de Vries Robbé, M., Van Kalmthout, W., & Place, C. (2012). Female Additional Manual (FAM). In *Additional guidelines to the HCR-20 for assessing risk for violence in women. English version.* Van der Hoeven Kliniek.

De Vogel, V., de Vries Robbé, M., Van Kalmthout, W., & Place, C. (2014). *Female additional manual (FAM). Additional guidelines to the HCR-20V3 for assessing risk for violence in women. English version.* Van der Hoeven Kliniek.

De Vogel, V., Stam, J., Bouman, Y. H. A., Ter Horst, P., & Lancel, M. (2016). Violent women: A multicentre study into gender differences in forensic psychiatric patients. *Journal of Forensic Psychiatry & Psychology, 27*(2), 145–168.

De Vogel, V., Bruggeman, M., & Lancel, M. (2019). Gender-sensitive violence risk assessment: Predictive validity of six tools in female forensic psychiatric patients. *Criminal Justice and Behaviour, 46*(4), 528–549.

Dolan, M., & Völlm, B. (2009). Antisocial personality disorder and psychopathy in women: A literature review on the reliability and validity of assessment instruments. *International Journal of Law and Psychiatry, 32*(1), 2–9.

Edens, J. F., Skeem, J. L., Cruise, K. R., & Cauffman, E. (2001). Assessment of 'juvenile psychopathy' and its association with violence: A critical review. *Behavioral Sciences & the Law, 19*, 53–80.

Efferson, L. M., & Glenn, A. L. (2018). Examining gender differences in the correlates of psychopathy: A systematic review of emotional, cognitive, and morality-related constructs. *Aggression and Violent Behaviour, 41*, 48–61.

Eisenbarth, H., Krammer, S., Edwards, B. G., Keihl, K. A., & Neumann, C. S. (2018). Structural analysis of the PCL-R and relationship to BIG FIVE personality traits and parenting characteristics in a Hispanic female offender sample. *Personality and Individual Differences, 129*, 59–65.

Espinosa, E. M., & Sorensen, J. R. (2015). The influence of gender and traumatic experiences on length of time served in juvenile justice settings. *Criminal Justice and Behavior, 43*(2), 187–203.

Falkenbach, D. M., Reinhard, E. E., & Roelofs Larson, R. (2017). Theory based gender differences in psychopathy subtypes. *Personality and Individual Differences, 105*, 1–6.

Fonagy, P., Target, M., Gergely, G., Allen, J. G., & Bateman, A. W. (2003). The developmental roots of borderline personality disorder in early attachment relationships: A theory and some evidence. *Psychoanalytic Inquiry, 23*(3), 412–459.

Forouzan, E. (2003). *Psychopathy among women: Conceptualisation and assessment problems*. Communication presented at the Third Annual International Association of Forensic Mental Health Services (IAFMHS), Miami, Florida.

Forouzan, E., & Cooke, D. J. (2005). Figuring out la femme fatale: Conceptual and assessment issues concerning psychopathy in females. *Behavioral Sciences & the Law, 23*(6), 765–778.

Forouzan, E., & Nicholls, T. L. (2015). Childhood and adolescent characteristics of women with high versus low psychopathy scores: Examining developmental precursors to the malignant personality disorder. *Journal of Criminal Justice, 43*(4), 307–320.

Forth, A. E., Hart, S. D., & Hare, R. D. (1990). Assessment of psychopathy in male young offenders. *Psychological Assessment: A Journal of Consulting and Clinical Psychology, 2*(3), 342–344. https://doi.org/10.1037/1040-3590.2.3.342

Forth, A. E., & Burke, H. C. (1998). Psychopathy in adolescent assessment, violence, and developmental precursors. In D. J. Cooke, A. D. Forth, & R. D. Hare (Eds.), *Psychopathy: Theory, research and implications for society* (pp. 205–230). Kluwer.

Forth, A. E., Kosson, D., & Hare, R. D. (2003). *Manual for the youth version of the Hare Psychopathy Checklist – Revised (PCL-YV)*. Multi-Health Systems.

Fremming, K. H. (1947). *Morbidity risk of mental disease and other mental abnormalities in an average Danish population*. Munksgaard.

Gacono, C. B., Loving, J. L., & Bodholdt, R. H. (2001). The Rorschach and psychopathy: Toward a more accurate understanding of the research findings. *Journal of Personality Assessment, 77*(1), 16–38.

Gilbert, P. (Ed.). (2005). *Compassion: Conceptualisations, research and use in psychotherapy*. Routledge.

Gobin, R. L., Reddy, M. K., Zlotnick, C., & Johnson, J. E. (2015). Lifetime trauma victimization and PTSD in relation to psychopathy and antisocial personality disorder in a sample of incarcerated women and men. *International Journal of Prisoner Health, 11*(2), 64–74.

Gottfried, E. D., Harrop, T. M., Anestis, J. C., Venables, N. C., & Sellbom, M. (2018). An examination of triarchic psychopathy constructs in female offenders. *Journal of Personality Assessment, 101*(5), 455–467.

Grann, M. (2000). The PCL-R and gender. *European Journal of Psychological Assessment, 16*(3), 147–149.

Grant, A., & Gadsby, J. (2018). The Power Threat Meaning Framework and international mental health nurse education: A welcome revolution in human rights. *Nurse Education Today, 68*, 1–3.

Gray, N. S., & Snowden, R. J. (2016). Psychopathy in women: Prediction of criminality and violence in UK and USA psychiatric patients resident in the community. *Psychiatry Research, 237*, 339–343.

Greenacre, P. (1945). Conscience in the psychopath. *American Journal of Orthopsychiatry, 15*(3), 495.

Grella, C. E. (2008). From generic to gender responsive treatment: Changes in social policies, treatment services, and outcomes for women in substance abuse treatment. *Journal of Psychoactive Drugs: Supplement, 5*, 327–343.

Guay, J. P., Knight, R. A., Ruscio, J., & Hare, R. D. (2018). A taxometric investigation of psychopathy in women. *Psychiatry Research, 261*, 565–573.

Hare, R. D. (1980). A research scale for the assessment of psychopathy in criminal populations. *Personality and Individual Differences, 1*(2), 111–119.

Hare, R. D. (1991). *The Hare PCL-R: Rating booklet*. Multi-Health Systems.

Hare, R. D. (2003). *Manual for the revised psychopathy checklist* (2nd ed.). Multi-Health Systems.

Hare, R. D. (2008). Psychological instruments in the assessment of psychopathy. In A. Felthous & H. Sass (Eds.), *International handbook of psychopathic disorders and the law* (pp. 41–68). Wiley.

Hare, R. D., & Neumann, C. S. (2005). The PCL-R assessment of psychopathy: Development, structural properties, and new directions. In C. J. Patrick (Ed.), *Handbook of psychopathy* (pp. 58–90). Guilford Press.

Hare, R. D., Hart, S. D., & Harpur, T. J. (1991). Psychopathy and the DSM-IV criteria for antisocial personality disorder. *Journal of Abnormal Psychology, 100*(3), 391–398.

Hemphill, J. F., & Hare, R. D. (2004). Some misconceptions about the Hare PCL-R and risk assessment: A reply to Gendreau, Goggin, and Smith. *Criminal Justice and Behavior, 31*(2), 203–243.

Henderson, D. K. (1939). *Psychopathic states*. Chapman & Hall.

Hicks, B. M., Markon, K. E., Patrick, C. J., Krueger, R. F., & Newman, J. P. (2004). Identifying psychopathy subtypes on the basis of personality structure. *Psychological Assessment, 16*(3), 276.

Hicks, B. M., Vaidyanathan, U., & Patrick, C. J. (2010). Validating female psychopathy subtypes: Differences in personality, antisocial and violent behavior, substance abuse, trauma, and mental health. *Personality Disorders, Theory, Research, and Treatment, 1*(1), 38.

Hunt, E., Bornovalova, M. A., & Patrick, C. J. (2015). Genetic and environmental overlap between borderline personality disorder traits and psychopathy: Evidence for promotive effects of factor 2 and protective effects of factor 1. *Psychological Medicine, 45*(07), 1471–1481.

Inciardi, J. A., Lockwood, D., & Pottieger, A. E. (1993). *Women and crack-cocaine*. Macmillan.

Jackson, R. L., Rogers, R., Neumann, C. S., & Lambert, P. L. (2002). Psychopathy in female offenders: An investigation of its underlying dimensions. *Criminal Justice and Behaviour, 29*(6), 692–704.

Johnstone, L., & Boyle, M. (2018). The power threat meaning framework: An alternative nondiagnostic conceptual system. *Journal of Humanistic Psychology*. https://doi.org/10.1177/0022167818793289

Johnstone, L., & Dallos, R. (2013). *Formulation in psychology and psychotherapy: Making sense of people's problems*. Routledge.

Johnstone, L., Boyle, M., Cromby, J., Dillon, J., Harper, D., Kinderman, P., & Read, J. (2018). *The power threat meaning framework*. British Psychological Society. Retrieved from https://www.bps.org.uk/sites/bps.org.uk/files/Policy

Karpman, B. (1941). On the need of separating psychopathy into two distinct clinical types: The symptomatic and the idiopathic. *Journal of Criminal Psychopathology, 3*, 112–137.

Karpman, B. (1948). The myth of the psychopathic personality. *American Journal of Psychiatry, 104*(9), 523–534.

Klein Tuente, S., Vogel, V. D., & Stam, J. (2014). Exploring the criminal behavior of women with psychopathy: Results from a multicenter study into psychopathy and violent offending in female forensic psychiatric patients. *International Journal of Forensic Mental Health, 13*(4), 311–322.

Kreis, M. K. F., & Cooke, D. J. (2011). Capturing the psychopathic female: A prototypicality analysis of the Comprehensive Assessment of Psychopathic Personality (CAPP) across gender. *Behavioural Sciences and the Law, 29*, 634–648.

Kreis, M. K., & Cooke, D. J. (2012). The manifestation of psychopathic traits in women: An exploration using case examples. *International Journal of Forensic Mental Health, 11*(4), 267–279.

Kreis, M. K. F., Cooke, D. J., Michie, C., Hoff, H. A., & Logan, C. (2012). The Comprehensive Assessment of Psychopathic Personality (CAPP): Content validation using prototypical analysis. *Journal of Personality Disorders, 26*(3), 402–413.

Kruepke, M. D. (2015). *Revisiting borderline personality disorder as a female expression of psychopathy: A facet level analysis and meta-analysis*. Doctoral dissertation. Verona, University.

Leichsenring, F., Leibing, E., Kruse, J., New, A. S., & Leweke, F. (2011). Borderline personality disorder. *The Lancet, 377*(9759), 74–84.

Linehan, M. M. (2014). *Cognitive-behavioral treatment of borderline personality disorder* (p. 1993). Guilford.

Logan, C. (2009). Psychopathy in women: Conceptual issues, clinical presentation and management. *Neuropsychiatrie: Klinik, Diagnostik, Therapie und Rehabilitation, 23*(1), 25–33.

Logan, C. (2014). The HCR-20 version 3: A case study in risk formulation. *International Journal of Forensic Mental Health, 13*(2), 172–180.

Logan, C. (2017). Forensic case formulation for violence and aggression. In P. Sturmey (Ed.), *The Wiley handbook of violence and aggression*. Wiley.

Logan, C., & Blackburn, R. (2009). Mental disorder in violent women in secure settings: Potential relevance to risk for future violence. *International Journal of Law and Psychiatry, 32*(1), 31–38.

Logan, C., & Weizmann-Henelius, G. (2012). Psychopathy in women: Presentation, assessment and management. In H. Häkkänen-Nyholm & J. O. Nyholm (Eds.), *Psychopathy and law: A Practitioner's guide* (pp. 99–125). Wiley.

Lunbeck, E. (2006). Narrating nymphomania between psychiatry and the law. In A. Sarat, L. Douglas, & M. Umphrey (Eds.), *Law's madness* (pp. 49–77). University of Michigan Press.

Lynam, D. R., & Gudonis, L. (2005). The development of psychopathy. *Annual Review of Clinical Psychology, 1*, 381–407.

McKeown, A. (2010). Female offenders: Assessment of risk in forensic settings. *Aggression and Violent Behavior, 15*(6), 422–429.

McKeown, A., & Harvey, E. (2018). Violent women: Treatment approaches and psychodynamic considerations. *Journal of Criminological Research, Policy and Practice, 4*(2), 124–135.

Motz, A. (2016). *The psychology of female violence: Crimes against the body*. Routledge.

Motz, A. (2019). Engaging women in forensic clinical interviews: The impact of gender. *International Journal of Forensic Mental Health, 18*(1), 21–34.

Neumann, C. S., Hare, R. D., & Pardini, D. A. (2015). Antisociality and the construct of psychopathy: Data from across the globe. *Journal of Personality, 83*(6), 678–692.

Nicholls, T. L., Ogloff, J. R., Brink, J., & Spidel, A. (2005). Psychopathy in women: A review of its clinical usefulness for assessing risk for aggression and criminality. *Behavioural Sciences and the Law, 23*(6), 779–802.

Odgers, C. L., Reppucci, D. N., & Moretti, M. M. (2005). Nipping psychopathy in the bud: An examination of the convergent, predictive, and theoretical utility of the PCL-YV among adolescent girls. *Behavioural Sciences and the Law, 23*(6), 743–763.

Patrick, C. J. (Ed.). (2005). *Handbook of psychopathy*. Guilford Press.

Pauli, M., Essemyr, K., Sorman, K., Howner, K., Gustavsson, P., & Liljeberg, J. (2018). Gendered expressions of psychopathy: Correctional staffs' perceptions of the CAPP and CAPB models. *International Journal of Forensic Mental Health, 17*(2), 97–110.

Penney, S. R., & Moretti, M. M. (2007). The relation of psychopathy to concurrent aggression and antisocial behavior in high-risk adolescent girls and boys. *Behavioral Sciences & the Law, 25*, 21–41.

Polaschek, D. L. L., & Daley, T. E. (2013). Treatment and psychopathy in forensic settings. *Aggression and Violent Behaviour, 18*(5), 592–603.

Rogstad, J. E., & Rogers, R. (2008). Gender differences in contributions of emotion to psychopathy and antisocial personality disorder. *Clinical Psychology Review, 28*(8), 1472–1484.

Rorschach, H. (1942). *Psychodiagnostics*. Hans Huber.

Salekin, R. T., Rogers, R., & Sewell, K. W. (1996). A review and meta-analysis of the Psychopathy Checklist–Revised: Predictive validity of dangerousness. *Clinical Psychology: Science and Practice, 3*, 203–213.

Salekin, R. T., Rogers, R., & Sewell, K. W. (1997). Construct validity of psychopathy in a female offender sample: A multitrait–multimethod evaluation. *Journal of Abnormal Psychology, 106*(4), 576–585.

Salisbury, E. J., & Van Voorhis, P. (2009). Gendered pathways: A quantitative investigation of women probationers' paths to incarceration. *Criminal Justice and Behavior, 36*(6), 541–566.

Seagrave, D., & Grisso, T. (2002). Adolescent development and the measurement of juvenile psychopathy. *Law and Human Behavior, 26*, 219–239.

Sellbom, M., Cooke, D. J., & Hart, S. D. (2015). Construct validity of the Comprehensive Assessment of Psychopathic Personality (CAPP) concept map: Getting closer to the core of psychopathy. *International Journal of Forensic Mental Health, 14*(3), 172–180.

Sevecke, K., Franke, S., Kosson, D., & Krischer, M. (2016). Emotional dysregulation and trauma predicting dimensions in female and male juvenile offenders. *Child and Adolescent Psychiatry and Mental Health, 10*(43). https://doi.org/10.1186/s13034-016-0130-7

Simpson, S. S., Yanher, J. L., & Dugan, L. (2008). Understanding women's pathways to jail: Analysing the lives of incarcerated women. *Australian & New Zealand Journal of Criminology, 41*, 84–108.

Skeem, J., Johansson, P., Andershed, H., Kerr, M., & Louden, J. E. (2007). Two subtypes of psychopathic violent offenders that parallel primary and secondary variants. *Journal of Abnormal Psychology, 116*(2), 395.

Southard, E. E. (1916). *Southard papers, 1892–1940*. Harvard Medical Library in the Francis A. Countway Library of Medicine.

Spataro, J., Mullen, P. E., Burgess, P. M., Wells, D. L., & Moss, S. A. (2004). Impact of child sexual abuse on mental health: Prospective study in males and females. *The British Journal of Psychiatry, 184*(5), 416–421.

Sprague, J., Javdani, S., Sadeh, N., Newman, J. P., & Verona, E. (2012). Borderline personality disorder as a female phenotypic expression of psychopathy? *Personality Disorders, Theory, Research, and Treatment, 3*(2), 127–139.

Strachan, C. E. (1993). *The assessment of psychopathy in female offenders*. Doctoral dissertation. Retrieved from https://open.library.ubc.ca/cIRcle/collections/ubctheses/831/items/1.0099215

Strand, S. J. M., & Selenius, H. (2019). Assessing risk for inpatient physical violence in a female forensic psychiatric sample – Comparing HCR-20v2 with the Female Additional Manual to the HCR-20v2. *Nordic Journal of Psychiatry, 73*(4–5), 248–256.

Thornton, D., & Blud, L. (2007). The influence of psychopathic traits on response to treatment. In H. Hervé & J. C. Yuille (Eds.), *The psychopath: Theory, research, and practice* (pp. 505–539). Lawrence Erlbaum.

Trippany, R. L., Helm, H. M., & Simpson, L. (2006). Trauma reenactment: Rethinking borderline personality disorder when diagnosing sexual abuse survivors. *Journal of Mental Health Counseling, 28*(2), 95–110.

Vablais, C. M. (2007). Toward a new model of psychopathy in women: A qualitative analysis of the Psychopathy Checklist–revised and the construct of psychopathy in female offenders. *Dissertation Abstracts International: Section B: The Sciences and Engineering, 68*(2-B), 1323.

Van der Kolk, B. A. (2015). *The body keeps the score: Brain, mind, and body in the healing of trauma*. Penguin Books.

Verona, E., & Vitale, J. (2006). Psychopathy in women: Assessment, manifestations, and etiology. In C. Patrick (Ed.), *Handbook of psychopathy* (pp. 415–436). Guilford Press.

Verona, E., Hicks, B. M., & Patrick, C. J. (2005). Psychopathy and suicidality in female offenders: Mediating influences of personality and abuse. *Journal of Consulting and Clinical Psychology, 73*(6), 1065–1073.

Verona, E., Sprague, J., & Javdani, S. (2012). Gender and factor-level interactions in psychopathy: Implications for self-directed violence risk and borderline personality disorder symptoms. *Personality Disorders, Theory, Research, and Treatment, 3*(3), 247–262.

Viljoen, S., Cook, A. N., Lim, Y. L., Layden, B. K., Bousfield, N. K., & Hart, S. D. (2015). Are psychopathic and borderline personality disorder distinct, or differently gendered expressions of the same disorder? An exploration using concept maps. *International Journal of Forensic Mental Health, 14*(4), 267–279.

Vincent, G. M., & Hart, S. D. (2002). Psychopathy in childhood and adolescence: Implications for the assessment and management of multi-problem youths. In R. R. Corrado, R. Roesch, S. D. Hart, & J. K. Gierowski (Eds.), *Multiproblem violent youth: A foundation for comparative research on needs, interventions and outcomes,* (pp.150–163). Amsterdam: IOS Press

Vitale, J. E., Smith, S. S., Brinkley, C. A., & Newman, J. P. (2002). The reliability and validity of the Psychopathy Checklist-Revised in a sample of female offenders. *Criminal Justice and Behavior, 29*(2), 202–231.

Warren, F., McGauley, G., Norton, K., Dolan, B., Preedy-Fayers, K., Pickering, A., & Geddes, J. R. (2003). *Review of treatments for severe personality disorder.* Home Office Online Report 30/03.

Webster, C. D., Douglas, K. S., Eaves, D., & Hart, S. D. (1997). HCR-20. Assessing the risk of violence. Version, 2.

Weizmann-Henelius, G., Grönroos, M., Putkonen, H., Eronen, M., Lindberg, N., & Häkkänen-Nyholm, H. (2010). Psychopathy and gender differences in childhood psychosocial characteristics in homicide offenders – A nationwide register based study. *Journal of Forensic Psychiatry and Psychology, 21*(6), 801–814.

Weizmann-Henelius, G., Virkkunen, M., Gammelgard, M., Eronen, M., & Putkonene, H. (2015). The PCL-R and violent recidivism in a prospective follow-up of a nationwide sample of female offenders. *Journal of Forensic Psychiatry & Psychology, 26*(5), 667–685.

Willmott, P., & Evershed, S. (2018). Interviewing people given a diagnosis of personality disorder in forensic settings. *International Journal of Forensic Mental Health, 17*(4), 338–350.

Wynn, R., Høiseth, M. H., & Pettersen, G. (2012). Psychopathy in women: Theoretical and clinical perspectives. *International Journal of Women's Health, 4*, 257–263.

Chapter 5
Psychopathy and Violence

Nicholas D. Thomson, Salpi Kevorkian, and Adelaide A. Verdugo-Thomson

Abstract Psychopathy is well-established as a risk-factor and predictor of violent and aggressive behavior. Psychopathic individuals, though an estimably small portion of the population, comprise a large portion of all violent crime committed. Psychopathic individuals display not only criminal versatility, but versatility in their approaches to violent and aggressive behavior. This chapter argues that understanding the association between the distinct facets of psychopathy and types of violent behavior and the mechanisms linking psychopathy to violence, and further establishing evidence-based strategies for men and women, should be a global public health priority in order to effectively break the psychopathy-violence link. Within this chapter, the similarities and differences of violent and aggressive behavioral outcomes, their distinct relations to the construct of psychopathy, implications, and recommendations for future research are explored.

Keywords Psychopathy · Psychopathic traits · Violence · Aggression · Offenders · Violent offending

5.1 An Introduction to Psychopathy and Violence

During the early hours of June 5th, 2002, 14-year old Elizabeth Smart awoke to Brian Mitchell holding a knife to her throat. For the next 9 months, numerous search parties would look tirelessly for Elizabeth, who was held hostage in a makeshift camp on the outskirts of Salt Lake City. There, she was held captive by Mitchell and his wife Wanda Barzee. During Elizabeth's captivity, Mitchell kept Elizabeth under the influence of drugs and alcohol, starved her, and fed her garbage, all while being tied by a 15-foot cable between two trees. Multiple times a day, Mitchell raped Elizabeth and regularly threatened her and her family's lives. Mitchell boasted that he was an angel

N. D. Thomson (✉) · S. Kevorkian · A. A. Verdugo-Thomson
Virginia Commonwealth University, Richmond, VA, USA
e-mail: Nicholas.Thomson@vcuhealth.org

J. E. Vitale (ed.), *The Complexity of Psychopathy*, Dangerous Behavior in Clinical and Forensic Psychology, https://doi.org/10.1007/978-3-030-83156-1_5

and a Davidic King, telling Elizabeth that in 7 years he would be stoned by a mob and lie dead in the streets for 3 days, and then rise up and kill the Antichrist. To help Mitchell defeat the Antichrist he would need to kidnap several more virgin brides. After months of gaining Mitchell's trust, he would eventually allow Elizabeth out in public to steal provisions. Under the religious disguise of a headdress and veil, Elizabeth eventually escaped captivity when two witnesses had recognized Mitchell and his wife after watching an episode of "America's Most Wanted."

Although Mitchell presented with religious delusion, his religious beliefs were an attempt to gain dominance and authority over others. Mitchell used the religious cloak as a mask to manipulate others for personal gain. Drawing from multiple testimonies and interviews, it was clear that Mitchell held grandiose views, regarded himself as a prophet, and asserted himself as an authority on all topics. Mitchell was manipulative and a pathological liar. Elizabeth recalled that he had an "ability to adapt to his surrounding and talk his way out of any situation… he took pleasure in getting away with things" (Mitchell & Kimball, 2010, p. 130). Mitchell did manage to talk his way out of trouble on multiple occasions, including during an arrest in San Diego, confrontation by a suspicious officer in the Salt Lake City library, and a run-in with the police in Las Vegas.

Mitchell parasitically lived off others by panhandling and stealing, which he preferred to do rather than work. He was callous and engaged in sadistic behaviors. During adolescence, Mitchell was physically and verbally abusive to his mother and sister; his own family described him as "cruel and sadistic" (Mitchell & Kimball, 2010, p. 25). After being arrested for soliciting sexual activity from a 4-year old neighbor, Mitchell told his psychologist that he knew the psychological vulnerabilities of his family, and he got satisfaction from upsetting others by using physical and psychological threats. During his first marriage, Mitchell kidnapped and sexually abused his children. As Mitchell's finances ran low he put his children up for adoption, prohibiting the children from having any contact with their biological family. During his second marriage, he discovered his wife was terrified of mice, so he neatly lined 50 mice on a cookie sheet in the oven "just so she could open up the oven door and have… a panic-stricken reaction and did the same not only with mice but with roaches during the course of their marriage" (Mitchell & Kimball, 2010, p. 133). Mitchell served his step-daughter her pet rabbit for dinner, later gloating that he tricked her into thinking it was chicken. Mitchell was a callous, cruel, and manipulative psychopathic individual that violated the rights of others, including those of his own children. During his court trial, psychiatrists found Mitchell to have a score of 34 on the Psychopathy Checklist-Revised, placing him well within the diagnostic threshold of psychopathy.

5.1.1 The Importance of Psychopathy for Preventing Violence

The community prevalence of psychopathy is low (men = 1–2%; women = 0.3–0.7%), yet, psychopathic individuals are responsible for a large proportion (20–40%) of all violent crime (Coid & Yang, 2011; Hare & Neumann, 2008; Thomson, 2019). As a result, it is estimated that psychopathy costs society $460 billion annually, making it one of the most expensive psychiatric disorders (Kiehl & Hoffman, 2011). Psychopathic individuals who engage in violence are found to be more gratuitously violent (e.g., overkill), cruel, and sadistic (Robertson & Knight, 2014). In hopes to break the cycle of violence, researchers have begun to explore the mechanisms linking psychopathy to violence. This is an important endeavor because by targeting a small group of individuals (~1%), the global number of violent crimes can drastically be reduced by 20–40%. Violence is a multifarious construct, where contextual factors play a major role. Psychopathic individuals display not only criminal versatility, but versatility in their violence. As psychopathic individuals are opportunistic in their violence, it is important to understand the association between psychopathic traits and different forms of violence to fully appreciate the utility of psychopathy as a construct for violence risk assessment.

The present chapter aims to provide an overview of the research linking psychopathy to aggression. First, we will provide a brief introduction to the dimensional construct of clinical psychopathy, which will be referenced throughout this chapter. It is important to recognize that not all violence is prosecuted and many acts of violence go unreported. To address this, we provide an overview of the association between psychopathy and aggression forms and subtypes in both community and institutional populations. Next, the chapter focuses on four major types of violent crime: homicide, sexual assault and rape (including stalking), assault (including intimate partner violence and institutional violence), and robbery. Lastly, because of the association between psychopathy and reoffending, recommendations for future research directions in the nexus of psychopathy, aggression, and violence are included.

5.1.2 The Construct of Psychopathy

Psychopathy is most widely studied using the Psychopathy Checklist-Revised (Hare, 2003), which remains the gold standard for clinical assessment of psychopathy (Thomson, 2019). The PCL-R includes 20 personality and behavioral symptoms, with each symptom rated using a three-point scale from, "item does not apply" (0) to "item definitely applies" (2). A PCL-R score of 30 or above in the US is used for a diagnosis, however, a score of 25 or above is often used in Europe and for women. The 40 items of the PCL-R map on to a 2-factor model, which includes Interpersonal-Affective psychopathic traits (Factor 1) and Impulsive-Antisocial psychopathic traits (Factor 2). The 2-factor model can be further broken into a 4-facet model (Hare, 2003; see Fig. 5.1), which includes the following facets: (1) Interpersonal (e.g., charming, manipulative), (2) Affective (e.g., callous lack of empathy, lack of remorse), (3) Lifestyle (e.g., impulsive, parasitic lifestyle), and (4) Antisocial facets (e.g., juvenile delinquency, criminal versatility). The 2-factor and the 4-facet models are the most commonly used constructs for determining risk for violent behavior. More recently, the 4-facet model has demonstrated more

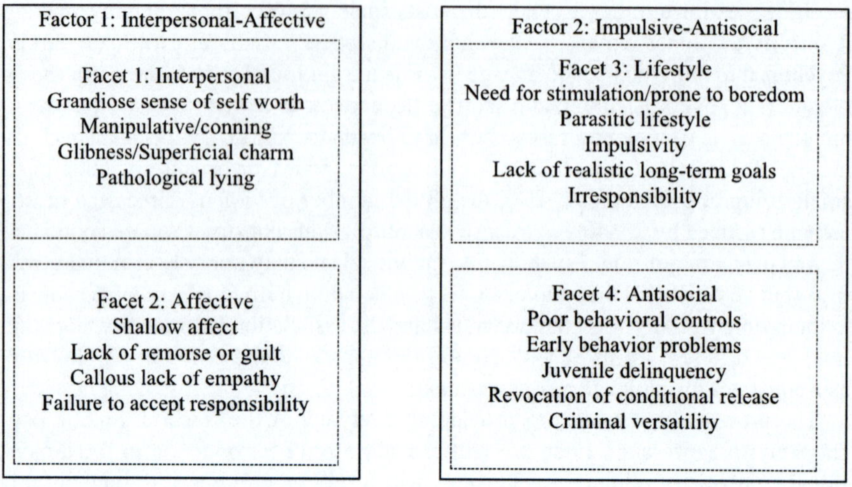

Fig. 5.1 2-Factor and 4-Facet Models
Caption: *Note.* **The items "promiscuous sexual behavior" and "many short-term relationships" are not included in factor or facet models but are included in total PCL-R scores (Hare, 2003)**

sensitivity in detecting sex differences in the psychopathy-violence link (Thomson et al., 2019a, b). Given the variance in functional utility of these models, and the widespread use of various PCL-R based measures within the extant literature, this chapter will seek to provide a comprehensive overview of both factor and facet model correlates. To better understand the predictors and outcomes of violence associated with psychopathy in both men and women, it is important to first examine the construct of aggression and its relation to the facets and factors of psychopathy in further detail.

5.2 Forms of Aggression

Aggression is an umbrella term used to describe behaviors that cause harm to others or oneself, but aggression does not always present in violence. Within the construct of aggression, there is further classification based on the function, such as proactive or reactive, and form, such as overt (e.g., physical, verbal) or covert (e.g., indirect/relational), and physical (e.g., acts of causing physical harm to another person or property) or verbal (e.g., verbal abuse, mocking, profanity, and character attacks). Indirect aggression, also termed "relational aggression," causes harm through various means such as gossiping and spreading rumors behind someone's back, ignoring and excluding someone purposely, defaming someone's character, and turning others against someone. It is thought that people generally use covert aggression when the costs of overt aggression are deemed too high (Archer & Coyne, 2005;

Björkqvist, 1994). Similarly, research has shown that men more often engage in overt forms of aggression, whereas women more often engage in levels of covert, or indirect, aggression (Thomson et al., 2019b).

The extant literature has well documented the associations between the facets of psychopathy and the manifestations of aggressive behavior, arguing that distinctive facets may be related to certain forms of aggression (Reidy et al., 2016). For example, research involving U.S. service members showed that the Antisocial and Interpersonal facets of psychopathy were related to higher levels of overt aggression (verbal and physical; Anestis et al., 2017). Similarly, when compared to adults who scored low on all psychopathy facets, adults who scored highest on the Antisocial and Interpersonal facets were found to have higher levels of verbal aggression (Colins et al., 2017). Also of interest are the notable sex differences that have been documented, suggesting that certain facets of psychopathy may predict disparate forms of aggressive behavior in men and women. For example, in a community sample of men and women, the Affective facet was associated with physical aggression but only for women, while the Antisocial facet was related to higher indirect aggression, but only for men (Thomson et al., 2019b). Further, a follow-up study found the association between higher Affective facet scores and higher physical aggression in women was moderated by exposure to physical abuse (Thomson et al., 2019a). For both men and women, the Antisocial facet was associated with higher physical aggression, and the Interpersonal facet was associated with higher verbal aggression, suggesting that the 4-facet model of psychopathy may provide both gender-neutral, and female-specific, risk assessments (Thomson et al., 2019b).

5.2.1 *Subtypes of Aggression*

Reactive aggression is an aggressive response to provocation or threat, and is viewed as a loss of emotional and behavioral control (Barratt, 1991; Berkowitz, 1993). In contrast, proactive aggression is calculated, predatory, and used for personal gain (Dodge, 1991; Dodge & Coie, 1987). Proactive aggression shares common features with psychopathy, such as the callous use of others to achieve some form of a personal goal (e.g., obtain money or sex). Further, research assessing biological correlates of proactive aggression and psychopathy show common predictors of the two, such as low anxiety, physiological hyporeactivity, and positive appraisal of threat (see Thomson, 2019, for a full review). It is not surprising, then, that results from violent offenders suggest that psychopathy is related to proactive violent crime (Cornell et al., 1996) and to proactive homicide (Woodworth & Porter, 2002).

Several studies to date have detailed findings of the aggression correlates of the factor and facet models in men and women. Cima and Raine (2009) showed that higher total psychopathy scores in male offenders predicted proactive aggression but not reactive aggression. In addition, using the 2-factor model of the Psychopathic Personality Inventory-Revised (PPI-R), the study showed that while both factors predicted proactive aggression, only the Impulsive-Antisociality factor was related to reactive aggression. A study by Declercq et al. (2012) showed the Interpersonal facet was the best predictor of predatory violence in male offenders, whereas the Antisocial facet was the least predictive facet of predatory violence. In partial support of this finding, a meta-analysis involving 53 studies found that the Interpersonal facet was the best predictor of proactive aggression, although the same study also found that the Lifestyle facet was most strongly related to both proactive and reactive aggression (Blais et al., 2014).

In a study using the PPI-R and the Levenson Self-Report Psychopathy Scale (LSRP) in a community sample of young men and women, important sex differences in the psychopathy-aggression link were found. Specifically, high scores on PPI-R Self-Centered Impulsivity (e.g., poor impulse control, manipulativeness) were associated with higher rates of proactive aggression in men, but not women. Conversely, higher LSRP Factor 2 scores (e.g., impulsive and uncontrolled behavior) were associated with higher reactive aggression in women than in men (Hecht et al., 2015). An explanation of these findings may be that, compared to men, women with higher Factor 2 traits may exhibit higher levels of emotional reactivity, which leads to greater reactive aggression.

Indeed, research including detained female adolescents found higher reactive aggression was associated with poorly regulated emotion and anger to perceived provocation (Marsee & Frick, 2007). Recent evidence in a cohort of young women extends this finding. In a community sample of young women, the Interpersonal, Affective, and Antisocial facets were associated with proactive aggression, and the Lifestyle facet was associated with reactive aggression (Thomson et al., 2018). However, when the authors assessed the moderating role of a biological vulnerability of emotion dysregulation on the psychopathy-aggression link, it was found that the Affective and Antisocial facets were related to reactive aggression for those with poor emotion regulation capability (Thomson et al., 2018). Thus, it seems that psychopathic traits are generally related to proactive aggression, especially the personality features of psychopathy, but the link between psychopathy and reactive aggression seems to be contingent on poor emotion regulation capability.

5.2.2 Summary of Psychopathy Factor and Facet Model Predictors of Aggression

The extant literature highlights key differences in facet and factor model predictors of the function and form of aggression within psychopathic individuals. Overall, several studies support the notion that the Interpersonal facet is, in particular, important for explaining proactive aggression (i.e., predatory, or instrumental, violence) across community and institutional samples (Blais et al., 2014; Declercq et al., 2012), while there is little evidence that the Lifestyle facet predicts proactive aggression. However, the Lifestyle facet is generally related to higher reactive aggression, and any association between psychopathy and reactive aggression is likely explained by poor emotion regulation capability (Thomson et al., 2019a, b, c). There is more overlap between the personality facets (i.e., Interpersonal) and behavioral facets (i.e., Antisocial) for forms of aggression. For example, the Antisocial and Interpersonal facets were both found to be related to overt aggression – more specifically, overt verbal aggression in (Colins et al., 2017), and overt verbal and physical aggression (Anestis et al., 2017; Thomson et al., 2019a, b, c). It is clear that more research is needed to expand on the present findings using the 4-facet model across population types. This, we believe, would lead to greater understanding of the contribution of each facet to the etiology and maintenance of aggressive behavior. Similarly, as manifestations of aggression have been found to be contingent on sex (i.e., men generally engage in overt behaviors, women generally engage in covert behaviors; Thomson et al., 2019a, b, c), it can be reasonably concluded that evaluating extraneous variables (e.g., history of potential physical abuse, emotional regulating capabilities, etc.) would also prove beneficial in understanding the differences that characterize the relationships between these constructs in both men and women.

5.3 Violent Crimes

Psychopathy is commonly understood as a well-established risk factor for violence and violent recidivism. The following section will present research findings that detail the link between psychopathy and specific categories of violent crimes (e.g., homicide, assault, sexual offending, intimate partner violence, robbery, future violent recidivism, and prison and inpatient violence). This will allow for further exploration of the different types of associations between these constructs. It will also provide an examination of the limitations of the existing literature.

5.3.1 Homicide

There is limited research exploring the link between psychopathy and homicide, and what exists is somewhat conflicting. Some findings, for example, demonstrate a weak association between psychopathy and homicide offending. For example, research from the Dangerous and Severe Personality Disordered (DSPD) unit in the United Kingdom found that psychopathic individuals were not significantly overrepresented in the homicide offender group when compared to non-psychopathic individuals (Casey et al., 2013). Consistent with this finding in men, in a sample of female forensic psychiatric patients from the Netherlands, Klein Tuente et al. (2014) found that homicide offenders were less likely to meet the diagnostic cutoff score for psychopathy (PCL-R > 25) than non-homicide offenders. In contrast with non-psychopathic homicide offenders, psychopathic females were more likely to have strangers as their victims, and their crimes were more often motivated by power, dominance, and personal gain (Klein Tuente et al., 2014). Another study found that female maximum security prisoners in the US who committed homicide generally had lower overall total psychopathy scores (Warren et al., 2005).

Several studies that use self-report measures of psychopathy have reported similar findings in demonstrating a weak link between homicide and psychopathy. For example, a study using self-report measures of psychopathy in a sample of 61 male serial murderers (Culhane et al., 2019) found that there was no significant difference in psychopathic traits between the serial murderers and community samples on the PPI-R (Lilienfeld & Widows, 2005) and LSRP (Levenson et al., 1995). However, in a study using the Self-Report Psychopathy Scale (SRP-III; Paulhus et al., 2016), the authors found that serial murderers had higher scores on all four facets (Interpersonal, Affective, Lifestyle, and Antisocial) than both community and college samples. Yet, when compared to other psychopathic offenders, serial murderers scored lower on all four facets, suggesting that, at least as measured by these self-report assessments, serial homicide is not necessarily indicative of psychopathy (Culhane et al., 2019). Another study using the SRP found that male murderers were not more psychopathic than other offending groups (e.g., first-time incarcerated offenders and recidivists; Sherretts et al., 2017). Using the facet structure of the SRP, the authors also found that homicide offenders scored lower than recidivists on the Interpersonal and Lifestyle facets (Sherretts et al., 2017).

The research presented so far suggests psychopathy is either not linked to homicide or is negatively associated with homicide. However, a recent meta-analysis by Fox and DeLisi (2019), which included 2603 homicide offenders, found higher psychopathy scores among homicide offenders (PCL-R = 21.1) as compared to nonoffenders (PCL-R = 5.2). The study also reported that 72% of homicide offenders met the PCL-R cut off score of 30, which is much higher than community rates (~1%). The authors found notable differences across countries. For instance, American murderers (PCL-R = 26.2) scored the highest when compared to Canadian murderers (PCL-R = 23.7), Finnish murderers (PCL-R = 20.3), Swedish murderers (PCL-R = 20.2), and German murderers (PCL-R = 17.4). In support of the positive link between psychopathy and homicide, youth who committed homicide scored higher on psychopathy total score and across all four facets of the PCL:Youth Version (PCL:YV) when compared to non-homicide juvenile offenders (Cope et al., 2014). One difference in this study was that 80% of the homicides were self-reported and the individual had not been convicted of the crime. Thus, the methods by which homicide is measured might impact its association with psychopathy. For example, those who commit homicide and get away with it may be more psychopathic, whereas those *convicted* of homicide are not overly represented as psychopathic. However, this line of inquiry needs to be further investigated.

What is clear is that psychopathic individuals who kill differ from non-psychopathic individuals in their motives and how they behave during and after the crime. Research has shown homicides committed by psychopathic individuals are likely to be planned and goal-directed for personal gain (Woodworth & Porter, 2002). Similarly, the victims of homicidal acts by psychopathic individuals are more likely to be strangers (Pajevic et al., 2017; Porter et al., 2003). Whereas most domestic homicide cases are driven by intense emotion (e.g., anger, jealousy, etc.), psychopathic individuals are more dispassionate and gratuitously violent (Juodis et al., 2014). Porter and Woodworth (2007) evaluated psychopathic individuals' levels of instrumentality and/or reactivity during the homicide using official criminal records and found that psychopathic individuals' homicides were more often instrumental than reactive. However, in their descriptions of the crime, psychopathic individuals were more likely to minimize or leave out important information to make the crime seem more reactive and less instrumental (Porter & Woodworth, 2007).

In summary, a significant amount of research indicates that psychopathy is not related to conviction of homicide. The extant literature would benefit from further examination of this association, however, as limitations in the present research include the lack of differentiation between types and motives of homicides, small samples sizes, and a lack of distinction between the subtypes of homicidal offenders (e.g., domestic homicide). Lastly, there is a need to evaluate the association between psychopathy and self-reports of homicide. It is possible, as found in youth, that the association between psychopathy and homicide is greater when homicide is self-reported. This may be because psychopathic individuals exaggerate their crimes to researchers; however, but it could also be argued that psychopathic individuals would be less likely to take responsibility for crimes for which they have not been convicted. If the self-reports are accurate, one explanation would be that psychopathic individuals are more likely to commit murder and have gotten away with it. At this stage, much more research is needed.

Research also suggests that psychopathic individuals may kill with premeditation and instrumentality. With time to plan and coordinate the murder, there is likely to be a greater chance of remaining undetected by police than with an unplanned and highly emotional murder. Psychopathic murders are crueler in their crimes, often torturing their victims before killing them. At the same time, psychopathic individuals who get caught for murder may minimize the instrumentality and embellish the reactive nature of their crime to feign socially desirable responses, or "fake good," particularly during high-stakes circumstances, such as forensic evaluations (Edens & Ruiz, 2006).

5.3.2 Assault

Most studies exploring the link between psychopathy and violence do not disentangle types of violence (e.g., homicide, assault, robbery). Thus, there remains a scarcity of research testing the association between psychopathy and assault, specifically. Recently, Reidy et al. (2016) explored the association between the 3- and 4-facet model of psychopathy, simple assault (without a weapon), and aggravated assault (with a weapon) in two community samples of men – one sample with an arrest history and the other without an arrest history. In the sample without a criminal history, the authors found that the frequency of physical fights was positively associated with the Affective and Lifestyle facets, yet, simple (without a weapon) and aggravated (with a weapon) assaults were only associated with the Affective facet. In their ex-criminal sample of men and using the 3-facet model, the authors found the Affective facet was associated with physical fights, simple assault, and aggravated assault, while the Lifestyle facet was associated only with simple assault. These results were largely consistent with the noncriminal sample of men. However, when exploring the 4-facet model (which includes the Antisocial facet), the Affective facet was no longer associated with physical fights or simple and aggravated assault. Instead, the Antisocial facet predicted all three forms of violence, and the Lifestyle facet predicted simple assault. This study indicates that psychopathic traits increase the risk of assault, however, this association may be different based on the individual's criminal history, and if the statistical model considers past criminal behavior and delinquency (e.g., Antisocial facet: criminal versatility, adult and juvenile delinquency). It is interesting that in the noncriminal sample, or when the Antisocial facet is not included in the model, the Affective facet is most predictive of all forms of violence. This is typically not found in male samples, especially in studies assessing prison violence (Chakhssi et al., 2014a; Walters & Heilbrun, 2010). In female prisoners, similar results have been found. Using institutional files to categorize convicted violent crime as either drug-related or not drug-related, Thomson (2017) found that women with higher scores on the Lifestyle facet were more likely to have been convicted of a drug-related violent assault. In contrast, women with higher scores on the Affective facet were more likely to have been convicted for a non-drug related violent assault.

Collectively, these studies show that psychopathic traits provide an important contribution to assessing risk for violent assault in both men and women. This research highlights the need to include the facet structure of psychopathy to fully understand which features of psychopathy drive the greatest risk of assault across context and samples types. Indeed, from the limited research to date, it seems that the affective and antisocial facets are most predictive of assault for men and women, with and without criminal histories. However, research that disentangles types of violent crime is limited, therefore much more research is needed in this area.

5.3.3 Intimate Partner Violence

Intimate partner violence (IPV) is defined as physical, sexual, psychological aggression, or stalking perpetrated by a current or former partner or spouse (CDC, 2020). Research linking psychopathy to IPV has been growing, and this research shows that psychopathic traits are related to a host of strategies to gain dominance and control over current, former, and potential partners. Indeed, psychopathic individuals are more likely to engage in IPV perpetration than non-psychopathic individuals (Grann & Wedin, 2002), and these associations will be explored in further detail within this section.

Psychopathy has become one of the most robust predictors of IPV, even when accounting for sex of the perpetrator or drug and alcohol use (Okano et al., 2016). For example, even accounting for a history of violence, including a history of IPV, psychopathy was associated with a greater frequency of IPV in a sample of male IPV perpetrators (Cunha et al., 2018). At the facet level, IPV frequency was associated with higher Affective facet scores, which is similar to findings for assault and sexual offending. Comparing the effects of psychopathy on IPV in men and women, research suggests Factor 2 is equally predictive of IPV for men and women, whereas Factor 1 was more strongly predictive of IPV for men than for women (Mager et al., 2014). Perpetrators may use physical, sexual, and psychological aggression to dominate their partners for their own gain. These characteristics overlap with the symptoms of the prototypical psychopath (e.g., affective and interpersonal psychopathic features). However, as we have seen thus far, these traits seem to be related to multiple forms of violence that may be used for the psychopathic individual's own gain.

Drawing from one of the longest-running longitudinal studies (i.e., the Cambridge Study in Delinquent Development), men were categorized based on the victims of their violence and then differentiated by their levels of psychopathy (Theobald et al., 2016). The groups included a violent conviction only group, a generally violent group who committed IPV and violence outside of IPV, an IPV only group, and a nonviolent group. The men who committed both IPV and other forms of violence had the highest psychopathy scores, whereas men who committed IPV only had lower scores when compared to both the generally violent men and violent conviction-only men. Again, total psychopathy scores seem to differentiate men who engage in a wide range of violence, rather than a specific form of violence.

There is mixed evidence linking cut off scores of psychopathy to stalking. For example, in a sample of 78 male and female stalking offenders, 15% were classified as psychopathic (Reavis et al., 2008). In contrast, Storey et al. (2009) identified only one psychopathic individual in their sample of 61 stalking offenders. However, using continuous psychopathy scores, the authors did find psychopathy correlated with three stalking domains: nature of stalking (e.g., intimidates victim), perpetrator risk factors (e.g., obsessed), and victim vulnerability (e.g., inconsistent behavior toward perpetrator). The authors acknowledged the low prevalence of psychopathy in their sample but highlighted that individuals with elevated psychopathy scores showed greater frequency, severity, and diversity in their stalking behaviors, and often took advantage of their victims' circumstances. Of the 4-facets, the Affective facet was most reliably associated with stalking behaviors. This has since been replicated in a sample of 109 convicted stalkers (Kropp et al., 2011), and psychopathy scores have been linked to stalking re-offending (Foellmi et al., 2016). Thus, it is evident that psychopathic traits increase the risk of stalking but that not all stalkers are psychopathic.

5.3.4 Sexual Offending

To date, most research assessing the association between psychopathy and sexual offending does not differentiate "serious sexual offenses," such as rape or sexual assault, from "other sexual offenses." As such, the authors use "sexual offending" as a catch-all term for all forms of sexual offending, unless stated otherwise. Research involving community samples has found those with higher levels of psychopathic traits endorse supportive beliefs about rape and place greater blame on the victim for the rape (Willis et al., 2017). Research also demonstrates the associations between particular facets of psychopathy and types of sexual offending. Using the 2-factor model, Factor 1 (Interpersonal-Affective) is associated with blaming the victim, while both Factors 1 and 2 are related to minimization of rape (Mouilso & Calhoun, 2013). Sexual offenders scoring high on all psychopathy facets have been found to have more sexual offenses, whereas scores on the Affective and Antisocial facets were related to sexually violent crimes (Krstic et al., 2018). The Interpersonal facet, specifically, was associated with paraphilic history (Krstic et al., 2018). Thus, it seems that higher psychopathy scores are generally related to more opportunistic sexual offending (i.e., sexual offending that victimizes indiscriminately, spanning a wider range of victims).

Studies of psychopathy have further conceptualized sex offenders based on their victim type. For example, mixed sex offenders who victimized both adults and children scored higher on psychopathy scores than sex offenders who targeted only adults or only children (Brown et al., 2015). In a sample of 229 sex offenders, a larger proportion of psychopathic individuals (PCL-R > 30) were mixed sex offenders (64%) when compared to rapists (36%), incest offenders (6%), child molesters (9%), and non-sex offenders (36%; Porter et al., 2000). This pattern has also been found in a sample of adolescent sex offenders. Parks and Bard (2006) found mixed sex offenders scored highest on total psychopathy scores when compared to child-only or adult-only sex offenders.

Using the 4-facet model, the Affective facet was most predictive being a mixed sex offender (Parks & Bard, 2006). In another adolescent sample, sex offenders scored higher on psychopathy than non-sex offenders and this difference was largely due to higher scores on the Interpersonal and Affective facets of psychopathy (Cale et al., 2015). However, when the sex offenders were compared to chronic violent offenders, there was no significant difference in Affective facet scores. That said, adolescent sex offenders with high levels of callous-unemotional traits (a similar construct to the Affective facet) have been found to have a greater number of sexual offense victims, to have engaged in more planning in the sexual offense, and to have used more violence against their victims (Lawing et al., 2010). Thus, it seems that in youth, higher levels of callous-unemotional traits, or higher levels of Affective facet scores, elicit patterns of chronic and violent sexual offending.

Once caught for sexual offending, psychopathic individuals continue to pose a greater risk for sexual recidivism (Reidy et al., 2013). In a meta-analysis involving 20 studies, psychopathy was found to be a strong predictor of sexual recidivism, but psychopathy was also the best predictor of all forms of violence (sexual and non-sexual violence; Hawes et al., 2013). In the case of sexual offending, the psychopathic individual is opportunistic, non-discriminant, and more sadistic (Mokros et al., 2011), making the psychopathic individual a more dangerous sexual predator.

5.3.5 *Robbery*

Robbery is defined as using physical force, coercion, and/or intimidation to take property from another person (Bureau of Justice Statistics, 2017; Thomson, 2018). In contrast, theft is defined as intentionally and dishonestly taking property from another person. Although robbery costs the US about $74 billion each year (DeLisi et al., 2017; Thomson, 2018), there is a lack of research assessing the link between psychopathy and robbery. Early research by Haapasalo (1994) showed psychopathic individuals are more likely to be convicted for robbery (43.3%) when compared to offenders scoring low on psychopathy (24.1%). Drawing from two Mexican samples, a prisoner and a student sample, Cirilo et al. (2018) found stealing (a combined measure of robbery and theft) was associated with higher levels of psychopathy. Although it seems logical to find an association between psychopathy and robbery, much more research is needed before evidence-based conclusions can be drawn.

5.3.6 *Violent Recidivism*

The aims of prison are deterrence, punishment, and rehabilitation. However, some men and women continue to engage in violence when they leave prison. In both men and women, psychopathy is a predictor for violent recidivism (Dhingra & Boduszek, 2013). In a large sample of male and female released offenders, Factor 1 was found to predict violent reoffending in women but not men, and Factor 2 was found to be predictive of violence for men and women (Coid et al., 2009). In a sample of male ex-offenders, the Comprehensive Assessment of Psychopathic Personality (CAPP) was found to predict violent recidivism over a 6-year period (Pedersen et al., 2010). Thus, among former prisoners, men and women with psychopathic traits are at a higher risk for violent re-offending, and it seems that the Affective facet is a specific risk factor for women. In contrast, psychiatric inpatients' violent recidivism is associated with higher levels of Factor 1 and 2 for both men and women.

5.3.7 *Prison and Inpatient Violence*

Psychopathic individuals continue to be violent during incarceration (Thomson, 2019), and research has shown that the Antisocial facet predicts prison violence in both men and women (Warren et al., 2017). This suggests, similar to past findings, that the Antisocial facet is a gender-neutral risk factor. By contrast, the Affective facet seems to be female-specific in its association with violence. For example, the Affective facet has not been found to be associated with prison violence in men (Chakhssi et al., 2014b; Edens et al., 2008; Walters & Heilbrun, 2010), however female prisoners with higher levels of affective psychopathic traits engaged in more prison violence over a period of 9-months and 12-months (Thomson et al., 2016, 2019c).

Psychopathy also emerges as an important violence risk factor for forensic inpatients, although some research suggests there are sex differences in these associations (de Vries Robbé et al., 2016; Heilbrun et al., 1998; Hildebrand et al., 2004). Research using the 2-factor model has shown that psychopathy is unrelated to institutional violence in women, but total psychopathy scores and Factor 2 scores predict institutional violence for men (de Vogel & de Ruiter, 2005). Using the facet model, female violence was predicted by Lifestyle and Antisocial facets, and for men, all facets predicted violence (de Vogel & Lancel, 2016). In a specialist sample of personality disordered male offenders, Factor 1 and both the Interpersonal and Affective facets were found to predict institutional violence (Langton et al., 2011), further illustrating the variability of findings between men and women.

It is possible that the range in findings may be due to variation in motives or function of violence. For example, it may be that predatory or goal-directed forms of violence, which are more characteristic of psychopathy, are more reliably predicted by the personality features of psychopathy. Indeed, research from the U.S. has found that inpatients who prospectively engaged in predatory violence had higher scores on the Interpersonal and Lifestyle facets (McDermott et al., 2008). Smith et al. (2013) found that both factors on the Psychopathic Personality Inventory-Revised (PPI-R), Fearless Dominance and Impulsive-Antisociality, predicted predatory inpatient aggression, but did not predict impulsive or psychotic aggression. Collectively, this research shows psychopathy is an important construct for better understanding inpatient violence.

5.3.8 Summary

The research detailing the associations between psychopathy and the major types of violent crime covered in this chapter clearly presents limitations in the overall assessment and evaluation of critical risk factors for violence in psychopathic individuals. First, a significant amount of research documents a weak association between homicide and total psychopathy scores – making it difficult to infer a direct link between the two, namely due to discrepancies in the classification of index homicides and knowledge gaps in undiscovered and non-convicted offenses. Second, findings are relatively consistent in demonstrating that Antisocial and Lifestyle facets are strong predictors of physical assault, but interestingly enough, additional research has demonstrated variability in these findings depending on the facet model (i.e., 3-facet model or 4-facet model) and on the sample type (i.e., community or institutional) used for evaluation (Reidy et al., 2016). It is well-established that psychopathy is a strong predictor of intimate partner violence, with associations to greater total scores, Factor 1 and 2 scores, and Affective facet scores – but these associations present differently in men versus women. To further highlight divergent findings within the literature, there is a lack of association between the Affective facet and prison violence for men, which is somewhat contrary to expectation. As seen throughout this chapter, the Affective facet is most frequently associated with a wide range of violent crimes in the community. One possible explanation for this might be that the Affective facet is only predictive of violence for men without an outstanding criminal history, as evidenced by Reidy et al. (2016). Third, there is a paucity of significant findings for the connection between psychopathy and robbery. More general support for this link between total scores and likelihood of robbery exists with limited evidential support on which specific facets link to, and are likely to predict, this crime. Fourth, the extant literature on sexual offending, which is predicated on a classification system that does not disentangle types of sexual offenses by severity, demonstrates associations with higher total psychopathy scores and presents specific links to the Antisocial and Affective facets in regards to sexually violent crimes (Krstic et al., 2018). However, it is difficult to infer whether these findings would be corroborated in studies that parse these offenses.

The Antisocial facet, a critical gender-neutral predictor, has been found to predict prison violence in both men and women, and warrants further exploration in its role in both institutional and prison-related violence given the fundamental link between psychopathy and criminal recidivism. As stated throughout the chapter, these findings further highlight the need for replication and extension of existing research using the 4-facet model to bolster further the evidential support for these associations between and across categories of violent behavior, sample populations, and sexes. Furthermore, given the heavy reliance on factor structures for predicting violent recidivism, future research using facet structures to predict violent recidivism among prisoners and psychiatric inpatients is critical to better understanding risk factors.

5.4 Chapter Summary and Recommendations for Future Investigation

It is clear that psychopathy is an important risk factor for aggression and violence, making it one of the most dangerous and detrimental psychiatric disorders to public health (Thomson, 2019). Homicide convictions are not indicative of intent, nor do they provide sufficient understanding of risk for or predictors of homicide. Although conviction records are widely used, they do not capture all cases of homicide. In 2017, 38% of homicides were unsolved (FBI, 2017). It is likely that many of the nearly 6000 unsolved homicide cases were not heat of the moment killings, but predatory and calculated killings. This method of killing is consistent with the profile of psychopathy. The evidence presented in this chapter demonstrates that psychopathic individuals engage in instrumental violence, however, it is clear that psychopathic individuals are opportunistic and versatile in their crimes, as well. For example, psychopathic individuals are more likely to sexually offend against children and adults, rather than selectively offending against either adults-only or children-only. They are also more likely to be violent against both family members and strangers, and continue to engage in violence while incarcerated or receiving mental health treatment. This evidence highlights the importance of research to begin exploring the mechanisms linking psychopathy to violence.

Violence research aims to improve our understanding of what causes a person to become violent. This knowledge helps prevention scientists develop models for treatment and early interventions. The same reasoning applies to psychopathy-related violence. Although there is mixed evidence for the treatability of psychopathy, treatment efforts would be better focused on violence risk-reduction. To effectively achieve this, three core research priorities to help increase of our understanding of psychopathy-violence link and to reduce the risk of psychopathy-related violence are proposed:

1. Continue to test the predictive utility of psychopathy for different forms and functions of violence, while being more specific about the construct of violence.

This chapter has presented findings from the past 30 years establishing psychopathy as a major risk factor for violence. However, there are key areas that warrant further attention to provide a deeper understanding of psychopathy-related violence. First, researchers need to strategize and promote greater specificity within the existing methods of classifying violence. A great deal of the mixed findings in the present chapter are likely due to the variability of how violence has been characterized or measured. Future researchers are encouraged to conduct exploratory studies on specific forms of violent crime (e.g., assault, robbery). Even within a violent crime domain, such as homicide, there are contextual factors that greatly impact risk assessment. Although this chapter shows that psychopathic individuals are opportunistic in their violence, this opportunistic behavior is often goal-directed. Therefore, studies assessing violent crimes are encouraged to explore the offenders' motive for the crime. Though this may be a time-consuming task with regards to data collection, generating a more comprehensive approach to classifying these crimes will greatly enhance our understanding and treatment approach for psychopathy-related violence. An additional recommendation is for research to include self-report data on the types of violent crime. This is important, as a significant proportion of all violent crimes go unreported and unsolved, and it is likely that a cunning and manipulative psychopathic individual is going to be the most successful at either "getting away" with their violence, or being prosecuted for fewer crimes than they commit.

2. Assess mediators that link psychopathy to violence, and focus intervention efforts to target the psychopathy-violence link.

Many symptoms of psychopathy seem inherently tied to violence. For instance, it seems only logical to expect that a person who is callous, and lacks empathy and remorse, is more likely to engage in violent behaviors. However, emerging research has found contributive factors that strengthen the association between psychopathy facets and violence. Future research should explore a battery of mediators/

moderators linking psychopathy to violence so treatment strategies can be applied to break, or at least reduce, this link. The authors agree with Sewall and Olver (2018, p. 2) in their statement that: "it is not illegal to be an unpleasant person, but it is clearly illegal to commit a violent sexual assault." The personality features of psychopathy are challenging to treat and manage during treatment. Psychopathic patients are manipulative and coercive – therefore, they can be disruptive and antagonistic. However, the aim of treatment should not be a battle with these personality features, as this will increase the risk of treatment drop out (Sewall & Olver, 2019). Instead, the focus for the treatment provider should be to manage and tolerate these personality traits to keep the individual in treatment to provide enough time for the intervention to address more malleable traits (e.g., impulsive-antisocial traits) and risk factors linking psychopathy to violence (Thomson, 2019).

3. Prioritize investigating sex differences in psychopathy.

The study of psychopathy and violence has increased in recent years, yet, there is still a lack of comparative data on women. Existing research suggests notable differences and similarities, between psychopathic men and women. This research highlights the need for future investigations to confirm, and expand on, sex differences across contexts (e.g., prison, community) and measures (e.g., self-report, clinical). It is well-established that there are sex differences in violence, therefore, it should be expected that psychopathic men and women will also differ in the etiology of violent behavior (i.e., the mechanisms that link psychopathy to violence are contingent on sex). Understanding sex-specific models of psychopathy and psychopathy-related violence is integral to the development of fair and effective treatment strategies for both sexes. Thus, researchers and clinicians are encouraged to take a sex-specific approach to help better understand, and eradicate, the link between psychopathy and violence for men and women.

5.5 Conclusion

Regardless of the setting or location (e.g., community, military, university, prison), or circumstances (e.g., receiving treatment or recently released from incarceration), men and women with high levels of psychopathic traits are more likely to perpetrate violence and recidivate. Thus, understanding the association between the distinct facets of psychopathy and types of violent behavior, the mechanisms linking psychopathy to violence, and establishing evidence-based strategies for men and women to break the psychopathy-violence link should be a global public health priority. By targeting a small percentage of the population (1–2%), it is possible that there could be a substantial reduction in the overall global burden of violent, criminal behavior.

References

Anestis, J. C., Green, B. A., Arnau, R. C., & Anestis, M. D. (2017). Psychopathic personality traits in the military: An examination of the Levenson Self-Report Psychopathy Scales in a novel sample. *Assessment, 26*, 670–683.

Archer, J., & Coyne, S. M. (2005). An integrated review of indirect, relational, and social aggression. *Personality and Social Psychology Review, 9*(3), 212–230.

Barratt, E. S. (1991). Measuring and predicting aggression within the context of a personality theory. *The Journal of Neuropsychiatry and Clinical Neurosciences, 3*(2), S35–S39.

Berkowitz, L. (1993). *Aggression: Its causes, consequences, and control*. McGraw-Hill.

Björkqvist, K. (1994). Sex differences in physical, verbal, and indirect aggression: A review of recent research. *Sex Roles, 30*(3–4), 177–188.

Blais, J., Solodukhin, E., & Forth, A. E. (2014). A meta-analysis exploring the relationship between psychopathy and instrumental versus reactive violence. *Criminal Justice and Behavior, 41*(7), 797–821.

Brown, A. R., Dargis, M. A., Mattern, A. C., Tsonis, M. A., & Newman, J. P. (2015). Elevated psychopathy scores among mixed sexual offenders: Replication and extension. *Criminal Justice and Behavior, 42*(10), 1032–1044.

Bureau of Justice Statistics. (2017). *Violent crime*.

Cale, J., Lussier, P., McCuish, E., & Corrado, R. (2015). The prevalence of psychopathic personality disturbances among incarcerated youth: Comparing serious, chronic, violent and sex offenders. *Journal of Criminal Justice, 43*(4), 337–344.

Casey, H., Rogers, R. D., Burns, T., & Yiend, J. (2013). Emotion regulation in psychopathy. *Biological Psychology, 92*(3), 541–548.

CDC. (2020). *Preventing intimate partner violence*. https://doi.org/10.15585/mmwr.ss6711a1external

Chakhssi, F., Bernstein, D., & de Ruiter, C. (2014a). Early maladaptive schemas in relation to facets of psychopathy and institutional violence in offenders with personality disorders. *Legal and Criminological Psychology, 19*(2), 356–372.

Chakhssi, F., Kersten, T., de Ruiter, C., & Bernstein, D. P. (2014b). Treating the untreatable: A single case study of a psychopathic inpatient treated with Schema Therapy. *Psychotherapy, 51*(3), 447–461.

Cima, M., & Raine, A. (2009). Distinct characteristics of psychopathy relate to different subtypes of aggression. *Personality and Individual Differences, 47*(8), 835–840.

Cirilo, H. G., Adrián, V., Leopoldo, D., Norma, G., Brenda, G., & Chriztian, C. (2018). Psychopathy as a predictor variable of the disposition to steal. *Revista Iberoamericana de Psicologia y Salud, 9*(2), 137–148.

Coid, J., & Yang, M. (2011). The impact of psychopathy on violence among the household population of Great Britain. *Social Psychiatry and Psychiatric Epidemiology, 46*(6), 473–480.

Coid, J., Yang, M., Ullrich, S., Zhang, T., Sizmur, S., Roberts, C., Farrington, D. P., & Rogers, R. D. (2009). Gender differences in structured risk assessment: Comparing the accuracy of five instruments. *Journal of Consulting and Clinical Psychology, 77*(2), 337–348.

Colins, O. F., Fanti, K. A., Salekin, R. T., & Andershed, H. (2017). Psychopathic personality in the general population: Differences and similarities across gender. *Journal of Personality Disorders, 31*(1), 49–74.

Cope, L. M., Ermer, E., Gaudet, L. M., Steele, V. R., Eckhardt, A. L., Arbabshirani, M. R., Caldwell, M. F., Calhoun, V. D., & Kiehl, K. A. (2014). Abnormal brain structure in youth who commit homicide. *NeuroImage: Clinical, 4*, 800–807.

Cornell, D. G., Warren, J., Hawk, G., Stafford, E., Oram, G., & Pine, D. (1996). Psychopathy in instrumental and reactive violent offenders. *Journal of Consulting and Clinical Psychology, 64*(4), 783–790.

Culhane, S. E., Walker, S., & Hildebrand, M. M. (2019). Serial homicide perpetrators' self-reported psychopathy and criminal thinking. *Journal of Police and Criminal Psychology, 34*(1), 1–13.

Cunha, O., Braga, T., & Gonçalves, R. A. (2018). Psychopathy and intimate partner violence. *Journal of Interpersonal Violence, 36*, 3–4.

de Vogel, V., & de Ruiter, C. (2005). The HCR-20 in personality disordered female offenders: A comparison with a matched sample of males. *Clinical Psychology & Psychotherapy, 12*(3), 226–240.

de Vogel, V., & Lancel, M. (2016). Gender differences in the assessment and manifestation of psychopathy: Results from a multicenter study in forensic psychiatric patients. *International Journal of Forensic Mental Health, 15*(1), 97–110.

de Vries Robbé, M., de Vogel, V., Wever, E. C., Douglas, K. S., & Nijman, H. L. I. (2016). Risk and protective factors for inpatient aggression. *Criminal Justice and Behavior, 43*(10), 1364–1385.

Declercq, F., Willemsen, J., Audenaert, K., & Verhaeghe, P. (2012). Psychopathy and predatory violence in homicide, violent, and sexual offences: Factor and facet relations. *Legal and Criminological Psychology, 17*(1), 59–74.

DeLisi, M., Reidy, D. E., Heirigs, M. H., Tostlebe, J. J., & Vaughn, M. G. (2017). Psychopathic costs: A monetization study of the fiscal toll of psychopathy features among institutionalized delinquents. *Journal of Criminal Psychology, 8*, 112–124.

Dhingra, K., & Boduszek, D. (2013). Psychopathy and criminal behaviour: A psychosocial research perspective. *Journal of Criminal Psychology, 3*(2), 83–107.

Dodge, K. A. (1991). The structure and function of reactive and proactive aggression. In D. Peppler & K. Rubin (Eds.), *The development and treatment of childhood aggression* (pp. 201–218). Erlbaum.

Dodge, K. A., & Coie, J. D. (1987). Social-information-processing factors in reactive and proactive aggression in children's peer groups. *Journal of Personality and Social Psychology, 53*(6), 1146–1158.

Edens, J. F., & Ruiz, M. A. (2006). On the validity of validity scales: The importance of defensive responding in the prediction of institutional misconduct. *Psychological Assessment, 18*(2), 220–224.

Edens, J. F., Poythress, N. G., Lilienfeld, S. O., Patrick, C. J., & Test, A. (2008). Further evidence of the divergent correlates of the Psychopathic Personality Inventory factors: Prediction of institutional misconduct among male prisoners. *Psychological Assessment, 20*(1), 86–91.

FBI. (2017). *Percent of offenses cleared by arrest or exceptional means.*

Foellmi, M. C., Rosenfeld, B., & Galietta, M. (2016). Assessing risk for recidivism in individuals convicted of stalking offenses. *Criminal Justice and Behavior, 43*(5), 600–616.

Fox, B., & DeLisi, M. (2019). Psychopathic killers: A meta-analytic review of the psychopathy-homicide nexus. *Aggression and Violent Behavior, 44*, 67–79.

Grann, M., & Wedin, I. (2002). Risk factors for recidivism among spousal assault and spousal homicide offenders. *Psychology, Crime & Law, 8*(1), 5–23.

Haapasalo, J. (1994). Types of offense among the Cleckley psychopaths. *International Journal of Offender Therapy and Comparative Criminology, 38*(1), 59–67.

Hare, R. D. (2003). *The Hare Psychopathy Checklist—Revised* (2nd ed.). Multi-Health Systems.

Hare, R. D., & Neumann, C. S. (2008). Psychopathy as a clinical and empirical construct. *Annual Review of Clinical Psychology, 4*(1), 217–246.

Hawes, S. W., Boccaccini, M. T., & Murrie, D. C. (2013). Psychopathy and the combination of psychopathy and sexual deviance as predictors of sexual recidivism: Meta-analytic findings using the Psychopathy Checklist—Revised. *Psychological Assessment, 25*(1), 233–243.

Hecht, L. K., Berg, J. M., Lilienfeld, S. O., & Latzman, R. D. (2015). Parsing the heterogeneity of psychopathy and aggression: Differential associations across dimensions and gender. *Personality Disorders, Theory, Research, and Treatment, 7*, 2–14.

Heilbrun, K., Hart, S. D., Hare, R. D., Gustafson, D., Nunez, C., & White, A. J. (1998). Inpatient and postdischarge aggression in mentally disordered offenders. *Journal of Interpersonal Violence, 13*(4), 514–527.

Hildebrand, M., De Ruiter, C., & Nijman, H. (2004). PCL-R psychopathy predicts disruptive behavior among male offenders in a Dutch forensic psychiatric hospital. *Journal of Interpersonal Violence, 19*(1), 13–29.

Juodis, M., Starzomski, A., Porter, S., & Woodworth, M. (2014). A comparison of domestic and non-domestic homicides: Further evidence for distinct dynamics and heterogeneity of domestic homicide perpetrators. *Journal of Family Violence, 29*(3), 299–313.

Kiehl, K. A., & Hoffman, M. B. (2011). The criminal psychopath: History, neuroscience, treatment, and economics. *Jurimetrics, 51*, 355–397.

Klein Tuente, S., de Vogel, V., & Stam, J. (2014). Exploring the criminal behavior of women with psychopathy: Results from a multicenter study into psychopathy and violent offending in female forensic psychiatric patients. *International Journal of Forensic Mental Health, 13*(4), 311–322.

Kropp, P. R., Hart, S. D., Lyon, D. R., & Storey, J. E. (2011). The development and validation of the guidelines for stalking assessment and management. *Behavioral Sciences & the Law, 29*(2), 302–316.

Krstic, S., Neumann, C. S., Roy, S., Robertson, C. A., Knight, R. A., & Hare, R. D. (2018). Using latent variable- and person-centered approaches to examine the role of psychopathic traits in sex offenders. *Personality Disorders, Theory, Research, and Treatment, 9*(3), 207.

Langton, C. M., Hogue, T. E., Daffern, M., Mannion, A., & Howells, K. (2011). Personality traits as predictors of inpatient aggression in a high-security forensic psychiatric setting: Prospective evaluation of the PCL-R and IPDE dimension ratings. *International Journal of Offender Therapy and Comparative Criminology, 55*(3), 392–415.

Lawing, K., Frick, P. J., & Cruise, K. R. (2010). Differences in offending patterns between adolescent sex offenders high or low in callous-unemotional traits. *Psychological Assessment, 22*(2), 298–305.

Levenson, M. R., Kiehl, K. A., & Fitzpatrick, C. M. (1995). Assessing psychopathic attributes in a noninstitutionalized population. *Journal of Personality and Social Psychology, 68*(1), 151–158.

Lilienfeld, S. O., & Widows, M. R. (2005). *Psychopathic Personality Inventory—Revised (PPI-R) professional manual*. Psychological Assessment Resources.

Mager, K. L., Bresin, K., & Verona, E. (2014). Gender, psychopathy factors, and intimate partner violence. *Personality Disorders, 5*(3), 257–267.

Marsee, M. A., & Frick, P. J. (2007). Exploring the cognitive and emotional correlates to proactive and reactive aggression in a sample of detained girls. *Journal of Abnormal Child Psychology, 35*(6), 969–981.

McDermott, B. E., Quanbeck, C. D., Busse, D., Yastro, K., & Scott, C. L. (2008). The accuracy of risk assessment instruments in the prediction of impulsive versus predatory aggression. *Behavioral Sciences & the Law, 26*(6), 759–777.

Mokros, A., Osterheider, M., Hucker, S. J., & Nitschke, J. (2011). Psychopathy and sexual sadism. *Law and Human Behavior, 35*(3), 188–199.

Mouilso, E. R., & Calhoun, K. S. (2013). The role of rape myth acceptance and psychopathy in sexual assault perpetration. *Journal of Aggression, Maltreatment & Trauma, 22*(2), 159–174.

Okano, M., Langille, J., & Walsh, Z. (2016). Psychopathy, alcohol use, and intimate partner violence: Evidence from two samples. *Law and Human Behavior, 40*(5), 517–523.

Pajevic, M., Batinic, B., & Stevanovic, N. (2017). Subtypes of homicide offenders based on psychopathic traits. *International Journal of Law and Psychiatry, 55*, 45–53.

Parks, G. A., & Bard, D. E. (2006). Risk factors for adolescent sex offender recidivism: Evaluation of predictive factors and comparison of three groups based upon victim type. *Sexual Abuse: A Journal of Research and Treatment, 18*(4), 319–342.

Paulhus, D. L., Neumann, C. S., & Hare, R. D. (2016). *Hare self-report psychopathy scale: Technical manual* (4th ed.). Multi-Health Systems.

Pedersen, L., Kunz, C., Rasmussen, K., & Elsass, P. (2010). Psychopathy as a risk factor for violent recidivism: Investigating the Psychopathy Checklist Screening Version (PCL:SV) and the Comprehensive Assessment of Psychopathic Personality (CAPP) in a forensic psychiatric setting. *International Journal of Forensic Mental Health, 9*(4), 308–315.

Porter, S., & Woodworth, M. (2007). "I'm sorry I did it…but he started it" A comparison of the official and self-reported homicide descriptions of psychopaths and non-psychopaths. *Law and Human Behavior, 31*(1), 91–107.

Porter, S., Fairweather, D., Drugge, J., Herve, H., Birt, A., & Boer, D. P. (2000). Profiles of psychopathy in incarcerated sexual offenders. *Criminal Justice and Behavior, 27*(2), 216–233.

Porter, S., Woodworth, M., Earle, J., Drugge, J., & Boer, D. (2003). Characteristics of sexual homicides committed by psychopathic and nonpsychopathic offenders. *Law and Human Behavior, 27*(5), 459–470.

Reavis, J. A., Allen, E. K., & Meloy, J. R. (2008). Psychopathy in a mixed gender sample of adult stalkers. *Journal of Forensic Sciences, 53*(5), 1214–1217.

Reidy, D. E., Kearns, M. C., & DeGue, S. (2013). Reducing psychopathic violence: A review of the treatment literature. *Aggression and Violent Behavior, 18*(5), 527–538.

Reidy, D. E., Lilienfeld, S. O., Berke, D. S., Gentile, B., & Zeichner, A. (2016). Psychopathy traits and violent assault among men with and without history of arrest. *Journal of Interpersonal Violence, 34*, 2438–2457.

Robertson, C. A., & Knight, R. A. (2014). Relating sexual sadism and psychopathy to one another, non-sexual violence, and sexual crime behaviors. *Aggressive Behavior, 40*(1), 12–23.

Sewall, L. A., & Olver, M. E. (2018). Sexual offender treatment outcomes among psychopathy subtypes. *Journal of Criminological Research, Policy and Practice*. Chicago.

Sewall, L. A., & Olver, M. E. (2019). Psychopathy and treatment outcome: Results from a sexual violence reduction program. *Personality Disorders, Theory, Research, and Treatment, 10*, 59–69.

Sherretts, N., Boduszek, D., Debowska, A., & Willmott, D. (2017). Comparison of murderers with recidivists and first time incarcerated offenders from U.S. prisons on psychopathy and identity as a criminal: An exploratory analysis. *Journal of Criminal Justice, 51*, 89–92.

Smith, S. T., Edens, J. F., & McDermott, B. E. (2013). Fearless dominance and self-centered impulsivity interact to predict predatory aggression among forensic psychiatric inpatients. *International Journal of Forensic Mental Health, 12*(1), 33–41.

Storey, J. E., Hart, S. D., Meloy, J. R., & Reavis, J. A. (2009). Psychopathy and stalking. *Law and Human Behavior, 33*(3), 237–246.

Theobald, D., Farrington, D. P., Coid, J. W., & Piquero, A. R. (2016). Are male perpetrators of intimate partner violence different from convicted violent offenders? Examination of psychopathic traits and life success in males from a community survey. *Journal of Interpersonal Violence, 31*(9), 1687–1718.

Thomson, N. D. (2017). An exploratory study of female psychopathy and drug-related violent crime. *Journal of Interpersonal Violence, 35*, 794–808.

Thomson, N. D. (2018). Psychopathy and violent crime. In M. DeLisi (Ed.), *Routledge international handbook of psychopathy and crime* (pp. 508–525). Routledge.

Thomson, N. D. (2019). *Understanding psychopathy: The biopsychosocial perspective*. Routledge.

Thomson, N. D., Towl, G. J., & Centifanti, L. C. M. (2016). The habitual female offender inside: How psychopathic traits predict chronic prison violence. *Law and Human Behavior, 40*(3), 257–269.

Thomson, N. D., Kiehl, K. A., & Bjork, J. M. (2018). Predicting violence and aggression in young women: The importance of psychopathy and neurobiological function. *Physiology & Behavior, 201*, 130–138.

Thomson, N. D., Bozgunov, K., Aboutanos, M., Vasilev, G., & Vassileva, J. (2019a). Physical abuse moderates the psychopathy-violence link differently for men and women. *Journal of Interpersonal Violence*. https://doi.org/10.1177/0886260519865956

Thomson, N. D., Bozgunov, K., Psederska, E., & Vassileva, J. (2019b). Sex differences on the four-facet model of psychopathy predict physical, verbal, and indirect aggression. *Aggressive Behavior, 45*(3), 265–274.

Thomson, N. D., Vassileva, J., Kiehl, K. A., Reidy, D. E., Aboutanos, M. B., McDougle, R., & DeLisi, M. (2019c). Which features of psychopathy and impulsivity matter most for prison violence? New evidence among female prisoners. *International Journal of Law and Psychiatry, 64*, 26–33.

United States of America v. Brian David Mitchell, Memorandum Decision and Order, Case No. 2:08CR125DAK, 03/01/2010, pp. 1–149.

Walters, G. D., & Heilbrun, K. (2010). Violence risk assessment and Facet 4 of the Psychopathy Checklist: Predicting institutional and community aggression in two forensic samples. *Assessment, 17*(2), 259–268.

Warren, J., South, S. C., Burnette, M. L., Rogers, A., Friend, R., Bale, R., & Van Patten, I. (2005). Understanding the risk factors for violence and criminality in women: The concurrent validity of the PCL-R and HCR-20. *International Journal of Law and Psychiatry, 28*(3), 269–289.

Warren, J., Wellbeloved-Stone, J. M., Dietz, P. E., & Millspaugh, S. B. (2017). Gender and violence risk assessment in prisons. *Psychological Services, 15*, 543–552.

Willis, M., Birthrong, A., King, J. S., Nelson-Gray, R. O., & Latzman, R. D. (2017). Are infidelity tolerance and rape myth acceptance related constructs? An association moderated by psychopathy and narcissism. *Personality and Individual Differences, 117*, 230–235.

Woodworth, M., & Porter, S. (2002). In cold blood: Characteristics of criminal homicides as a function of psychopathy. *Journal of Abnormal Psychology, 111*(3), 436–445.

Chapter 6
Psychopathy and Neurodevelopmental Disorders

Greg Bohall, Jennifer E. Vitale, and Darren Lemon

Abstract Neurodevelopmental disorders, specifically intellectual disability (ID) and autism spectrum disorder (ASD), and psychopathy are completely separate and distinct diagnoses/conditions. Despite their drastic differences at the surface level, symptoms and behaviors associated with neurodevelopmental disorders and/or psychopathy are embedded in the very fabric of the individuals' life and significantly impacts their daily functioning. Lower intelligence and adaptive functioning deficits are symptoms of ID and intelligence quotient is seen as unchangeable due to the organic nature of ID. Social interaction deficits and engaging in repetitive behaviors are symptoms of ASD and significantly impair the individuals' ability to engage with others and their community. Lastly, psychopathic traits are deeply ingrained in the individuals' personality. This chapter explores the relationship between ID and psychopathy and ASD and psychopathy. More specifically, this chapter will provide an overview of each diagnosis/condition, assessment information for each diagnosis/condition, information on various comorbid relationships, and outline prominent interventions.

Keywords Psychopathy · Neurodevelopmental disorders · Intellectual disability · Mental retardation · Autism Spectrum disorder · Applied behavior analysis · Cognitive-behavioral therapy · Person-centered active support

G. Bohall (✉)
Innovative Psychological Solutions, A Professional Corporation, Los Angeles, CA, USA

J. E. Vitale
Hampden-Sydney College, Hampden-Sydney, VA, USA

D. Lemon
Applied Behavioral Alternatives, Inc., Arcadia, CA, USA

J. E. Vitale (ed.), *The Complexity of Psychopathy*, Dangerous Behavior in Clinical and Forensic Psychology, https://doi.org/10.1007/978-3-030-83156-1_6

6.1 Introduction

Neurodevelopmental disorders, specifically intellectual disability (ID) and autism spectrum disorder (ASD), and psychopathy are separate and distinct diagnoses/conditions. Despite their drastic differences at the surface level, symptoms and behaviors associated with neurodevelopmental disorders and/or psychopathy are embedded in the very fabric of the individuals' life and significantly impacts their daily functioning. Lower intelligence and adaptive functioning deficits are symptoms of ID and intelligence quotient is seen as unchangeable due to the organic nature of ID. Social interaction deficits and engaging in repetitive behaviors are symptoms of ASD and significantly impair the individuals' ability to engage with others and their community. Lastly, psychopathic traits are deeply ingrained in the individuals' personality. This chapter explores the relationship between ID and psychopathy and ASD and psychopathy. More specifically, this chapter will provide an overview of each diagnosis/condition, assessment information for each diagnosis/condition, information on various comorbid relationships, and outline prominent interventions.

6.2 Overview of Psychopathy

Although not currently recognized in DSM-5 (American Psychiatric Association [APA], 2013) and often mistakenly equated with Antisocial Personality Disorder, psychopathy represents a distinct condition, characterized not only by impulsive, antisocial behavior, but also by characteristic deficits in interpersonal and emotional functioning (Cleckley 1941/1988; Crego & Widiger, 2015; Hare, 1996). The first thorough clinical description of psychopathy was presented by Cleckley (1941/1988) in *The Mask of Sanity*. His sixteen criteria, including superficial charm and good intelligence, unreliability, pathologic egocentricity and incapacity for love, untruthfulness and insincerity, and failure to follow any life plan, have provided a conceptualization of the psychopathy syndrome that has served as the basis for the subsequent development of both explanatory models and theories as well as assessment tools.

In 1991, Hare published the Psychopathy Checklist-Revised (PCL-R), a 20-item rating scale that assesses the interpersonal, affective, and behavioral aspects of psychopathy. Each item is scored on the basis of a clinical interview, as well as a corroborating file review, on a scale from 0 (not present) to 2 (definitely present). Thus, scores range from 0 to 40, and a clinical cut score of 30 has been recommended (Hare, 1991). Using this cut score, rates of psychopathy among North American male offenders range from 15% to 49% (Herve et al., 2004; Salekin et al., 1998), whereas rates among female offenders have been somewhat lower (e.g., Salekin et al., 1997; Vitale et al., 2002). Since the introduction of the PCL-R, other measures have emerged, including self-report and rating scales developed for alternative settings/populations (e.g., the Psychopathy Checklist: Youth Version (Forth et al., 2003), the Antisocial Process Screening Device [APSD; Frick & Hare, 2001], and the Psychopathic Personality Inventory [PPI; Lilienfeld & Andrews, 1996]). Although these measures have demonstrated utility in clinical and research contexts (e.g., Salekin et al., 2018; Sellbom et al., 2019), the PCL-R remains the predominant measure of psychopathy in most settings.

PCL-R based psychopathy has been associated with abnormalities in emotion functioning (e.g., Dargis et al., 2018; Ermer et al., 2012; Hansen et al., 2008; Herba et al., 2007), attentional functioning (e.g., Hiatt et al., 2004; Newman et al., 1997; Zeier et al., 2009), and psychophysiological and neural responding (e.g., Blair et al., 2018; Decety et al., 2013; Patrick et al., 1993; Vermeij et al., 2018). It is reliably associated with deficits in empathy (e.g., Domes et al., 2013; Vitale et al., 2002) and with impulsivity (e.g., de Tribolet-Hardy et al., 2014; Gray et al., 2019; Pauli et al., 2019). Further, PCL-R assessed psychopathy is related to criminal offending and recidivism (e.g., Hare & Hart, 1993; Hemphill et al., 1998), and treatment resistance in the form of noncompliance and higher attrition rates (e.g., Berger et al., 2012; Richards et al., 2003).

Originally described as a measure with a two-factor structure, Hare and colleagues (e.g, Hare et al., 2018; Hare & Neumann, 2008), currently promote a two-factor model that encompasses four underlying facets (Facet 1: Interpersonal; Facet 2: Affective; Facet 3: Lifestyle; Facet 4: Antisocial). The factor/facet structure of the instrument has important implications for the use of the measure. For example, it has become apparent that the different components of the measure do not always relate in similar ways to external criterion (e.g., Gardner et al., 2018; Gray et al., 2019; Jeandarme et al., 2017). Such patterns may also be relevant when the relations between PCL-R assessed psychopathy and the symptoms/characteristics of other mental disorders are examined.

6.3 Overview of Neurodevelopmental Disorders

The neurodevelopmental disorders are a group of conditions where the onset is in the developmental period and are characterized by developmental deficits that impair social, personal, academic, and/or occupational functioning (APA, 2013). Developmental deficits vary from specific limitations such as learning or executive function control to global impairments such as intelligence or social skills; these disorders frequently co-occur (APA, 2013). Neurodevelopmental disorders include intellectual disability (ID), communication disorders, autism spectrum disorders (ASD), attention deficit/hyperactivity disorder, motor disorders, and specific learning disorders. In a study by Boyle et al. (2011) through the United States Department of Health and Human Services Centers for Disease Control and Prevention, an analysis of trends of neurodevelopmental disorders found that 1 in 6 children in the United States had a neurodevelopmental disability (between 2006 and 2008), parent reported neurodevelopmental disability diagnoses had increased 17.1% (between 1997 and 2008), and the prevalence of any neurodevelopmental disability was 13.9% (between 1997 and 2008). Additionally, the authors found that males had twice the prevalence of any neurodevelopmental disability compared to females, Hispanic children had lower prevalence of several disorders when compared to Caucasian and African American children, and children from families with income below the federal poverty line had a higher prevalence of neurodevelopmental disabilities.

6.4 Intellectual Disability

ID is a neurodevelopmental disorder with (1) an onset occurring in the developmental period, (2) deficits in intellectual functioning, and (3) conceptual (executive functioning, academic skills), social (social interaction), and practical (functional living skills) adaptive functioning deficits (APA, 2013). In the previous DSM-IV-TR, this diagnosis was termed mental retardation and severity was determined by IQ score. In the present DSM-5, the various levels of severity are based on adaptive functioning as this determines the levels of supports required in rehabilitation efforts. Deficits in problem solving, planning, abstract thinking, learning from experience, academic learning, and general mental abilities are characteristics of this disorder and result in impairments in adaptive functioning (APA, 2013).

There are numerous maladaptive behaviors that are associated with ID. These behaviors include self-injurious behaviors, stereotypic movements, anger and aggression, food intake problems, and issues sleeping. Of individuals diagnosed with ID, approximately 10–12% exhibit self-injurious behaviors (Van Ingen et al., 2010). Examples of self-injurious behaviors include but are not limited to biting, skin picking, punching/slapping, trichotillomania, cutting, and eye poking. The most common stereotypic movements exhibited by individuals with ID include making noises or some other vocalization, abnormal posturing, hand waving, hand flapping, hand mouthing, and rocking back and forth. Stereotypic movements are oftentimes conceptualized similarly to self-injurious behaviors; however, stereotypic movements do not normally cause tissue damage and are automatically reinforcing whereas self-injurious behaviors cause bodily damage and only a small percentage is automatically reinforced (Vollmer et al., 2014). For many individuals with ID, life experiences from childhood onward are conducive to the stimulation of anger (Taylor & Novaco, 2013). When considering that individuals with ID experience deficiencies in adaptive functioning, environmental and social circumstances can trigger anger and cognitive deficits can impair effective coping. Anger control has long been theoretically and empirically linked to aggressive behavior (Berkowitz et al., 1969; Megargee, 1966); aggressive behavior is frequently cited as the most prevalent problem behavior for individuals with ID (Benson & Brooks, 2008). Emerson et al. (2001) found that 42% of people with ID exhibit some form of interpersonal aggression. Approximately 30% of adults with ID struggle with food intake (Gravestock, 2000). Some of these food intake issues include the refusal of food and drink, pica, rumination, and rapid eating. Problems sleeping include insomnia, hypersomnia, and parasomnias. When compared to individuals without a disability, children and adults with ID and/or other neurodevelopmental disabilities are more likely to experience one or more of these sleeping problems (Didden et al., 2014).

Among adults, prevalence of ID in the general population is approximately 1% (Maulik et al., 2013). Of this prevalence, approximately 85% of cases have mild disabilities, 10% of cases have moderate disabilities, 4% of cases have severe disabilities, and 2% have profound disabilities (King et al., 2009). Individuals diagnosed with ID have higher levels of unmet needs and receive less effective treatment (Taylor & Knapp, 2013). This is clinically concerning as this population experiences an inequality of access to services and limited access to effective treatment options. These reasons include a lack of knowledge and awareness of cognitive and emotional problems experienced by people with ID, reluctance on behalf of the therapists to provide services to this population, and lack of quality evidence to guide practice with this population (Taylor & Knapp, 2013). When considering that a majority of individuals with ID are in the mild range, it can be reasonably concluded that if they receive appropriate care, they can achieve improved treatment outcomes. However, when considering that this population has higher levels of unmet needs, they receive less effective treatment, they have a lack of awareness of their condition, and therapists are often reluctant to provide services, individuals with ID have a significant disadvantage in terms of access to and quality of effective interventions.

6.4.1 *Clinical Assessment of Intellectual Disability*

The diagnostic criteria for ID includes deficits in intellectual functioning, deficits in adaptive functioning, and the onset of these deficits occur in the developmental period; levels of severity is based on adaptive functioning as it determines the level of support(s) needed (APA 2013). In order to diagnose ID, the assessor must utilize standardized assessments to determine intellectual functioning (intelligence quotient) and level of adaptive functioning. Additionally, determining the age of onset requires a rigorous review of available records and collateral contacting in order to verify information. Lastly, although not yet strongly supported in the academic literature, assessment tools for psychopathology and/or challenging behaviors for individuals with ID have been developed.

6.4.1.1 Assessment of Intellectual Functioning

The evaluation of the intellectual functioning prong includes clinical assessment and the use of individualized, global, standardized intelligence testing. The intelligence tests that are generally accepted in practice are the *Wechsler Adult Intelligence Scale-4th Edition* (*WAIS-IV:* 2008) and the *Stanford-Binet Intelligence Scales-5th Edition* (*SB-5:* 2003). As with any form of standardized testing, there are numerous factors that impact the interpretation of results in intellectual assessment. The standard error of measurement, practice effects, the Flynn Effect, mental health symptoms, and cultural and linguistic factors are factors that impact the interpretation of the intelligence quotient (IQ; Macvaugh & Cunningham, 2009). Oftentimes, IQ is conceptualized as a specific number when it should be viewed as existing within a range of error for the given test. The standard error of measurement is a standard deviation score that provides this range to indicate how extensive that error in assessment is likely to be.

As previously mentioned, the severity of the diagnosis shifted from being based on IQ scores to levels of adaptive functioning; this change was needed as the specific "cutoff score" is no longer as relevant and IQ can be considered based on a range. A practice effect can occur when an individual is completing the same intelligence test in a relatively short period of time. When this occurs, IQ ranges can be artificially increased due to exposure to the same test as opposed to actual improvements in intellectual ability. In order to avoid practice effect issues, avoid administration of the same intellectual assessment within a 12-month duration. The Flynn Effect is the well-supported finding that IQ scores elevate by approximately .31 points per year from the date of the standardization of the intelligence test to the date of administration. The Flynn Effect further supports that IQ is not an absolute number. Although the specific reason(s) for this artificial elevation has not been pinpointed, factors such as improved medical practices (e.g., prenatal care, improved prevention), increased access to education and the emphasis on higher education, improved technology (e.g., technological applications to improve deficiencies), and emphasis on maturity (earlier acquisition of intelligence) may explain this inflation. For example, if an individual is being tested in 2021 with the *Wechsler Adult Intelligence Scale- 4th Edition* (2008), multiply .31 by the number of years (13) from the date of standardization to determine the Flynn Effect. To account for the Flynn Effect, you would deduct 4 (4.03) from the Full Scale IQ. Despite the level of severity shifting from the intellectual prong to the adaptive prong, in clinical and forensic cases, authors recommend that assessors provide both the observed Full Scale IQ and the Flynn-corrected score to the referral source. Lastly, below are some of the more common assessment measures used to assess the intellectual prong of intellectual disability:

Wechsler Adult Intelligence Scale-4th Edition (WAIS-IV: 2008): The Wechsler family of intelligence scales have had a significant impact on intellectual assessment. In adult intellectual assessment, the WAIS-IV is seen as the "gold standard." Despite its regular use, it has been criticized as the scales do not have a strong theoretical underpinning. However, Wechsler was influenced by Charles Spearman and Edward Thorndike; two prominent theorists at the time. The WAIS-IV has 15 subtests that comprise of the following indices: Verbal Comprehension Index (VCI), Perceptual Reasoning Index (PRI), Working Memory Index (WMI), Processing Speed Index (PSI), and Full Scale IQ (FSIQ). Of the 15 subtests included in the WAIS-IV, the first 10 are the standard battery and the remaining 5 are supplemental. Lastly, the WAIS-IV is being updated and is currently in the data collection and validation phase; the updated version will be called the WAIS-V.

Stanford-Binet Intelligence Scales-5th Edition (SB5: 2003): The SB5 is somewhat of an offshoot of the Cattell-Horn-Carroll Theory of Cognitive Abilities. CHC theory normally lists 8–10 factors whereas the SB5 has the following 5 factors:

fluid reasoning, knowledge, quantitative reasoning, visual-spatial processing, and working memory. These five cognitive factors were based on research on school achievement and ratings from experts of the importance of these factors in the assessment of reasoning. The SB5 has 10 subtests that include Verbal IQ (VIQ), Nonverbal IQ (NVIQ), and Full Scale IQ (FSIQ) as indices.

Kaufman Adolescent and Adult Intelligence Test (KAAIT: 1993): The KAAIT utilizes the original, dichotomous Horn-Cattell model of fluid intelligence and crystallized intelligence. This inventory has 10 subtests in the Expanded Battery and the indices include the crystallized scale and the fluid scale. Although this inventory is still being used, caution should be exercised as it is quite dated (1993) for current use.

Woodcock-Johnson IV Tests of Cognitive Abilities *(WJ-IV COG: 2014):* The WJ-IV COG is based on the evolution of the Cattell-Horn-Carroll Theory of Cognitive Abilities and contains 18 tests. Of these 18, the first 10 are the standard battery and the remaining 8 are the extended battery. These tests are designed to measure verbal attention, letter-pattern matching, phonological processing, visualization, and non-word repetition.

Reynolds Intellectual Assessment Scales-2nd Edition (RIAS-2: 2015): The RIAS-2 is theoretically guided by the Cattell-Horn-Carroll theory of Cognitive Abilities and also divided intelligence into verbal and nonverbal domains. This inventory has 8 subtests that make up the following indices: Verbal Intelligence Index (VIX), Nonverbal Intelligence Index (NIX), Composite Intelligence Index (CIX), Composite Memory Index (CMX), and the Speed Processing Index (SPI).

6.4.1.2 Assessment of Adaptive Functioning

Adaptive deficits impact the individual's functioning in one or more areas of daily life such as social interaction, independent living, and communication across different environments such as home, school, or work (APA, 2013). Although the term adaptive functioning appears to be somewhat straightforward, psychologists and legal professionals struggle with this given the wide range of possibilities for the term. For example, adaptive behavior can range from functional living skills such as toileting and clothing oneself, to more complex skills such as appropriate interpersonal interactions and financial management. Furthermore, questions regarding the conceptualization of adaptive functioning increases the complicated nature of this prong as some measure adaptive functioning as knowledge of the skill and others measure actual performance. Although a consensus in the field exists where the individual's actual performance is to be measured as opposed to knowledge of the skill, these two conceptualizations do exist and may further complicate understanding of adaptive functioning (Everington & Olley, 2008). The DSM-5 does elucidate adaptive functioning into practical, conceptual, and social domains, however, the determination of this prong is still quite broad and subjective. Adaptive functioning is most reliably evaluated when the individual's normal daily behavioral patterns across a variety of environments and contexts are assessed.

Similar to the intellectual functioning prong, the use of standardized instruments are recommended for assessing the adaptive functioning prong. A majority of instruments used to measure adaptive functioning assess the individual's present functioning in the community. A methodological problem exists when the individual to be assessed is incarcerated for numerous years as adaptive functioning in the community is far more demanding than in a highly-structured correctional environment. Furthermore, actual performance of the adaptive functioning is near impossible to assess when the individual to be assessed is institutionalized. In these instances, the assessor undertakes an assessment based on historical data (previous service providers, arrest records, clinical documentation) and clinical judgment. Although validity of retrospective assessment is a concern, adaptation in a correctional institution should generally not be viewed as congruent to adaptive functioning in the community (Macvaugh & Cunningham, 2009).

The clinical interview to determine adaptive functioning of individuals with ID is a complicated procedure as well. When completing the clinical interview to assess adaptive functioning, recommended actions include building an alliance, creating a relaxed environment, outlining the process, reviewing expectations, progressing from less demanding to more demanding questions, beginning with open questions followed by "either-or" questions and then utilizing closed questions to clarify details, using simple language, anchoring questions to memorable events, and summarizing periodically (Carr & O'Reilly, 2016). Record review is also an important component of determining adaptive functioning. Information such as employment and educational history, family history, medical history, social and environmental history, substance use history, mental health history, psychiatric history, criminal background, and previous incarcerations can provide insight into historical adaptive functioning. Another valuable source of information can be obtained from collateral interviews. This communication may include interviewing former employers, members in the community, teachers, and others who could be familiar with the individual across different settings. In the aforementioned retrospective assessments, these interviews with collateral contacts may be the only source of information to assess adaptive behavior. However, as with any interview situation, validity of the information and potential bias is a concern that must be considered. Authors recommend that these interviews be done individually so the focus can be on the individual contact and information can be compared across contacts. Lastly, below are some of the more common assessment measures used to assess adaptive functioning:

Vineland Adaptive Behavior Scales-3rd Edition (Vineland-3: 2016): The Vineland-3 is appropriate for use in individuals from birth to 90 years of age and assesses adaptive functioning in individuals with intellectual disability, autism spectrum disorder, and attention-deficit/hyperactivity disorder. This inventory has the following domains: communication, daily living skills, socialization, motor skills, and maladaptive behavior. The combination of these domains comprises 13 subdomains. The Vineland series has a history of being the leading measure assessing personal and social skills needed for everyday living.

Adaptive Behavior Assessment System-3rd Edition (ABAS-3: 2015): The ABAS-3 is useful in the assessment of individuals with developmental delays, intellectual disability, autism spectrum disorder, neuropsychological disorders, learning disabilities, and sensory or physical impairments. This inventory is appropriate for assessing adaptive functioning for individuals from birth up until 89 years of age. Adaptive functioning is assessed through eleven skill areas in practical, conceptual, and social domains.

Scales of Independent Behavior-Revised (SIB-R: 1996): The SIB-R is appropriate for use in individuals from birth up to 80 years of age. It contains 14 subscales that group into motor, social interaction and communication, personal living, and community living domains to assess adaptive behavior. Furthermore, the SIB-R has 8 maladaptive behavior subscales grouped in the following 3 domains: internalized behavior problems, externalized behavior problems, and asocial maladaptive behavior.

Assessment of Functional Living Skills (AFLS: 2012): The AFLS is a comprehensive inventory that assesses 735 functional skills in the following life areas: basic living skills, community participation, home skills, school skills, independent living skills, and vocational skills.

Adaptive Behavior Scale-Residential and Community Version-2nd Edition (1993): This inventory was standardized on a sample aged 3–69 years and provides data on personal self-sufficiency, community self-sufficiency, personal-social responsibility, social adjustment, and personal adjustment.

Diagnostic Adaptive Behavior Scale (DABS: 2013): The DABS is appropriate for individuals aged 4 to 21. This inventory assesses adaptive functioning in the following domains: conceptual, social, and practical skills. The DABS provides diagnostic information around the cutoff point where an individual is deemed to have "significant limitations" in adaptive functioning.

6.4.1.3 Assessment of the Onset of Intellectual Disability

The third prong of the ID diagnosis is that the onset of the intellectual and adaptive deficits is during the developmental period. The benefit of this component of the diagnosis is that it rules out other conditions such as traumatic brain injury which may cause confusion when diagnosing. Clinically, "developmental period" refers to the onset taking place in childhood or adolescence. In forensic instances, the age of onset may be established by the State or jurisdiction. For example, some States define developmental period as occurring prior to age 18 whereas others have extended the age to 22 (Ellis, 2003).

To determine the age of onset of this diagnosis, school records are perhaps the most valuable source of knowledge (school behaviors, individualized education plan, diagnostic assessments, involvement in Individuals with Disabilities Education Act special education, school counseling, etc.). Parents/legal guardian may also seek clinical intervention services outside the school setting in conjunction with or separately from any school-based interventions. Therefore, the importance of accuracy in documentation (current practice and for future record requests) and retention of records after termination (for future record requests) is paramount for establishing the diagnosis of ID for a child or adolescent or if an adult is seeking services (State Developmental Services, eligibility for State disability benefits, Americans with Disability Act reasonable accommodations, etc.), has current legal involvement (capacity to waive Miranda rights, fitness to proceed with trial, parental capacity and child evaluations, decisional capacity evaluations, assessment for grave disability/conservatorship, etc.), or requires documentation surrounding a childhood clinical concern or assessment of future risk (future diagnosis of intellectual disability, future risk of violence, future risk of sexual offending, child abuse, depression/suicide, etc.). According to the American Psychological Association (2007) *Record Keeping Guidelines (Guideline 7)*, "In the absence of a superseding requirement, psychologists may consider retaining full records until 7 years after the last date of service delivery for adults or until 3 years after a minor reaches the age of majority, whichever is later" (p. 199). According to this guideline, psychologists are to carefully assess the importance of this clinical information as it relates to making decisions about retaining or disposing of records. The Behavior Analyst Certification Board (BACB) concurs with this guideline. In the BACB (2014) *Professional and Ethical Compliance Code for Behavior Analysts (Standard 2.11: Records and Data),* behavior analysts are required to retain data and records for 7 years post-termination. Although the APA and BACB are in agreement, the BACB is more stringent as record keeping is an enforceable ethical standard whereas APA has put forth this as a guideline (unenforceable). Additionally, according to the American Counseling Association (2014) *ACA Code of Ethics (Standard B.6.h),* counselors are to "apply careful discretion and deliberation before destroying records that may be needed by a court of law, such as notes on child abuse, suicide, sexual harassment, or violence" (p. 8). The ACA Code of Ethics does not identify a timeframe for retaining such records, however, they are explicitly in agreement with the APA in that the determination is based on the clinicians' assessment of the importance of such clinical information. Authors recommend adherence to the 2007 APA Record Keeping Guidelines as it provides a timeframe for retaining records as well as an assessment and determination by the clinician on whether to retain or destroy a record after this timeframe for future purposes (diagnosis, seeking services, legal involvement, and childhood clinical concerns).

6.4.1.4 Clinical Assessment of Comorbid Psychopathology in Individuals with Intellectual Disability

As previously reviewed, individuals diagnosed with ID are more likely to have a psychiatric diagnosis than those without ID (see Cooper & van der Speck, 2009). Also, individuals with ID tend to have maladaptive behaviors such as anger and aggression, food intake issues, problems sleeping, stereotypic movements, and self-injurious behaviors. However, diagnosing these comorbid mental health conditions and maladaptive behaviors is complicated as the diagnostic criteria is based on individuals without ID and issues such as atypical presentations of psychiatric disorders, error by the interviewer, language to report symptoms, and recognizing changes in functioning (Jopp & Keys, 2001) impact the accuracy of diagnosing. Furthermore, mental health assessment tools for adults with ID is in its developmental stages as inventories have been created, however, minimal supportive evidence on its use has been discovered (Mohr & Costello, 2007). Although strong support has not yet been established, and may not be necessarily recommended at this time, we have included information on mental health assessments that are specific for individuals diagnosed with ID:

Developmental Behavior Checklist 2 (DBC2: 2018): The DBC2 is an inventory completed by the informant. This inventory focuses on emotional and behavioral problems that is most likely to be experienced by individuals with intellectual disability or individuals with other neurodevelopmental disabilities.

Psychopathology Checklist for Adults with Intellectual Disability (P-AID: 2008): The P-AID is completed by the informant and areas assessed includes mania, psychosis, depression, dementia, anxiety disorders, and obsessive-compulsive disorder. Furthermore, maladaptive behaviors that are assessed include verbal and physical aggression, self-injurious behavior, sexually inappropriate behavior, demanding behavior, wandering behavior, oppositional behavior, and destructive behavior.

Assessment of Dual Diagnosis (ADD: 1997): The ADD is an inventory that is completed by the informant. The ADD screens for mental health conditions in the following categories: mania, depression, anxiety, PTSD, eating disorders, personality disorders, sexual disorders, schizophrenia, pervasive developmental disorder, conduct disorders, somatoform disorders, substance abuse disorders, and dementia.

Complicated Grief Questionnaire for People with Intellectual Disabilities (CGQ-ID: 2009): The CGQ-ID is completed by the informant and assesses complicated grief reactions (separation distress and traumatic grief) of the individual with an intellectual disability.

Glasgow Depression *Scale (2003):* The Glasgow Depression Scale is completed by the informant or is completed by the individual. This scale is designed to measure depression in individuals with a learning disability.

Glasgow Anxiety Scale for People with an Intellectual Disability (GAS-ID: 2003): The GAS-ID is a self-report scale designed to measure anxiety in individuals with intellectual disability.

*Aberrant Behavior Checklist-2nd Edition (ABC-2: 2017):*The ABC-2 is completed by the informant and assesses problem behaviors of individuals diagnosed with intellectual disability, cerebral palsy, epilepsy, and autism spectrum disorder. This inventory includes 58 items that fall into the following five subscales: hyperactivity/noncompliance, inappropriate speech, stereotypic behavior, irritability, and social withdrawal.

Mood, Interest & Pleasure Questionnaire (MIPQ: 2003): The MIPQ is completed by the informant and was designed for use with individuals with severe or profound intellectual disabilities. As the title would suggest, this questionnaire has a mood subscale as well as an interest and pleasure subscale.

Mini PAS-ADD (1997): The Mini PAS-ADD is an assessment tool designed to evaluate mental health conditions in individuals with intellectual disability. This inventory assesses psychosis, dementia, autism, anxiety/phobias, depression, expansive mood, and obsessions and compulsions.

Challenging Behaviour Interview (CBI: 2003): The CBI is completed by the informant and consists of two parts. In the first, the informant determines whether the individual has shown self-injury, physical aggression, verbal aggression, disruption in the environment, or inappropriate vocalizations. The second part requires informant to answer questions to identify the severity of the identified challenging behavior(s).

Diagnostic Assessment for the Severely Handicapped- II (DASH-II: 1995): The DASH-II is completed by the informant and measures comorbid psychopathology in individuals with severe and profound intellectual disabilities. The 13 subscales of this inventory include: Mania, anxiety, depression, autism spectrum disorder, schizophrenia, self-injury, stereotypic behaviors, sleep disorders, elimination disorders, eating disorders, psychosexual disorders, organic conditions, and impulsive control.

Mood and Anxiety Semi-Structured Interview (MASS: 2007): The MASS is completed by the informant and the areas assessed include anxiety disorders, major depressive disorder, and mania.

Reiss Screen for Maladaptive Behavior (The Reiss Screen: 1988): The Reiss Screen is completed by the informant and is normed on adolescents and adults with all levels of severity of intellectual disability. The inventory assesses the probability that individual has autism, aggression, dependent personality, avoidant behavior, depression, psychosis, paranoia, overactivity, drug abuse, sexual problems, self-injury, stealing, and suicidal tendencies.

Anger *Inventory (AI: 2009):* The AI is either completed as a self-report inventory or by the informant. Questions on this inventory assess anger. More specifically, the individual's reactivity across potentially provoking situations is tested.

6.4.2 Diagnostic Comorbidity

Individuals diagnosed with ID are three to four times more likely to experience psychiatric disorders than those not diagnosed (Cooper & van der Speck, 2009). Risk factors for mental illness for those diagnosed with ID include adult abuse, parental divorce in childhood, historical adverse life events, and type of accommodation and support (Smiley et al., 2007). Cooper et al. (2007) found that 40.9% of individuals diagnosed with ID (mental retardation at the time) had a psychiatric disorder as well. Moreover, Emerson and Hatton (2007) reported that 36% of children and adolescents with ID more than likely exhibited a psychiatric disorder. Psychiatric diagnosing is complicated as diagnostic criteria for disorders is based on individuals without ID and problems such as language to report symptoms, atypical presentation of psychiatric disorders, interviewer error, and accurately recognizing changes in functioning of individuals with an existing disability (Jopp & Keys, 2001) impact diagnostic assessment. Under-diagnosis and over-diagnosis of mental health conditions is also an issue with this population. Clinical intervention is complicated as well as most psychotherapeutic interventions require appropriate interpersonal skills, insight to identify thoughts and feelings, a cognitive capacity to complete tasks (homework, memory skills, self-reflection, etc.), and ability to understand the model of treatment. In this section, common psychiatric conditions that are comorbid to ID will be reviewed.

According to the Centers for Disease Control and Prevention (2020), 31% of children who are diagnosed with ASD have also been diagnosed with ID. The behavioral symptom overlap between the two disorders has long been known. For example, individuals with severe intellectual difficulties impact accurate diagnosing as it is difficult to determine if an absence of socialization and/or repetitive behaviors are attributable to gross cognitive impairment(s) or an additional diagnosis of ASD (Bradley et al., 2004). Additionally, social skills impairment is not just associated with ASD or ID; it has also been associated with substance use disorders, anxiety, conduct problems, and psychotic disorders (Bellack & Hersen, 1998). Moreover, repetitive behaviors are not only associated with ASD or ID as it is also found in psychiatric disorders (e.g. schizophrenia) and neurological disorders (e.g. Parkinson's disease; Lecavalier et al., 2011). In reviewing this information, it can be reasonably concluded that ASD and ID are highly comorbid and the behavioral symptoms make it difficult for accurate diagnosing of both conditions as well as potentially comorbid psychiatric conditions.

Anxiety disorders stem from perceived environmental threats or the perception of danger which trigger the fight or flight response. Disorders in this category are the most prevalent type of psychiatric disorders in the general population; repeated studies have reported that anxiety disorders in people with ID are, at the minimum, comparable to those in the general population (Sturmey et al., 2014). Genetic factors as well as exposure to traumas, parent-child relationship, degree of attachment, and prolonged periods of separation are clinical factors associated with anxiety disorders. When considering how prominent disorders in this category are and the complex nature of ID, expertise in different assessment and intervention strategies is required.

Mood disorders are common in individuals with ID, however, they are difficult to recognize and assess as they are oftentimes masked by problem behavior. For example, anger and aggression are common presentations that may overshadow underlying mood disorders such as major depressive disorder. Abandonment and/or poor relationships between child and parent can predispose the child to depression; this situation is exacerbated by ID (Hollins, 2003). Furthermore, negative self-image and lack of autonomy may contribute to the onset of mood disorders in individuals with ID (Hollins & Sinason, 2000). Poor social conditions, such as lack of employment, limited access to mental health services, low socioeconomic status, and lack of meaningful relationships has long been associated with depression. When considering the historical preference for institutionalized interventions for individuals with ID, it can be reasonably concluded that this exacerbates depressive symptoms for this population. Despite this information, much is known about intervention for mood disorders but less is known on its applicability to individuals with ID.

The association between ID and psychotic disorders is unclear, however, there is evidence that supports abnormal development of the nervous system predisposes individuals to disorders in this diagnostic category (Sawa & Kamiya, 2003).

Although it is likely that there is more than one cause for the onset of psychotic disorders, it can be reasonably concluded that early neurodevelopmental influences impact the onset of these disorders. Diagnosing psychotic disorders in this population proves difficult as individuals with ID struggle differentiating between internal and external events and may misinterpret events to an external source (Stenfert Kroese et al., 1998). Furthermore, appropriate behaviors and communication in more severe and profound intellectual disability is quite limited, therefore, the ability to diagnose any disorder, including psychotic disorders, may be overshadowed by ID. When considering the potential of diagnostic overshadowing, psychotic disorders in this population may not be appropriately treated.

Since individuals with ID are significantly more prone to experiencing other comorbid conditions and when considering barriers to clinical assessment and therapist reluctance to intervene with this population, this represents a significant clinical issue. Furthermore, the aforementioned maladaptive behaviors associated with the ID diagnosis (self-injurious behaviors, stereotypic movements, anger and aggression, food intake problems, issues sleeping) further complicate clinical assessment and psychotherapy. Since there is no clear clinical response, the clinical psychology field is at an impasse. Although anxiety disorders, mood disorders, and psychotic disorders were highlighted, this does not preclude other conditions, such as substance-related and addictive disorders or personality disorders, from being clinically relevant for intervention.

6.4.3 *Intellectual Disability and Psychopathy*

There has been relatively little research examining the associations between ID and psychopathy traits, particularly among offenders. This is likely due, in part, to a general paucity of research on forensic ID populations (Morrisey & Hollin, 2011; Torr, 2003). However, it may also be attributable to a clinical tradition that presents psychopathy as incompatible with ID (e.g., Cleckley, 1941/1988; Karpman, 1941). Despite this conceptualization, however, there is not a strong, negative relationship between psychopathy traits and IQ (Forth et al., 1990; Morrisey et al. 2005) and there are individuals who exhibit both ID and psychopathy traits (Morrisey et al. 2005). Further, examinations of the PCL-R facets within non-ID populations show a varied pattern of associations between psychopathy and IQ (Salekin et al., 2004; Vitacco et al., 2008). For example, whereas IQ is positively correlated with the interpersonal facet—a pattern consistent with Cleckley's (1941/1988) conceptualization—intelligence is negatively correlated with the affective and lifestyle facets.

Rayner et al. (2015) highlighted the relative dearth of research within forensic ID populations in their review of research on the relation between ID and personality disorders. They found that, within forensic ID populations, Borderline Personality Disorder (BPD) and Antisocial Personality Disorder (ASPD) were the most common personality disorders (Rayner et al., 2015). This may be due, in part, to the association between these disorders and criminal offending (e.g., Robitaille et al.,

2017). However, it may also be attributed to the overlap between certain features of these disorders (e.g., affective lability, self-harm, and impulsivity for BPD and impulsive and sometimes aggressive behavior for ASPD) and some characteristics of ID (Morrisey & Hollin, 2011).

One of the key findings to emerge from Rayner et al.'s (2015) review was that individuals with comorbid ID and personality disorders were different from individuals with ID alone. Importantly, within these ID offender populations, the combination of ID and personality disorder was associated with higher rates of prior conviction, greater likelihood of placement in a high security setting, greater number of comorbid psychiatric diagnoses, and higher rates of medication prescription (Rayner et al., 2015). The ID/personality disorder group also had a higher IQ than the ID group without personality disorder (Rayner et al., 2015). Consistent with these findings, the presence of psychopathy traits within forensic ID populations has been associated with less positive treatment progress (Morrisey & Hollin 2011). Taken together, these data suggest that the presence of a personality disorder among offenders with ID may have important implications for risk assessment, placement, and treatment considerations.

Whereas Rayner et al. (2015) examined the relations between ID and personality disorders more generally, Morrisey and Hollin (2011) focused specifically on studies of psychopathy in ID populations. Within their review, the authors noted several key points of overlap between ID and psychopathy that are worth further consideration. These include the associations that both psychopathy and ID have with negative early environmental experiences, such as abuse and neglect (Fournier et al., Chap. 9 this volume; Hatton & Emerson, 2004), the associations that both psychopathy and ID have with conduct disorder diagnoses in adolescence, and longitudinal data that connects low verbal IQ, attention difficulties, and impulsivity in childhood with psychopathy ratings in adulthood (Morrisey & Hollin, 2011).

Although there is some limited evidence to support the predictive validity of psychopathy in ID populations for treatment progress and recidivism (e.g., Morrisey & Hollin, 2011), the number of studies is small and the findings not always consistent. For example, in their review, Morrisey and Hollin (2011) did not find strong evidence for an association between psychopathy and aggressive institutional behavior. Further, there are no large-scale, well-controlled studies of treatment response for individuals with both ID and psychopathy traits.

Future studies examining psychopathy and ID are needed, and will need to take into account two considerations. First, they will need to address the still limited understanding of the development of personality disorders within ID populations (Rayner et al., 2015), which complicates the application of models of personality disorder developed in non-ID populations to this group. Second, the generalizability of personality disorder assessments, such as the PCL-R, is not yet well understood in ID populations. For example, some PCL-R items (e.g., shallow affect) may be challenging to apply to individuals with deficits in their ability to identify or express their emotional experiences (Morrisey & Hollin, 2011). Similarly, the limited occupational and social functioning of individuals with ID may interfere with ratings of several of the antisocial lifestyle items (e.g., parasitic lifestyle, irresponsibility; Morrissey et al., 2010). In support of the possibility that psychopathy assessment may be more challenging in this population, Morrisey et al. (2010) found that PCL-R interrater reliability was related to IQ within the ID sample, with lower IQ scores (i.e., below the sample median) associated with lower reliability. It will be important for future studies of psychopathy in ID populations to consider these limitations, so that the field can develop a more clear understanding of the ways in which these conditions interact, and their implications for management and treatment.

6.4.4 Intellectual Disability and Criminal Offending

Individuals diagnosed with ID have problems learning and tend to learn more slowly than those without the diagnosis. Furthermore, this population tends to exhibit cognitive rigidity, struggles with maintaining attention, processes information slowly, and experiences difficulty in planning and implementing complex behaviors (Salekin et al., 2010). Individuals with ID oftentimes learn through imitation of others and often complete behaviors to please others or to fit in with a group. This desire to conform leads to problems with self-direction which includes adapting to change, decision-making, and planning for the future. Adaptive deficits include struggles with employment or education, social relationships and interaction, and independent living skills. Although these adaptive impairments exist, individuals with ID do experience successes in these conceptual, practical, and social adaptive functions. Achievements in adaptive functioning may be partly attributed to the repetitive nature of these tasks and their applicability to everyday life.

Prevalence rates of offenders with ID is in question as methods of data collection across studies varies considerably. However, data does suggest that between 4% and 10% of incarcerated persons in the United States have a diagnosis of ID (Petersilia, 2000). Furthermore, comorbidity of psychiatric disorders and offenders with ID is 89% (Mannynsalo et al., 2009). These offenders oftentimes exhibit a pattern of aimlessness, tend to focus on the present day, and struggle maintaining employment (Salekin et al., 2010). Similarly to the general population, offenders with ID are likely to be functioning in the mild level and would be expected to have some successes in having a social network, employment in labor jobs or positions that require limited cognitive skill, and independent living skills (Salekin et al., 2010). Since most offenders would be functioning in the mild level, they are less likely to be identified as having ID as their outward appearance and presentation is not significantly different from those not diagnosed. Lastly, when considering deficits in cognitive functioning, desire to fit in with a group, and learning through imitation, incarcerated offenders with ID are more vulnerable to negative influences that are inherent to correctional environments.

6.4.5 Clinical Intervention for Intellectual Disability

In order to effectively provide clinical intervention for this population, understanding the diagnosis of ID and associated clinical issues, knowing how to accurately assess and diagnose ID, and understanding how comorbid conditions can lead to various presentations of ID are all important aspects to consider when providing clinical intervention. In this section, descriptions of clinical interventions for ID based on this information will provided.

6.4.5.1 Applied Behavior Analysis

Applied behavior analysis (ABA) is the science that is derived from the principles of behavior that are applied systematically in order to improve socially significant behavior; experimentation is also utilized in order to identify the variables responsible for behavioral change (Cooper et al., 2020). ABA has made significant contributions in developing instructional strategies for individuals with ID (O'Reilly et al., 2016). In ABA, the functional behavior assessment (FBA) enables assessor to develop hypotheses surrounding the relations among environmental events and behavior. The FBA is a systematic, evidence-based process for assessing the relationship between the environment and behavior (Blair et al., 1999) in order to guide the development of positive interventions based off the function(s) of the behavior (Horner, 1994). The five functions of behavior are social positive reinforcement (immediate attention gained from others after the problem behavior), tangible reinforcement (behaviors result due to the access to reinforcing materials), automatic positive reinforcement (social reinforcers are ruled out and the behavior occurs when they are alone), social negative reinforcement (learned behaviors as a result of their effectiveness in terminating/postponing aversive events), and automatic negative reinforcement (when pain or an uncomfortable condition makes its termination reinforcing; Cooper et al., 2020). When the function(s) of the problem behavior(s) has been identified, client-specific proactive and reactive behavioral strategies can be implemented to decrease the frequency and severity of the behavior(s) for reduction. Additionally, task analyses (complex sequence of behaviors are broken down to determine appropriate support) are developed in order to support consumer by improving functional living skills.

The development of procedures to determine and understand the complexities surrounding the function of behavior(s) and teaching the individual alternative behaviors that serve the same function is central to ABA practice. Through the use of this intervention, individuals can be rehabilitated so they can prosper in all areas of life, including with their non-disabled peers. Therefore, (1) creating environments that are sensitive to the individuals' needs, (2) increasing engagement in meaningful activity, (3) increasing interpersonal contact and community engagement, (4) increasing the individuals' repertoire of functional living skills, and (5) overall improvement of an individuals' quality of life all support the idea that behavioral interventions make the greatest contribution to individuals with ID

(Jones & Dowey, 2013). Sturmey (2014a) completed a meta-analysis of (1) interventions aimed to increase adaptive behaviors (conceptual, social, and practical skills), and (2) interventions used to increase specific adaptive behaviors (grooming, safety measures, managing money, cleaning, and communication as examples). In this meta-analysis, author found that the evidence-based interventions were almost all behavioral methods. In a separate meta-analysis by Sturmey (2014b), (1) interventions for broadly defined "maladaptive behaviors," (2) interventions for specific maladaptive behaviors (self-injurious behavior, aggression, pica, etc.), (3) specific intervention methods, and (4) interventions for specific populations were assessed. In this meta-analysis, Sturmey (2014b) found (1) the most support was for behavioral and behavior analytic interventions, and (2) there was some support for CBT and other psychosocial interventions. Lastly, in their systematic review of 49 studies on the use of behavior analytic interventions to develop skills in young children with ID between the years 2000 (January) to 2020 (April), Ho et al. (2020) concluded that behavioral analytic interventions that targeted academic skills met criteria as an emerging intervention based on the use of the Scientific Merit Rating Scale (developed by the National Autism Center), therefore, these interventions can be used effectively to support skill development in children with intellectual disability.

Person-Centered Active Support

Although not specific to ABA, person-centered active support shares fundamental aspects of ABA that includes the correct implementation of instructional strategies prescribed by behavior analyst, the emphasis of the relationship between environment and behavior (creating environments based on individuals' needs, increase community engagement and interpersonal contact, and increase engagement in meaningful activity), and the prescribed positive interventions from behavior analyst are enacted by individuals' support system (family, social support in the community, and/or staff of a facility). For individuals with ID who are receiving services in a facility, staff adherence to the behavioral intervention plan is imperative. However, various research on facility services has shown that staff provide minimal assistance, approximately 10% of the total time (i.e. less than 6 min per hour; Mansell et al., 2013; Netten et al., 2010). Additionally, on average, individuals with severe disabilities spend at least half of their time *not* involved in meaningful activities (Mansell et al., 2013); this contradicts some of the core fundamentals of ABA. Person-centered active support recognizes that for individuals who are diagnosed with ID, their quality of life depends on the support provided by others; this intervention is a response to the aforementioned staff support and minimal engagement in meaningful activities.

The foundation of person-centered active support is on the engagement of meaningful activities and relationships as well as active support (Beadle-Brown & Hutchinson, 2016). In the context of this intervention, engagement is defined as (1) completing a constructive activity with materials (art, washing dishes, weight lifting, etc.), (2) interacting with others, and (3) joining in group activities (group sports, playing a board game, joining a special interest group, etc.; Mansell et al., 2005). The key principles of active support include (1) every moment has potential to make the most of it, (2) "little and often" moments for individuals with ID to engage briefly in meaningful activities and relationships, (3) graded assistance so ensure success (appropriate level of support), and (4) maximizing choice and control (Mansell et al., 2005). Successful implementation of this approach has been shown to increase engagement in positive interpersonal relationships and meaningful activities (Beadle-Brown et al., 2012; Stancliffe et al., 2007), increase and improve individuals' adaptive functioning skills (Mansell et al., 2002), and reduce maladaptive behavior(s) where the function is for social positive reinforcement (attention) or automatic positive reinforcement (self-stimulatory behavior; Koritsas et al., 2008). When an individual with ID is engaged in meaningful activities, receives active support, and is receiving ABA services, the individual may experience an overall improvement in their quality of life.

6.4.5.2 Cognitive-Behavioral Therapies

For many psychiatric disorders, the evidence base supports the use of the cognitive-behavioral therapies (CBTs). CBTs share the following three fundamental propositions: (1) cognitive activity impacts behavior, (2) cognitive activity may be monitored and changed, and (3) desired behavior change can be impacted through cognitive change (Dobson & Dozois, 2010). CBTs have the following three classes of interventions: (1) problem-solving therapies, (2) cognitive restructuring methods, and (3) coping skills therapies (Mahoney & Arnkoff, 1978). The more prominent CBTs include rational emotive behavior therapy, cognitive therapy, self-instructional training, self-control treatments, stress inoculation training, problem-solving therapy, structural and constructivist psychotherapy, and acceptance and commitment therapy. Epp and Dobson (2010) reviewed outcome literature for 20 disorders/conditions in adults; for each, they examined the efficacy of CBT as an intervention. In this review, authors found that the following disorders/conditions indicated positive evidence for absolute efficacy of CBT use:

Unipolar Depression	Bipolar Disorder
Generalized Anxiety Disorder	Bulimia Nervosa
Binge-Eating Disorder	Anorexia Nervosa
Schizophrenia	Marital Distress
Anger/Violent Offending	Sexual Offending
Chronic Pain	Borderline Personality Disorder
Substance Use Disorders	Somatoform Disorders
Sleep difficulties	

Moreover, authors found that the use of exposure and cognitive restructuring was the treatment of choice for specific phobia, social phobia, and panic disorder. Lastly, Epp and Dobson (2010) found that the use of exposure, response prevention, and cognitive restructuring showed positive evidence for absolute efficacy for their use with individuals with obsessive-compulsive disorder and exposure and cognitive techniques showed positive evidence for absolute efficacy for their use with those diagnosed with panic disorder. Therefore, when considering the sheer number of diagnoses and clinical issues listed, the use of the CBTs has become a prominent intervention for various diagnoses in the DSM-5 as well as for common clinical issues.

The evidence base for individuals with a psychiatric disorder *without* ID definitively supports the use of the CBTs (Dagnan, 2007). Despite the expansive uses of the CBTs for psychiatric diagnoses and various clinical issues, its use for individuals with intellectual disability is not as efficacious. However, CBT techniques have been adapted in order to be used as an intervention for individuals with ID. Despite these adaptations, no guidelines exist for developing the therapeutic relationship with individuals diagnosed with ID; the development of these skills occurs through supervision, practice, and modeling (Lindsay et al., 2013). Therefore, practicing clinicians may not be able to adjust their interpersonal and therapeutic style to develop rapport with individuals diagnosed with ID. Behavior analytic interventions appear to have the strongest foundation for rehabilitation for individuals diagnosed with ID. However, as previously reviewed, Cooper et al. (2007) found that 40.9% of individuals diagnosed with ID also had a psychiatric disorder and Emerson and Hatton (2007) reported that 36% of children diagnosed with ID had a comorbid psychiatric disorder. Due to this high comorbidity between ID and psychiatric disorders across the lifespan, the combination of ABA and CBT (with potential pharmacological interventions) may provide the best prognosis for overall rehabilitation.

6.5 Autism Spectrum Disorder

ASD is characterized by persistent deficits in social communication and interaction across multiple contexts as well as having restrictive, repetitive patterns of interests, behavior, or activities (APA, 2013). Impairment in social interactions/communication and restricted and repetitive behaviors and interests can vary in severity; the severity level is based on level of support(s) needed. Although some individuals with ASD can live independently, others may experience an impact on their education and employment, their families may not be able to supply the required support, and societal attitudes towards individuals with ASD are all factors that impact the quality of life for individuals diagnosed with ASD (World Health Organization [WHO], 2021).

Due to ASD being a behaviorally defined disorder, the determination of its prevalence is difficult; some of the data provided should be interpreted with caution. Approximately 1 in 54 children has been diagnosed with ASD in the United States;

boys are more than four times more likely to be diagnosed with ASD, minority groups tend to be less often diagnosed and if diagnosed, it is oftentimes later in life (Centers for Disease Control and Prevention, 2020). Worldwide, it is estimated that about 1 in 270 people are diagnosed with ASD; individuals with this disorder often experience stigma, discrimination, and violations of human rights (WHO, 2021).

Challenging behaviors are common clinical concerns in individuals diagnosed with ASD; they can have a devastating impact on the individual's family/social support network, their educational and employment opportunities, their personal safety (self-injury), acquisition of legal involvement (others are harmed), and medical and mental health stability. Many of these challenging/maladaptive behaviors were provided and elaborated on earlier (self-injurious behaviors, stereotypic movements, anger/aggression, food intake problems, and sleeping issues). Through the reduction/elimination of identified challenging behaviors and the strengthening of prosocial behaviors, the individual can improve their overall quality of life.

6.5.1 Clinical Assessment of Autism Spectrum Disorder

The diagnostic criteria for ASD include (1) persistent deficits in social communication and social interaction across multiple contexts, (2) restricted, repetitive patterns of behavior, interests, and/or activities, (3) symptoms occurring in the early developmental period, (4) symptoms cause clinically significant impairment in social, occupational, or other areas of functioning, and (5) is not better explained by intellectual disability (APA 2013). Therefore, clinical assessment must take all of these areas into account for an accurate diagnosis of ASD. In Table 6.1, the name of the

Table 6.1 Clinical assessment measures for autism spectrum disorders

Clinical assessment measure	Age group	Diagnostic criteria
Autism behavior checklist	3 years old through school age	1, 2, 3, 4
Autism diagnostic interview-revised	Children/adults with years years	1, 2, 3, 4
Autism diagnostic observation schedule-2	12 months through Adulthood	1, 2, 4
Autism observation scale for infants	6 months old through 18 months old	1, 2, 3, 4
Behavior observation scale for autism	Children	1, 2, 3, 4, 5
Childhood autism rating scale-2	2 years old and older	1, 2, 4
Developmental dimensional and diagnostic interview	Not specified	1, 2
Diagnostic interview for social and communication disorders	All ages	1, 2, 4
Gilliam autism rating scale-3	3 years old through 22 years old	1, 2
Modified checklist for autism in toddlers-revised	Toddlers between 16 months and 30 months	1, 3

clinical assessment measure, age group, and diagnostic criteria addressed (1–5 from above) are provided:

The amount of measures provided indicates that there have been advancements in ASD assessment over time. The *diagnostic criteria* heading in Table 6.1 may be somewhat limited in terms of knowing the onset of symptoms, degree of impairment, and if the symptoms are not better explained by ID. Since authors have not reviewed all items in each measure, some of them may actually provide some of this information. For example, as it relates to the age of onset of symptoms in the developmental period, if it is a measure designed only for children (e.g. Autism Observation Scale for Infants), it would only be providing information on if symptoms were present or not for a diagnosis of ASD in the developmental period. However, for adult measures or for measures where the age range is expansive (e.g. Autism Diagnostic Observation Schedule-2), the age of onset and degree of impairment would need to be investigated further.

Similar to diagnosing ID, the age of onset of symptoms of ASD is important as it helps rule out other conditions. As previously reviewed, "developmental period" may be established by the state of residence or jurisdiction and therefore could impact this criterion. School, medical, and clinical records continue to be the most important components in establishing the presence of ASD symptoms (or lack thereof) for a diagnosis of ASD in adulthood (if not diagnosed in childhood). Assessors and psychotherapists should continue to be mindful of retaining records in the event where a client requests them for future requests when seeking financial services, disability services, and/or historical records that may impact present legal involvement.

When assessing the degree of impairment in school, social, or occupational areas of current functioning, information may be obtained through direct observation, school/work records, clinical records, medical records, and/or informant/collateral interviews. If possible, direct observation is preferred as the assessor can see if client is impaired in any life areas and to what extent. Additionally, informant/collateral interviews provide a wealth of information when assessor is unable to be present. Although determining the individual's impairment in these various life areas is subjective, documentation (school/work, clinical, and medical) can help as assessor determines if this criterion is met.

6.5.1.1 Clinical Assessment of Comorbid Psychopathology in Individuals with Autism Spectrum Disorder

There are few clinical measures for comorbid psychopathology in individuals with ASD. Additionally, evidence supporting their usage is scant. Although research has lagged in completing scientific studies in order to provide greater details on the efficacy of their use, these measures may have utility. The subsequent measures should be utilized with caution.

The Autism Spectrum Disorder- Comorbid for Children Scale (ASD-CC; Matson et al., 2009) and the Autism Comorbidity Interview- Present and Lifetime Version

(ACI-PL; Leyfer et al., 2006) were specifically designed for children with ASD. The ASD-CC is a rating scale that is designed to assess symptoms of emotional difficulties. The goal of the ASD-CC is to differentiate symptoms that are usual for children with ASD from those that constitute co-occurring psychopathology (Matson & Wilkins, 2008). The ACI-PL is a semi-structured diagnostic measure to be used by trained assessors when interviewing an informant. Extreme caution should be used when utilizing this measure as authors (Leyfer et al., 2006) reported that they did not attempt to differentiate between symptoms of ASD from those of co-occurring psychopathologies and have stated that further testing is needed.

The Stress Survey Schedule for Persons with Autism and Other Developmental Disabilities (SSS; Groden et al., 2001) and the Schedule for the Assessment of Psychiatric Problems Associated with Autism (and Other Developmental Disorders; SAPPA; Bolton & Rutter, 1994). The SSS is a rating scale that measures the intensity of symptoms that are associated with the experience of stress. In a study by Groden et al. (2001) where the SSS was administered to children and adults aged 3–40 years old who were diagnosed with ASD and/or other developmental disabilities, content validity was established. Additionally, in a study by Goodwin et al. (2007) where children and adults aged 3–41 years old with ASD were given the SSS, results indicated that the SSS is a valid tool to discern which dimensions of stress are perceived to be the least and most stressful for individuals with ASD. The SAPPA is a semi-structured diagnostic measure utilized by trained assessors when interviewing an informant. The SAPPA has been used in multiple studies (see Bradley & Bolton, 2006; Hutton et al., 2008; Raznahan et al., 2006), however, no studies have reported validity and reliability data for use (Underwood et al., 2011).

For adults, the Peters Delusional Inventory (Peters et al., 1999), Yale-Brown Obsessions and Compulsions Scale (Goodman et al., 1989), Hospital Anxiety and Depression Scales (Zigmond & Snaith, 1983), Beck Depression Inventory (Beck et al., 1961), and the Beck Anxiety Inventory (Beck, 1993) has been utilized successfully in research and clinical work with individuals with ASD (Hare, 2013). Measures designed to assess psychopathology in adults diagnosed with ASD and severe or profound ID include the Psychopathology in Autism Checklist (PAC; Helverschou et al., 2009) and the Autism Spectrum Disorders- Comorbidity for Adults (ASD-CA; Matson & Boisjoli, 2008). The PAC is completed by the informant whereas for the ASD-CA is completed by a trained clinician during an interview with an informant. Helverschou et al. (2009) completed a pilot study where individuals with ASD and severe or profound ID (with and without psychiatric disorders) were included and informants completed the PAC. The PAC exhibited good reliability as participants with a psychiatric diagnosis scored higher on all subscales than those without. However, since numerous participants scored higher on a number of subscales the PAC was minimally able to distinguish between psychiatric conditions. Reliability and validity data on each subscale of the ASD-CA has varied widely (Underwood et al., 2011), therefore, it should be used with caution.

6.5.2 Diagnostic Comorbidity

The prevalence of psychiatric disorders are higher for individuals with ASD when compared to the general population (Simonoff et al., 2008). Despite this information, psychiatric disorders within this population are oftentimes overlooked as the symptoms are attributed to ASD (Matson & Boisjoli, 2008) as opposed to being diagnosed accordingly. For example, when considering the restrictive and repetitive behaviors as a symptom of ASD and the behavioral compulsions (washing hands, ordering, checking, etc.) as a symptom of obsessive-compulsive disorder, an individual may be solely diagnosed with ASD, solely diagnosed with obsessive-compulsive disorder, or diagnosed with both. The difficulty in distinguishing ASD from psychiatric disorders is due to (1) the diagnostic criteria for diagnosing a psychiatric condition may be set too low, (2) the characteristics of individuals diagnosed with ASD can hinder the employment of standard assessment procedures, (3) the traits of autism and psychiatric disorders oftentimes co-occur, and (4) the various types of psychiatric disorders that co-occur can further complicate diagnosing (Helverschou et al., 2011). Due to this symptom overlap (restrictive/repetitive behaviors and behavioral compulsions) and co-occurrences (ASD and other psychiatric conditions), it has led to a contentious debate within clinical psychology (obsessive-compulsive disorder as a discrete diagnosis or symptoms as part of ASD). It has proven to be difficult to provide accurate estimations as prevalence rate estimates range between 9% and 89% (Howlin, 2002). With all considered, it can be reasonably concluded that estimates of psychiatric comorbidity for individuals with ASD is on the higher end, however, caution should be exercised when reviewing the provided data due to these various factors.

In a study on psychiatric comorbidity in children with ASD, Romero et al. (2016) identified that 85% of the sample of children diagnosed with ASD had a comorbid psychiatric diagnosis and 35% of those were taking at least one psychotropic medication. Additionally, authors found that attention-deficit/hyperactivity disorder (ADHD), generalized anxiety disorder, and major depressive disorder as being the most commonly diagnosed comorbidities. In a national study assessing the needs of individuals with ASD in the United Kingdom, approximately 32% of parents identified that their child with ASD experienced significant psychological and emotional disturbances (Barnard et al., 2001). Although this data is not specific to a psychiatric disorder, this distress obviously warrants clinical attention as the wide range of emotions, their management, and resulting issues (e.g., sleep disturbances, substance usage, interpersonal conflict, etc.) are important clinical concerns for an individual's overall stability.

Between 30% and 50% of individuals diagnosed with ASD manifest ADHD symptoms (Davis & Kollins, 2012). The co-occurrence of these disorders has resulted in a lower overall quality of life and poorer adaptive functioning (Vora & Sikora, 2011) as well as significant behavioral, emotional, adaptive, and academic problems in the home and the community (including school; Rao & Landa, 2014). ASD and ADHD are more commonly found in males than in females and typically present, even just symptoms, at preschool age (Leitner, 2014). The co-occurrence of these disorders is also difficult to diagnose (similar to comorbid obsessive-compulsive disorder) as interpersonal communication, maintaining attention, impulsive behavior, and varying degrees of hyperactivity manifest in both disorders. In cases where both diagnoses exist, the DSM-5 recognizes the co-occurrence and allows for both diagnoses when the previous DSM-IV-TR did not.

Individuals with psychiatric disorders oftentimes exhibit symptoms of more than one disorder and co-occurrence of these conditions has been found in individuals with ASD (Ghaziuddin, 2005). For example, in two separate studies that were conducted with community samples, Simonoff et al. (2008) identified two or more psychiatric diagnoses in 41% of the sample and Leyfer et al. (2006) reported a median of three psychiatric conditions in their sample. Of these psychiatric diagnoses, depression and anxiety disorders are the most frequent comorbid psychiatric condition diagnosed in individuals with ASD (Hutton et al., 2008; Melville et al., 2008). Additionally, depression and anxiety disorders oftentimes co-occur (Howlin, 2000), therefore, this further complicates the emotional responses that an individual with ASD may have when they struggle in interpersonal situations. The rates of development of a psychotic disorder for individuals with ASD was on par with those in the general population (Cederlund et al., 2008); there appears to be no increased risk. Although an individual can have ASD with no psychiatric disorders, the evidence supports that there are issues in diagnosing (diagnostic overshadowing), and that in many cases, an individual with ASD will likely have a comorbid psychiatric disorder.

6.5.3 Autism Spectrum Disorder and Psychopathy

Both psychopathy and ASD have been described as involving dysfunctions of empathy (e.g. Bird & Viding, 2014; Blair, 2005; Jones et al., 2009a; Lockwood, 2016). Evidence for psychopathy as involving empathy dysfunction is drawn from many sources. In addition to those traits that are represented in the PCL-R (Hare, 1991) and reflect the individual's lack of understanding or appreciation of others' emotional experience (i.e., lack of guilt/remorse, shallow affect, callous/unempathic), psychopathic individuals also show decreased physiological responses to others' distress (e.g., Blair et al., 1997) and deficits in the recognition of others' distress expressions (e.g., Blair et al., 2001; Kosson et al., 2002). Individuals high in psychopathic traits exhibit atypical neural activation in response to others' emotional experiences, including abnormalities in orbitofrontal (OFC) activation (e.g., Decety et al., 2013; Lockwood et al. 2013a, b) and reduced amygdala responsivity to others' emotional facial expressions (e.g., Jones et al., 2009b). ASD has also been associated with abnormalities in empathic responding, especially in performance on tasks related to cognitive perspective taking (e.g., Baron-Cohen et al., 1985; Dziobek et al., 2008; Frith & Happé, 2005). Individuals with ASD also show lower scores on both self-report (Baron-Cohen & Wheelwright, 2004) and parent report (Hudry & Slaughter, 2009) assessments of empathy and sensitivity to the emotional situations of others.

Although both psychopathy and ASD have been associated with deficits in empathic responding, and some neuroimaging work shows abnormalities for both groups in amygdala (e.g., Ashwin et al., 2007; Jones et al., 2009b), anterior cingulate cortex (ACC) and anterior insula (AI) responses (see Lockwood, 2016 for a review), there is considerable evidence to suggest that the deficits in empathy exhibited by individuals high in psychopathic traits and those exhibited by individuals with ASD are not the same. Empathy is not a unidimensional concept and can be further differentiated into cognitive and emotional/affective types (e.g., Bird & Viding, 2014; Blair, 2005, 2008;Cox et al., 2012 ; Lockwood, 2016). Cognitive empathy involves understanding the emotional states of others, and is captured by concepts such as mentalizing, perspective taking, and Theory of Mind, whereas emotional/affective empathy involves sharing the emotional state of another person as a result of direct or indirect observation of their experience (e.g., Blair, 2005, 2008; Lockwood, 2016). These different components of empathy are dissociable on the basis of distinct neurocognitive circuits (Cox et al., 2012; Lockwood, 2016) and are separately assessed on self-report or behavioral measures of empathy. Neither ASD nor psychopathy are associated with global deficits in empathy. Rather, deficits appear to be relatively specific to either cognitive empathy—in the case of ASD—or emotional empathy—in the case of psychopathy (e.g., Blair, 2005, 2008; Jones et al., 2010; Lockwood et al. 2013a, b; Oliver et al., 2016).

Consistent with this, on self-report measures of empathy such as the Interpersonal Reactivity Index (IRI; Davis, 1983), the pattern of associations for high and low psychopathic personality traits and high and low ASD characteristics are dissimilar in key ways. For example, in a sample of 79 college students assessed using the Psychopathic Personality Inventory- Short Form (PPI-SF; Lilienfeld & Hess, 2001) and the Autism-Spectrum Quotient (AQ; Baron-Cohen et al., 2001), found that high vs. low ASQ scorers differed significantly only in their ratings on the Perspective Taking subscale of the IRI, whereas high vs. low ASQ scorers differed significantly only in their ratings on the Empathic Concern scale. Dissimilarities are also apparent on tasks assessing the components of empathy. For example, where individuals with ASD typically show some deficits in Theory of Mind function (e.g., Baron-Cohen et al., 1985; Frith & Happé, 2005; Jones et al., 2010), psychopathic individuals do not (e.g., Blair et al., 1996; Jones et al., 2010). Conversely, individuals with ASD show normal neural and physiological responses to others' experience of distress (Blair, 1999; Fan et al., 2014).

Gillespie et al. (2014) emphasized the differences between the abnormalities in neural responses to social interactions exhibited by ASD versus psychopathic individuals. For example, research has shown abnormalities in psychopathic individuals' neural responses to observed social interactions—although these abnormalities can be reduced when participants are instructed to "feel" the experience (Meffert et al., 2013). In contrast, individuals with ASD appear able to show both normal social and empathy activations when they are observing social or personally relevant individuals—although they show abnormalities in responding when the targets are unfamiliar (Oberman et al., 2008; Pierce & Redcay, 2008). These patterns suggest that in the presence of empathy-relevant stimuli, the abnormal neural responding of individuals with ASD traits is moderated by factors that do not influence the responses of psychopathic individuals. Specifically, among individuals with ASD, but not psychopathy, deficits in spontaneous vicarious representation occur primarily when the observation targets are unfamiliar (Gillespie et al., 2014).

Beyond these well-documented differences in the empathy deficits exhibited by these two groups, the literature provides consistent evidence to show that, while psychopathy and ASD may sometimes co-occur, they do not represent different expressions of a shared underlying deficit or process. For example, Rogers et al. (2006) examined the co-occurrence of ASD traits as assessed by the Social Communication Questionnaire and psychopathy traits as assessed by the ASPSD (Frick & Hare, 2001) in a sample of 28 adolescent boys with DSM-IV diagnoses of either Autism Spectrum Disorder or Asperger's Disorder. The results showed that the severity of ASD traits was unrelated to the level of Callous/Unemotional traits. In addition, participants who were high versus low in CU traits did not differ from each other on either mentalizing or executive function tests (i.e., abilities that represent core cognitive deficits in ASD), indicating that psychopathy traits were unrelated to the core ASD deficits. Consistent with findings in psychopathy, those participants with high CU traits did show deficits on a moral-conventional distinction task, and on an emotion facial recognition task (Rogers et al., 2006).

Jones, Larsson, et al. (2009a) further explored the co-occurrence of psychopathy and ASD traits within the Twin Early Development Study sample (Oliver & Plomin, 2007). Their study comprised 642 twin pairs aged 8 to 10. The authors examined both the extent of phenotypic overlap between psychopathic personality characteristics and ASD traits and the relative contributions of genetic versus environmental influences to this overlap. The results showed moderate phenotypic associations between psychopathy and ASD traits, as well as high heritability for psychopathic and ASD traits individually. Further, although there was some genetic overlap between psychopathic and ASD traits, this overlap did not meaningfully account for individual differences in psychopathic characteristics, demonstrating a genetic influence for psychopathic characteristics independent of the overlap between psychopathic traits and autism traits (Jones et al., 2009a). The results also showed that whereas the shared environmental influences associated with psychopathic characteristics were the same influences associated with ASD traits, there was no overlap in non-shared environmental influences. Thus, whereas some of the shared environmental influences that contribute to psychopathy also contribute to ASD (e.g., prenatal and obstetric risk factors), the non-shared environmental influences associated with psychopathy were specific to that syndrome. Similar results were found by O'Nions et al. (2015) in a study of 7- to 8-year-old twins that examined the overlap in ASD (as reflected in social communication and social interaction) and CU traits. As in Jones et al. (2009a), the results showed some moderate phenotypic overlap between ASD and CU traits. Importantly, however, the majority of the genetic variance in CU traits was explained by independent genetic influences, supporting the conclusion that the genetic influences on CU and ASD traits are distinct (O'Nions et al., 2015).

When considering the overlap or co-occurrence of psychopathy and ASD, some authors have suggested that it may be necessary to consider the role of alexithymia (Bird & Viding, 2014; Lockwood et al., 2013a, b; Takamatsu & Takai, 2019). Alexithymia is a syndrome characterized by deficits in the identification, description, and differentiation of emotion states, as well as a tendency towards externally-oriented thinking (Nemiah et al., 1976). Alexithymia is associated with ASD and psychopathy (Bird & Cook, 2013; Lockwood et al. 2013) and is related to deficits in affective empathy (Patil & Silani, 2014). Although some studies suggest that the associations between empathy deficits and ASD, psychopathy, and alexithymia may be separable (e.g., Lockwood et al., 2013a, b; Takamatsu & Takai, 2019), it may nevertheless be useful to include assessments of alexithymia traits in studies that compare empathy and emotional responding in individuals with ASD and psychopathy traits (Bird & Viding, 2014).

6.5.4 Autism Spectrum Disorder and Criminal Offending

Despite the advantages of media outlets providing the greater public with needed information for health and safety, it also has its downfalls. Media coverage has oftentimes insinuated that a perpetrator has been diagnosed with ASD without credible evidence that supports this claim. These proclamations can lead to unwarranted negative reactions from the public (stigmatization) toward those diagnosed with ASD. Furthermore, in some of these high profile cases presented in the media, there is little evidence of a formal ASD diagnosis (Brewer et al., 2017; Maras et al., 2015) and extensive reviews of the scientific literature have not found a direct link between ASD and violent behavior or criminality (Bjorkly, 2009; Lerner et al., 2012). Therefore, despite these media conjectures, there is no causal link between the diagnosis of ASD and criminality. However, researchers have shifted their attention to trying to understand criminal behavior amongst individuals with ASD (Slaughter et al., 2019).

6.5.5 Clinical Intervention for Autism Spectrum Disorder

Clinical intervention for ASD, similarly to intervention for ID, is complex and multifaceted. Understanding the diagnosis of ASD, associated clinical issues, accurate assessment and diagnosis, and the impact of comorbid conditions are all important aspects to consider when providing clinical intervention. In this section, clinical interventions for ASD will be provided. Also, clinical interventions for comorbid ASD and psychopathy will be reviewed.

6.5.5.1 Applied Behavior Analysis and Person Centered Active Support

The key components of ABA as an intervention for ID were provided in detail earlier in this chapter. Therefore, the foundations of this intervention will not be re-reviewed in this section. The use of ABA-based interventions for individuals with ASD is strongly supported in the academic literature (e.g., Matson et al., 1996; Wolery et al., 2005). A common challenge for individuals with ASD is the transition from school to adulthood where the skills in the classroom have minimal applicability in the adult world (Gerhardt et al., 2014). Therefore, improving adaptive functioning is an important clinical focus even though it is not a part of the diagnosis of ASD (however, is a criterion for ID). ABA interventions are applied systematically in order to improve socially significant behavior (Cooper et al., 2020) by remediating delays in social skills, improving functional living skills, and managing challenging behaviors. In utilizing ABA for individuals with ASD, reinforcement is used to strengthen appropriate behaviors (e.g., play, social skills, gestures, etc.) in order to alleviate the core deficits of the disorder (remediate delays) and to help individuals integrate into activities and settings with non-disabled peers.

Person centered active support, as previously reviewed, shares fundamental aspects of ABA. The core emphasis is on the correct implementation of instructional strategies (behavioral interventions), creating environments based on the individuals' needs, increase community engagement and interpersonal contact, and use of staff/family to enact the interventions across various settings. Successful implementation of this approach has been shown to increase engagement in positive interpersonal relationships and meaningful activities (Beadle-Brown et al., 2012; Stancliffe et al., 2007), increase and improve individuals' adaptive functioning skills (Mansell et al., 2002), and reduce maladaptive behavior(s) where the function is for social positive reinforcement (attention) or automatic positive reinforcement (self-stimulatory behavior; Koritsas et al., 2008). The science-driven instructional strategies coupled with a supportive environment, timely prompts, and appropriate guidance can increase the efficacy of this intervention and improve the overall quality of life for individuals with ASD.

6.5.5.2 Verbal Behavior and Clinical Communication Training

Skinner's (1957) approach to verbal behavior focused on the functional properties of language and proposed that language was a conditioned behavior and is subject to the same principles of conditioning, reinforcement, and punishment. Furthermore, Skinner (1957) termed echoics, mands, tacts, and intraverbals as "elementary verbal operants" that are relevant to teaching language to individuals with ASD. Echoic behavior is defined as instances where verbal behavior is controlled by the verbal stimuli. For example, if a child wants a cookie and the parent states "say please" and the child responds with "please" (echo). Mands include verbal behaviors that are under the control of motivational variables. For example, if a child wants the cookie, they may ask, "May I have a cookie?" The reason for the use of this mand is due to the child's motivation to receive a cookie. Tacts occur when an individual states objects and actions in their environment. For example, if at the beach, a tact would be stating "water" in the presence of the ocean. Lastly, intraverbals are situations where the verbal behavior occurs as a result of other instances of verbal behavior; the verbal stimulus and verbal response do not directly match each other. Responding to a question such as, "What is your favorite food?" by stating "pizza" is an intraverbal behavior.

Verbally restating words spoken by others (echoic) is a fundamental verbal behavior that can support the acquisition of other forms of verbal behavior (Higbee & Sellers, 2011). The primary use of echoic training is to establish more complex verbal operants. Socially appropriate manding provides individuals the opportunity to create change in their environment. Initially in mand training, utilizing the individuals' motivation to obtain a highly desired desired/preferred item (child asking for a cookie from above) is usually implemented. Oftentimes the desired item (cookie jar with cookies in it) is visible and the individual is prompted to request. Much of our communication is tacting objects. In tact training, if an individual has a well-developed echoic repertoire, the instructor/clinician would present the item followed by a tact prompt. Intraverbal training is a more complex; if taught too early (based on the individual's developmental level) it may be problematic (Sundberg, 2007). Intraverbal training should not be employed until echoic, mand, and tact training repertoires have been developed (Sundberg & Partington, 1998). An example of intraverbal training would be if an individual was highly reinforced by a song, the training may be to fill in the word or line after instructor/clinician begins. Since communication across multiple contexts is a core deficit for individuals with ASD, clinical communication training is an important intervention to address this area.

6.5.5.3 Cognitive-Behavioral Therapies

As previously reviewed, CBTs are efficacious for numerous psychiatric disorders and/or clinical issues (marital distress, anger, etc.; see Epp & Dobson, 2010); the foundations of these interventions were previously provided so they will not be elaborated upon in this section. Despite the expansive uses of the CBTs, its use for individuals with ASD in and of themselves is not as efficacious if it is the primary modality for intervention. The use of CBT techniques can be adapted to the ADS population if the clinician does not engage as much on long discussions on its efficacy, but focus on the practical goals of adapting to and coping with various aspects of the world around them (Hare, 2013). Similar to clinicians utilizing adapted CBT interventions for individuals with ID, the adapted uses of CBT techniques for individuals with ASD may be effective if the individual has a comorbid psychiatric disorder. As it relates to ASD, broad ongoing support is favored as opposed to specific "treatment" (CBT) and CBT techniques may be a very small part of the broader psychosocial support system developed (Powell, 2002) with a particular emphasis on behavioral techniques.

6.6 The Impact of Psychopathy on Clinical Interventions for ID or ASD

Following a long period of therapeutic pessimism (e.g., Hare et al., 2000; Lykken, 1995), there is growing interest in determining the interventions that may be most effective when working with individuals with high levels of psychopathic traits (see Blais et al., Chap. 13, this volume; de Ruiter & Hildebrand, Chap. 14, this volume). For example, emphases on the application of the RNR model (Andrews & Bonta, 1994) and on the possibilities of early intervention (e.g., Caldwell, 2011; Salekin et al., 2012) are changing how the antisocial behaviors of psychopathic individuals are conceptualized and addressed. However, it is apparent that individuals with psychopathy traits represent a significant therapeutic challenge. These individuals are more disruptive and noncompliant when in treatment (Hare et al., 2000; Hildebrand & de Ruiter, 2012) and are also more likely to drop out of treatment (e.g., Berger et al., 2012; Hobson et al., 2000; Wong et al., 2012). Thus, no matter what intervention approach is used, clinicians will also need to address these additional challenges.

These issues may be especially relevant when working with individuals who have high levels of psychopathy traits and meet criteria for another clinical disorder. As described above, ABA has demonstrated efficacy for individuals with ASD and ID (Matson et al., 1996; Sturmey, 2014b; Wolery et al., 2005). However, there have not been studies examining treatment for individuals with either ASD and psychopathy traits or ID and psychopathy traits. As a result, it is unclear how the presence psychopathy might impact the efficacy of this – or other—interventions. There is some evidence that the presence of personality disorders could complicate interventions among individuals with ID. For example, among forensic populations, the co-occurrence of ID and a personality disorder is associated with higher security settings (Hogue et al., 2006) and greater likelihood of reoffending and repeat offending (Alexander et al., 2006; Torr, 2008).

In addition to the increased risks that high levels of psychopathy traits may confer on individuals with either ASD or ID, there are also some characteristics of the syndromes that may be relevant when considering how psychopathy traits could impact interventions within these populations. For example, as noted earlier, both ASD and psychopathy are associated with empathy deficits and a well-established literature shows that these deficits are distinguishable, with ASD associated with deficits in perspective-taking and cognitive empathy, and psychopathy traits associated with deficits in affective empathy. When ASD and psychopathy traits co-occur, therefore, that individual would be expected to show deficits in both domains, which would likely affect treatment and management of this group.

Potential similarities in some of the effects of ID and psychopathy are also likely to complicate treatment in a high psychopathy/ID group. ID and psychopathy are both associated with impulsivity, which can also be linked to greater risk for antisocial and criminal behavior. Further, as previously noted, criminal offenders with ID have difficulty with long-term planning and maintaining employment (Salekin et al., 2010), which are also characteristics of individuals with high levels of psychopathy traits. These overlaps can create difficulties in the assessment of these syndromes, and, if both ID and psychopathy are present, may potentially exacerbate these negative behaviors among these individuals.

There is limited research examining the co-occurrence of psychopathy and either ASD or ID and the impacts of co-occurrence on treatment outcomes. However, given evidence that psychopathy is associated with higher rates of in-treatment non-compliance and attrition, that the presence of a personality disorder diagnosis is associated with higher risk among individuals with ID, and that psychopathy confers additional limitations on empathy among individuals with ASD, it is likely that the presence of psychopathy traits will make effective treatment for these individuals more difficult.

6.7 Conclusion

Although there are some limitations, there is a robust literature addressing both the assessment and treatment of ID and ASD. A number of standardized assessment instruments have been developed for use with these groups, and ABA has emerged as a treatment of choice. However, while there is evidence that both ID and ASD are comorbid with other psychiatric conditions, there is only limited research on the overlap between these disorders and psychopathy. Further, in contrast to the treatment literature for ID and ASD, effective treatments for psychopathy have yet to be fully identified. Because the comorbidity of psychopathy and either ID or ASD has only minimally been explored, it is not yet clear what the impacts are of co-occurring psychopathy/ID or psychopathy/ASD on assessment and treatment. Thus, systematic research is recommended in order to (1) learn more about the relationships that exist between each disorder and psychopathy, (2) identify and implement assessment procedures that are sensitive to psychopathy and ID/ASD, (3) develop assessment measures that are sensitive to psychopathy and ID/ASD, and (4) develop and implement clinical interventions to address comorbid psychopathy and ID/ASD.

References

Alexander, R. T., Crouch, K., Halstead, S., & Pichaud, J. (2006). Long-term outcome from a medium secure service for people with ID. *Journal of Intellectual Disability Research, 50*, 305–315.

American Counseling Association. (2014). *2014 American counseling association code of ethics*. Author.

American Psychiatric Association. (2013). *Diagnostic and statistical manual of mental disorders* (5th ed.). Author.

American Psychological Association. (2007). Record keeping guidelines. *American Psychologist, 62*(9), 993–1004. https://doi.org/10.1037/0003-066X.62.9.993

Andrews, D. A., & Bonta, J. (1994). *The psychology of criminal conduct*. Anderson.

Ashwin, C., Baron-Cohen, S., Wheelwright, S., O'Riordan, M., & Bullmore, E. T. (2007). Differential activation of the amygdala and the "social brain" during fearful face-processing in Asperger syndrome. *Neuropsychologia, 45*, 2–14.

Barnard, J., Harvard, V., Potter, D., & Prior, A. (2001). *Ignored or ineligible? The reality for adults with autism spectrum disorders*. The National Autistic Society.

Baron-Cohen, S., & Wheelwright, S. (2004). The empathy quotient: An investigation of adults with Asperger syndrome or high functioning autism and normal sex differences. *Journal of Autism and Developmental Disorders, 34*, 163–175.

Baron-Cohen, S., Leslie, A. M., & Frith, U. (1985). Does the autistic child have a "theory of mind"? *Cognition, 21*, 37–46.

Baron-Cohen, S., Wheelwright, S., Skinner, R., Martin, J., & Clubley, E. (2001). The autism spectrum quotient (AQ): Evidence from Asperger syndrome/high functioning autism, males and females, scientists and mathematicians. *Journal of Autism and Developmental Disorders, 31*, 5–17.

Beadle-Brown, Julie, Hutchinson, Aislinn, Whelton, Beckie (2012) Person-Centred Active Support-Increasing Choice, Promoting Independence and Reducing Challenging Behaviour. *Journal of Applied Research in Intellectual Disabilities, 25*(4). pp. 291–307. ISSN 1360-2322. https://doi.org/10.1111/j.1468-3148.2011.00666.x

Beadle-Brown, J., & Hutchinson, A. (2016). Person-centered active support; The cake not the icing. In A. Carr, C. Linehan, G. O'Reilly, P. Noonan-Walsh, & J. McEvoy (Eds.), *The handbook of intellectual disability and clinical psychology practice* (2nd ed., pp. 211–239). Routledge.

Beck, A. T. (1993). *Beck anxiety inventory*. Pearson.

Beck, A. T., Ward, C. H., Mendelson, M., Mock, J., & Erbaugh, J. (1961). An inventory for measuring depression. *Archives of General Psychiatry, 4*, 561–571. https://doi.org/10.1001/archpsyc.1961.01710120031004

Behavior Analyst Certification Board. (2014). *Professional and ethical compliance code for behavior analysts*. Author.

Bellack, A. S., & Hersen, M. (1998). *Behavioral assessment: A practical handbook* (4th ed.). Allyn & Bacon.

Benson, B. A., & Brooks, W. T. (2008). Aggressive challenging behaviour and intellectual disability. *Current Opinion in Psychiatry, 21*(5), 454–458. https://doi.org/10.1097/YCO.0b013e328306a090

Berger, K., Rotermund, P., Vieth, E. R., & Hohnhorst, A. (2012). The prognostic value of the PCL-R in relation to the SUD treatment ending. *International Journal of Law and Psychiatry, 35*, 198–201.

Berkowitz, L., Lepinski, J. P., & Argulo, E. J. (1969). Awareness of own anger level and subsequent aggression. *Journal of Personality and Social Psychology, 11*, 293–300. https://doi.org/10.1037/h0027037

Bird, G., & Cook, R. (2013). Mixed emotions: The contribution of alexithymia to the emotional symptoms of autism. *Translational Psychiatry, 3*, e285. https://doi.org/10.1038/tp.2013.61

Bjorkly, S. (2009). Risk and dynamics of violence in Asperger's syndrome: A systematic review of the literature. *Aggression and Violent Behavior, 14*(5), 306–312. https://doi.org/10.1016/j.avb.2009.04.003

Blair, R. J. R. (1999). Psychophysiological responsiveness to the distress of others in children with autism. *Personality and Individual Differences, 26*, 477–485.

Blair, R. J. R. (2005). Responding to the emotions of others: Dissociating forms of empathy through the study of typical and psychiatric populations. *Consciousness and Cognition, 14*, 698–718.

Blair, R. J. R. (2008). Fine cuts of empathy and the amygdala: Dissociable deficits in psychopathy and autism. *The Quarterly Journal of Experimental Psychology, 61*, 157–170.

Blair, R. J. R., Sellars, C., Strickland, I., Clark, F., Williams, A., Smith, M., et al. (1996). Theory of mind in the psychopath. *Journal of Forensic Psychiatry, 7*, 15–25.

Blair, R. J., Jones, L., Clark, F., & Smith, M. (1997). The psychopathic individual: A lack of responsiveness to distress cues? *Psychophysiology, 34*, 192–198.

Blair, K. C., Umbreit, J., & Bos, C. S. (1999). Using functional assessment and children's preferences to improve the behavior of young children with behavioral disorders. *Behavioral Disorders, 24*(2), 151–166. https://doi.org/10.1177/019874299902400202

Blair, R., Colledge, E., Murray, L., & Mitchell, D. (2001). A selective impairment in the processing of sad and fearful expressions in children with psychopathic tendencies. *Journal of Abnormal Child Psychology, 29*, 491–498.

Blair, R. J. R., Meffert, H., Hwang, S., & White, S. F. (2018). Psychopathy and brain function: A review of brain imaging findings. In C. J. Patrick (Ed.), *Handbook of psychopathy* (2nd ed., pp. 401–421). The Guilford Press.

Bolton, P. F., & Rutter, M. (1994). *Schedule for assessment of psychiatric problems associated with autism (and other developmental disorders)*. University of Cambridge.

Boyle, C. A., Boulet, S., Schieve, L. A., Cohen, R. A., Blumberg, S. J., Yeargin-Allsopp, M., Visser, S., & Kogan, M. D. (2011). Trends in the prevalence of developmental disabilities in US children, 1997-2008. *Pediatrics, 127*(6), 1034–1042. https://doi.org/10.1542/peds.2010-2989

Bradley, E., & Bolton, P. (2006). Episodic psychiatric disorders in teenagers with learning disabilities with and without autism. *British Journal of Psychiatry, 189*, 361–366. https://doi.org/10.1192/bjp.bp.105.018127

Bradley, E. A., Summers, J. A., Wood, H. L., & Bryson, S. E. (2004). Comparing rates of psychiatric and behavior disorders in adolescents and young adults with severe intellectual disability with and without autism. *Journal of Autism and Developmental Disorders, 34*(2), 151–161. https://doi.org/10.1023/b:jadd.0000022606.97580.19

Brewer, N., Zoanetti, J., & Young, R. L. (2017). The influence of media suggestions about links between criminality and autism spectrum disorder. *Autism, 21*(1), 117–121. https://doi.org/10.1177/1362361316632097

Caldwell, M. F. (2011). Treatment-related changes in behavioral outcomes of psychopathy facets in adolescent offenders. *Law and Human Behavior, 35*, 275–287.

Carr, A., & O'Reilly, G. (2016). Consultation, interviewing, and report writing. In A. Carr, C. Linehan, G. O'Reilly, P. Noonan-Walsh, & J. McEvoy (Eds.), *The handbook of intellectual disability and clinical psychology practice* (2nd ed., pp. 161–207). Routledge.

Cederlund, M., Hagberg, B., Billstedt, E., Gillberg, C., & Gillberg, C. (2008). Asperger syndrome and autism: A comparative longitudinal follow-up study more than 5 years after original diagnosis. *Journal of Autism and Developmental Disorders, 38*(1), 72–85. https://doi.org/10.1007/s10803-007-0364-6

Centers for Disease Control and Prevention. (2020). *Autism and developmental disabilities monitoring (ADDM) network*. Retrieved from https://www.cdc.gov/ncbddd/autism/addm.html

Cleckley, H. (1941/1996). *The mask of sanity*. Mosby.

Cooper, S., & van der Speck, R. (2009). Epidemiology of mental ill health in adults with intellectual disability. *Current Opinion in Psychiatry, 22*(5), 431–439. https://doi.org/10.1097/YCO.0b013e32832e2a1e

Cooper, S., Smiley, E., Morrison, J., Williamson, A., & Allan, L. (2007). Mental ill-health in adults with intellectual disabilities: Prevalence and associated factors. *British Journal of Psychiatry, 190*, 27–35. https://doi.org/10.1192/bjp.bp.106.022483

Cooper, J. O., Heron, T. E., & Heward, W. L. (2020). *Applied behavior analysis* (3rd ed.). Pearson Education.

Cox, C. L., Uddin, L. Q., Di Martino, A., Castellanos, F. X., Milham, M. P., & Kelly, C. (2012). The balance between feeling and knowing: Affective and cognitive empathy are reflected in the brain's intrinsic functional dynamics. *Social Cognitive and Affective Neuroscience, 7*, 727–737.

Crego, C., & Widiger, T. A. (2015). Psychopathy, DSM-5, and a caution. *Personality Disorders: Theory, Research, and Treatment, 5*, 335–347.

Dagnan, D. (2007). Psychosocial interventions for people with intellectual disabilities and mental ill-health. *Current Opinion in Psychiatry, 20*(5), 456–460. https://doi.org/10.1097/YCO.0b013e3282ab9963

Dargis, M., Wolf, R. C., & Koenigs, M. (2018). Psychopathic traits are associated with reduced fixations to the eye region of fearful faces. *Journal of Abnormal Psychology, 127*(1), 43–50.

Davis, M. H. (1983). Measuring individual differences in empathy: Evidence for a multidimensional approach. *Journal of Personality and Social Psychology, 44*, 113–126.

Davis, N. O., & Kollins, S. H. (2012). Treatment for co-occurring attention-deficit/hyperactivity disorder and autism spectrum disorder. *Neurotherapeutics, 9*(3), 518–530. https://doi.org/10.1007/s13311-012-0126-9

de Tribolet-Hardy, F., Vohs, K., Mokros, A., & Habermeyer, E. (2014). Psychopathy, intelligence, and impulsivity in German violent offenders. *International Journal of Law and Psychiatry, 37*, 238–244.

Decety, J., Skelly, L. R., & Kiehl, K. A. (2013). Brain response to empathy-eliciting scenarios involving pain in incarcerated individuals with psychopathy. *JAMA Psychiatry, 70*, 638–645.

Didden, R., Braam, W., Maas, A., Smits, M., Sturmey, P., Sigafoos, J., & Curfs, L. (2014). Sleep problems. In P. Sturmey & R. Didden (Eds.), *Evidence-based practice and intellectual disabilities* (pp. 219–234). Wiley.

Dobson, K. S., & Dozois, D. J. A. (2010). Historical and philosophical bases of the cognitive-behavioral therapies. In K. S. Dobson (Ed.), *Handbook of cognitive-behavioral therapies* (3rd ed., pp. 3–38). The Guilford Press.

Domes, G., Hollerbach, P., Vohs, K., Mokros, A., & Habermeyer, E. (2013). Emotional empathy and psychopathy in offenders: An experimental study. *Journal of Personality Disorders, 27*, 67–84.

Dziobek, I., Rogers, K., Fleck, S., Bahnemann, M., Heekeren, H. R., Wolf, O. T., & Convit, A. (2008). Dissociation of cognitive and emotional empathy in adults with Asperger syndrome using the multifaceted empathy test (MET). *Journal of Autism and Developmental Disorders, 38*, 464–473.

Ellis, J. W. (2003). Mental retardation and the death penalty: A guide to state legislative issues. *Mental and Physical Disability Law Reporter, 27*(1), 11–24.

Emerson, E., & Hatton, C. (2007). Mental health of children and adolescents with intellectual disabilities in Britain. *British Journal of Psychiatry, 191*, 493–499. https://doi.org/10.1192/bjp.bp.107.038729

Emerson, E., Kiernan, C., Alborz, A., & Reeves, D. (2001). The prevalence of challenging behaviors: A total population study. *Research in Developmental Disabilities, 22*(1), 77–93. https://doi.org/10.1016/S0891-4222(00)00061-5

Epp, A. M., & Dobson, K. S. (2010). The evidence base for cognitive-behavioral therapy. In K. S. Dobson (Ed.), *Handbook of cognitive-behavioral therapies* (3rd ed., pp. 39–73). The Guilford Press.

Ermer, E., Kahn, R. E., Salovey, P., & Kiehl, K. A. (2012). Emotional intelligence in incarcerated men with psychopathic traits. *Journal of Personality and Social Psychology, 103*(1), 194–204.

Everington, C., & Olley, J. G. (2008). Implications of *Atkins v. Virginia:* Issues in defining and diagnosing mental retardation. *Journal of Forensic Psychology Practice, 8*(1), 1–23. https://doi.org/10.1080/15228930801947278

Fan, Y. T., Chen, C., Chen, S. C., Decety, J., & Cheng, Y. (2014). Empathic arousal and social understanding in individuals with autism: Evidence from fMRI and ERP measurements. *Social and Cognitive Affective Neuroscience, 9*, 1203–1213.

Forth, A. E., Hart, S. D., & Hare, R. D. (1990). Assessment of psychopathy in male young offenders. *Psychological Assessment: A Journal of Consulting and Clinical Psychology, 2*, 342–344.

Forth, A. E., Kosson, D. S., & Hare, R. D. (2003). *The psychopathy checklist: Youth version*. Multi-Health Systems.

Frick, P. J., & Hare, R. D. (2001). *The antisocial process screening device*. Multi-Health Systems.

Frith, U., & Happé, F. (2005). Autism spectrum disorder. *Current Biology, 15*, 786–790.

Gardner, B. O., Boccaccini, M. T., & Murrie, D. C. (2018). Which PCL-R scores best predict forensic clinicians' opinions of offender risk? *Criminal Justice and Behavior, 45*, 1404–1419.

Gerhardt, P. F., Garcia, M. F., & Foglia, A. (2014). Skill-building interventions for adolescents and adults with autism spectrum disorders. In M. Tincani & A. Bondy (Eds.), *Autism spectrum disorders in adolescents and adults: Evidence-based and promising interventions* (pp. 164–181). The Guilford Press.

Ghaziuddin, M. (2005). *Mental health aspects of autism and Asperger syndrome*. Jessica Kingsley Publishers.

Gillespie, S. M., McCleery, J. P., & Oberman, L. M. (2014). Spontaneous versus deliberate vicarious representations: Different routes to empathy in psychopathy and autism. *Brain, 137*, 1–3.

Goodman, W. K., Price, L. H., Rasmussen, S. A., Mazure, C., Fleischman, R. L., Hill, C. L., Heninger, G. R., & Charney, D. S. (1989). The Yale-Brown obsessive compulsive scale. *Archives of General Psychiatry, 46*(11), 1006–1111. https://doi.org/10.1001/archpsyc.1989.01810110048007

Goodwin, M. S., Groden, J., Velicer, W. F., & Diller, A. (2007). Brief report: Validating the stress survey schedule for persons with autism and other developmental disabilities. *Focus on Autism and Other Developmental Disabilities, 22*(3), 183–189. https://doi.org/10.1177/10883576070220030501

Gravestock, J. (2000). Eating disorders in adults with intellectual disability. *Journal of Intellectual Disability Research, 44*(6), 625–637. https://doi.org/10.1046/j.1365-2788.2000.00308.x

Gray, N., Weidacker, K., & Snowden, R. J. (2019). Psychopathy and impulsivity: The relationship of psychopathy to different aspects of UPPS-P impulsivity. *Psychiatry Research, 272*, 474–482.

Groden, J., Diller, A., Bausman, M., Velicer, W., Norman, G., & Cautela, J. (2001). The development of a stress survey schedule for persons with autism and other developmental disabilities. *Journal of Autism and Developmental Disorders, 31*(2), 207–217. https://doi.org/10.1023/a:1010755300436

Hansen, A. L., Johnsen, B. H., Hart, S., Waage, L., & Thayer, J. F. (2008). Brief communication: Psychopathy and recognition of facial expressions of emotion. *Journal of Personality Disorders, 22*(6), 639–644.

Hare, R. D. (1991). *Manual for the Hare psychopathy checklist–revised* (1st ed.). Multi-Health Systems.

Hare, R. D. (1996). Psychopathy: A clinical construct whose time has come. *Criminal Justice and Behavior, 23*, 25–54.

Hare, D. J. (2013). Developing psychotherapeutic interventions for people with autism spectrum disorders. In J. L. Taylor, W. R. Lindsay, R. P. Hastings, & C. Hatton (Eds.), *Psychological therapies for adults with intellectual disabilities* (pp. 193–206). John Wiley & Sons, Ltd.

Hare, R. D., & Hart, S. D. (1993). Psychopathy, mental disorder, and crime. In S. Hodgins (Ed.), *Mental disorder and crime* (pp. 104–115). Sage Publications.

Hare, R. D., & Neumann, C. S. (2008). Psychopathy as a clinical and empirical construct. *Annual Review of Clinical Psychology, 4*, 217–246.

Hare, R. D., Clark, D., Grann, M., & Thornton, D. (2000). Psychopathy and the predictive validity of the PCL-R: An international perspective. *Behavioral Sciences & the Law, 18*, 623–645.

Hare, R. D., Neumann, C. S., & Mokros, A. (2018). The PCL-R assessment of psychopathy: Development, properties, debates, and new directions. In C. J. Patrick (Ed.), *Handbook of psychopathy* (2nd ed., pp. 39–79). The Guilford Press.

Hatton, C., & Emerson, E. (2004). The relationship between life events and psychopathology amongst children with intellectual disabilities. *Journal of Applied Research in Intellectual Disabilities, 17*, 109–117.

Helverschou, S. B., Bakken, T. L., & Martinsen, H. (2009). The psychopathology in autism checklist (PAC): A pilot study. *Research in Autism Spectrum Disorders, 3*(1), 179–195. https://doi.org/10.1016/j.rasd.2008.05.004

Helverschou, S. B., Bakken, T. L., & Martinsen, H. (2011). Psychiatric disorders in people with autism spectrum disorders: Phenomenology and recognition. In J. L. Matson & P. Sturmey (Eds.), *International handbook of autism and pervasive developmental disorders* (pp. 53–76). Springer.

Hemphill, J. F., Templeman, R., Wong, S., & Hare, R. D. (1998). Psychopathy and crime: Recidivism and criminal careers. In D. J. Cooke, R. D. Hare, & A. Forth (Eds.), *Psychopathy: Theory, research and implications for society* (pp. 375–399). Kluwer Academic Publishers.

Herba, C., Sheilagh, H., Blackwood, N., Kumari, V., Naudts, K., & Phillips, M. (2007). The neurobiology of psychopathy: A focus on emotion processing. In H. Hervé & J. C. Yuille (Eds.), *The psychopath: Theory, research, and practice* (pp. 253–283). Lawrence Erlbaum Associates Publishers.

Herve, H., Mitchell, D., & Cooper, B. S. (2004). Psychopathy and unlawful confinement: An examination of perpetrator and event characteristics. *Canadian Journal of Behavioural Science, 36*, 137–145.

Hiatt, K. D., Schmitt, W. A., & Newman, J. P. (2004). Stroop tasks reveal abnormal selective attention among psychopathic offenders. *Neuropsychology, 18*, 50–59.

Higbee, T. S., & Sellers, T. P. (2011). Verbal behavior and communication training. In J. L. Matson & P. Sturmey (Eds.), *International handbook of autism and pervasive developmental disorders* (pp. 367–379). Springer.

Hildebrand, M., & de Ruiter, C. (2012). Psychopathic traits and change on indicators of dynamic risk factors during inpatient forensic psychiatric treatment. *International Journal of Law & Psychiatry, 35*, 276–288.

Ho, H., Perry, A., & Koudys, J. (2020). A systematic review of behaviour analytic interventions for young children with intellectual disabilities. *Journal of Intellectual Disability Research, 65*(1), 11–31. https://doi.org/10.1111/jir.12780

Hobson, J., Shine, J., & Roberts, R. (2000). How do psychopaths behave in a prison therapeutic community? *Psychology, Crime and Law, 6*, 139–154.

Hogue, T., Steptoe, L., Taylor, J. L., Lindsay, W. R., Mooney, P., Pinkney, L., Johnston, S., Smith, A. H. W., & O'Brien, G. (2006). A comparison of offenders with intellectual disability across three levels of security. *Criminal Behavior and Mental Health, 16*, 13–28.

Hollins, S. (2003). Counselling and psychotherapy. In W. Fraser & M. Kerr (Eds.), *Seminars in the psychiatry of learning disabilities* (pp. 186–200). Gaskell.

Hollins, S., & Sinason, V. (2000). Psychotherapy, learning disabilities and trauma: New perspectives. *British Journal of Psychiatry, 176*(1), 32–36. https://doi.org/10.1192/bjp.176.1.32

Horner, R. H. (1994). Functional assessment: Contributions and future directions. *Journal of Applied Behavior Analysis, 27*(2), 401–404. https://doi.org/10.1901/jaba.1994.27-401

Howlin, P. (2000). Outcome in adult life for more able individuals with autism or Asperger syndrome. *Autism, 4*(1), 63–83. https://doi.org/10.1177/1362361300004001005

Howlin, P. (2002). Autistic disorders. In P. Howlin & O. Udwin (Eds.), *Outcomes in neurodevelopmental and genetic disorders* (pp. 136–168). Cambridge University Press.

Hudry, K., & Slaughter, V. (2009). Agent familiarity and emotional context influence the everyday empathic responding of young children with autism. *Research in Autism Spectrum Disorders, 3*, 74–85.

Hutton, J., Goode, S., Murphy, M., Couteur, A. L., & Rutter, M. (2008). New-onset psychiatric disorders in individuals with autism. *Autism, 12*(4), 373–390. https://doi.org/10.1177/1362361308091650

Jeandarme, I., Pouls, C., Oei, T. I., & Bogaerts, S. (2017). Forensic psychiatric patients with comorbid psychopathy: Double trouble? *The International Journal of Forensic Mental Health, 16*, 149–160.

Jones, R. S. P., & Dowey, A. (2013). Behavioral approaches to working with mental health problems. In J. L. Taylor, W. R. Lindsay, R. P. Hastings, & C. Hatton (Eds.), *Psychological therapies for adults with intellectual disabilities* (pp. 223–236). John Wiley & Sons, Ltd..

Jones, A. P., Larsson, H., Ronald, A., Rijsdijk, F., Busfield, P., McMillan, A., Plomin, R., & Viding, E. (2009a). Phenotypic and aetiological associations between psychopathic tendencies, autistic traits, and emotion attribution. *Criminal Justice and Behavior, 36*, 1198–1212.

Jones, A. P., Laurens, K., Herba, C., Barker, G., & Viding, E. (2009b). Amygdala hypoactivity to fearful faces in boys with conduct problems and callous-unemotional traits. *American Journal of Psychiatry, 166*, 95–102.

Jones, A. P., Happé, F. G., Gilbert, F., Burnett, S., & Viding, E. (2010). Feeling, caring, knowing: Different types of empathy deficit in boys with psychopathic tendencies and autism spectrum disorder. *Journal of Child Psychology and Psychiatry, 51*, 1188–1197.

Jopp, D. A., & Keys, C. B. (2001). Diagnostic overshadowing reviewed and reconsidered. *American Journal on Mental Retardation, 106*(5), 416–433. https://doi.org/10.1352/0895-8017(2001)106<0416:DORAR>2.0.CO;2

Karpman, B. (1941). On the need of separating psychopathy into two distinct clinical types: The symptomatic and the idiopathic. *Journal of Criminology and Psychopathology, 3*, 112–137.

King, B., Toth, K., Hodapp, R., & Dykens, E. (2009). Intellectual disability. In B. J. Sadock, V. A. Sadock, & P. Ruiz (Eds.), *Comprehensive textbook of psychiatry* (9th ed., pp. 3444–3474). Lippincott Williams & Wilkins.

Koritsas, S., Iacono, T., Hamilton, D., & Leighton, D. (2008). The effect of active support training on engagement, opportunities for choice, challenging behavior and support needs. *Journal of Intellectual and Developmental Disability, 33*(3), 247–256. https://doi.org/10.1080/13668250802282944

Kosson, D. S., Suchy, Y., Mayer, A. R., & Libby, J. (2002). Facial affect recognition in criminal psychopaths. *Emotion, 2*, 398–411.

Lecavalier, L., Snow, A. V., & Norris, M. (2011). Autism spectrum disorders and intellectual disability. In J. L. Matson & P. Sturmey (Eds.), *International handbook of autism and pervasive developmental disorders* (pp. 37–52). Springer.

Leitner, Y. (2014). The co-occurrence of autism and attention deficit hyperactivity disorder in children- What do we know? *Frontiers in Human Neuroscience, 8*, 268. https://doi.org/10.3389/fnhum.2014.00268

Lerner, M. D., Haque, O. S., Northrup, E. C., Lawer, L., & Bursztajn, H. J. (2012). Emerging perspectives on adolescents and young adults with high-functioning autism spectrum disorders, violence, and criminal law. *Journal of the American Academy of Psychiatry and the Law, 40*(2), 177–190.

Leyfer, O. T., Folstein, S. E., Bacalman, S., Davis, N. O., Dinh, E., Morgan, J., Tager-Flusberg, H., & Lainhart, J. E. (2006). Comorbid psychiatric disorders in children with autism: Interview development and rates of disorders. *Journal of Autism and Developmental Disorders, 36*(7), 849–861. https://doi.org/10.1007/s10803-006-0123-0

Lilienfeld, S. O., & Andrews, B. P. (1996). Development and preliminary validation of a self- report measure of psychopathic personality traits in noncriminal populations. *Journal of Personality Assessment, 66*, 488–524.

Lilienfeld, S. O., & Hess, T. (2001). Psychopathic personality traits and somatization: Sex differences and the mediating role of negative emotionality. *Journal of Psychopathology and Behavioral Assessment, 23*, 11–24.

Lindsay, W. R., Jahoda, A. J., & Willner, P. (2013). Adapting psychological therapies for people with intellectual disabilities II: Treatment approaches and modifications. In J. L. Taylor, W. R. Lindsay, R. P. Hastings, & C. Hatton (Eds.), *Psychological therapies for adults with intellectual disabilities* (pp. 85–100). John Wiley & Sons, Ltd.

Lockwood, P. L. (2016). The anatomy of empathy: Vicarious experience and disorders of social cognition. *Behavioral Brain Research, 311*, 255–268.

Lockwood, P. L., Bird, G., Bridge, M., & Viding, E. (2013a). Dissecting empathy: High levels of psychopathic and autistic traits are characterized by difficulties indifferent social information processing domains. *Frontiers in Human Neuroscience, 7*, 1–6.

Lockwood, P. L., Sebastian, C. L., McCrory, E. J., Hyde, Z. H., Gu, X., De Brito, S. A., & Viding, E. (2013b). Association of callous traits with reduced neural response to others' pain in children with conduct problems. *Current Biology, 23*, 901–905.

Lykken, D. T. (1995). *The antisocial personalities*. Erlbaum.

Macvaugh, G. S. & Cunningham, M. D. (2009). *Atkins v. Virginia:* Implications and recommendations for forensic practice. *The Journal of Psychiatry & Law, 37*(2–3), 131–187. https://doi.org/10.1177/009318530903700203

Mahoney, M. J., & Arnkoff, D. B. (1978). Cognitive and self-control therapies. In S. L. Garfield & A. E. Bergin (Eds.), *Handbook of psychotherapy and behavior change: An empirical analysis* (pp. 689–722). Wiley.

Mannynsalo, L., Putkonen, H., Lindberg, N., & Kotilainen, I. (2009). Forensic psychiatric perspective on criminality associated with intellectual disability: A nationwide register-based study. *Journal of Intellectual and Developmental Disability Research, 53*(3), 279–288. https://doi.org/10.1111/j.1365-2788.2008.01125.x

Mansell, Jim, Elliott, Teresa, Beadle-Brown, Julie, Ashman, Bev, Macdonald, Susan (2002) Engagement in meaningful activity and 'active support' of people with intellectual disabilities in residential care. *Research in Developmental Disabilities, 23*(5). 342–352. ISSN 0891-4222. https://doi.org/10.1016/S0891-4222(02)00135-X

Mansell, J., Beadle-Brown, J., Ashman, B., & Ockenden, J. (2005). *Person-centred active support: A multimedia training resource for staff to enable participation, inclusion and choice for people with learning disabilities*. Pavilion.

Mansell, J., Beadle-Brown, J., & Bigby, C. (2013). Implementation of active support in Victoria, Australia: An exploratory study. *Journal of Intellectual and Developmental Disability, 38*(1), 48–58. https://doi.org/10.3109/13668250.2012.753996

Maras, K., Mulcahy, S., & Crane, L. (2015). Is autism linked to criminality? *Autism, 19*(5), 515–516. https://doi.org/10.1177/1362361315583411

Matson, J. L., & Boisjoli, J. A. (2008). Autism spectrum disorders in adults with intellectual disability and comorbid psychopathology: Scale development and reliability of the ASD-CA. *Research in Autism Spectrum Disorders, 2*(2), 276–287. https://doi.org/10.1016/j.rasd.2007.07.002

Matson, J. L., & Wilkins, J. (2008). Reliability of the autism spectrum disorders- comorbid for children (ASD-CC). *Journal of Developmental and Physical Disabilities, 20*, 327–336. https://doi.org/10.1007/s10882-008-9100-1

Matson, J. L., Benavidez, D. A., Compton, L. S., Paclawskyj, T., & Baglio, C. (1996). Behavioral treatment of autistic persons: A review of research from 1980 to the present. *Research in Developmental Disabilities, 17*(6), 433–465. https://doi.org/10.1016/s0891-4222(96)00030-3

Matson, J. L., LoVullo, S. V., Rivet, T. T., & Boisjoli, J. A. (2009). Validity of the autism spectrum disorder- comorbid for children (ASD-CC). *Research in Autism Spectrum Disorders, 3*(2), 345–357. https://doi.org/10.1016/j.rasd.2008.08.002

Maulik, P. K., Mascarenhas, M. N., Mathers, C. D., Dua, T., & Saxena, S. (2013). Prevalence of intellectual disability: A meta-analysis of population-based studies. *Research in Developmental Disabilities, 32*(2), 419–436. https://doi.org/10.1016/j.ridd.2010.12.018

Meffert, H., Gazzola, V., den Boer, J. A., Bartels, A. A., & Keysers, C. (2013). Reduced spontaneous but relatively normal deliberate vicarious representations in psychopathy. *Brain, 136*, 2550–2562.

Megargee, E. (1966). Undercontrolled and overcontrolled personality types in extreme antisocial aggression. *Psychological Monographs, 80*, 1–29. https://doi.org/10.1037/h0093894

Melville, C. A., Cooper, S., Morrison, J., Smiley, E., Allan, L., Jackson, A., Finlayson, J., & Mantry, D. (2008). The prevalence and incidence of mental ill-health in adults with autism and intellectual disabilities. *Journal of Autism and Developmental Disorders, 38*(9), 1676–1688. https://doi.org/10.1007/s10803-008-0549-7

Mohr, C., & Costello, H. (2007). Mental health assessment and monitoring tools for people with intellectual disabilities. In N. Bouras & G. Holt (Eds.), *Psychiatric and behavioural disorders in intellectual and developmental disabilities* (2nd ed., pp. 24–41). Cambridge University Press.

Morrissey, C., & Hollin, C. (2011). Antisocial and psychopathic personality disorders in forensic intellectual disability populations: What do we know so far? *Psychology, Crime, & Law, 17*, 133–149.

Morrissey, C., Cooke, D., Michie, C., Hollin, C., Hogue, T., Lindsay, W. R., & Taylor, J. L. (2010). Structural, item, and test generalizability of the psychopathy checklist-revised to offenders with intellectual disabilities. *Assessment, 17*, 16–29.

Nemiah, J. C., Freyberger, H., & Sifneos, P. E. (1976). Alexithymia: A view of the psychosomatic process. In O. W. Hill (Ed.), *Modern trends in psychosomatic medicine* (pp. 430–439). Butterworths.

Netten, A., Beadle-Brown, J., Trukeschitz, B., Towers, A., Welch, E., Forder, J., et al. (2010). *Measuring the outcomes of care homes: Final report*. Personal Social Services Research Unit.

Newman, J. P., Schmitt, W. A., & Voss, W. (1997). Processing of contextual cues in psychopathic and nonpsychopathic offenders. *Journal of Abnormal Psychology, 106*, 563–575.

O'Nions, E., Tick, B., Rijsdijk, F., Happé, F., Plomin, R., Ronald, A., et al. (2015). Examining the genetic and environmental associations between autistic social and communication deficits and psychopathic callous-unemotional traits. *PLoS One, 10*, e0134331. https://doi.org/10.1371/journal.pone.0134331

O'Reilly, M., Gevarter, C., Falcomata, T., Sigafoos, J., & Lancioni, G. E. (2016). Applied behavior analysis and positive behaviour supports. In A. Carr, C. Linehan, G. O'Reilly, P. Noonan-Walsh, & J. McEvoy (Eds.), *The handbook of intellectual disability and clinical psychology practice* (2nd ed., pp. 241–263). Routledge.

Oberman, L. M., Ramachandran, V. S., & Pineda, J. A. (2008). Modulation of mu suppression in children with autism spectrum disorders in response to familiar or unfamiliar stimuli: The mirror neuron hypothesis. *Neuropsychologia, 46*, 1558–1565.

Oliver, B. R., & Plomin, R. (2007). Twins' Early Development Study (TEDS): Amultivariate, longitudinal genetic investigation of language, cognition and behavior problems from childhood through adolescence. *Twin Research and Human Genetics, 10*, 96–105.

Oliver, L. D., Neufeld, R. W. J., Dziobek, I., & Mitchel, D. G. V. (2016). Distinguishing the relationship between different aspects of empathic responding as a function of psychopathic, autistic, and anxious traits. *Personality and Individual Differences, 99*, 81–88.

Patil, I., & Silani, G. (2014). Reduced empathic concern leads to utilitarian moral judgments in trait alexithymia. *Frontiers in Psychology, 5*, 1–12.

Patrick, C. J., Bradley, M. M., & Lang, P. J. (1993). Emotion in the criminal psychopath: Startle reflex modulation. *Journal of Abnormal Psychology, 102*, 82–92.

Pauli, M., Liljeberg, J., Gustavsson, P., Kristiansson, M., & Howner, K. (2019). Assessing the relevance of self-reported ADHD symptoms and cognitive functioning for psychopathy using the PCL-R and the TriPM. *The Journal of Forensic Psychiatry & Psychology, 30*(4), 642–657.

Peters, E. R., Joseph, S. A., & Garety, P. A. (1999). Measurement of delusional ideation in the normal population: Introducing the PDI (Peters et al. Delusions inventory). *Schizophrenia Bulletin, 25*(3), 553–576. https://doi.org/10.1093/oxfordjournals.schbul.a033401

Petersilia, J. (2000). *Doing justice? The criminal justice system and offenders with developmental disabilities*. University of California, Berkeley, California Policy Research Center.

Pierce, K., & Redcay, E. (2008). Fusiform function in children with an autism spectrum disorder is a matter of 'who'. *Biological Psychiatry, 64*, 552–560.

Powell, A. (2002). *Taking responsibility: Good practice guidelines for services-adults with asperger syndrome*. The National Autistic Society.

Rao, P. A., & Landa, R. J. (2014). Association between severity of behavioral phenotype and comorbid attention deficit hyperactivity disorder symptoms in children with autism spectrum disorders. *Autism, 18*(3), 272–280. https://doi.org/10.1177/1362361312470494

Rayner, K., Wood, H., Beail, N., & Nagra, M. K. (2015). Intellectual disability, personality disorder and offending: A systematic review. *Advances in Mental Health and Intellectual Disabilities, 9*, 50–61.

Raznahan, A., Joinson, C., O'Callaghan, F., Osborne, J. P., & Bolton, P. F. (2006). Psychopathology in tuberous sclerosis: An overview and findings in a population-based sample of adults with tuberous sclerosis. *Journal of Intellectual Disability Research, 50*(Pt 8), 561–569. https://doi.org/10.1111/j.1365-2788.2006.00828.x

Richards, H., Casey, J., & Lucente, S. (2003). Psychopathy and treatment response in incarcerated female substance abusers. *Criminal Justice and Behavior, 30*, 251–276.

Robitaille, M.-P., Checknita, D., Vitaro, F., Tremblay, R. E., Paris, J., & Hodgins, S. (2017). A prospective, longitudinal, study of men with borderline personality disorder with and without comorbid anti-social personality disorder. *Borderline Personality Disorder and Emotion Dysregulation, 4*, 25. https://doi.org/10.1186/s40479-017-0076-2

Rogers, J., Viding, E., Blair, R. J. R., Frith, U., & Happé, F. (2006). Autism spectrum disorder and psychopathy: Shared cognitive underpinnings or double hit? *Psychological Medicine, 36*, 1789–1798.

Romero, M., Aguilar, J. M., Del-Rey-Mejìas, A., Mayoral, F., Rapado, M., Peciña, M., Barbancho, M. A., Ruiz-Veguilla, M., & Lara, J. P. (2016). Psychiatric comorbidities in autism spectrum disorder: A comparative study between DSM-IV-TR and DSM-5 diagnosis. *International*

Journal of Clinical and Health Psychology, 16(3), 266–275. https://doi.org/10.1016/j.ijchp.2016.03.001

Salekin, R. T., Rogers, R., & Sewell, K. W. (1997). Construct validity of psychopathy in a female offender sample: A multitrait-multimethod evaluation. *Journal of Abnormal Psychology, 106*, 576–585.

Salekin, R. T., Rogers, R., Ustad, K. L., & Sewell, K. W. (1998). Psychopathy and recidivism among female inmates. *Law and Human Behavior, 22*, 109–128.

Salekin, R. T., Neumann, C. S., Leistico, A. R., & Zalot, A. A. (2004). Psychopathy in youth and intelligence: An investigation of Cleckley's hypothesis. *Journal of Clinical Child and Adolescent Psychology, 33*, 731–742.

Salekin, K. L., Olley, J. G., & Hedge, K. A. (2010). Offenders with intellectual disability: Characteristics, prevalence, and issues in forensic assessment. *Journal of Mental Health Research in Intellectual Disabilities, 3*, 97–116. https://doi.org/10.1080/19315861003695769

Salekin, R. T., Tippey, J. G., & Allen, A. D. (2012). Treatment of conduct problem youth with interpersonal callous traits using mental models: Measurement of risk and change. *Behavioral Sciences & the Law, 30*, 470–486.

Salekin, R. T., Andershed, A., Batky, B. D., & Bontemps, A. P. (2018). Are callous unemotional (CU) traits enough? *Journal of Psychopathology and Behavioral Assessment, 40*, 1–5.

Sawa, A., & Kamiya, A. (2003). Elucidating the pathogenesis of schizophrenia. *British Medical Journal, 327*(7416), 632–633. https://doi.org/10.1136/bmj.327.7416.632

Sellbom, M., Cooke, D. J., & Shou, Y. (2019). Development and initial validation of the comprehensive assessment of psychopathic personality-self-report (CAPP-SR). *Psychological Assessment, 31*, 878–894. https://doi.org/10.1037/pas0000714

Simonoff, E., Pickles, A., Charman, T., Chandler, S., Loucas, T., & Baird, G. (2008). Psychiatric disorders in children with autism spectrum disorders: Prevalence, comorbidity, and associated factors in a population-derived sample. *Journal of the American Academy of Child and Adolescent Psychiatry, 47*(8), 921–929. https://doi.org/10.1097/CHI.0b013e318179964f

Skinner, B. F. (1957). *Verbal behavior*. Copley.

Slaughter, A. M., Hein, S., Hong, J. H., Mire, S. S., & Grigorenko, E. L. (2019). Criminal behavior and school discipline in juvenile justice-involved youth with autism. *Journal of Autism and Developmental Disorders, 49*(6), 2268–2280. https://doi.org/10.1007/s10803-019-03883-8

Smiley, E., Cooper, S. A., Finlayson, J., Jackson, A., Allan, L., Mantry, D., … Morrison, J. (2007). Incidence and predictors of mental ill-health in adults with intellectual disabilities: Prospective study. *British Journal of Psychiatry, 191*, 313–319. https://doi.org/10.1192/bjp.bp.106.031104

Stancliffe, R. J., Harman, A. D., Toogood, S., & McVilly, K. R. (2007). Australian implementation and evaluation of active support. *Journal of Applied Research in Intellectual Disabilities, 20*(3), 211–227. https://doi.org/10.1111/j.1468-3148.2006.00319.x

Stenfert Kroese, B., Cushway, D., & Hubbard, C. (1998). The conceptualization of dreams by people with intellectual disabilities. *Journal of Applied Research in Int2ellectual Disabilities, 11*(2), 146–155. https://doi.org/10.1111/j.1468-3148.1998.tb00056.x

Sturmey, P. (2014a). Adaptive behavior. In P. Sturmey & R. Didden (Eds.), *Evidence-based practice and intellectual disabilities* (pp. 29–61). John Wiley & Sons.

Sturmey, P. (2014b). Maladaptive behavior. In P. Sturmey & R. Didden (Eds.), *Evidence-based practice and intellectual disabilities* (pp. 62–84). John Wiley & Sons.

Sturmey, P., Lindsay, W. R., & Vause, & Neil, N. (2014). Anxiety disorders. In P. Sturmey & R. Didden (Eds.), *Evidence-based practice and intellectual disabilities* (pp. 235–260). John Wiley & Sons, Ltd.

Sundberg, M. L. (2007). Verbal behavior. In J. O. Cooper, T. E. Heron, & W. L. Heward (Eds.), *Applied behavior analysis* (2nd ed., pp. 526–547). Pearson/Merrill Prentice Hall.

Sundberg, M. L., & Partington, J. W. (1998). *Teaching language to children with autism or other developmental disabilities (7.1)*. Behavior Analysts, Inc.

Takamatsu, R., & Takai, J. (2019). With or without empathy: Primary psychopathy and difficulty in identifying feelings predict utilitarian judgment in sacrificial dilemmas. *Ethics & Behavior, 29*, 71–85.

Taylor, J. L., & Knapp, M. (2013). Mental health and emotional problems in people with intellectual disabilities. In J. L. Taylor, W. R. Lindsay, R. P. Hastings, & C. Hatton (Eds.), *Psychological therapies for adults with intellectual disabilities* (pp. 1–14). Wiley.

Taylor, J. L., & Novaco, R. W. (2013). Anger control problems. In J. L. Taylor, W. R. Lindsay, R. P. Hastings, & C. Hatton (Eds.), *Psychological therapies for adults with intellectual disabilities* (pp. 133–156). John Wiley & Sons, Ltd..

Torr, J. (2003). Personality disorder in intellectual disability. *Current Opinion in Psychiatry, 16*, 517–521.

Torr, J. (2008). Personality disorder and offending in people with learning disabilities. *Advances in Mental Health and Learning Disabilities, 2*, 4–10.

Underwood, L., McCarthy, J., & Tsakanikos, E. (2011). Assessment of comorbid psychopathology. In J. L. Matson & P. Sturmey (Eds.), *International handbook of autism and pervasive developmental disorders* (pp. 287–294). Springer.

Van Ingen, D. J., Moore, L. L., Zaja, R. H., & Rojahn, J. (2010). The behavior problems inventory (BPI-01) in community-based adults with intellectual disabilities: Reliability and concurrent validity Vis-à-Vis the inventory for client and agency planning (ICAP). *Research in Developmental Disabilities, 31*(1), 97–107. https://doi.org/10.1016/j.ridd.2009.08.004

Vermeij, A., Kempes, M. M., Cima, M. J., Mars, R. B., & Brazil, I. A. (2018). Affective traits of psychopathy are linked to white-matter abnormalities in impulsive male offenders. *Neuropsychology, 32*(6), 735–745. deficits in empathy.

Vitacco, M. J., Neumann, C. S., & Wodushek, T. (2008). Differential relationships between the dimensions of psychopathy and intelligence: Replication with adult jail inmates. *Criminal Justice and Behavior, 35*, 48–55.

Vitale, J. E., Smith, S. S., Brinkley, C. A., & Newman, J. P. (2002). The reliability and validity of the psychopathy checklist–revised in a sample of female offenders. *Criminal Justice and Behavior, 29*, 202–231.

Vollmer, T. R., Bosch, A. B., Ringdahl, J. E., & Rapp, J. T. (2014). Stereotypic behavior. In P. Sturmey & R. Didden (Eds.), *Evidence-based practice and intellectual disabilities* (pp. 163–197). John Wiley & Sons, Ltd.

Vora, P., & Sikora, D. (2011). *Society for Developmental and Behavioral*. Pediatrics.

Wolery, M., Barton, E. E., & Hine, J. F. (2005). Evolution of applied behavior analysis in the treatment of individuals with autism. *Exceptionality, 13*(1), 11–23. https://doi.org/10.1207/s15327035ex1301_3

Wong, S. C. P., Gordon, A., Gu, D., Lewis, K., & Olver, M. E. (2012). The effectiveness of violence reduction treatment for psychopathic offenders: Empirical evidence and a treatment model. *International Journal of Forensic Mental Health, 11*, 336–349.

World Health Organization. (2021). *Autism spectrum disorders*. Retrieved from https://www.who.int/news-room/fact-sheets/detail/autism-spectrum-disorders

Zeier, J. D., Maxwell, J. S., & Newman, J. P. (2009). Attention moderates the processing of inhibitory information in primary psychopathy. *Journal of Abnormal Psychology, 118*, 554–563.

Zigmond, A. S., & Snaith, R. P. (1983). The hospital anxiety and depression scale. *Acta Psychiatrica Scandinavica, 67*(6), 361–370. https://doi.org/10.1111/j.1600-0447.1983.tb09716.x

Chapter 7
Psychopathy and Psychotic Disorders

John R. Anderson and David Kosson

Abstract Psychopathy and psychosis are often misunderstood and incorrectly conflated. We examine the relationship between psychopathy and various psychotic and psychotic-spectrum disorders. The paucity of literature exploring the intersection of psychopathic traits and psychosis is surprising given that each domain is the subject of a rich clinical research literature. We first examine the relationship between psychopathy and psychotic-spectrum disorders, with emphases on schizophrenia, metacognition, violence, and patients within secure forensic settings. Most current literature focuses specifically on the relationship between psychopathy and schizophrenia. We also explore the relationship between psychopathy and personality disorders related to psychosis including Cluster A personality disorders. Lastly, we provide recommendations for future research. Specifically, more etiological factors should be considered and the possible link between psychopathy and a broader range of psychotic disorders should be examined. The relationship between psychopathy and schizotypal personality appears to be a particularly informative avenue for future research.

Keywords Metacognition · Psychopathy · Psychosis · Schizophrenia · Schizotypal · Violence

7.1 Introduction

Psychopathy and psychotic disorders are both typically debilitating lifetime diagnoses that are costly for society. In tangible terms, the economic burden of schizophrenia, one psychotic disorder, was estimated at $155.7 billion per year in the United States alone (Cloutier et al., 2016), and the economic burden for psychopathy in the United States has been estimated at about $460 million per year (Kiehl & Hoffman,

J. R. Anderson (✉) · D. Kosson
Rosalind Franklin University of Medicine and Science, North Chicago, IL, USA
e-mail: John.Anderson@courts.state.mn.us

J. E. Vitale (ed.), *The Complexity of Psychopathy*, Dangerous Behavior in Clinical and Forensic Psychology, https://doi.org/10.1007/978-3-030-83156-1_7

2011). Psychopathy, psychosis, and their association are often misunderstood. As exemplified in Albert Hitchcock's 1960 film *Psycho*, lay conceptualizations of severely mentally ill people often link violent behavior, typically murder, with thought disorders including delusions and hallucinations. Such antisocial behavior is often misleadingly conflated with psychopathy and/or psychotic disorders. In fact, in one recent survey of people attending jury duty, a large sample misidentified psychotic symptoms as a prototypical feature of psychopathy (Smith et al., 2014).

This chapter examines the relationship between psychopathy and various psychotic and psychotic-spectrum disorders. The paucity of literature exploring the intersection of psychopathic traits and psychosis is surprising given that each domain is the subject of a rich clinical research literature. The first half of this chapter will explore the relationship between psychopathy and psychotic-spectrum disorders, with emphases on schizophrenia and patients within secure forensic settings. The second half will explore the relationship between psychopathy and other personality disorders commonly conceptualized as related to psychosis or existing on a spectrum with overt psychosis. Lastly, we provide recommendations for future research.

7.2 Psychopathy

Psychopathy is a cluster of pathological personality traits characterized by interpersonal, affective, lifestyle, and antisocial dimensions. Psychopathy is associated with many traits such as callousness and impulsivity, as well as transgressive behaviors (Cleckley, 1941). Hervey Cleckley, an early theorist, considered psychopathy to be distinct from psychosis, stating (1988):

> Fanatics and false prophets who show real but not so obvious signs of classic psychosis, as everyone must by now have learned, sometimes attract hundreds or thousands of followers who contribute large funds to projects founded on delusion. … Even those showing plain evidence of very serious disorder, persons as fully psychotic as many on the wards of the state hospitals, also succeed in appearing to large groups not only as sage leaders or men with supernatural powers but also as God. The psychopath, on the other hand is free of all technical signs of this sort. There are no demonstrable defects in theoretical reasoning. (p. 247)

Cleckley's description of "theoretical reasoning" refers to thought more broadly, and he describes thought processes within the psychopathic individual as free of delusions or hallucinations or other signs of psychosis.

Long before Cleckley's (1941) seminal work, *The Mask of Sanity*, psychiatrists in Europe described early conceptualizations of what would evolve into to the syndrome of psychopathy. In 1801, French psychiatrist Philippe Pinel described *manie sans délire* or mania without delirium as "perversion of the active faculties, marked by sanguinary fury, with a blind propensity to acts of violence" (Pinel, 1806, p. 151). Pinel's student, Jean-Étienne Dominique Esquirol, postulated that these serious antisocial acts were driven by a hidden impulse not easily detectible to a diagnostician (Goldstein, 1998; Jones, 2017). In England, James Cowles Prichard coined the term *moral insanity* to denote a syndrome which left intellectual or reasoning abilities intact but in which moral principles became perverted or depraved (Prichard, 1837). Emil Kraepelin, the preeminent German psychiatrist, included in his psychiatric textbook a section on moral insanity in a chapter on what he termed psychopathic personalities (Kraepelin, 1913; Wetzel, 2000).

In recent decades, psychopathy has been viewed as an increasingly important construct to assess in a variety of settings. People high in psychopathic traits make up only approximately 1% of the general population (Coid et al., 2009a, b) and 10–15% of offender populations (Hare, 2003). Yet their behavior has been shown to have an outsized impact on the criminal justice system. They commit crime at a substantially higher rate than nonpsychopathic individuals (Anderson et al., 2018; Hare, 2003; Walsh, 2013). Psychopathy is also associated with a variety of cognitive deficits (e.g., Newman et al., 2010; Smith & Lilienfield, 2015), affective deficits (e.g., Bagley et al., 2009; Christianson et al., 1996) and physiological anomalies.

Clinical psychopathy has been most commonly measured using Hare's Psychopathy Checklist- Revised (PCL-R; Hare, 2003) and its derivatives including the Psychopathy Checklist Screening Version (PCL-SV; Hart et al., 1995), and the Psychopathy Checklist: Youth Version (PCL: YV; Forth et al., 2003). The PCL-R is a 20-item scale that can be divided into two broad factors, which measure the interpersonal and affective features of the construct (Factor 1) and the chronic antisocial behavior and lifestyle features (Factor 2; Harpur et al., 1988; Harpur et al., 1989). These two factors have been further subdivided into facets reflecting interpersonal, affective, lifestyle, and antisocial features (Hare, 2003; Hare & Neumann, 2008).

The interrelated facets and factors are important in understanding the traits that make up the cluster of personality traits associated with psychopathy. Factor 1 is sometimes considered the affective and interpersonal core of psychopathy and can be subdivided into an arrogant, deceitful interpersonal style (the Interpersonal Facet), and deficient affective experience (the Affective Facet). By contrast, Factor 2 is considered more broadly related to externalizing psychopathology and social deviance and has been subdivided into impulsive, irresponsible lifestyle (the Lifestyle Facet) and early, persistent, and versatile antisocial behavior (the Antisocial Facet; Hare, 2003; Hare et al., 1990). The intercorrelations between ratings on these facets have been conceptualized as reflecting a superordinate psychopathy factor (Neumann et al., 2007). In studies throughout the world, the four-facet model shows good model fit independent of sample, assessment, or method of assessment (see Neumann et al., 2014 for a review). Although some have argued that the behaviors encapsulated in the antisocial facet are solely a consequence of elevated levels of the interpersonal, affective, and lifestyle facets (e.g, Cooke & Michie, 1997; Skeem & Cooke, 2010), longitudinal structural equation modeling (SEM) studies have provided evidence that such versatile and persistent antisocial behavior is as strongly implicated in the factor structure of psychopathy as the interpersonal, affective, and lifestyle features (Neumann et al., 2014). In fact, many consider it to be an essential component of psychopathy (Hare, 2016; Lynam & Miller, 2012; Miller & Lynam, 2015; Neumann et al., 2014, 2016).

Relatedly, psychopathy reflects a multifaceted disorder distinct from the externalizing antisocial behavior associated with Antisocial Personality Disorder (ASPD). Given the evidence that ASPD with psychopathy and ASPD without psychopathy differ on a variety of behavioral (Rogers & Rogstad, 2010), laboratory (Riser & Kosson, 2013), and brain indices (Gregory et al., 2012), we will not review research addressing ASPD in general or findings on ASPD in the absence of psychopathy in this chapter.

In summary, psychopathy is a well-validated syndrome of personality pathology. Psychopathy is present in a minority of the members of community and incarcerated samples. Even so, psychopathic individuals are responsible for a disproportionately high level of violent and nonviolent crime.

7.3 Psychosis

Central to any definition of psychosis is the concept of impaired reality testing. The *Diagnostic and Statistical Manual, 5th Edition* (APA, 2013) criteria require hallucinations, delusions, or both to be present in order to label symptoms as psychotic. Hallucinations refer to sensory perception in the absence of a stimulus; insight as to the source of the perception may be present or not (Arciniegas, 2015). Delusions refer to fixed false beliefs and could include many types of delusions such as persecutory, grandiose, and referential among others (Arciniegas, 2015). Psychotic disorders are considered severe psychopathology and are commonly characterized by major impairment in psychosocial functions as well as impairments on laboratory measures of cognitive and affective functioning (Bora et al., 2009; Daros et al., 2014). Individuals with psychotic disorders exhibit physiological anomalies (Greenhalgh et al., 2017; Raz & Raz, 1990), and these disorders have also been linked with antisocial behavior (Arseneault et al., 2003).

7.3.1 Schizophrenia

Schizophrenia is a complex, chronic, and often debilitating disorder which affects men and women at roughly equal rates; onset is typically in the early twenties with slightly earlier onset in men (Hochman & Lewine, 2004), and prevalence is generally estimated to be about 1% of the population (Arajärvi et al., 2005; Kulhara & Chakrabarti, 2001). Kraepelin is often credited with first identifying the disorder (Cornblatt et al., 2008). He described *dementia praecox* as having an early onset followed by deteriorating course and symptoms which were seemingly unrelated to emotion (Kraepelin & Robertson, 1919). Eugen Bleuler renamed Kraepelin's disorder schizophrenia after proposing that many patients did not exhibit a deteriorating course (Cornblatt et al., 2008). Further, the use of the term schizophrenia, stemming from the Greek words *schizo*, meaning split, and *phren*, meaning mind, conveyed

Bleuler's perspective that the essence of the disorder was a splitting or lack of connectedness between psychological functions.

With regard to current nosology, the *Diagnostic and Statistical Manual, 5th Edition* (*DSM 5*; American Psychiatric Association; APA, 2013) lists symptoms which are often conceptualized as "positive" symptoms including hallucinations and delusions, "negative" symptoms, including diminished emotional expression, anhedonia, and avolition, and disorganized symptoms related to speech, thought, and motor movements. The diagnosis describes a disorder characterized by thoughts or experiences that seem out of touch with reality, disorganized speech or behavior, and decreased participation in daily activities. Psychosis is also present in other syndromes such as delusional disorder, schizoaffective disorder, and affective disorders such as major depressive disorder with psychosis, and bipolar disorder. However, very little research has been conducted examining the links between these disorders and psychopathy. Therefore, they are not considered further in this chapter.

7.4 Psychopathy in Forensic Psychiatric Settings

Reasons for commitment to forensic psychiatric settings include, but are not limited to, assessment of competency to stand trial and/or mental state at the time of an alleged offense, competency restoration services, commitment of people adjudicated not guilty by reason of insanity (legal language varies by state or nation), and inpatient hospitalization of inmates or accused offenders who pose a threat to themselves or others. No matter the reason for commitment to a high security hospital setting, psychotic symptoms are prevalent. At the same time, not every patient included in studies of secure forensic samples will have a history of psychosis. Assessing psychopathy among psychotic forensic patients is important with regard to assessing risk and potential responsivity to treatment, among other outcomes.

The PCL-R (Hare, 2003) is routinely used in correctional and forensic settings around the world to inform risk assessments (Archer et al., 2006; DeMatteo et al., 2014; Viljoen et al., 2010). Psychopathy, as assessed by the PCL-R and PCL: SV, is often used to assess dangerousness in secure forensic settings (DeMatteo et al., 2014). The question of whether the basic structure of psychopathy is retained in these settings is important to consider. Hill et al. (2004) reported that the four-facet model including interpersonal, affective, lifestyle, and antisocial facets achieved good overall fit in a confirmatory factor analysis (CFA) and better prediction of violence than two and three-factor models.

Estimates of the proportion of offenders exhibiting high levels of psychopathic features in secure forensic facilities vary widely in different parts of the world, with prevalence rates ranging from around 7% (Heilbrun et al., 1998) to about 30% (Hill et al., 2004) in American forensic hospitals. Psychopathic traits appear to be comorbid with psychotic disorders at a small, but significant rate, with the proportion of overlap varying somewhat for patients in different countries and different settings.

For example, regarding overlap with specific psychotic disorders among patients at English and Scottish forensic hospitals, psychopathy was comorbid with a nonspecific diagnosis of psychosis in 11% of cases examined (Blackburn et al., 2003). Notably, in this study, psychopathy ratings over 25 were associated with a lower rate of psychotic disorder diagnoses, and it has sometimes been suggested that a cutoff of 25 in European forensic settings is analogous to a cutoff of 30 in North American forensic settings (see Cooke, 1998). However, some have criticized the use of this cutoff as based on a flawed use of the Item Response Theory (IRT) approach (Bolt et al., 2007).

In a sample of American maximum security psychiatric patients, 68% of the patients were diagnosed with a psychotic disorder, and 30% met clinical criteria for psychopathy (Hill et al., 2004). The comorbidity between psychopathy and schizophrenia specifically is explored in greater detail later in this chapter. Therefore, factors outside of those related to psychosis or psychopathy specifically could have played a role in the ability of these models to fit the data. Skeem et al. (2003) found that the use of Cooke and Michie's (1997) three-factor model, which excludes the antisocial facet, resulted in a reduced ability of overall psychopathy ratings to predict violence among patients.

More sophisticated methods have been implemented to determine which aspects of psychopathy are most central to its diagnosis within psychiatric hospitals. Both IRT and network analysis are methods for identifying the most central items in measures of constructs. However, IRT explorations within forensic hospitals have been rare. Network analysis is a more recently employed method of graphically and quantitatively representing the centrality, or influence, that symptoms of a disorder have on the presence of other symptoms. Preszler et al. (2018) used an adaptive LASSO (Least Absolute Shrinkage and Selection Operator) network to represent partial correlations among PCL-R item scores in a sample of patients committed to a psychiatric hospital in California. The majority of the sample was diagnosed with schizophrenia-spectrum disorders including schizophrenia (40%) and schizoaffective disorder (29%, Preszler et al., 2018). In this sample, affective symptoms, especially lack of remorse and failure to accept responsibility, were more central or integral to maintaining the structure of the psychopathy network than symptoms related to the interpersonal, lifestyle and antisocial facets. This finding suggests that in a sample in which the majority of the patients have been diagnosed with a psychotic disorder, affective features may be especially important for diagnosing psychopathy (Preszler et al., 2018).

A network analysis of the PCL-R in a large Dutch forensic psychiatric sample yielded somewhat different findings (Verschuere et al., 2018). This sample consisted of offenders under mandatory inpatient treatment following commission of violent crimes determined to be the result of psychopathology. Callousness/lack of empathy (an affective feature) was a somewhat central psychopathic symptom, but impulsivity and parasitic lifestyle (both part of the Lifestyle Fact) were the most central features of psychopathy in this sample (Verschuere et al., 2018). Unfortunately, interpretations of these findings for this review are limited because the authors did not provide a breakdown regarding the proportion of offenders who had experienced psychosis or been diagnosed with psychotic disorders.

Other researchers have conducted person-centered analyses to examine whether psychopathic traits are associated with one or more distinct profiles within clinical forensic settings. In a Dutch forensic psychiatric sample, Klein Haneveld et al. (2018) used latent profile analysis (LPA; Masyn, 2013; Oberski, 2016) to identify unobserved, or latent, profile (or class) membership for individuals rated on PCL-R items. In a sample of 190 offenders, 11 offenders were diagnosed with psychosis as their primary presenting illness and a further 45 were diagnosed with a mixture of psychosis and personality pathology as primary diagnoses. Findings provide evidence of heterogeneity among offenders, particularly offenders diagnosed with severe mental illnesses and psychopathic traits. Specifically, the analyses identified one group of "prototypical" or highly psychopathic offenders and two groups of offenders moderately high in psychopathic traits. Prototypical psychopathic offenders were especially likely to drop out of treatment following release from the hospital or to have treatment deemed inefficacious and be transferred to another hospital. Approximately 97% of the prototypical psychopathy group had been diagnosed with a personality disorder, and 22% of this group had been diagnosed with a comorbid psychotic disorder.

In clinical settings, differentiation of psychopathic traits from other psychological disorders is crucial to treatment and eventual release; however, some studies have raised questions about the reliability of PCL-R ratings among forensic examiners. Jeandarme et al. (2017) examined interrater reliability of PCL-R scores in a Belgian sample which included both forensic hospital patients and prisoners. Scores did not significantly differ between the two samples. However, interrater reliability was poor across item, facet, and total scores. The authors suggested that, although the psychometrics of the PCL-R are often quite good in controlled research settings (see Cooke et al., 2004; Gacono & Hutton, 1994; Hare, 2003; Ismail & Looman, 2016; Kroner & Mills, 2001; Laurell & Daderman, 2007; Porter et al., 2003), the reliability of the measure may not always be adequate in prison and hospital settings. Given evidence of discrepancies in PCL-R ratings in other contexts (e.g., Blais et al., 2017), it is plausible that the lower reliability in Jeandarme et al. (2017) may reflect the need for greater adherence to training or administration recommendations rather than a fundamental difficulty in using the PCL-R reliably in forensic hospital settings (e.g., Boccaccini et al., 2017).

In summary, the assessment of psychopathy is important in settings with elevated rates of psychotic disorders, such as forensic psychiatric settings. Rates of psychopathy are higher in settings with higher rates of psychotic disorders (Heilbrun et al., 1998; Hill et al., 2004). In these settings, a four-factor structure for psychopathy has sometimes been reported to fit the data better than a three-factor structure (Hill et al., 2004; Vitacco et al., 2005). Moreover, impulsivity and parasitic lifestyle may be especially important to consider in settings with increased rates of psychosis (Verschuere et al., 2018). In at least one sample, researchers have reported that a subgroup of patients with both psychopathic traits and psychosis symptoms were characterized by reduced treatment responsiveness (Klein Haneveld et al., 2018).

Finally, in light of evidence for lower interrater agreement in at least one sample (Jeandarme et al., 2017), clinicians must be cognizant of potential obstacles to accurate diagnosis.

7.5 Psychopathy and Schizophrenia

Perhaps somewhat surprisingly, clinical research examining the intersection of psychopathy and schizophrenia (and the intersection of psychopathy and psychotic disorders broadly) could be considered budding at best. In this section, we consider both the likelihood that the specific syndromes of psychopathy and schizophrenia or the features comprising these syndromes co-occur, and the implications of these syndromes co-occurring in some individuals. These can be conceptualized as two different kinds of questions: variable-centered questions, which address relationships among scores on variables in samples (as a whole), and person-centered questions, which address how subsets of samples differ from each other with respect to their scores on the variables measured.

Let us first consider the question of the associations, on average, between psychopathy and schizophrenia (and schizophrenia-spectrum disorders). Several studies have examined comorbidity rates between psychopathic traits and schizophrenia symptoms. The rates of comorbidity most commonly reported for elevated levels of psychopathic traits and schizophrenia range between 17% and 19% (Rasmussen & Levander, 1996; Nolan et al., 1999). At this time, we are not aware of any studies that have directly examined relationships between the components of schizophrenia and the specific components of psychopathy.

In addition to exploring comorbidity, several recent studies have examined the correlates of the presence of both schizophrenia and psychopathy. Whereas some of these studies explored below have focused on the impact of differences in levels of psychopathic traits on relationships between schizophrenia and various potential correlates among individuals with schizophrenia, others have focused on the impact of differences in rates of schizophrenia among offenders. Specifically, most researcher have focused on the impact of schizophrenia and psychopathy features on cognitive functioning, particularly for constructs related to metacognition, as well as for externalizing behaviors such as violence. Several of the correlates of both schizophrenia and psychopathy have also been postulated as mechanisms that may underlie the violence seen in a minority of patients with schizophrenia.

Metacognitive abilities are a subset of executive functions sometimes described as essential for social interactions and resolving dilemmas in daily life. Although people with psychopathy have been generally characterized by an unimpaired ability to understand the cognitive states of others (also referred to as theory of mind, ToM; Blair et al., 1996; Dolan & Fullam, 2004; Fertuck et al., 2009; Lyons et al., 2013; Richell et al., 2003; Wai & Tiliopoulos, 2012) they do show impairments in understanding the affective states of others (cognitive empathy; e.g., Brook & Kosson, 2013; Decety et al., 2013; Fan et al., 2011) and a lack of affective responsiveness to the affective states of others (affective empathy; Blair, 2005; Meffert et al., 2013). In addition, efficacious metacognition has been shown to inhibit violence among individuals high in psychopathy (Blair, 1995). Conversely, metacognitive deficits, especially those related to recognition of affective states, have been linked to violence among patients with schizophrenia (Abu-Akel & Abushua'leh, 2004; Bo et al., 2011, 2014).

Abu-Akel et al. (2015) found that the relationships among metacognition, psychopathy, and schizophrenia were complex. In a sample of 79 patients with schizophrenia and a history of criminal offending, they obtained evidence that psychopathic traits were negatively related to metacognitive abilities in general. However, they also found evidence, for two of three metacognition subscales, that the overall relationship between psychopathic traits and awareness of one's own and others' mental states reflected two distinct relationships for different subgroups of participants. Higher levels of psychopathic traits were associated with higher levels of metacognition in patients rated at 24 and higher on the PCL-R. However, higher levels of psychopathic traits were associated with lower levels of metacognition among patients with lower scores on the PCL-R (e.g., below 24). Abu-Akel et al. (2015) surmised that this group of patients with schizophrenia obtaining high ratings of clinical psychopathy constitutes a unique group in which psychopathic traits help to improve metacognition among offenders with schizophrenia; however, the authors did not examine relations to facet scores which might also explain the pattern.

Similarly, Bo et al. (2014) have proposed that "mentalizing" may be a potential mediator between psychopathy and aggression. Mentalizing, closely related to metacognition and ToM, refers to the ability to think about and attribute cognitive and affective states to oneself and to others (Dimaggio et al., 2011; Frith & Frith, 2012). In their study of 108 patients with schizophrenia, Bo et al. (2014) found that premeditated aggressive behavior among patients with schizophrenia was associated with relatively weaker mentalizing ability and relatively higher ratings on psychopathic traits. Moreover, they noted that the ability to understand the mental states of others was a significant mediator of the relationship between psychopathy and type of aggression (premeditated versus impulsive) in patients with schizophrenia. Further, they found that having a deficient emotional and intact cognitive mentalizing profile in relation to others was associated with a pattern of predominantly premeditated aggression, accounting for 60% of the total effect.

Theory of mind (ToM) is sometimes used interchangeably with mentalizing (Brothers & Ring, 1992) and has been described as the ability to infer others' knowledge, needs, intentions and beliefs (Premack & Woodruff, 1978). In a small, nonclinical sample, Gillespie et al. (2017) found that the combination of self-reported psychopathic traits and positive psychotic experiences was associated with increased ability to judge cognitive mental states of others but not affective states. In comparison, the combination of psychopathy and autistic traits was associated with a comparatively reduced ability to judge both the cognitive and affective mental states of others.

The associations between schizophrenia, psychopathy, and meta-cognitive processes have been examined only relatively recently; much of the earlier research focused primarily on links between psychopathy, schizophrenia (or other forms of major mental illness), and violence and aggressive behaviors (e.g., Abushua'leh & Abu-Akel, 2006; Fullam & Dolan, 2008; McGregor et al., 2012; Nolan et al., 1999; Tengström et al., 2000). For example, earlier studies suggested that people with diagnoses of major mental illnesses, including schizophrenia, are four to six times more likely than those in the general population to commit violent acts (Hodgins, 1992; Lindqvist & Allebeck, 1990; Swanson et al., 1990). However, more recent findings have suggested that it is the presence of psychosis, as opposed to the historical diagnosis of a major mental illness, that predicts violence (Douglas et al., 2009; Skeem et al., 2016; Taylor et al., 2008). Consistent with this perspective, Douglas et al.'s (2009) meta-analysis demonstrated that the presence of psychosis substantially increases risk for violence compared to the absence of any mental disorder but that psychosis itself does not increase the risk for violence among individuals with externalizing disorders.

There is one additional correlate of schizophrenia that merits at least brief attention. A small number of studies have investigated the possibility that psychopathy, like schizophrenia, is characterized by disorganized speech, a construct closely related to the disorganization component of schizophrenia. As noted above, Cleckley (1941) emphasized that psychopathic individuals were not characterized by the usual signs of irrationality associated with psychosis. Nevertheless, reportedly, in at least one edition of The Mask of Sanity (according to Gillstrom & Hare, 1988), Cleckley also noted anomalous speech patterns in his case descriptions of psychopathy, which he suggested might reflect deceptive tactics such as those used by advertisers and politicians but which others have interpreted as reflecting cognitive disorganization (e.g., Gillstrom & Hare, 1988; Hamilton et al., 2015). Both studies summarized here were conducted on samples of general inmates rather than on forensic samples, although Williamson (1991) excluded four participants due to diagnoses of schizophrenia or schizoaffective disorder. In her initial study, psychopathic traits were positively related to a lack of cohesion in speech as well as clinical ratings of disorganized speech. Notably, the mistakes were as apparent in a neutral story as in an affective story, ruling out an emotional dysfunction explanation for the impairment. Later, Brinkley et al. (1999) replicated some of these findings, including the lack of cohesion in personal narratives, in a sample of United States prisoners (Brinkley et al., 1999). Whereas Williamson (1991) reported that all but one of her high psychopathy participants exhibited at least one sign of clinically significant speech impairment, Brinkley et al. (1999) did not address the issue of severity.

Several researchers have argued that levels of psychopathy may help to explain the violence and aggression exhibited by people with schizophrenia (Abushua'leh & Abu-Akel, 2006; Nolan et al., 1999; Rasmussen & Levander, 1996; Tengström et al., 2004). The finding that psychopathy, better than some other factors, predicts violence among people with major mental illnesses like schizophrenia has been replicated several times in multiple samples in different countries (e.g., Skeem & Mulvey, 2001; Tengström et al., 2000, 2004). For instance, Skeem and Mulvey (2001) found in a large civil psychiatric sample that the predictive power of the PCL:SV for future violence remained robust after controlling for covariates such as recent violence, criminal history, substance abuse, and other personality disorders. In their sample, they reported that the predictive power of the PCL:SV was based principally on the antisocial facet of psychopathy. In another study, psychopathy as assessed by the PCL-R has also been shown to predict violent acts among offenders specifically diagnosed with schizophrenia, with ratings on both Factors 1 and 2 predicting future violent crime (Tengström et al., 2000). In this sample, psychopathy predicted violent recidivism as well as or better than other risk factors such as age and previous violence (Tengström et al., 2000). Finally, in another study, offenders with schizophrenia and high psychopathy scores were shown to commit more crimes than those with low psychopathy scores, and psychopathy was a better predictor of future violence than substance use (Tengström et al., 2004).

Bo et al. (2013) examined the utility of the components of psychopathy in predicting violence among psychiatric patients with schizophrenia in forensic and nonforensic settings. They found that overall levels of psychopathic traits as well as ratings on both factors and all four facets were predictive of premeditated aggression. Similarly, in a community sample of individuals with schizophrenia-related diagnoses McGregor et al. (2012) found that psychopathy total scores, ratings for both factors and for Facets 2, 3, and 4, as well as substance misuse were all predictive of membership in a violent versus nonviolent group. In this study, psychopathy remained predictive of violence after controlling for substance misuse (see also Tengström et al., 2004).

Self-reported psychopathy ratings have been shown to predict the majority of the variance in self-reported reactive (impulsive) and proactive (instrumental) aggression when examined along with measures of substance use and persecutory ideation among inpatients diagnosed with schizophrenia (van Dongen et al., 2016). In this study, persecutory ideations explained most of the variance in observed aggression in a hospital unit, and paranoia was related to reactive aggression but not proactive aggression. The use of drugs or alcohol was unrelated to aggression in this sample. These findings provide evidence consistent with claims that paranoid ideation may contribute to violence in schizophrenia-spectrum disorders and that psychopathy is important to understanding violence among people diagnosed with schizophrenia (van Dongen et al., 2016).

Recently, researchers have examined whether individual differences in trait impulsivity and related cognitive and executive functions can help to account for relationships between schizophrenia, psychopathy, and violence. Among the many aspects of cognition that are often impaired in schizophrenia, inhibitory control is a cognitive function that has been shown to be impaired among people diagnosed with schizophrenia (Hill et al., 2004) and linked to impulsivity (Logan et al., 1997; Visser et al., 1996). A recent meta-analysis including 110 studies and over 45,000 individuals diagnosed with some form of psychosis (87.7% with schizophrenia) reported poorer impulse control, along with other factors such as substance use and previous violence, to be associated with increased risk for violence (Witt et al., 2013).

Violence among people diagnosed with schizophrenia is often described as multidetermined or having many roots. Several distinct mechanisms have been postulated to underlie the violence seen in a minority of patients with schizophrenia, and some of these also appear promising candidates for explaining relationships between psychopathy, psychosis, and violent behavior. Impulsivity has been identified along with other psychopathic traits and with psychotic symptoms as primary causes of violence among schizophrenic patients (Stahl, 2014). Impulsivity appears promising as a potential mediator of relationships between psychopathy among patients with schizophrenia given that impulsivity has sometimes been proposed as a specific component of schizotypal traits (Chapman et al., 1984; Kendler & Hewitt, 1992; Raine, 2006), and impulsivity is a recognized feature of psychopathy (Hare, 2003). Moreover, although a plurality of factors including psychopathy are often associated with aggression among individuals with schizophrenia in inpatient settings (McDermott & Holoyda, 2014), impulsivity has often been implicated as at least partially accounting for violence (Nolan et al., 1999). Consistent with this perspective, Wisconsin Card Sorting Task (WCST) performance has been associated with a poor response to some pharmacological anti-aggression treatments among people diagnosed with schizophrenia (Krakowski & Czobor, 2012), and dysfunctional frontotemporal circuitry in impulsivity and aggression in schizophrenia has been offered as one explanation for the link between schizophrenia, impulsivity, and violence (Hoptman, 2015).

Krakowski and Czobor (2017) argued that neurocognitive impairments are important to consider in examining violence among people with schizophrenia. Employing canonical discriminant analysis, they identified two distinct patterns of relationships between proneness to aggression in schizophrenia and neuropsychological impairments: the found relationships between impulsivity, cognitive and executive deficits, impairment in fear recognition, and higher levels of aggression, and relationships between WCST perseverative errors, facial affect processing impairment, and lower levels of aggression. These findings suggest that, among the patients with schizophrenia in this study, excitement and poor impulse control, along with executive dysfunction, were associated with heightened risk for violence, whereas blunted affect and motor retardation were associated with reduced risk for violence.

Paranoia has also been proposed to be a possible mediator of the violent behavior displayed by a minority of people diagnosed with schizophrenia. Specifically, Raine (2013) has proposed that, because paranoid patients with schizophrenia are overly suspicious of the actions of others, a seemingly reasonable defense, in their minds, would be to act violently toward others before a perceived threat could be carried out. Relatedly, delusions of grandeur could provide a righteous feeling of power or control over others, also potentially contributing to violence (Raine, 2013).

In summary, research explicitly exploring the relationship between psychopathy and schizophrenia is scarce, but some recent findings shed light on their associations. Psychopathy has been shown to predict violent acts among people diagnosed with schizophrenia (Abushua'leh & Abu-Akel, 2006; Nolan et al., 1999; Rasmussen & Levander, 1996; Tengström et al., 2004), with ratings on both psychopathy factors (Skeem & Mulvey, 2001; Tengström et al., 2000), and ratings on most psychopathy facets predicting future violent crime (Bo et al., 2013; McGregor et al., 2012). Several clinical features associated with psychosis also appear to be promising candidates for understanding links between schizophrenia, psychopathy, and violence.

Among patients with schizophrenia, psychopathy and metacognitive abilities are negatively related in patients rated relatively low in psychopathy. However, among patients with high scores on the PCL-R, this relationship became positive (Abu-Akel et al., 2015). Further, an interaction of self-reported psychopathic traits and positive psychotic experiences was associated with increased ability to judge mental states of others (Gillespie et al., 2015). Premeditated aggressive behavior among patients with schizophrenia was associated with relatively weaker mentalizing ability and relatively higher ratings on psychopathic traits (Bo et al., 2014).

Impulsivity, one trait of psychopathy, has been clearly implicated in violence among patients with schizophrenia (Enticott et al., 2008; Witt et al., 2013). Impairments in executive functioning related to disinhibition have also been demonstrated in patients with schizophrenia (Krakowski & Czobor, 2017), and such impairments are potentially related to psychopathy. Paranoia has also been identified as a construct that contributes to violence among psychotic and delusional schizophrenic patients in at least one sample (Raine, 2013), and paranoid ideation has been related to reactive aggression but not proactive aggression among patients diagnosed with schizophrenia (van Dongen et al., 2016). Importantly, impulsivity and paranoia may be important to consider in working to understand violence and aggression among people diagnosed with schizophrenia who also exhibit psychopathic traits.

7.6 Psychopathy and Personality Disorders Related to Psychosis

There has been substantial attention paid to relationships between psychopathic traits and symptoms of other personality disorders. Examination of the Cluster A personality disorders, which are characterized by impaired reality testing and rigidity and share some features with schizophrenia and delusional disorder, may provide valuable insights into the relationships between psychopathy and the psychotic disorders. Several studies have reported relationships between the symptoms of these personality disorders and the features of psychopathy.

Paranoid personality disorder describes a pervasive distrust of others beginning by early adulthood that is associated with a variety of expressions of doubts, suspicions, and grudges, including attributions of hostility or danger to the actions of others (APA, 2013). Prevalence estimates in the general population have ranged between 2% and 4% (Grant et al., 2004; Torgersen et al., 2001). Hildebrand and de Ruiter (2004), in a sample of Dutch forensic psychiatric patients, reported ratings on Factors 1 and 2 of the PCL-R were positively correlated with symptoms of paranoid personality disorder. In a sample of forensic psychiatric patients from England and Scotland, Blackburn (2007) reported paranoid personality symptoms were positively correlated with ratings on both the Lifestyle and Antisocial Facets of psychopathy. In contrast, Warren and Burnette (2013) showed paranoid personality disorder was positively associated with ratings on all four facets of psychopathy among US prisoners. Recently, Klipfel et al. (2017) found that paranoid personality disorder symptoms were associated with PCL-R total scores and Antisocial Facet scores at the zero-order level among United States county jail inmates. Further, residualized indices of paranoid personality disorder symptoms (controlling for the effect of ratings on other psychopathy facets and for ratings on symptoms of other personality disorders) were uniquely related to Antisocial Facet ratings. A recent analysis of two additional samples slightly complicated the interpretation of these findings. In an independent sample of United States offenders, Klipfel (2018) observed significant zero-order correlations between paranoid personality disorder symptoms and ratings on all four PCL-R facets but obtained a significant partial correlation (after controlling for other facet scores) only for ratings on the Lifestyle facet. In contrast, in a sample of United Kingdom forensic hospital patients, only Lifestyle and Antisocial facet correlations were significant at the zero-order level, and there were no unique relationships with paranoid personality disorder symptoms, suggesting that most of the variance related to paranoid personality disorder was shared among the psychopathy facets (Klipfel, 2018; see also Coid et al., 2009a, b). Unfortunately, most prior studies of this issue have not investigated the possibility of unique versus shared relationships with paranoid personality disorder. Thus, paranoid personality ratings appear to be related to psychopathy ratings, but the components of psychopathy associated with this disorder may vary across samples or may partly reflect shared variance among the psychopathy facets.

Schizoid personality disorder, another Cluster A personality disorder, refers to a pervasive pattern of detachment from social relationships and a restricted range of expression of emotions in interpersonal settings, beginning by early adulthood, that appears consistent with a lack of interest in or lack of enjoyment of interpersonal relationships (APA, 2013). Estimates of prevalence in community samples have ranged from less than 1% to about 3% (Grant et al., 2004; Wiessman, 1993). The simple relationship between symptoms of schizoid personality disorder and psychopathy may be somewhat less consistent than that observed for both paranoid personality disorder and schizotypal personality disorder (discussed below). Warren and Burnette (2013) found symptoms of schizoid personality were positively related to ratings of the Affective, Lifestyle, and Antisocial Facets of psychopathy in United States prisoners. However, Klipfel et al. (2017) reported there were no zero-order correlations or partial correlations between schizoid personality symptoms and PCL-R total or facet scores. Interestingly, in a follow-up study, Klipfel (2018) reported unique correlations between the number of schizoid personality disorder symptoms and Affective Facet ratings in both a United States prison sample and a European forensic hospital sample. Similarly, Coid et al. (2009a, b) reported unique correlations between schizoid personality disorder symptoms and Affective Facet ratings in a representative sample of prisoners from England and Wales. In summary, although zero-order correlations between schizoid personality disorder and psychopathy component scores were reliable (for Affective and Interpersonal

Facets) only in one of two United States forensic samples examined, the replication of unique relationships in both European psychiatric and prison samples and United States prison samples suggests a relatively robust relationship between core affective features of psychopathy and symptoms of schizoid personality disorder. Even so, it is important to note here that there have been relatively few investigations of empirical relations between psychopathy and schizoid personality.

7.7 Schizotypy

Schizotypy is a multidimensional construct referring to a range of pathological personality and behavioral factors (Barrantes-Vidal et al., 2010, 2013; Green et al., 2008; Kwapil & Barrantes-Vidal, 2012). The term is most often used to refer to symptoms of schizotypal personality disorder and is sometimes used to refer to a syndrome or constellation of cognitive and perceptual experiences and psychotic-like behaviors, which has been linked to psychotic disorders but which has also been described as a nonclinical constellation of personality traits with specific cognitive, affective, and psychophysiological correlates (Claridge & Broks, 1984). The prevalence of schizotypal personality disorder is estimated to be 4.6% in the United States (APA, 2013). Males are more likely than females to be diagnosed with schizotypal personality disorder (Kotsafitis & Neale, 1993). Because schizotypal personality appears important both as a significant personality disorder in its own right and also as a condition that may provide insight into the development of schizophrenia (e.g., see Raine, 2006), it is cross-listed in the *DSM* 5 under both Personality Disorders and Schizophrenia Spectrum and Other Psychotic Disorders. There are a variety of different manifestations of schizotypy, and there are no necessary or sufficient features.

Schizotypy and schizotypy-like features, have long been considered to exist on a schizophrenia or psychosis continuum (Kwapil & Barrantes-Vidal, 2015). Meehl (1962) first introduced the construct to specify an inherited vulnerability to schizophrenia-spectrum disorders which is expressed as a multidimensional personality organization. Recent research studies, including epidemiological examinations, provide reliable evidence that current operationalizations of the schizotypal personality construct are related to schizophrenia (Kendler, 1988; Parnas et al., 2005). One study demonstrated a genetic linkage between symptoms of schizotypy and schizophrenia (e.g., Yasuda et al., 2011). There is also evidence linking symptoms of schizotypy more broadly to the prospective development of psychotic disorders (Chapman et al., 1994).

Like schizophrenia, schizotypal personality has been conceptualized as consisting of positive, negative, and disorganized components in both clinical and nonclinical samples (Arndt et al., 1991; Barrantes-Vidal et al., 2013, 2015; Bilder et al., 1985; Gruzelier, 1996; Liddle & Barnes, 1990; Kwapil et al., 2012; Suhr & Spitznagel, 2001). Suhr and Spitznagel (2001) describe factor analytic evidence for these three dimensions (Arndt et al., 1991; Bilder et al., 1985; Lenzenweger et al.,

1991; Liddle, 1987; Liddle & Barnes, 1990; Peralta et al., 1992). In these three-factor models, positive symptoms are those related to hallucinations and delusions; negative symptoms such as anhedonia, avolition, and restricted affect comprise a second dimension; and disorganized symptoms represents a third dimension. Positive and negative schizotypy are the dimensions most commonly replicated across samples and assessment measures (e.g. Kwapil et al., 2012; Raine et al., 1994; Vollema & van den Bosch, 1995; Stefanis et al., 2002).

Negative symptoms associated with schizotypy require further discussion and consideration. Although early theorists described schizoidia as a broad construct important for conceptualizing schizophrenia which subsumed modern concepts of schizotypal traits (Hoch & Polatin, 1949; Kretschmer, 1920, 1922), the modern diagnostic category of schizoid personality disorder focuses on a more narrow set of symptoms or features that is considered to be related to the negative symptoms of schizophrenia. Positive schizotypy has been uniquely related to psychotic-like experiences, substance abuse, mood disorders, and mental health treatment (Kwapil et al., 2008). Both dimensions have been linked to poorer overall and social functioning, but negative schizotypy has also been associated with decreased likelihood of intimate relationships (Kwapil et al., 2008).

From a person-centered perspective, clusters of people with positive symptoms and with negative symptoms have been identified, and those in the negative symptom cluster have exhibited schizoid personality disorder-like symptoms, impaired social adjustment, high conscientiousness and low agreeableness (Barrantes-Vidal et al., 2010). Assessments of schizotypy which include a negative symptom component, it seems, can account to some degree for findings based on more modern and narrow operationalizations of schizoid personality disorder symptoms. In summary, schizotypal traits broadly and schizotypal personality describe a complex cluster of symptoms related to odd perceptual experiences and interpersonal behavior (APA, 2013; Barrantes-Vidal et al., 2010, 2013; Green et al., 2008; Kwapil & Barrantes-Vidal, 2012). Many consider schizotypy to represent a predisposition to schizophrenia, though others approach the construct as an independent personality disorder, or as existing on a continuum including normal personality variation.

7.7.1 Associations Between Psychopathy and Schizotypy

We now consider the question of whether there are relationships between psychopathy and schizotypy and the implications of the syndromes co-occurring in some individuals through both variable-centered and person-centered approaches. Studies have provided relatively more evidence for relationships between psychopathy and schizotypy than for relationships between psychopathy and other Cluster A personality disorders. One notable change from our earlier discussion of psychopathy and schizophrenia is that we could locate no published studies that have explicitly probed for violence as a correlate of the combination of psychopathic traits and schizotypy.

As noted above, the existence of people with symptoms or features of both psychopathy and schizotypy has a long history within psychiatry. "Schizoid psychopaths" who were relatives of people diagnosed with schizophrenia were first described by Kallmann (1938) as exhibiting predominantly 'psychopathic' features while also displaying schizophrenic-like traits. Dunaif and Hoch (1955) wrote about pseudopsychopathic or pseudoneurotic schizophrenia in patients who were not overtly psychotic, but who displayed some schizophrenia symptoms (such as altered self-perception and difficulty discerning fantasy from reality) and antisociality. Similarly, Heston (1970) described some children of mothers diagnosed with schizophrenia as being "schizoid psychopaths" who were impulsive and illogical in the crimes they committed, indicating, he believed, that some schizotypal and psychopathic traits may co-occur. Notably, although these authors employed the term 'schizoid' to refer to the broader notion of schizoidia, it appears that their clinical descriptions emphasized traits which, today, would be considered consistent with both the negative symptom and disorganization dimensions of schizotypy, respectively. In short, it appears that the term schizoid psychopaths was used to refer to people exhibiting both psychopathic and schizotypal traits. Some years later, Raine (2013) highlighted the anecdotal finding that people who are high in both schizotypal and psychopathic traits tend to have only relatively superficial friendships and often display emotional blunting.

Taking a variable-centered approach, Raine (1992) explored the association between psychopathy and schizotypal traits. Hare and Forth (1985) had previously reported that criminals scoring in the middle range of psychopathy had showed some signs of paranoid schizophrenia and schizotypal personality, along with some neuropsychological abnormalities. Consequently, Raine (1992) hypothesized that inmates scoring in a middle (or intermediate) group in terms of levels of psychopathy would show higher levels of schizotypal traits. Partly consistent with this hypothesis, elevated levels of schizotypal traits were found among those in middle and high psychopathy groups compared to people placed in the low group (Raine, 1992). These findings appear consistent with Heston's (1966) proposal that unstable, impulsive lifestyle can co-occur with features of psychopathy.

More recently, in an undergraduate sample, Ragsdale and Bedwell (2013) examined comorbidity between self-reported schizotypal features as assessed by the Schizotypal Personality Questionnaire (SPQ) and self-reported psychopathic personality traits as measured by the Psychopathic Personality Inventory – Revised (PPI-R; Lilienfeld et al., 2005). The authors postulated that impulsivity would explain the shared variance between psychopathy and schizotypy. Consistent with Raine's (1992) findings for subgroups of inmates examined with the original PCL, they found dimensional indices of psychopathic and schizotypal personality traits to be related at total levels (Ragsdale & Bedwell, 2013), and this association was apparently driven by the antisocial lifestyle (or Factor 2) features of psychopathy. Interestingly, in this study, schizotypy appeared to be negatively related to the affective-interpersonal features of psychopathy. However, the implications of these findings are constrained by the very modest associations between the indices of Factor 1 traits as measured by the PPI and ratings on the interpersonal and affective features of psychopathy using clinical measures such as the PCL-R (Miller & Lynam, 2011; Poythress et al., 2010).

Findings are somewhat different for studies using clinical measures of schizotypy and psychopathy. There have been several studies of these relationships. Examining zero-order correlations between ratings of PCL-R-rated psychopathy and clinical measures of *DSM* criteria for personality disorders, Rogers et al. (2007) found scores for schizotypal personality disorder were positively correlated only with scores on the interpersonal facet of psychopathy. Coid et al. (2009a, b) found no unique correlations between ratings on the psychopathy facets and the symptoms of schizotypal personality disorder, after controlling for scores on the other facets and on the other symptoms of personality disorder. Klipfel (2018) have examined these relationships in several samples (which are discussed above). In Klipfel et al. (2017), schizotypal personality disorder ratings were correlated with total psychopathy scores, as well as with ratings on the lifestyle and antisocial facets ratings – but only at the zero-order level. That is, after controlling for symptoms of other personality disorders and other psychopathy facets, the association was no longer evident, suggesting that the variance shared among different personality disorders and psychopathy facets was responsible for this apparent association. In a follow-up study, Klipfel (2018) found that, among the United States prisoners, psychopathy and schizotypy total scores were positively correlated, as were schizotypy and scores on each facet, though effects were small; however, there were no unique correlations after controlling for the shared variance among symptoms of personality disorders. In contrast, in a UK forensic psychiatric sample, schizotypal and psychopathic features were uncorrelated at both the level of zero-order and partial correlations (Klipfel, 2018). Considering the patterns of findings in all of the samples, the zero-order relationship between schizotypal personality disorder symptoms and PCL-R ratings was somewhat inconsistent across samples. In addition, findings suggest the shared variance between personality disorders is important in examining their relationships between schizotypal personality disorder and psychopathy (Klipfel, 2018).

Ragsdale et al. (2013) investigated the associations of PPI-R and SPQ scores along with skin conductance measures in an independent sample of undergraduates viewing affectively valenced pictures. They replicated positive relationships between schizotypy and indices of the antisocial-lifestyle features and negative relationships between schizotypy and affective-interpersonal features of psychopathy (Ragsdale et al., 2013). In addition, they reported that schizotypal traits were associated with increased autonomic responses to emotional and neutral pictures, in contrast to the autonomic hypo-responsiveness often found in clinical psychopathy (e.g., Raine & Venables, 1988). However, Ikezawa et al. found (2012) distinct subgroups of patients with schizophrenia who were characterized by electrodermal hyporesponsivness versus hyperresponsiveness. Consistent with this distinction is evidence that some antisocial individuals are characterized by both electrodermal hyporesponsiveness and schizotypal traits (Raine & Venables, 1984). Taken together, these findings suggest that there may be more than one important relationship between schizotypal features and psychopathic features. That is, there may be a relationship between schizotypy and the antisocial lifestyle features of psychopathy in general, and there may also be a relationship between schizotypy and psychopathic traits and reduced electrodermal responsiveness in a subset of individuals characterized by both kinds of traits. Even so, the lack of studies of relevant clinical samples limits confidence in the generalizability of these findings.

Evidence reviewed above suggests psychopathy and schizotypy may share common associations, such as impulsivity in lifestyle (Ragsdale & Bedwell, 2013; Ragsdale et al., 2013). Early theoretical conceptualizations (e.g., Heston, 1966, 1970; Kallman, 1938; Kraepelin, 1913) have led researchers to conduct a handful of studies, and findings have shown those scoring moderately high on measures of clinical psychopathy also have elevated scores on clinical measures of schizotypal traits (Raine, 1992). Of course, such findings do not address the distinction between shared and unique variance. Moreover, the studies that have examined both shared and unique variance between psychopathy and schizotypal traits suggest that, in some samples, the disorders associated with both positive and negative aspects of schizotypy may be related to psychopathy (Klipfel et al., 2017; Klipfel, 2018; Rogers et al., 2007). Negative symptom schizotypy (sometimes called narrowly defined schizoidia) appears to be relatively robustly and negatively related to the interpersonal facet and positively related to the affective facet of psychopathy. Conversely, the lifestyle and antisocial facets of psychopathy appear to be uniquely associated with positive aspects of schizotypy in some samples, but these relationships appear to reflect shared variance between psychopathy and symptoms of other personality disorders. In summary, our review suggests psychopathy may be related to unique manifestations of schizotypal traits.

7.8 Conclusion and Recommendations

Psychopathy is a well-validated syndrome comprising interpersonal, affective, lifestyle, and antisocial traits which has been identified and studied for two centuries. Rates of psychopathy are elevated not only in prison settings but also in settings characterized by many patients with psychotic disorders. Among patients with schizophrenia, psychopathy and metacognitive abilities are positively related in patients rated as medium and low on psychopathy. However, among patients with high scores on the PCL-R, psychopathic traits are associated with impaired metacognition. To our knowledge, no prior studies have addressed interactions between psychopathic traits and symptoms of schizophrenia. Psychopathy predicts violence among people diagnosed with schizophrenia. Impulsivity and paranoia have been proposed as possible mechanisms to explain violence among some psychotic and delusional patients with schizophrenia.

Many consider schizotypy a predisposition to schizophrenia, whereas others approach the construct as an independent personality disorder. Studies examining subsets of offenders who are rated as moderately high on measures of psychopathy suggest that such offenders have elevated scores on clinical measures of schizotypal traits. The robust relationships between psychopathy and schizotypal traits suggest the possibility that the disorders may be related at the level of total scores and this relationship has been replicated in several offender samples, although it was not found in at least one forensic hospital sample. Our review also suggests some specific associations between positive symptom schizotypy and the antisocial lifestyle (Factor 2) features of psychopathy and between negative symptom schizotypy and the core affective features of psychopathy, although studies directly addressing symptoms of schizotypal personality disorder and components of psychopathy have been somewhat inconsistent and suggest that much of the relationship between positive symptom schizotypy and psychopathy may reflect variance shared among different forms of personality pathology. As noted above, a large proportion of the research examining psychopathy and psychosis has focused on violence and externalizing behaviors with relatively little exploration of cognitive and affective processes. Therefore, the current review reflects this overrepresentation with the caveat that, although violence prediction is clearly important, more vigorous exploration of other correlates of these syndromes also appears critical to understanding, preventing and treating these syndromes.

We briefly mention the construct of schizopathy, a term which has sometimes been used to refer to a form of psychopathology characterized by traits of both psychopathy and schizophrenia. As reviewed above, psychopathy has heretofore been associated with both schizophrenia (Abushua'leh & Abu-Akel, 2006; Bo et al., 2013; Nolan et al., 1999; Rasmussen & Levander, 1996; Tengström et al., 2004) and schizotypal personality (Heston, 1970; Kallman, 1938; Klipfel, 2018; Klipfel et al., 2017; Kraepelin, 1913; Raine, 1991, 1992; Ragsdale & Bedwell, 2013; Ragsdale et al., 2013; Rogers et al., 2007). Clinical reports and studies of individuals with both psychopathic and schizotypal/psychotic features and reports of commonalities outlined in the development (e.g.. impulsivity) and their correlates of the separate syndromes (e.g., violence), it may be possible to identify a specific personality pathology syndrome to understand better the clinical characteristics and impact of such combinations of features. Although included in this review are some studies purporting to examine schizoid psychopaths, there has been to our knowledge little to no systematic inquiry into the validity of the schizopathy construct or the nature of its correlates. In addition, very little research has examined the association between psychopathy and disorders with psychotic symptoms outside of schizophrenia-spectrum disorders. Aside from schizoaffective disorder, which is often grouped with schizophrenia for research purposes, we were unable to identify studies examining the relationship between comorbid mood and psychotic symptoms (such as those sometimes noted in bipolar disorder or major depressive disorder with psychotic features) with psychopathic features.

In closing, we make several recommendations regarding relationships between psychopathy and psychosis. First, correlates beyond those related to metacognition and violence should be investigated. The host of etiologically relevant factors and clinically relevant outcomes that merit investigation include heritability, exposure to trauma, psychophysiology, proneness to emotion, emotion processing and emotion regulation, and neural activation. Second, the possible relationships between psychopathy and a broader range of psychotic disorders (e.g., delusional disorder, affective disorders with psychosis) should be examined. Third, the evidence of associations between negative symptom schizotypy and affective features of psychopathy and the inconsistent associations between positive symptom schizotypy and the antisocial lifestyle features of psychopathy may help to inform studies of the etiology of both psychopathy and schizophrenia, and additional attention to the shared variance among personality disorders may help to uncover important mechanisms in the development and maintenance of these syndromes. Lastly, the small number of individuals who are relatively high in psychopathic and schizotypal traits appear to comprise an important subgroup, and further study of the characteristics associated with elevations of both kinds of traits may help illuminate the relationship between psychopathy and psychosis.

References

Abu-Akel, A., & Abushua'leh, K. (2004). 'Theory of mind' in violent and nonviolent patients with paranoid schizophrenia. *Schizophrenia Research, 69*, 45–53.

Abu-Akel, A., Heinke, D., Gillespie, S. M., Mitchell, I. J., & Bo, S. (2015). Metacognitive impairments in schizophrenia are arrested at extreme levels of psychopathy: The cut-off effect. *Journal of Abnormal Psychology, 124*(4), 1102.

Abushua'leh, K., & Abu-Akel, A. (2006). Association of psychopathic traits and symptomatology with violence in patients with schizophrenia. *Psychiatry Research, 143*(2), 205–211.

American Psychiatric Association. (2013). *Diagnostic and statistical manual of mental disorders, 5th edition: DSM-5*. American Psychiatric Association.

Anderson, J. R., Walsh, Z., & Kosson, D. S. (2018). Psychopathy, self-identified race/ethnicity and nonviolent recidivism: A longitudinal study. *Law and Human Behavior, 42*(6), 531–544.

Arajärvi, R., Suvisaari, J., Suokas, J., Schreck, M., Haukka, J., Hintikka, J., Partonen, T., & Lönnqvist, J. (2005). Prevalence and diagnosis of schizophrenia based on register, case record and interview data in an isolated Finnish birth cohort born 1940–1969. *Social Psychiatry and Psychiatric Epidemiology, 40*(10), 808–816.

Archer, R. P., Buffington-Vollum, J. K., Stredny, R. V., & Handel, R. W. (2006). A survey of psychological test use patterns among forensic psychologists. *Journal of Personality Assessment, 87*, 84–94. https://doi.org/10.1207/s15327752jpa8701_07

Arciniegas D. B. (2015). Psychosis. *Continuum (Minneapolis, Minn.), 21*(3 Behavioral Neurology and Neuropsychiatry), 715–736. https://doi.org/10.1212/01.CON.0000466662.89908.e7

Arndt, S., Alliger, R. J., & Andreasen, N. C. (1991). The distinction of positive and negative symptoms: The failure of a two-dimensional model. *The British Journal of Psychiatry, 158*(3), 317–322.

Arseneault, L., Cannon, M., Murray, R., Poulton, R., Caspi, A., & Moffitt, T. E. (2003). Childhood origins of violent behaviour in adults with schizophreniform disorders. *British Journal of Psychiatry, 183*, 520–525.

Bagley, A. D., Abramowitz, C. S., & Kosson, D. S. (2009). Vocal affect recognition and psychopathy: Converging findings across traditional and cluster analytic approaches to assessing the construct. *Journal of Abnormal Psychology, 118*(2), 388.

Barrantes-Vidal, N., Lewandowski, K. E., & Kwapil, T. R. (2010). Psychopathology, social adjustment and personality correlates of schizotypy clusters in a large nonclinical sample. *Schizophrenia Research, 122*(1), 219–225.

Barrantes-Vidal, N., Gross, G. M., Sheinbaum, T., Mitjavila, M., Ballespí, S., & Kwapil, T. R. (2013). Positive and negative schizotypy are associated with prodromal and schizophrenia-spectrum symptoms. *Schizophrenia Research, 145*(1), 50–55.

Barrantes-Vidal, N., Grant, P., Kwapil, T.R. (2015). The role of schizotypy in the study of the etiology of schizophrenia spectrum disorders. Schizophrenia Bulletin, 41 (2), S408–S416, https://doi.org/10.1093/schbul/sbu191

Bilder, R. M., Mukherjee, S., Rieder, R. O., & Pandurangi, A. K. (1985). Symptomatic and neuropsychological components of defect states. *Schizophrenia Bulletin, 11*(3), 409.

Blackburn, R. (2007). Personality disorder and antisocial deviance: Comments on the debate on the structure of the psychopathy checklist-revised. *Journal of Personality Disorders, 21*(2), 142–159.

Blackburn, R., Logan, C., Donnelly, J., & Renwick, S. (2003). Personality disorders, psychopathy and other mental disorders: Co-morbidity among patients at English and Scottish high-security hospitals. *The Journal of Forensic Psychiatry & Psychology, 14*(1), 111–137.

Blair, R. J. (1995). A cognitive developmental approach to mortality: Investigating the psychopath. *Cognition, 57*, 1–29.

Blair, R. J. (2005). Responding to the emotions of others: Dissociating forms of empathy through the study of typical and psychiatric populations. *Consciousness and Cognition, 14*, 698–718.

Blair, J., Sellars, C., Strickland, I., Clark, F., Williams, A., Smith, M., & Jones, L. (1996). Theory of mind in the psychopath. *Journal of Forensic Psychiatry, 7*, 15–25.

Blais, J., Forth, A. E., & Hare, R. D. (2017). Examining the interrater reliability of the Hare Psychopathy Checklist – Revised across a large sample of trained raters. *Psychological Assessment, 29*(6), 762–775.

Bo, S., Abu-Akel, A., Kongerslev, M., Haahr, U. H., & Simonsen, E. (2011). Risk factors for violence among patients with schizophrenia. *Clinical Psychology Review, 31*, 711–726.

Bo, S., Forth, A., Kongerslev, M., Haahr, U. H., Pedersen, L., & Simonsen, E. (2013). Subtypes of aggression in patients with schizophrenia: The role of personality disorders. *Criminal Behaviour and Mental Health, 23*(2), 124–137.

Bo, S., Abu-Akel, A., Kongerslev, M., Haahr, U. H., & Bateman, A. (2014). Mentalizing mediates the relationship between psychopathy and type of aggression in schizophrenia. *Journal of Nervous and Mental Disease, 202*, 55–63.

Boccaccini, M. T., Rufino, K. A., Jeon, H., & Murrie, D. C. (2017). Does the predictive validity of psychopathy ratings depend on the clinical experience of the raters? *International Journal of Forensic Mental Health, 16*(2), 130–138.

Bolt, D. M., Hare, R. D., & Neumann, C. S. (2007). Score metric equivalence of the psychopathy checklist–revised (PCL-R) across criminal offenders in north america and the United Kingdom: A critique of Cooke, Michie, Hart, and Clark (2005) and new analyses. *Assessment, 14*(1), 44–56.

Bora, E., Yucel, M., & Pantelis, C. (2009). Cognitive functioning in schizophrenia, schizoaffective disorder and affective psychoses: Meta-analytic study. *The British Journal of Psychiatry, 195*(6), 475–482.

Brinkley, C. A., Newman, J. P., Harpur, T. J., & Johnson, M. M. (1999). Cohesion in texts produced by psychopathic and nonpsychopathic criminal inmates. *Personality and Individual Differences, 26*(5), 873–885.

Brook, M., & Kosson, D. S. (2013). Impaired cognitive empathy in criminal psychopathy: Evidence from a laboratory measure of empathic accuracy. *Journal of Abnormal Psychology, 122*(1), 156.

Brothers, L., & Ring, B. (1992). A neuroethological framework for the representation of minds. *Journal of Cognitive Neuroscience, 4*(2), 107–118.

Chapman, L. J., Chapman, J. P., Numbers, J. S., Edell, W. S., Carpenter, B. N., & Beckfield, D. (1984). Impulsive nonconformity as a trait contributing to the prediction of psychotic-like and schizotypal symptoms. *Journal of Nervous and Mental Disease, 172*(11), 681–691.

Chapman, L. J., Chapman, J. P., Kwapil, T. R., Eckblad, M., & Zinser, M. C. (1994). Putatively psychosis-prone subjects 10 years later. *Journal of Abnormal Psychology, 103*(2), 171–183.

Christianson, S., Forth, A. E., Hare, R. D., Strachan, C., Lidberg, L., & Thorell, L. (1996). Remembering details of emotional events: A comparison between psychopathic and non-psychopathic offenders. *Personality and Individual Differences, 4*, 437–443. https://doi.org/10.1016/0191-8869(95)00220-0

Claridge, G., & Broks, P. (1984). Schizotypy and hemisphere function: Theoretical considerations and the measurement of schizotypy. *Personality and Individual Differences, 5*(6), 633–648.

Cleckley, H. (1941). *The Mask of Sanity*. Mosby.

Cleckley, H. (1988). *The Mask of Sanity* (5th ed.). CV Mosby Company.

Cloutier, M., Aigbogun, M. S., Guerin, A., Nitulescu, R., Ramanakumar, A. V., Kamat, S. A., DeLucia, M., Duffy, R., Legacy, S. N., Henderson, C., & François, C. (2016). The economic burden of schizophrenia in the United States in 2013. *The Journal of Clinical Psychiatry, 77*(6), 764–771.

Coid, J., Yang, M., Ullrich, S., Roberts, A., & Hare, R. D. (2009a). Prevalence and correlates of psychopathic traits in the household population of Great Britain. *International Journal of Law and Psychiatry, 32*, 65–73. https://doi.org/10.1016/j.ijlp.2009.01.002

Coid, J., Yang, M., Ullrich, S., Roberts, A., Moran, P., Bebbington, P., Brugha, T., Jenkins, R., Farrell, M., Lewis, G., Singleton, N., & Hare, R. (2009b). Psychopathy among prisoners in England and Wales. *International Journal of Law and Psychiatry, 32*(3), 134–141.

Cooke, D. J. (1998). Cross-cultural aspects of psychopathy. In T. Millon, E. Simonsen, M. Birket Smith, & R. D. Davis (Eds.), *Psychopathy: Antisocial, criminal, and violent behavior* (pp. 260–276). Guilford.

Cooke, D. J., & Michie, C. (1997). An item response theory analysis of the Hare Psychopathy Checklist--Revised. *Psychological Assessment, 9*(1), 3–14.

Cooke, D. J., Hart, S. D., & Michie, C. (2004). Cross-national differences in the assessment of psychopathy: Do they reflect variations in raters' perceptions of symptoms? *Psychological Assessment, 16*, 335–339.

Cornblatt, B. A., Green, M. F., Walker, E. F., & Mittal, V. A. (2008). Schizophrenia: Etiology and neurocognition. In *Oxford textbook of psychopathology* (pp. 298–332). Oxford University Press.

Daros, A. R., Ruocco, A. C., Reilly, J. L., Harris, M. S., & Sweeney, J. A. (2014). Facial emotion recognition in first-episode schizophrenia and bipolar disorder with psychosis. *Schizophrenia Research, 153*(1–3), 32–37.

Decety, J., Chen, C., Harenski, C. L., & Kiehl, K. A. (2013). An fMRI study of affective perspective taking in individuals with psychopathy: Imagining another in pain does not evoke empathy. *Frontiers in Human Neuroscience, 7*(September), 1–12.

DeMatteo, D., Edens, J. F., Galloway, M., Cox, J., Smith, S. T., Koller, J. P., & Bersoff, B. (2014). Investigating the role of the psychopathy checklist-revised in United States case law. *Psychology, Public Policy, and Law, 20*(1), 96–107. https://doi.org/10.1037/a0035452

Dimaggio, G., Nicolo, G., Bru¨ne, M, & Lysaker, P. H. (2011). Mental state understanding in adult psychiatric disorders: Impact on symptoms, social functioning and treatment. *Psychiatry Research, 190*(1), 1–2.

Dolan, M., & Fullam, R. (2004). Theory of mind and mentalizing ability in antisocial personality disorders with and without psychopathy. *Psychological Medicine, 34*, 1093–1102.

Douglas, K. S., Guy, L. S., & Hart, S. D. (2009). Psychosis as a risk factor for violence to others: A meta-analysis. *Psychological Bulletin, 135*(5), 679.

Dunaif, S., & Hoch, P. (1955). Pseudoneurotic schizophrenia. In P. Hoch & P. Zubin (Eds.), *Psychiatry and the law* (pp. 169–195). Grune and Stratton.

Enticott, P. G., Ogloff, J. R., Bradshaw, J. L., & Fitzgerald, P. B. (2008). Cognitive inhibitory control and selfreported impulsivity among violent offenders with schizophrenia. *Journal of Clinical and Experimental Neuropsychology, 30(2), 157–162.*

Fan, Y., Duncan, N. W., de Greck, M., & Northoff, G. (2011). Is there a core neural network in empathy? An fMRI based quantitative meta-analysis. *Neuroscience and Biobehavioral Reviews, 35*(3), 903–911.

Fertuck, E. A., Jekal, A., Song, I., Wyman, B., Morris, M. C., Wilson, S. T., Brodsky, B. S., & Stanley, B. (2009). Enhanced 'reading the mind in the eyes' in borderline personality disorder compared to healthy controls. *Psychological Medicine, 39*, 1979–1988.

Forth, A. E., Kosson, D. S., & Hare, R. D. (2003). *Hare PCL: Youth Version (PCL: YV) rating booklet*. MHS.

Frith, C. D., & Frith, U. (2012). Mechanisms of social cognition. *Annual Review of Psychology, 63*, 287–313.

Fullam, R. S., & Dolan, M. C. (2008). Executive function and in-patient violence in forensic patients with schizophrenia. *The British Journal of Psychiatry, 193*(3), 247–253.

Gacono, C. B., & Hutton, H. E. (1994). Suggestions for the clinical and forensic use of the Hare Psychopathy checklist-revised (PCL-R). *International Journal of Law and Psychiatry, 17*, 303–317.

Gillespie, S. M., Rotshtein, P., Wells, L. J., Beech, A. R., & Mitchell, I. J. (2015). Psychopathic traits are associated with reduced attention to the eyes of emotional faces among adult male non-offenders. *Frontiers in human neuroscience, 9, 552.*

Gillespie, S. M., Mitchell, I. J., & Abu-Akel, A. M. (2017). Autistic traits and positive psychotic experiences modulate the association of psychopathic tendencies with theory of mind in opposite directions. *Scientific Reports, 7*(1), 6485.

Gillstrom, B. J., & Hare, R. D. (1988). Language related hand gestures in psychopaths. *Journal of Personality Disorders, 2*, 21–27.

Goldstein, J. (1998). Professional knowledge and professional self-interest. The rise and fall of monomania in 19th-century France. *International Journal of Law and Psychiatry, 21*(4), 385–396.

Grant, B. F., Hasin, D. S., Stinson, F. S., Dawson, D. A., Chou, S. P., Ruan, W. J., & Pickering, R. P. (2004). Prevalence, correlates, and disability of personality disorders in the United States: Results from the National Epidemiologic Survey on alcohol and related conditions. *The Journal of Clinical Psychiatry, 65*(7), 948–958.

Green, M. J., Raine, A., & Boyle, G. J. (2008). Schizotypal personality models. *Humanities Social Sciences Papers*. Paper 296.

Greenhalgh, A. M., Gonzalez-Blanco, L., Garcia-Rizo, C., Fernandez-Egea, E., Miller, B., Arroyo, M. B., & Kirkpatrick, B. (2017). Meta-analysis of glucose tolerance, insulin, and insulin resistance in antipsychotic-naive patients with nonaffective psychosis. *Schizophrenia Research, 179*, 57–63.

Gregory, S., Simmons, A., Kumari, V., Howard, M., Hodgins, S., & Blackwood, N. (2012). The antisocial brain: Psychopathy matters: A structural MRI investigation of antisocial male violent offenders. *Archives of General Psychiatry, 69*(9), 962–972.

Gruzelier, J. H. (1996). The factorial structure of schizotypy: Part I Affinities with syndromes of schizophrenia. *Schizophrenia Bulletin, 22*(4), 611–620. https://doiorg.ezproxy.rosalindfranklin.edu/10.1093/schbul/22.4.611

Hamilton, R. K., Hiatt Racer, K., & Newman, J. P. (2015). Impaired integration in psychopathy: A unified theory of psychopathic dysfunction. *Psychological Review, 122*(4), 770–791.

Hare, R. D. (2003). *Manual for the psychopathy checklist-revisited* (2nd ed.). Multi-Health Systems.

Hare, R. D. (2016). Forward. In C. B. Gacono (Ed.), *The clinical and forensic assessment of psychopathy: A practitioner's guide* (2nd ed., pp. xvi–xviii). Routledge.

Hare, R. D., & Forth, A. E. (1985). Psychopathy and lateral preference. *Journal of Abnormal Psychology, 94*(4), 541.

Hare, R. D., & Neumann, C. S. (2008). Psychopathy as a clinical and empirical construct. *Annual Review of Clinical Psychology, 4*, 217–246.

Hare, R. D., Harpur, T. J., Hakstian, A. R., Forth, A. E., Hart, S. D., & Newman, J. P. (1990). The revised psychopathy checklist: Reliability and factor structure. *Psychological Assessment: Journal of Consulting and Clinical Psychology, 2*, 338–341.

Harpur, T. J., Hakstian, A. R., & Hare, R. D. (1988). Factor structure of the psychopathy checklist. *Journal of Consulting and Clinical Psychology, 56*, 741–747.

Harpur, T. J., Hare, R. D., & Hakstian, R. (1989). A two-factor conceptualization of psychopathy: Construct validity and implications for assessment. *Psychological Assessment. Journal of Consulting and Clinical Psychology, 1*, 6–17.

Hart, S. D., Cox, D. N., & Hare, R. D. (1995). *The Hare psychopathy checklist: Screening version*. Multi-Health Systems.

Heilbrun, K., Hart, S. D., Hare, R. D., Gustafson, D., Nunez, C., & White, A. J. (1998). Inpatient and postdischarge aggression in mentally disordered offenders: The role of psychopathy. *Journal of Interpersonal Violence, 13*(4), 514–527.

Heston, L. L. (1966). Psychiatric disorders in foster home reared children of schizophrenic mothers. *The British Journal of Psychiatry, 112*(489), 819–825.

Heston, L. L. (1970). The genetics of schizophrenic and schizoid disease. *Science, 167*(3916), 4, 249–256.

Hildebrand, M., & de Ruiter, C. (2004). PCL-R psychopathy and its relation to DSM-IV axis I and II disorders in a sample of male forensic psychiatric patients in the Netherlands. *International Journal of Law and Psychiatry, 27*(3), 233–248.

Hill, C. D., Neumann, C. S., & Rogers, R. (2004). Confirmatory factor analysis of psychopathy checklist: Screening version in offenders with axis I disorders. *Psychological Assessment, 16*(1), 90.

Hoch, P., & Polatin, P. (1949). Pseudoneurotic forms of schizophrenia. *Psychiatric Quarterly, 23*(2), 248–276.

Hochman, K. M., & Lewine, R. R. (2004). Age of menarche and schizophrenia onset in women. *Schizophrenia Research, 69*(2–3), 183–188.

Hodgins, S. (1992). Mental disorder, intellectual deficiency, and crime. Evidence from a birth cohort. *Archives of General Psychiatry, 49*, 476–483.

Hoptman, M. J. (2015). Impulsivity and aggression in schizophrenia: A neural circuitry perspective with implications for treatment. *CNS Spectrums, 20*(3), 280–286.

Ikezawa, S., Corbera, S., Liu, J., & Wexler, B. E. (2012). Empathy in electrodermal responsive and nonresponsive patients with schizophrenia. *Schizophrenia Research, 142*(1–3), 71–76.

Ismail, G., & Looman, J. (2016). Field inter-rater reliability of the psychopathy checklist-revised. *International Journal of Offender Therapy and Comparative Criminology*. Advance online publication.

Jeandarme, I., Edens, J. F., Habets, P., Bruckers, L., Oei, K., & Bogaerts, S. (2017). PCL-R field validity in prison and hospital settings. *Law and Human Behavior, 41*(1), 29–43.

Jones, D. W. (2017). Moral insanity and psychological disorder: The hybrid roots of psychiatry. *History of Psychiatry, 28*(3), 263–279.

Kallman, F. J. (1938). *The genetics of schizophrenia*. Augustin.

Kendler, K. S. (1988). Familial aggregation of schizophrenia and schizophrenia spectrum disorders. *Archives of General Psychiatry, 45*, 377–386.

Kendler, K. S., & Hewitt, J. (1992). The structure of self-report schizotypy in twins. *Journal of Personality Disorders, 6*(1), 1–17.

Kiehl, K. A., & Hoffman, M. B. (2011). The criminal psychopath: History, neuroscience, treatment, and economics. *Jurimetrics, 51*, 355.

Klein Haneveld, E., Neumann, C. S., Smid, W., Wever, E., & Kamphuis, J. H. (2018). Treatment responsiveness of replicated psychopathy profiles. *Law and Human Behavior, 42*(5), 484.

Klipfel, K. M. (2018). *Psychopathy and its relations with other personality disorders: An extension of findings in two distinct samples*. Unpublished doctoral dissertation. Rosalind Franklin University of Medicine and Science, North Chicago, Illinois.

Klipfel, K. M., Garofalo, C., & Kosson, D. S. (2017). Clarifying associations between psychopathy facets and personality disorders among offenders. *Journal of Criminal Justice, 53*, 83–91.

Kotsaftis, A., & Neale, J. M. (1993). Schizotypal personality disorder 1: The clinical syndrome. *Clinical Psychology Review, 13*(5), 451–472.

Kraepelin, E. (1913). *Clinical psychiatry: A textbook for physicians*. Macmillam.

Kraepelin, E., & Robertson, G. M. (1919). *Dementia praecox and paraphrenia, together with manic-depressive insanity and paranoia*. Classics of Medicine Library.

Krakowski, M. I., & Czobor, P. (2012). Executive function predicts response to antiaggression treatment in schizophrenia: A randomized controlled trial. *The Journal of Clinical Psychiatry, 73*(1), 74–80.

Krakowski, M. I., & Czobor, P. (2017). Proneness to aggression and its inhibition in schizophrenia: Interconnections between personality traits, cognitive function and emotional processing. *Schizophrenia Research, 184*, 82–87.

Kretschmer, E. (1920). der sensitive beziehungswahn. ein beitrag zur paranoiafrage und zur psychiatrischen charakterlehre. *The Journal of Nervous and Mental Disease, 52*(5), 461–462.

Kretschmer, E. (1922). Körperbau und Charakter. Untersuchungen zum Konstitutionsproblem und zur Lehre von den Temperamenten. *Zeitschrift für Induktive Abstammungs- und Vererbungslehre, 30*(1), 139–144.

Kroner, D. G., & Mills, J. F. (2001). The accuracy of five risk appraisal instruments in predicting institutional misconduct and new convictions. *Criminal Justice and Behavior, 28*, 471–489.

Kulhara, P., & Chakrabarti, S. (2001). Culture and schizophrenia and other psychotic disorders. *Psychiatric Clinics of North America, 24*(3), 449–464.

Kwapil, T. R., & Barrantes-Vidal, N. (2012). Schizotypal personality disorder: An integrative review. In *The Oxford handbook of personality disorders* (pp. 437–477). Oxford University Press.

Kwapil, T. R., Barrantes-Vidal, N., & Silvia, P. J. (2008). The dimensional structure of the Wisconsin schizotypy scales: Factor identification and construct validity. *Schizophrenia Bulletin, 34*(3), 444–457.

Kwapil, T. R., Brown, L. H., Silvia, P. J., Myin-Germeys, I., & Barrantes-Vidal, N. (2012). The expression of positive and negative schizotypy in daily life: an experience sampling study. Psychological Medicine, 42(12), 2555–2566.

Kwapil, T. R., & Barrantes-Vidal, N. (2015). Schizotypy: Looking back and moving forward. *Schizophrenia Bulletin, 41*(2), S366–S373. https://doi.org/10.1093/schbul/sbu186

Laurell, J., & Dåderman, A. M. (2007). Psychopathy (PCL-R) in a forensic psychiatric sample of homicide offenders: Some reliability issues. *International Journal of Law and Psychiatry, 30*, 127–135.

Lenzenweger, M. F., Dworkin, R. H., & Wethington, E. (1991). Examining the underlying structure of schizophrenic phenomenology: Evidence for a three-process model. *Schizophrenia Bulletin, 17*(3), 515.

Liddle, P. F. (1987). The symptoms of chronic schizophrenia. A re-examination of the positive negative dichotomy. *The British Journal of Psychiatry, 151*(2), 145–151.

Liddle, P. F., & Barnes, T. R. (1990). Syndromes of chronic schizophrenia. *The British Journal of Psychiatry, 157*(4), 558–561.

Lilienfeld, S. O., Widows, M. R., & Staff, P. A. R. (2005). Psychopathic personality inventory TM-revised. *Social Influence (SOI), 61*(65), 97.

Lindqvist, P., & Allebeck, P. (1990). Schizophrenia and crime. A longitudinal follow-up of 644 schizophrenics in Stockholm. *British Journal of Psychiatry, 157*, 345–350.

Logan, G. D., Schachar, R. J., & Tannock, R. (1997). Impulsivity and inhibitory control. *Psychological Science, 8*, 60–64.

Lynam, D. R., & Miller, J. D. (2012). Fearless dominance and psychopathy: A response to Lilienfeld et al. *Personality Disorders, 3*, 341–353.

Lyons, M., Healy, N., & Bruno, D. (2013). It takes one to know one: Relationship between lie detection and psychopathy. *Personality and Individual Differences, 55*(6), 676–679.

Masyn, K. E. (2013). Latent class analysis and finite mixture modeling. In *The Oxford handbook of quantitative methods* (pp. 551–611). Oxford University Press.

McDermott, B. E., & Holoyda, B. J. (2014). Assessment of aggression in inpatient settings. *CNS Spectrums, 19*(5), 425–431.

McGregor, K., Castle, D., & Dolan, M. (2012). Schizophrenia spectrum disorders, substance misuse, and the four-facet model of psychopathy: The relationship to violence. *Schizophrenia Research, 136*(1), 116–121.

Meehl, P. E. (1962). Schizotaxia, schizotypy, schizophrenia. *American Psychologist, 17*, 827–838.

Meffert, H., Gazzola, V., den Boer, J. A., Bartels, A. A., & Keysers, C. (2013). Reduced spontaneous but relatively normal deliberate vicarious representations in psychopathy. *Brain: A Journal of Neurology, 136*(Pt 8), 2550–2562.

Miller, J. D., & Lynam, D. R. (2011). An examination of the psychopathic personality inventory's nomological network: A meta-analytic review. *Personality Disorders, Theory, Research, and Treatment, 3*(3), 305–326.

Miller, J. D., & Lynam, D. R. (2015). Psychopathy and personality: Advances and debates. *Journal of Personality, 83*, 585–592.

Neumann, C. S., Hare, R. D., & Newman, J. P. (2007). The super-ordinate nature of the psychopathy checklist-revised. *Journal of Personality Disorders, 21*, 102–117.

Neumann, C. S., Hare, R. D., & Pardini, D. A. (2014). Antisociality and the construct of psychopathy: Data from across the globe. *Journal of Personality, 83*, 678–692.

Neumann, C. S., Vitacco, M. J., & Mokros, A. S. (2016). Using both variable-centered and person-centered approaches to understanding psychopathic personality. In C. B. Gacono (Ed.), *The clinical and forensic assessment of psychopathy: A practitioner's guide* (2nd ed., pp. 14–31). Routledge.

Newman, J. P., Curtin, J. J., Bertsch, J. D., & Baskin-Sommers, A. R. (2010). Attention moderates the fearlessness of psychopathic offenders. *Biological Psychiatry, 67*(1), 66–70.

Nolan, K. A., Volavka, J., Mohr, P., & Czobor, P. (1999). Psychopathy and violent behavior among patients with schizophrenia or schizoaffective disorder. *Psychiatric Services, 50*(6), 787–792.

Oberski, D. L. (2016). A review of "latent variable modeling with R". *Journal of Educational and Behavioral Statistics, 41*, 226–233.

Parnas, J., Licht, D., & Bovet, P. (2005). Chapter 8: Cluster a personality disorders: A review. In M. Maj, H. S. Akiskal, J. E. Mezzich, & A. Okasha (Eds.), *Personality disorders. WPA series evidence and experience in psychiatry* (pp. 1–74). Wiley.

Peralta, V., De Leon, J., & Cuesta, M. J. (1992). Are there more than two syndromes in schizophrenia? A critique of the positive-negative dichotomy. *The British Journal of Psychiatry, 161*(3), 335–343.

Pinel, P. (1806). *A treatise on insanity: In which are contained the principles of a new and more practical nosology of maniacal disorders than has yet been offered to the public* (Vol. 1806). W. Todd.

Porter, S., Woodworth, M., Earle, J., Drugge, J., & Boer, D. (2003). Characteristics of sexual homicides committed by psychopathic and nonpsychopathic offenders. *Law and Human Behavior, 27*, 459–470.

Poythress, N. G., Lilienfeld, S. O., Skeem, J. L., Douglas, K. S., Edens, J. F., Epstein, M., & Patrick, C. J. (2010). Using the PCL-R to help estimate the validity of two self-report measures of psychopathy with offenders. *Assessment, 17*(2), 206–219.

Premack, D., & Woodruff, G. (1978). Does the chimpanzee have a theory of mind? *Behavioral and Brain Sciences, 1*(4), 515–526.

Preszler, J., Marcus, D. K., Edens, J. F., & McDermott, B. E. (2018). Network analysis of psychopathy in forensic patients. *Journal of Abnormal Psychology, 127*(2), 171.

Prichard, J. C. (1837). *A treatise on insanity: And other disorders affecting the mind* (Vol. 1837). Haswell, Barrington, and Haswell.

Ragsdale, K. A., & Bedwell, J. S. (2013). Relationships between dimensional factors of psychopathy and schizotypy. *Frontiers in Psychology, 4*, 1–7.

Ragsdale, K. A., Mitchell, J. C., Cassisi, J. E., & Bedwell, J. S. (2013). Comorbidity of schizotypy and psychopathy: Skin conductance to affective pictures. *Psychiatry Research, 210*(3), 1000–1007.

Raine, A. (1991). The SPQ: A scale for the assessment of schizotypal personality based on *DSM III-R* criteria. *Schizophrenia Bulletin, 17*(4), 555–564.

Raine, A. (1992). Schizotypal and borderline features in psychopathic criminals. *Personality and Individual Differences, 13*(6), 717–721.

Raine, A. (2006). Schizotypal personality: Neurodevelopmental and psychosocial trajectories. *Annual Review of Clinical Psychology*, 2, 291–326. https://doi.org/10.1146/annurev.clinpsy.2.022305.095318.

Raine, A. (2013). A recipe for violence: Malnutrition, metals, and mental health. In *The anatomy of violence: The biological roots of crime*. Vintage Books.
Raine, A., & Venables, P. (1984). Electrodermal nonresponding, antisocial behavior, and schizoid tendencies in adolescents. *Psychophysiology, 21*(4), 424–433.
Raine, A., & Venables, P. H. (1988). Skin conductance responsivity in psychopaths to orienting, defensive, and consonant-vowel stimuli. *Journal of Psychophysiology, 2*(3), 221–225.
Raine, A., Reynolds, C., Lencz, T., Scerbo, A., Triphon, N., & Kim, D. (1994). Cognitive perceptual, interpersonal, and disorganized features of schizotypal personality. *Schizophrenia Bulletin, 20*(1), 191–201.
Raine, A., Dodge, K., Loeber, R., Gatzke-Kopp, L., Lynam, D., Reynolds, C., Stouthamer-Loeber, M., & Liu, J. (2006). The reactive–proactive aggression questionnaire: Differential correlates of reactive and proactive aggression in adolescent boys. *Aggressive Behavior, 32*(2), 159–171.
Raine, A., Fung, A. L. C., & Lam, B. Y. H. (2011). Peer victimization partially mediates the schizotypy-aggression relationship in children and adolescents. *Schizophrenia Bulletin, 37*(5), 937–945.
Rasmussen, K., & Levander, S. (1996). Symptoms and personality characteristics of patients in a maximum security psychiatric unit. *International Journal of Law and Psychiatry, 19*, 27–37.
Raz, S., & Raz, N. (1990). Structural brain abnormalities in the major psychoses: A quantitative review of the evidence from computerized imaging. *Psychological Bulletin, 108*(1), 93.
Richell, R. A., Mitchell, D. G., Newman, C., Leonard, A., Baron-Cohen, S., & Blair, R. J. (2003). Theory of mind and psychopathy: Can psychopathic individuals read the 'language of the eyes'? *Neuropsychologia, 41*, 523–526.
Riser, R. E., & Kosson, D. S. (2013). Criminal behavior and cognitive processing in male offenders with antisocial personality disorder with and without comorbid psychopathy. *Personality Disorders, Theory, Research, and Treatment, 4*(4), 332.
Rogers, R., & Rogstad, J. E. (2010). Psychopathy and APD in non-forensic patients: Improved predictions or disparities in cut scores? *Journal of Psychopathology and Behavioral Assessment, 32*(3), 353–362.
Rogers, R., Jordan, M. J., & Harrison, K. S. (2007). Facets of psychopathy, axis II traits, and behavioral dysregulation among jail detainees. *Behavioral Sciences & the Law, 25*(4), 471–483.
Skeem, J. L., & Cooke, D. J. (2010). Is criminal behavior a central component of psychopathy? Conceptual directions for resolving the debate. *Psychological Assessment, 22*, 433–445.
Skeem, J. L., & Mulvey, E. P. (2001). Psychopathy and community violence among civil psychiatric patients: Results from the MacArthur Violence Risk Assessment Study. *Journal of Consulting and Clinical Psychology, 69*(3), 358.
Skeem, J. L., Mulvey, E. P., & Grisso, T. (2003). Applicability of traditional and revised models of psychopathy to the psychopathy checklist: Screening version. *Psychological Assessment, 15*, 41–55.
Skeem, J., Kennealy, P., Monahan, J., Peterson, J., & Appelbaum, P. (2016). Psychosis uncommonly and inconsistently precedes violence among high-risk individuals. *Clinical Psychological Science, 4*(1), 40–49.
Smith, S. F., & Lilienfeld, S. O. (2015). The response modulation hypothesis of psychopathy: A meta-analytic and narrative analysis. *Psychological Bulletin, 141*(6), 1145–1177.
Smith, S. T., Edens, J. F., Clark, J., & Rulseh, A. (2014). "So, what *is* a psychopath?" Venireperson perceptions, beliefs, and attitudes about psychopathic personality. *Law and Human Behavior, 38*(5), 490–500.
Stahl, S. M. (2014). Deconstructing violence as a medical syndrome: Mapping psychotic, impulsive, and predatory subtypes to malfunctioning brain circuits. *CNS Spectrums, 19*(5), 357–365.
Stefanis, N. C., Hanssen, M., Smirnis, N. K., Avramopoulos, D. A., Evdokimidis, I. K., Stefanis, C. N., Verdoux, H., & Van Os, J. (2002). Evidence that three dimensions of psychosis have a distribution in the general population. *Psychological Medicine, 32*, 347–358.
Suhr, J. A., & Spitznagel, M. B. (2001). Factor versus cluster models of schizotypal traits. I: A comparison of unselected and highly schizotypal samples. *Schizophrenia Research, 52*(3), 231–239.

Swanson, J. W., Holzer, C. E. D., Ganju, V. K., & Jono, R. T. (1990). Violence and psychiatric disorder in the community: Evidence from the Epidemiologic Catchment Area surveys. *Hospital and Community Psychiatry, 41*, 761–770.

Taylor, P. J., Hill, J., Bhagwagar, Z., Darjee, R., & Thomson, L. D. (2008). Presentations of psychosis with violence: Variations in different jurisdictions. A comparison of patients with psychosis in the high security hospitals of Scotland and England. *Behavioral Sciences & the Law, 26*(5), 585–602.

Tengström, A., Grann, M., Långström, N., & Kullgren, G. (2000). Psychopathy (PCL-R) as a predictor of violent recidivism among criminal offenders with schizophrenia. *Law and Human Behavior, 24*(1), 45–58.

Tengström, A., Hodgins, S., Grann, M., Langstrom, N., & Kullgren, G. (2004). Schizophrenia and criminal offending: The role of psychopathy and substance use disorders. *Criminal Justice and Behavior, 31*, 367–391.

Torgersen, S., Kringlen, E., & Cramer, V. (2001). The prevalence of personality disorders in a community sample. *Archives of General Psychiatry, 58*(6), 590–596.

van Dongen, J. D., Buck, N. M., & van Marle, H. J. (2016). Positive symptoms, substance use, and psychopathic traits as predictors of aggression in persons with a schizophrenia disorder. *Psychiatry Research, 237*, 109–113.

Verschuere, B., van Ghesel Grothe, S., Waldorp, L., Watts, A. L., Lilienfeld, S. O., Edens, J. F., Skeem, J. L., & Noordhof, A. (2018). What features of psychopathy might be central? A network analysis of the Psychopathy Checklist-Revised (PCL-R) in three large samples. *Journal of Abnormal Psychology, 127*(1), 51–65.

Viljoen, J. L., McLachlan, K., & Vincent, G. M. (2010). Assessing violence risk an psychopathy in juvenile and adult offenders: A survey of clinical practices. *Assessment, 17*, 377–395.

Visser, M., Das-Smaal, E., & Kwakman, H. (1996). Impulsivity and negative priming: Evidence for diminished cognitive inhibition in impulsive children. *British Journal of Psychology, 87*, 131–140.

Vitacco, M. J., Neumann, C. S., & Jackson, R. L. (2005). Testing a four-factor model of psychopathy and its association with ethnicity, gender, intelligence, and violence. *Journal of Consulting and Clinical Psychology, 73*(3), 466–476.

Vollema, M. G., & van den Bosch, R. J. (1995). The multidimensionality of schizotypy. *Schizophrenia Bulletin, 21*, 19–31.

Wai, M., & Tiliopoulos, N. (2012). The affective and cognitive empathic nature of the dark triad of personality. *Personality and Individual Differences, 52*, 794–799.

Walsh, Z. (2013). Psychopathy and criminal violence: The moderating effect of ethnicity. *Law and Human Behavior, 37*(5), 303.

Warren, J. I., & Burnette, M. (2013). The multifaceted construct of psychopathy: Association with APD, clinical, and criminal characteristics among male and female inmates. *International Journal of Forensic Mental Health, 12*(4), 265–273.

Weissman, M. M. (1993). The epidemiology of personality disorders: A 1990 update. *Journal of Personality Disorders, 7*, 44–62.

Wetzell, R. F. (2000). *Inventing the criminal: A history of German criminology, 1880–1945*. The University of North Carolina Press.

Williamson, S. E. (1991). *Cohesion and coherence in the speech of psychopathic criminals*. Unpublished thesis, University of British Columbia.

Witt, K., Van Dorn, R., & Fazel, S. (2013). Risk factors for violence in psychosis: Systematic review and meta-regression analysis of 110 studies. *PLoS One, 8*(2), e55942.

Yasuda, Y., Hashimoto, R., Ohi, K., Fukumoto, M., Umeda-Yano, S., Yamamori, H., Okochi, T., Iwase, M., Kazui, H., Iwata, N., & Takeda, M. (2011). Impact on schizotypal personality trait of a genome-wide supported psychosis variant of the ZNF804A gene. *Neuroscience Letters, 495*(3), 216–220.

Chapter 8
Psychopathy and Mood Disorders

Monika Dargis

Abstract Psychopathy is a personality disorder characterized by callous, reckless, and impulsive antisocial behavior (Hare R, The psychopathy checklist-revised. In: Encyclopedia of psychology and law. SAGE, 2003). Psychopathic individuals are routinely incarcerated for both violent and non-violent crimes, representing 15–25% of the adult prison population (Hart SD, Hare RD, Curr Opin Psychiatry 9(2):129–132, 1996), and commit a disproportionate amount of crime (Hare RD, Psychopaths and their nature: implications for the mental health and criminal justice systems. In: Psychopathy: antisocial, criminal, and violent behavior. Guilford, pp 188–212 1998). Kiehl and Hoffman (Jurimetrics, 51, 355, 2011) estimated that psychopathic offenders alone are responsible for $460 billion per year in societal costs (e.g., lost property, police, courts, prosecutors, public defenders, prisons). Psychopathy is thus a particularly severe disorder with devastating consequences and costs to society.

Keywords Psychopathy · Mood disorder · Depression · Antisocial · Treatment

8.1 Introduction to Psychopathy

Psychopathy is a personality disorder characterized by callous, reckless, and impulsive antisocial behavior (Hare, 2003). Psychopathic individuals are routinely incarcerated for both violent and non-violent crimes, representing 15–25% of the adult prison population (Hart & Hare, 1996), and commit a disproportionate amount of crime (Hare, 1998). Kiehl and Hoffman (2011) estimated that psychopathic offenders alone are responsible for $460 billion per year in societal costs (e.g., lost property, police, courts, prosecutors, public defenders, prisons). Psychopathy is thus a particularly severe disorder with devastating consequences and costs to society.

M. Dargis (✉)
New York Presbyterian- Weill Cornell Medical Center, New York, NY, USA

J. E. Vitale (ed.), *The Complexity of Psychopathy*, Dangerous Behavior in Clinical and Forensic Psychology, https://doi.org/10.1007/978-3-030-83156-1_8

8.2 Measurement of Psychopathy in Incarcerated Samples

The Psychopathy Checklist-Revised (PCL-R) is the most widely used assessment tool to measure psychopathic traits among criminal offenders (Hare, 2003). The PCL-R is a scale of 20 items rated 0–2 based on the degree to which the trait is present. Items are rated after thorough review of institutional files that detail criminal and social histories, as well as a semi-structured interview designed to assess the traits which comprise the scale. PCL-R scores range from 0 to 40, with a score greater or equal to 30 used to identify psychopathic individuals. The "average" inmate scores between 21 and 23 on the PCL-R, and it is estimated that an individual in the general population without a criminal record will score between 1 and 3 (Hare, 2003). Accordingly, a score of a 30 or greater is substantially higher than the typical antisocial personality found in prison settings. In line with this, almost all psychopathic offenders also meet criteria for antisocial personality disorder (ASPD), a personality disorder characterized by rule-breaking behavior, impulsivity and a disregard for others beginning before age 15 (American Psychiatric Association, 2013). The reverse, however, is not true: most people with antisocial personality disorder do not meet criteria for psychopathy. Accordingly, ASPD and psychopathy represent distinct disorders.

While PCL-R total scores indicate overall severity, psychopathy is considered a multifaceted disorder. Factor analyses have consistently shown that the PCL-R can be further broken into a two-Factor and a four-Facet model (Flores-Mendoza et al., 2008; Hare, 2003; Neumann et al., 2006, 2013). Factor 1 comprises the interpersonal-affective features of psychopathy (Facet 1: interpersonal [e.g., superficial charm, grandiosity]; Facet 2: affective [e.g., callousness, lack of remorse]) whereas Factor 2 comprises the lifestyle-antisocial features of psychopathy (Facet 3: lifestyle [e.g., impulsivity, irresponsibility]; Facet 4: antisocial [e.g., criminal versatility, juvenile delinquency]). Factor 2 traits are often present among individuals with ASPD, whereas Factor 1 traits appear to be unique to the construct of psychopathy.

8.3 Heterogeneity in Psychopathy

Although frequently discussed as a unitary construct, there is strong theoretical and empirical evidence indicating that there are two subtypes of psychopathic offenders who differ primarily on measures of anxiety and negative affect. Lykken (1996), for instance, theorized that psychopathy in the presence of low levels of anxiety and negative affect (primary, Low-NA) originates from biological abnormalities and is characterized by fearlessness and unemotionality. He proposed psychopathy in the presence of high levels of anxiety and negative affect (secondary, High-NA) as a distinct construct that, while phenotypically very similar to Low-NA psychopathy, differs drastically in experience of neuroticism, negative affect, and anxiety. Lykken argued that the secondary/High-NA psychopath often experiences tension and stress during and/or after the commission of crimes.

In line with this theoretical conjecture, data driven approaches such as model-based cluster analysis and latent class analysis have consistently differentiated groups of psychopathic individuals by anxiety/negative affect. (e.g., Blackburn et al., 2008; Claes et al., 2014; Gill & Stickle, 2016; Hicks et al., 2004). Although prior research has included only psychopathic individuals in their analyses (i.e., used a discrete cut off to form a "psychopath" group), recent work has shown that these two groups emerge using the same analytic strategies (i.e., cluster analysis) in a sample of offenders with a wide-range of psychopathic traits (Dargis & Koenigs, 2018). This work provides additional evidence of distinct subgroups of psychopathic offenders within the broader offender population.

There is some evidence that the Low-NA psychopathic group scores slightly higher on the interpersonal-affective traits of psychopathy, whereas the High-NA group scores higher on the lifestyle-antisocial traits (e.g., Hicks et al., 2010; Skeem et al., 2007). However, the two subtypes have not been reliably differentiated using clinical interviews alone, as the two groups largely present as phenotypically similar.

8.4 Introduction to Mood Disorders

Mood disorders include both bipolar and depressive disorders, and are characterized by distinct periods of elevated, irritable, and/or depressed mood (American Psychological Association, 2013). Mood disorders are quite prevalent in the United States (Gelenberg, 2010; Judd & Akiskal, 2003), and are associated with significant functional impairment (Marvel & Paradiso, 2004; Wittchen et al., 2011). For instance, symptoms associated with bipolar and depressive disorders often result in an inability to work (Wittchen et al., 2011), difficulty maintaining interpersonal relationships (Zlotnick et al., 2000), and elevated mortality rates (Angst et al., 2002). Below, specific diagnostic and clinical features of each mood disorder defined by the Diagnostic and Statistical Manual of Mental Disorders (DSM-5, American Psychiatric Association, 2013) are reviewed.

8.4.1 Bipolar I Disorder

The defining feature of bipolar I disorder is the presence of at least one manic episode: a period of unusually elevated or irritable mood, increased goal-directed behavior or energy that lasts for at least 1 week. During this period of mood disturbance, at least three of the following symptoms must also be present: grandiosity, deceased need for sleep, talkative/pressured talking, racing thoughts, distractibility, an increase in goal directed behavior, or risky behavior (American Psychiatric Association, 2013). Hypomanic episodes (manic episodes lasting at least 4 days) and depressive episodes (defined below) are also common in bipolar disorder, although they are not required for diagnosis.

12-month prevalence rates for bipolar disorder are approximately 1.5% (Blanco et al., 2017). On average, age of onset for a first manic, hypomanic or depressive episode is 18 years old. Bipolar I disorder is associated with an increased risk for suicide (approximately 15 times higher than the general population; American Psychiatric Association, 2013), and often results in significant functional impairment, including poor physical health, impairment in work ability, lower socioeconomic status, and interpersonal difficulties.

8.4.2 *Bipolar II Disorder*

Bipolar II disorder is characterized by at least one hypomanic episode (i.e., manic episode described above last for at least 4 days), *and* a current or past major depressive episode (described below). 12-month prevalence rates for bipolar II disorder are .8% in the United States. Average age-of onset for bipolar II disorder symptoms is the mid-20's (American Psychiatric Association, 2013). Bipolar II disorder is also associated with an increased risk of suicide, although there is some evidence of higher lethality of suicide attempts in bipolar II vs. bipolar I disorder. Functional impairment is significant in individuals with bipolar II disorder.

8.4.3 *Cyclothymic Disorder*

Cyclothymic disorder is characterized by a period of at least 2-years consisting of several periods of hypomanic and depressive symptoms that do not meet full criteria for hypomanic or major depressive episodes. The prevalence rate for cyclothymic disorder is .4–1%. Symptoms typically arise in adolescence or early adulthood (American Psychiatric Association, 2013).

8.4.4 *Disruptive Mood Dysregulation Disorder (DMDD)*

Disruptive Mood Dysregulation Disorder includes severe and recurrent verbal and/or physical (e.g., physical aggression towards people or property) outbursts that are "grossly out of proportion in intensity or duration to the situation" (American Psychiatric Association, 2013). The temper outbursts must be considered inconsistent with developmental level, and occur, on average, three or more times per week. In between temper outbursts, mood is generally irritable. Disruptive behavior must be present in at least two settings (e.g., home, school), and diagnoses should not be made before 6 years of age or after age 18. Prevalence estimates for DMDD are not established, and disruptive behavior must begin before age 10 in order to warrant diagnosis. Children diagnosed with DMDD are at risk of later developing major depressive episodes and/or anxiety disorders in adulthood.

8.4.5 *Major Depressive Disorder*

A major depressive episode is defined by a period lasting 2-weeks that includes either depressed mood and/or loss of interest or pleasure in activities, and four or more of the following symptoms: significant change in body weight or appetite (increase or decrease), insomnia or hypersomnia, psychomotor agitation or retardation, fatigue, feelings of worthlessness or inappropriate guilt, difficulty concentrating or making decisions, and recurrent thoughts of death (e.g., recurrent thoughts of suicide without a plan, with a specific plan, or attempts) (American Psychiatric Association, 2013).

12-month prevalence rates for major depression are approximately 7%, and age of onset tends to be during puberty, although it can occur at any age (American Psychiatric Association, 2013). Major depressive disorder is associated with an increased risk of suicide, particularly for men, individuals who are single or live alone, and those with prominent feelings of hopelessness. Depressive episodes often result in significant functional impairment, including complete inability to attend to basic needs (e.g., eating, showing), physical illness, and decrease role functioning.

8.4.6 *Persistent Depressive Disorder*

Persistent depressive disorder (formerly dysthymic disorder) is characterized by a period of at least 2 years with consistently depressed mood, in addition to at least two of the following symptoms: appetite changes, insomnia or hypersomnia, fatigue, low self-esteem, poor concentration, or feelings of hopelessness (American Psychiatric Association, 2013). 12-month prevalence rate for persistent depressive disorder are .5% (American Psychiatric Association, 2013). Age of onset is typically in childhood, and is associated with a range of mild to severe functional impairments.

8.4.7 *Premenstrual Dysphoric Disorder*

Premenstrual dysphoric disorder includes a series of affective symptoms present during the final week before the onset of menses, and must improve within a few days after the onset of a menstrual cycle. Symptoms include at least one of the following: affective lability, irritability, anger and/or interpersonal conflicts, depressed mood, and anxiety. In addition, at least one of the following symptoms must also be present: decreased interest in usual activities, difficulty concentrating, lethargic, change in appetite, hypersomnia or insomnia, feeling overwhelmed, or physical symptoms (e.g., muscle pain, weight gain. "bloating"). In total, 5 symptoms must be present to warrant diagnosis (American Psychiatric Association, 2013).

The 12-month prevalence estimates for premenstrual dysphoric disorder range from 1.8% to 5.8% (American Psychiatric Association, 2013). Onset of symptoms can occur at any age after the initiation of menses. Interpersonal difficulties are often associated with premenstrual dysphoric disorder symptoms (American Psychiatric Association, 2013).

8.5 Psychopathy and Mood Disorders

Largely, the research on the relationship between psychopathy and mood disorders has focused on symptoms (e.g., depressive symptoms, manic symptoms) rather than specific diagnoses. To date, there are no published studies available on the relationship between psychopathy and cyclothymic, persistent depressive, premenstrual dysphoric, or bipolar II disorders. Accordingly, the following sections will focus on depressive disorders and bipolar disorders.

8.5.1 Psychopathy and Depressive Disorders

Early theoretical conjecture suggested that psychopathy and depression are mutually exclusive disorders. This is consistent with Fowles' (1980) approach and avoidance model of human behavior, which suggested that the behavioral inhibition system (BIS) regulates inhibitory behaviors (e.g., avoidance) when faced with a punishment, whereas the behavioral activation system (BAS) motivates behavior (e.g., approach) in the face of reward. Following the BAS/BIS framework, internalizing disorders (e.g., depression, anxiety) are characterized by a strong BIS and weak BAS, contributing to low levels of approach behavior (e.g., anxiety-related avoidance) and increased withdrawal (e.g., disengagement from activities). In contrast, disorders falling on the externalizing spectrum are characterized by a strong BAS and weak BIS, resulting in excessive approach and dysregulated behavior (e.g., sensation seeking). Theoretically, this puts psychopathy and depression on opposite ends of a spectrum, with contradictory underlying systems contributing to their symptomology. This framework lead some (Lovelace & Gannon, 1999) to conclude that psychopathy cannot occur in the presence of depressive symptomology. Similarly, others have emphasized that the clinical symptomology that characterizes psychopathy and depression are in direct contrast, providing additional theoretical rationale for their mutual exclusivity (Cleckley, 1941; Lovelace & Gannon, 1999; Willemsen et al., 2011). While individuals with psychopathic traits tend to be socially dominant, uncaring, and grandiose (Hare, 2003), those with depression are typically socially withdrawn, ruminative, and experience low self-esteem (American Psychiatric Association, 2013).

Although theory suggests that psychopathy and depression cannot/should not co-occur, empirical studies on psychopathy and depression are overwhelmingly mixed. Several studies have shown that psychopathic traits and depression are *inversely* related, supporting aforementioned theory (Latzman et al., 2018; Lovelace & Gannon, 1999; Moeller & Hell, 2003; Sevecke et al., 2009; Stålenheim & Von Knorring, 1996; Willemsen et al., 2011; Willemsen & Verhaeghe, 2012). However, a similar number of studies have reported that depression is *positively* related to psychopathy (Blonigen et al., 2010; Hemphälä & Tengström, 2010; Love & Holder, 2014; Miller et al., 2010; Sram, 2017; Stinson et al., 2005), and several groups have failed to find a relationship between psychopathy and depression at all (Assadi et al., 2006; Blackburn et al., 2003; Pham & Saloppé, 2010; Rasmussen et al., 1999; Rutherford et al., 1997; Salekin et al., 2004). Still, others have documented significant interactive effects between psychopathy and depression (Pennington et al., 2015; Price et al., 2013; Smith et al., 2013), indicating that individuals who have both high levels of psychopathy and depression tend to have poorer outcomes (e.g., more aggressive, more significant drug use, great suicidal ideation).

There are likely several factors contributing to the complexity in defining the relationship between psychopathy and depression. The first is the differential, and oftentimes conflicting, association between the interpersonal-affective (Factor 1) features of psychopathy, lifestyle-antisocial (Factor 2) features of psychopathy, and external correlates. A number of studies have shown that PCL-R Factors and Facets have differential external correlates (Hicks et al., 2010). For instance, the interpersonal-affective features of psychopathy (e.g., grandiosity, superficial charm, callousness) are positively associated with measures of social dominance (e.g., Verona et al., 2001), and negatively associated with measures of anxiety (e.g., Blonigen et al., 2010). Conversely, the lifestyle-antisocial features of psychopathy (e.g., impulsivity, irresponsibility, sensation seeking) are negatively associated with social adjustment (Miller et al., 2010) and positively correlated with measures of anxiety (Blonigen et al., 2010). As a result, suppressor effects (Hicks & Patrick, 2006) between the two distinct symptom clusters can conflate overall relationships with global measures of psychopathy (e.g., PCL-R).

Considering suppressor effects in the context of psychopathy and depression may clarify some of the inconsistencies throughout the literature. Of the studies that have documented an inverse relationship between psychopathy and depression, most have shown that it is the interpersonal-affective features of psychopathy that are negatively related to depression, but not the lifestyle-antisocial traits (Latzman et al., 2018; Sevecke et al., 2009; Willemsen & Verhaeghe, 2012). Conversely, those studies showing positive associations between depression and psychopathy generally document a positive relationship between the lifestyle-antisocial traits of the disorder and depression, but not the interpersonal-affective (Blonigen et al., 2010; Miller et al., 2010). The few studies that have examined the unique variance of the interpersonal-affective and lifestyle-antisocial traits (i.e., included both variables in the same model to control for shared variance) and internalizing symptomology generally have mirrored these results (Hicks & Patrick, 2006). Accordingly, it may be that while the grandiose, charming and callous features of psychopathy are inversely related to depression, the impulsive and antisocial features are positively associated.

An additional factor that should be considered in the context of psychopathy and depression includes the heterogeneity within psychopathy. Of the studies that have identified subtypes of psychopathic offenders and compared the two groups on measures of internalizing, all have reported that the secondary or high-negative affect (High-NA) group of psychopathic individuals endorse significantly greater symptoms of depression than the primary or low-negative affect (Low-NA) group (Gill & Stickle, 2016; Hicks et al., 2010; Kimonis et al., 2011, 2012; Vaughn et al., 2009). This finding is consistent across age groups (juveniles vs. adults) as well as gender. Consequently, examining the relationship between psychopathy and depression with psychopathy operationalized as a unitary construct (e.g., PCL-R score vs. psychopathic subtype) may result in inconsistent findings due to the wide range of depression severities present among psychopathic subtypes. Indeed, even studies that documented an overall inverse relationship between psychopathy and depression noted that their sample included individuals who presented with clinically significant symptoms of both psychopathy and depression, suggesting the two constructs are not mutually exclusive (Willemsen et al., 2011).

While psychopathy and depression are seemingly a paradox of symptoms, it has been well-established that internalizing and externalizing disorders frequently co-occur (Lilienfeld, 2003). The notion that an individual could exhibit severe personality pathology (i.e., psychopathy) and another form of psychopathology (e.g., depression) is not particularly novel. In fact, a person presenting with a significant form of psychopathology is more likely to experience other forms of psychopathology (Newman et al., 1998). Accordingly, it may be that a subset of individuals with psychopathic traits experience elevated psychopathology more generally, including depression. While this certainly complicates the relationship between psychopathy and depression globally, it may account for the variation in findings across studies.

8.5.2 Psychopathy and Bipolar Disorder

Remarkably few studies have directly examined the co-occurrence of psychopathy and bipolar disorder. In fact, only one study to date has measured psychopathic traits in individuals with bipolar disorder. Demirel et al. (2014) investigated differences in facial emotion recognition and severity of psychopathy among delinquent and non-delinquent psychiatric patients in Istanbul with a diagnosis of bipolar disorder. The results indicated that the group of patients with a criminal history had significantly higher PCL-R scores than the patients without a criminal record. Additionally, the patient group with higher levels of psychopathy and delinquency displayed poorer emotion recognition ability than the non-delinquent group. The authors suggested that deficits in emotion recognition ability may be an important factor in differentiating individuals with bipolar disorder who engage in criminal behavior from those who do not.

It is worth noting that although the delinquent group scored higher on psychopathy than the non-delinquent group in this sample, average PCL-R scores in both groups were very low (8.6 and 6.3, respectively). Even using less stringent cut off criteria for psychopathy "diagnosis" (i.e., PCL-R score ≥ 25 vs. 30), the sample utilized in this study did not include any participants with clinical levels of psychopathy. Accordingly, it is plausible that the elevated PCL-R scores in the delinquent group reflect a higher level of general criminality, rather than psychopathic personality, per se, making it difficult to draw conclusions about the relationship between psychopathy and bipolar disorder in this sample.

Although the literature on psychopathy and bipolar disorder is limited, there is evidence of considerable comorbidity between bipolar disorder and personality disorders, especially "Cluster B" personality disorders (i.e., personality disorders characterized by dramatic and erratic behavior, including borderline, antisocial, narcissistic, and histrionic) (Fan & Hassell, 2008). Studies have shown that individuals with bipolar disorder comorbid with a personality disorder have poorer recovery times post-hospitalization, poorer functional outcomes, and greater substance abuse (Dunayevich et al., 2000; Kay et al., 2002). More specifically, Cluster B personality traits in individuals with a bipolar disorder diagnosis have been linked to a higher number of lifetime suicide attempts, and more severe depression (Garno et al., 2005). Others have reported a specific association between bipolar disorder and antisocial personality traits (Khemakhem et al., 2016), and have shown that individuals with comorbid bipolar disorder and antisocial personality disorder engage in more impulsive behavior (Swann et al., 2010). Similarly, individuals with bipolar disorder have a high risk for aggression (Látalová, 2009).

Specific comorbidity between bipolar disorder and antisociality has also been documented in childhood (i.e., childhood mania and conduct disorder). Conduct disorder is characterized by antisocial behaviors beginning before age 15 years, and is a necessary diagnostic precursor to diagnose antisocial personality disorder in adults. Comorbid bipolar disorder and conduct disorder may be a distinct type of psychopathology, requiring individualized intervention strategies. As in adulthood, comorbid bipolar and conduct disorders in adolescence is characterized by poorer functioning and increased risk of hospitalization (Biederman et al., 1997, 2018; Wozniak et al., 2001). Accordingly, although the relationship between psychopathy and bipolar disorder has not been delineated, there is evidence that manic episodes put individuals at risk of aggression, and that bipolar disorder in combination with a personality disorder is associated with poor clinical outcomes.

8.5.3 Psychopathy and Suicidality

Suicidal ideation, self-injurious behavior, and suicide attempts are common among individuals with mood disorders (Nierenberg et al., 2001). Perhaps not surprisingly, the available data on the relationship between psychopathy and suicidality largely mirrors the relationships between psychopathy and depression. Specifically, it has been shown that suicidality is negatively correlated with the interpersonal-affective traits of psychopathy, but positively associated with the lifestyle-antisocial traits of psychopathy (Douglas et al., 2006, 2008; Gunter et al., 2011; Patrick et al., 2005; Verona et al., 2001, 2005).

Studies that have compared suicidality between psychopathic subtypes have shown that the secondary/High-NA subtype endorses a greater degree of suicidal ideation than the primary/Low-NA subtype (Hicks et al., 2010). Notably, these relationships seem to be somewhat dependent on how suicidality is operationalized. For instance, Douglas et al. (2006) reported that, in a sample of 682 male offenders, total number of suicide *attempts* were positively associated with Factor 2 traits, but there was no relationship between suicide attempts and Factor 1 traits. However, the severity of suicidal *ideation* was inversely related to Factor 1 traits, and positively related to Factor 2 traits. Other studies that have operationalized suicidality as a number of suicide attempts, rather than suicidal ideation or self-injurious behavior, have also reported positive relationships with the Factor 2 features of psychopathy, but no relationships with the Factor 1 traits (Douglas et al., 2006; Patrick et al., 2005; Swogger et al., 2009; Verona et al., 2001). There are some inconsistencies in these findings. For instance, Verona et al. (2005) reported that suicide *attempts* were negatively associated with Factor 1 traits in female inmates. In contrast, Seveke et al. (2009) found positive associations with the affective features of psychopathy and suicidal *behavior* in adolescent female detainees, although these authors did not report a relationship between suicidal behavior and psychopathy in male detainees.

Interestingly, most studies that have reported no association with the Factor 1 traits of psychopathy and suicidal *behavior/attempts* have been entirely male samples (Douglas et al., 2008; Patrick et al., 2005; Smith et al., 2013; Verona et al., 2001), suggesting there may be gender differences in how suicidality relates to psychopathy. Furthermore, it seems that while the Factor 1 traits of psychopathy are generally a protective factor against suicidal *ideation* (i.e., inversely correlated), they are not as consistently a protective factor against suicidal *behavior*. It will be important for future research to clarify these relationships, identify if there are specific risk factors for suicide, and/or different assessment strategies needed to evaluate risk of suicide among high psychopathy individuals, particularly if high psychopathy individuals are less likely to report suicidal ideation.

8.6 Clinical Assessment Considerations

Although the relationships between psychopathy and mood disorders are complicated, there is certainly evidence that psychopathy and mood disorders are not mutually exclusive constructs. As such, thorough clinical assessment of mood symptoms and suicidality is critical when working with individuals with antisocial or psychopathic traits. Even studies that have documented an overall negative relationship between measures of depression and psychopathy have specifically noted that their sample included individuals with high levels of psychopathy and depression (Willemsen et al., 2011). In other words, high psychopathy individuals may endorse significant mood disturbances, despite presenting as otherwise grandiose.

Moreover, the psychopathic subtype literature has consistently shown that a subset of highly psychopathic individuals experience clinically significant psychological distress (e.g., anxiety, depression, PTSD), indicating that a subset of highly psychopathic individuals may be *expected* to endorse mood disorder symptoms.

The interpersonal features of psychopathy (e.g., glibness, superficial charm) may present some challenges for clinicians when conducting clinical assessment and evaluating mood disorder symptoms. For instance, high psychopathy individuals are characteristically interpersonally dominant, talkative, and tend to derail conversation with unrelated topics (Hare, 2003). It is likely helpful for clinicians evaluating individuals with psychopathic traits to incorporate self-report questionnaires in addition to clinical interviews to ensure they are adequately assessing all relevant symptomology. Although high psychopathy individuals tend to lie pathologically, they appear to provide valid self-report questionnaire responses (Neumann et al., 2008), and thus these may be helpful clinical tools to use during psychological evaluation.

8.7 Clinical Intervention Considerations

The relationships between psychopathy and mood disorder symptoms are complicated. It follows that clinical interventions may be impacted in important ways by these relationships. In the next sections, treatments for mood disorders, psychopathy, and for addressing the comorbidity between the two are discussed.

8.7.1 Treatment of Mood Disorders

Research on the treatment of depression suggests that both medication and psychotherapy can be helpful in managing symptomology (Cuijpers et al., 2007; Thase & Kupfer, 1996), although effect sizes, overall, are fairly small (Cuijpers et al., 2010). Psychopharmacological and psychotherapeutic interventions are equally as effective at reducing symptoms of depression (Amick et al., 2015; DeRubeis et al., 2005). Notably, there is some evidence that behavioral therapies may be more effective at preventing symptom relapse than medication (Dobson et al., 2008). There are several evidence-based treatments for depression, however most studies have not shown reliable differences in efficacy across therapy modalities (Barth et al., 2013). Rather, there is evidence that commonalities across psychotherapies (i.e., "common factors"; Messer & Wampold, 2002) may account for symptom change, regardless of the type of therapy being employed.

As with depression, bipolar disorder is often treated with medication, as well as psychotherapy. Mania associated with bipolar disorder is most commonly treated with psychotropic (e.g., Lithium) antipsychotic (e.g., Quetiapine) or anticonvulsant (e.g., divalproex) medication (Baldessarini et al., 2019; Geddes & Miklowitz,

2013). There are some inconsistencies in the literature regarding the type of medication that is most effective at stabilizing manic episodes, although generally Lithium appears to have the most evidence for long-term relapse prevention. Although there is evidence that antipsychotic and anticonvulsant medications are effective in the management of mania, there is less information available regarding the long-term benefits of these when compared to Lithium (Geddes & Miklowitz, 2013). In addition to psychiatric management, there is some evidence suggesting that psychosocial interventions can aid in long-term maintenance and relapse prevention of mood disturbances among individuals with bipolar disorder (Miziou et al., 2015).

8.7.2 Treatment of Psychopathy

Although there is a longstanding misconception that psychopathy is untreatable, the current lack of effective treatment strategies is likely more reflective of the lack of empirical studies examining treatments for high psychopathy individuals. In fact, the few studies that have sought to reduce psychopathic traits and/or behavioral problems associated with psychopathy have reported promising results. For instance, Baskin Sommers et al. (2015) implemented a laboratory-based cognitive remediation program designed to target psychopathy-specific attentional deficits (i.e., impairments in response modulation) and reported that high psychopathy individuals performed significantly better on various response modulation tasks post-intervention. Similarly, there is evidence that juveniles with psychopathic traits benefit from an intensive, secure treatment program that incentivizes prosocial behavior (Caldwell, 2011; Caldwell et al., 2006, 2007, 2012). Indeed, adolescents who have completed this program, regardless of psychopathy level, are less likely to reoffend upon release (Caldwell et al., 2007).

Several studies, while not specifically aiming to treat psychopathic traits, have examined the effect of PCL-R score on treatment outcomes as well as therapeutic alliance in corrections-based treatments (e.g., sexual offender treatment). There is some evidence that high psychopathy individuals are less likely to complete treatment (Olver & Wong, 2009), and have difficulty establishing productive relationships with therapists (DeSorcy et al., 2017; Walton et al., 2016). However, recent evidence has shown that high psychopathy individuals are capable of therapeutic change, and that therapeutic change is associated with reduced risk level, regardless of psychopathy level (Sewall & Olver, 2019). Accordingly, although a specific evidence-based treatment for psychopathy does currently not exist, the literature on treating psychopathy is promising and suggests that individuals with psychopathic traits can benefit from traditional treatment methods.

8.7.3 *Treating Comorbidity*

The effectiveness of treating psychopathic traits in the presence of a co-occurring mood disorder is unknown. Given that difficulty with interpersonal relationships is a key feature of most personality disorders, it has been documented that personality disorder symptoms (regardless of specific personality disorder) can complicate the development of the client-therapist working alliance (Lingiardi et al., 2005). Similarly, individuals with personality disorder symptoms generally show poorer treatment outcomes when seeking therapy for mood disorders (George et al., 2018). For example, Post et al. (2018) reported that the severity of personality disorder symptomology was associated with adverse treatment outcomes in patients with bipolar disorder. Similarly, George et al. (2018) reported that "Cluster B" personality traits (e.g., antisocial) were associated with poorer depression outcomes at a 6-month follow-up.

Although personality disorder symptomology tends to be associated with worse treatment outcomes overall, there is evidence that co-occurring mood symptoms can be effectively treated among individuals with antisocial personality disorder (ASPD). For instance, Dialectical Behavioral Therapy (DBT) (Linehan, 1987) reduces self-harm behavior and depression symptoms among men with borderline personality disorder and antisocial behavior (Wetterborg et al., 2018). Similarly, it has been reported that men with ASPD and depression benefit more from cognitive-based treatments than men with ASPD without depression (Woody et al., 1985). There is also evidence that children with bipolar disorder and co-occurring conduct disorder exhibit fewer symptoms of conduct disorder/behavioral problems when manic symptoms remit. The authors suggested that targeting manic symptoms in youth with conduct disorder might simultaneously improve the trajectory of manic and conduct disorder symptoms. In line with this suggestion, medication used to treat mania has been shown to reduce aggressive behavior (Correll, et al., 2017) and treatments targeting emotion regulation (e.g., DBT) can reduce antisocial behavior (Stadler et al., 2016).

8.8 Summary

The literature on psychopathy and depression is somewhat inconsistent. Although theoretical models suggest the two constructs are mutually exclusive, and there is empirical data indicating depression is inversely related to psychopathy, there is equally compelling data indicating that highly psychopathic individuals can experience depressive symptomology, and certain features of psychopathy may even be positively associated with depression. The inconsistencies reported are likely due to a combination of suppressor effects, such that the interpersonal and affective traits of psychopathy are negatively associated with depression, whereas the lifestyle and antisocial traits are positively associated with depression. Moreover, heterogeneity within the construct of psychopathy suggests that a subset of psychopathic individuals endorse significant depressive symptomology, muddling the overall relationships between psychopathy and depression. Although certain features of psychopathy seem to be inversely related to depression, there is evidence that psychopathic individuals do endorse symptoms of depression, and these individuals may be at particular risk for aggression and substance abuse.

Although the extant literature does not clearly delineate the specific relationship between psychopathic traits and bipolar disorder, there is considerable evidence for comorbidity between bipolar disorder and antisociality, more generally. This has been shown at different developmental time points. Moreover, individuals with bipolar disorder comorbid with disordered personality traits have worse clinical and functional outcomes. These results suggest that individuals with both psychopathic traits and bipolar disorder may be a particularly difficult patient population to treat.

The relationship between psychopathy and suicidality generally mirrors the findings reported for psychopathy and depression. While some studies have documented negative associations with certain features of psychopathy and suicidality, others have shown positive relationships. In addition to the suppressor and heterogeneity concerns discussed in relation to depression, a complication within the psychopathy-suicidality literature is that the associations seem to differ depending on how suicidality is operationalized (ideation vs. behavior). There is also some indication that the relationship between psychopathy and suicidality differs by gender, although more information is needed to state this conclusively.

8.9 Recommendations

Clinicians conducting psychological evaluations, risk assessments and/or intake interviews with high psychopathy individuals should include thorough assessment of depression symptomology and suicidality, even if the individual's interpersonal style suggests otherwise. In addition to the research showing that a subset of high psychopathy individuals experience significant emotional distress, there is some indication that psychopathy and internalizing symptoms interact, resulting in more significant clinical impairment (e.g., Price et al., 2013). As such, psychopathic traits alone should not be viewed as a protective factor against other psychopathology. Instead, the presence of psychopathic traits should encourage further assessment of internalizing symptoms, as those individuals with both psychopathy and emotional distress may be a particularly high risk clinical population.

Clinicians working with individuals who present with both psychopathic traits and mood disruption may consider conceptualizing the primary treatment need as a generally high level of dysregulation (e.g., emotional, behavioral, impulse control), versus "high psychopathy with comorbid mood disorder". While limited, the available data suggests that improving emotion regulation strategies more generally (rather than treating a personality disorder, per se) may provide the most benefit to individuals with co-occurring personality and mood disorders (Sauer-Zavala et al.,

2015). Accordingly, transdiagnostic treatment strategies (i.e., treatments that target symptomology rather than specific diagnosis) may be promising interventions for individuals with antisocial personality traits and comorbid mood disturbance. For instance, the Unified Protocol for the Transdiagnostic Treatment of Emotional Disorders (Ellard et al., 2010) has been used to effectively treat symptoms of depression and anxiety (Barlow et al., 2017; Sakiris & Berle, 2019), PTSD (Varkovitzky et al., 2017), and borderline personality traits (Lopez et al., 2015). Although theoretical, targeting emotion regulation among individuals with psychopathic traits who also endorse significant emotional distress may improve overall emotion-regulation strategies, resulting in fewer behavioral problems associated with psychopathy.

It will be important for researchers to study the efficacy of such interventions, including traditional evidence-based therapies (e.g., DBT), to treat psychopathology among individuals with psychopathic traits. Although psychopathy is not a contraindication for evidence-based or empirically-supported treatments, studies have not examined treatment response to well-established treatment protocols in the context of psychopathy. Utilizing treatment approaches that already have an evidence base with high psychopathy people could be an important first step towards identifying effective treatments for psychopathy, especially psychopathy with co-occurring mood disorder.

Finally, researchers and clinicians alike should consider the utility of common factors approaches to psychotherapy when working with individuals with psychopathic traits (Wampold, 2015). It is possible that a key to effective intervention with severely antisocial individuals is the ability to establish an effective therapeutic alliance, express empathy, and build trust. Although individuals with personality disorder traits may have difficulty establishing therapeutic alliance given oftentimes long histories of social dysfunction and chaotic relationships (Olesek et al., 2016), there is evidence that therapist, *not patient*, factors determine the strength of a therapeutic alliance (Baldwin et al., 2007). With this in mind, clinicians who plan to work in forensic or correctional settings should prioritize establishing an effective therapeutic alliance with their clients, and understand that although individuals with psychopathic traits may be challenging to work with, it is the therapist who ultimately controls the strength of their working relationship (Baldwin et al., 2007).

References

American Psychiatric Association. (2013). *Diagnostic and statistical manual of mental disorders (DSM-5®)*. American Psychiatric Pub.

Amick, H. R., Gartlehner, G., Gaynes, B. N., Forneris, C., Asher, G. N., Morgan, L. C., Coker-Schwimmer, E., Forneris, C., Boland, E., Lux, L. J., Gaylord, S., Bann, C., Pierl, C. B., & Lohr, K. N. (2015). Comparative benefits and harms of second generation antidepressants and cognitive behavioral therapies in initial treatment of major depressive disorder: Systematic review and meta-analysis. *BMJ, 351*, h6019. https://doi.org/10.1136/bmj.h6019

Angst, F., Stassen, H. H., Clayton, P. J., & Angst, J. (2002). Mortality of patients with mood disorders: Follow-up over 34–38 years. *Journal of Affective Disorders, 68*(2), 167–181. https://doi.org/10.1016/S0165-0327(01)00377-9

Assadi, S. M., Noroozian, M., Pakravannejad, M., Yahyazadeh, O., Aghayan, S., Shariat, S. V., & Fazel, S. (2006). Psychiatric morbidity among sentenced prisoners: Prevalence study in Iran. *British Journal of Psychiatry, 188*(2), 159–164. https://doi.org/10.1192/bjp.188.2.159

Baldessarini, R. J., Tondo, L., & Vázquez, G. H. (2019). Pharmacological treatment of adult bipolar disorder. *Molecular Psychiatry, 24*(2), 198–217. https://doi.org/10.1038/s41380-018-0044-2

Baldwin, S. A., Wampold, B. E., & Imel, Z. E. (2007). Untangling the alliance-outcome correlation: Exploring the relative importance of therapist and patient variability in the alliance. *Journal of Consulting and Clinical Psychology, 75*(6), 842–852. https://doi.org/10.1037/0022-006X.75.6.842

Barlow, D. H., Farchione, T. J., Bullis, J. R., Gallagher, M. W., Murray-Latin, H., Sauer-Zavala, S., Bentley, K. H., Thompson-Hollands, J., Conklin, L. R., Boswell, J. F., Ametaj, A., Carl, J. R., Boettcher, H. T., & Cassiello-Robbins, C. (2017). The Unified Protocol for Transdiagnostic Treatment of Emotional Disorders compared with diagnosis-specific protocols for anxiety disorders: A randomized clinical trial. *JAMA Psychiatry, 74*(9), 875–884. https://doi.org/10.1001/jamapsychiatry.2017.2164

Barth, J., Munder, T., Gerger, H., Nuesch, E., Trelle, S., Znoj, H., Jüni, P., & Cuijpers, P. (2013). Comparative efficacy of seven psychotherapeutic interventions for patients with depression: A network meta-analysis. *PLoS Medicine, 10*(5), e1001454. https://doi.org/10.1371/journal.pmed.1001454

Baskin-Sommers, A. R., Curtin, J. J., & Newman, J. P. (2015). Altering the cognitive-affective dysfunctions of psychopathic and externalizing offender subtypes with cognitive remediation. *Clinical Psychological Science, 3*(1), 45–57. https://doi.org/10.1177/2167702614560744

Biederman, J., Faraone, S. V., Hatch, M., Mennin, D., Taylor, A., & George, P. (1997). Conduct disorder with and without mania in a referred sample of ADHD children. *Journal of Affective Disorders, 44*(2), 177–188. https://doi.org/10.1016/S0165-0327(97)00043-8

Biederman, J., Fitzgerald, M., Woodworth, K. Y., Yule, A., Noyes, E., Biederman, I., Faraone, S. V., Wilens, T., & Wozniak, J. (2018). Does the course of manic symptoms in pediatric bipolar disorder impact the course of conduct disorder? Findings from four prospective datasets. *Journal of Affective Disorders, 238*, 244–249. https://doi.org/10.1016/j.jad.2018.05.020

Blackburn, R., Logan, C., Donnelly, J., & Renwick, S. (2003). Personality disorders, psychopathy and other mental disorders: Co-morbidity among patients at English and Scottish high-security hospitals. *The Journal of Forensic Psychiatry & Psychology, 14*(1), 111–137. https://doi.org/10.1080/1478994031000077925

Blackburn, R., Logan, C., Donnelly, J. P., & Renwick, S. J. (2008). Identifying psychopathic subtypes: Combining an empirical personality classification of offenders with the Psychopathy Checklist-Revised. *Journal of Personality Disorders, 22*(6), 604–622.

Blanco, C., Compton, W. M., Saha, T. D., Goldstein, B. I., Ruan, W. J., Huang, B., & Grant, B. F. (2017). Epidemiology of DSM-5 bipolar I disorder: Results from the National Epidemiologic Survey on Alcohol and Related Conditions – III. *Journal of Psychiatric Research, 84*, 310–317. https://doi.org/10.1016/j.jpsychires.2016.10.003

Blonigen, D. M., Patrick, C. J., Douglas, K. S., Poythress, N. G., Skeem, J. L., Lilienfeld, S. O., Edens, J. F., & Krueger, R. F. (2010). Multimethod assessment of psychopathy in relation to factors of internalizing and externalizing from the Personality Assessment Inventory: The impact of method variance and suppressor effects. *Psychological Assessment, 22*(1), 96–107. https://doi.org/10.1037/a0017240

Caldwell, M. (2011). Treatment-related changes in behavioral outcomes of psychopathy facets in adolescent offenders. *Law and Human Behavior, 35*(4), 275–287. https://doi.org/10.1007/s10979-010-9239-z

Caldwell, M., Skeem, J., Salekin, R., & Van Rybroek, G. (2006). Treatment response of adolescent offenders with psychopathy features: A 2-year follow-up. *Criminal Justice and Behavior, 33*(5), 571–596. https://doi.org/10.1177/0093854806288176

Caldwell, M., McCormick, D. J., Umstead, D., & Van Rybroek, G. J. (2007). Evidence of treatment progress and therapeutic outcomes among adolescents with psychopathic features. *Criminal Justice and Behavior, 34*(5), 573–587. https://doi.org/10.1177/0093854806297511

Caldwell, M., McCormick, D., Wolfe, J., & Umstead, D. (2012). Treatment-related changes in psychopathy features and behavior in adolescent offenders. *Criminal Justice and Behavior, 39*(2), 144–155. https://doi.org/10.1177/0093854811429542

Claes, L., Tavernier, G., Roose, A., Bijttebier, P., Smith, S. F., & Lilienfeld, S. O. (2014). Identifying personality subtypes based on the five-factor model dimensions in male prisoners: Implications for psychopathy and criminal offending. *International Journal of Offender Therapy and Comparative Criminology, 58*(1), 41–58.

Cleckley, H. (1941). *The mask of sanity; an attempt to reinterpret the so-called psychopathic personality*. Mosby.

Correll, C. U., Yu, X., Xiang, Y., Kane, J. M., & Masand, P. (2017). Biological treatment of acute agitation or aggression with schizophrenia or bipolar disorder in the inpatient setting. *Annals of Clinical Psychiatry, 29*(2), 92–107.

Cuijpers, P., van Straten, A., & Warmerdam, L. (2007). Behavioral activation treatments of depression: A meta-analysis. *Clinical Psychology Review, 27*(3), 318–326. https://doi.org/10.1016/j.cpr.2006.11.001

Cuijpers, P., van Straten, A., Bohlmeijer, E., Hollon, S. D., & Andersson, G. (2010). The effects of psychotherapy for adult depression are overestimated: A meta-analysis of study quality and effect size. *Psychological Medicine, 40*(2), 211–223. https://doi.org/10.1017/S0033291709006114

Dargis, M., & Koenigs, M. (2018). Personality traits differentiate subgroups of criminal offenders with distinct cognitive, affective, and behavioral profiles. *Criminal Justice and Behavior, 45*(7), 984–1007.

Demirel, H., Yesilbas, D., Ozver, I., Yuksek, E., Sahin, F., Aliustaoglu, S., & Emul, M. (2014). Psychopathy and facial emotion recognition ability in patients with bipolar affective disorder with or without delinquent behaviors. *Comprehensive Psychiatry, 55*(3), 542–546. https://doi.org/10.1016/j.comppsych.2013.11.022

DeRubeis, R. J., Hollon, S. D., Amsterdam, J. D., Shelton, R. C., Young, P. R., Salomon, R. M., O'Reardon, J. P., Lovett, M. L., Gladis, M. M., Brown, L. L., & Gallop, R. (2005). Cognitive therapy vs medications in the treatment of moderate to severe depression. *JAMA Psychiatry, 62*(4), 409–416. https://doi.org/10.1001/archpsyc.62.4.409

DeSorcy, D. R., Olver, M. E., & Wormith, J. S. (2017). Working alliance and psychopathy: Linkages to treatment outcome in a sample of treated sexual offenders. *Journal of Interpersonal Violence*, 0886260517698822. https://doi.org/10.1177/0886260517698822

Dobson, K. S., Hollon, S. D., Dimidjian, S., Schmaling, K. B., Kohlenberg, R. J., Gallop, R. J., Rizvi, S. L., Gollan, J. K., Dunner, D. L., & Jacobson, N. S. (2008). Randomized trial of behavioral activation, cognitive therapy, and antidepressant medication in the prevention of relapse and recurrence in major depression. *Journal of Consulting and Clinical Psychology, 76*(3), 468–477. https://doi.org/10.1037/0022-006X.76.3.468

Douglas, K. S., Herbozo, S., Poythress, N. G., Belfrage, H., & Edens, J. F. (2006). Psychopathy and suicide: A multisample investigation. *Psychological Services, 3*(2), 97–116. https://doi.org/10.1037/1541-1559.3.2.97

Douglas, K. S., Lilienfeld, S. O., Skeem, J. L., Poythress, N. G., Edens, J. F., & Patrick, C. J. (2008). Relation of antisocial and psychopathic traits to suicide-related behavior among offenders. *Law and Human Behavior, 32*(6), 511–525. https://doi.org/10.1007/s10979-007-9122-8

Dunayevich, E., Sax, K., Keck, P., McElroy, S., Sorter, M., McConville, B., & Strakowski, S. (2000). Twelve-month outcome in bipolar patients with and without personality disorders. *The Journal of Clinical Psychiatry, 61*(2), 134–139.

Ellard, K. K., Fairholme, C. P., Boisseau, C. L., Farchione, T. J., & Barlow, D. H. (2010). Unified Protocol for the Transdiagnostic Treatment of Emotional Disorders: Protocol development and initial outcome data. *Cognitive and Behavioral Practice, 17*(1), 88–101. https://doi.org/10.1016/j.cbpra.2009.06.002

Fan, A. H., & Hassell, J. (2008). Bipolar disorder and comorbid personality psychopathology: A review of the literature. *The Journal of Clinical Psychiatry, 69*(11), 1794–1803. https://doi.org/10.4088/JCP.v69n1115

Flores-Mendoza, C. E., Alvarenga, M. A. S., Herrero, Ó., & Abad, F. J. (2008). Factor structure and behavioural correlates of the Psychopathy Checklist-Revised [PCL-R] in a Brazilian prisoner sample. *Personality and Individual Differences, 45*(7), 584–590.

Fowles, D. C. (1980). The three arousal model: Implications of Gray's two-factor learning theory for heart rate, electrodermal activity, and psychopathy. *Psychophysiology, 17*(2), 87–104. https://doi.org/10.1111/j.1469-8986.1980.tb00117.x

Garno, J. L., Goldberg, J. F., Ramirez, P. M., & Ritzler, B. A. (2005). Bipolar Disorder with comorbid Cluster B personality disorder features: Impact on suicidality. *The Journal of Clinical Psychiatry, 66*(3), 339–345. https://doi.org/10.4088/JCP.v66n0310

Geddes, J. R., & Miklowitz, D. J. (2013). Treatment of bipolar disorder. *Lancet (London, England), 381*(9878), 1672–1682. https://doi.org/10.1016/S0140-6736(13)60857-0

Gelenberg, A. J. (2010). The prevalence and impact of depression. *The Journal of Clinical Psychiatry, 71*(3), e06. https://doi.org/10.4088/jcp.8001tx17c

George, M. P., Garrison, G. M., Merten, Z., Heredia, D., Gonzales, C., & Angstman, K. B. (2018). Impact of personality disorder cluster on depression outcomes within collaborative care management model of care. *Journal of Primary Care & Community Health, 9*, 2150132718776877. https://doi.org/10.1177/2150132718776877

Gill, A. D., & Stickle, T. R. (2016). Affective differences between psychopathy variants and genders in adjudicated youth. *Journal of Abnormal Child Psychology, 44*(2), 295–307. https://doi.org/10.1007/s10802-015-9990-1

Gunter, T. D., Chibnall, J. T., Antoniak, S. K., Philibert, R. A., & Hollenbeck, N. (2011). Predictors of suicidal ideation, suicide attempts, and self-harm without lethal intent in a community corrections sample. *Journal of Criminal Justice, 39*(3), 238–245. https://doi.org/10.1016/j.jcrimjus.2011.02.005

Hare, R. D. (1998). Psychopaths and their nature: Implications for the mental health and criminal justice systems. In *Psychopathy: Antisocial, criminal, and violent behavior* (pp. 188–212). Guilford.

Hare, R. (2003). The psychopathy checklist-revised. In *Encyclopedia of psychology and law*. SAGE.

Hart, S. D., & Hare, R. D. (1996). Psychopathy and antisocial personality disorder. *Current Opinion in Psychiatry, 9*(2), 129–132.

Hemphälä, M., & Tengström, A. (2010). Associations between psychopathic traits and mental disorders among adolescents with substance use problems. *British Journal of Clinical Psychology, 49*(1), 109–122. https://doi.org/10.1348/014466509X439216

Hicks, B. M., & Patrick, C. J. (2006). Psychopathy and negative emotionality: Analyses of suppressor effects reveal distinct relations with emotional distress, fearfulness, and anger-hostility. *Journal of Abnormal Psychology, 115*(2), 276–287. https://doi.org/10.1037/0021-843X.115.2.276

Hicks, B. M., Markon, K. E., Patrick, C. J., Krueger, R. F., & Newman, J. P. (2004). Identifying psychopathy subtypes on the basis of personality structure. *Psychological Assessment, 16*(3), 276.

Hicks, B. M., Vaidyanathan, U., & Patrick, C. J. (2010). Validating female psychopathy subtypes: Differences in personality, antisocial and violent behavior, substance abuse, trauma, and mental health. *Personality Disorders, 1*(1), 38–57. https://doi.org/10.1037/a0018135

Judd, L. L., & Akiskal, H. S. (2003). The prevalence and disability of bipolar spectrum disorders in the US population: Re-analysis of the ECA database taking into account subthreshold cases. *Validating the Biopolar Spectrum, 73*(1), 123–131. https://doi.org/10.1016/S0165-0327(02)00332-4

Kay, J. H., Altshuler, L. L., Ventura, J., & Mintz, J. (2002). Impact of axis II comorbidity on the course of bipolar illness in men: A retrospective chart review. *Bipolar Disorders, 4*(4), 237–242. https://doi.org/10.1034/j.1399-5618.2002.01165.x

Khemakhem, R., Homri, W., Karoui, D., Mezghani, M., Mouelhi, L., Bram, N., Romdhane, I. B., & Labbane, R. (2016). Mutual influence between mood disorders and personality disorders. *European Psychiatry, 33*, S250. https://doi.org/10.1016/j.eurpsy.2016.01.506

Kiehl, K. A., & Hoffman, M. B. (2011). The criminal psychopath: History, neuroscience, treatment, and economics. *Jurimetrics, 51*, 355.

Kimonis, E. R., Skeem, J. L., Cauffman, E., & Dmitrieva, J. (2011). Are secondary variants of juvenile psychopathy more reactively violent and less psychosocially mature than primary variants? *Law and Human Behavior, 35*(5), 381–391. https://doi.org/10.1007/s10979-010-9243-3

Kimonis, E. R., Frick, P. J., Cauffman, E., Goldweber, A., & Skeem, J. (2012). Primary and secondary variants of juvenile psychopathy differ in emotional processing. *Development and Psychopathology, 24*(3), 1091–1103. https://doi.org/10.1017/S0954579412000557

Látalová, K. (2009). Bipolar disorder and aggression. *International Journal of Clinical Practice, 63*(6), 889–899. https://doi.org/10.1111/j.1742-1241.2009.02001.x

Latzman, R. D., Palumbo, I. M., Sauvigné, K. C., Hecht, L. K., Lilienfeld, S. O., & Patrick, C. J. (2018). Psychopathy and internalizing psychopathology: A triarchic model perspective. *Journal of Personality Disorders, 33*(2), 262–287. https://doi.org/10.1521/pedi_2018_32_347

Lilienfeld, S. O. (2003). Comorbidity between and within childhood externalizing and internalizing disorders: Reflections and directions. *Journal of Abnormal Child Psychology, 31*(3), 285–291. https://doi.org/10.1023/A:1023229529866

Linehan, M. M. (1987). Dialectical Behavior Therapy for borderline personality disorder: Theory and method. *Bulletin of the Menninger Clinic, 51*(3), 261–276.

Lingiardi, V., Filippucci, L., & Baiocco, R. (2005). Therapeutic alliance evaluation in personality disorders psychotherapy. *Psychotherapy Research, 15*(1–2), 45–53. https://doi.org/10.1080/10503300512331327047

Lopez, M. E., Stoddard, J. A., Noorollah, A., Zerbi, G., Payne, L. A., Hitchcock, C. A., Meier, E. A., Esfahani, A. M., & Ray, D. B. (2015). Examining the efficacy of the Unified Protocol for Transdiagnostic Treatment of Emotional Disorders in the treatment of individuals with Borderline Personality Disorder. *Cognitive and Behavioral Practice, 22*(4), 522–533. https://doi.org/10.1016/j.cbpra.2014.06.006

Love, A. B., & Holder, M. D. (2014). Psychopathy and subjective well-being. *Personality and Individual Differences, 66*, 112–117. https://doi.org/10.1016/j.paid.2014.03.033

Lovelace, L., & Gannon, L. (1999). Psychopathy and depression: Mutually exclusive constructs? *Journal of Behavior Therapy and Experimental Psychiatry, 30*(3), 169–176. https://doi.org/10.1016/S0005-7916(99)00022-1

Lykken, D. T. (1996). Psychopathy, sociopathy, and crime. *Society, 34*(1), 29–38.

Marvel, C. L., & Paradiso, S. (2004). Cognitive and neurological impairment in mood disorders. *Psychiatric Clinics, 27*(1), 19–36. https://doi.org/10.1016/S0193-953X(03)00106-0

Messer, S. B., & Wampold, B. E. (2002). Let's face facts: Common factors are more potent than specific therapy ingredients. *Clinical Psychology: Science and Practice, 9*(1), 21–25. https://doi.org/10.1093/clipsy.9.1.21

Miller, J. D., Dir, A., Gentile, B., Wilson, L., Pryor, L. R., & Campbell, W. K. (2010). Searching for a vulnerable Dark Triad: Comparing Factor 2 psychopathy, vulnerable narcissism, and Borderline Personality Disorder. *Journal of Personality, 78*(5), 1529–1564. https://doi.org/10.1111/j.1467-6494.2010.00660.x

Miziou, S., Tsitsipa, E., Moysidou, S., Karavelas, V., Dimelis, D., Polyzoidou, V., & Fountoulakis, K. N. (2015). Psychosocial treatment and interventions for bipolar disorder: A systematic review. *Annals of General Psychiatry, 14*(1), 19. https://doi.org/10.1186/s12991-015-0057-z

Moeller, A. A., & Hell, D. (2003). Affective disorder and 'psychopathy' in a sample of younger male delinquents. *Acta Psychiatrica Scandinavica, 107*(3), 203–207. https://doi.org/10.1034/j.1600-0447.2003.02377.x

Neumann, C. S., Kosson, D. S., Forth, A. E., & Hare, R. D. (2006). Factor structure of the Hare Psychopathy Checklist: Youth Version (PCL: YV) in incarcerated adolescents. *Psychological Assessment, 18*(2), 142.

Neumann, C. S., Malterer, M. B., & Newman, J. P. (2008). Factor structure of the Psychopathic Personality Inventory (PPI): Findings from a large incarcerated sample. *Psychological Assessment, 20*(2), 169–174. https://doi.org/10.1037/1040-3590.20.2.169

Neumann, C. S., Johansson, P. T., & Hare, R. D. (2013). The Psychopathy Checklist-Revised (PCL-R), low anxiety, and fearlessness: A structural equation modeling analysis. *Personality Disorders, Theory, Research, and Treatment, 4*(2), 129.

Newman, D. L., Moffitt, T. E., Caspi, A., & Silva, P. A. (1998). Comorbid mental disorders: Implications for treatment and sample selection. *Journal of Abnormal Psychology, 107*(2), 305–311. https://doi.org/10.1037/0021-843X.107.2.305

Nierenberg, A. A., Gray, S. M., & Grandin, L. D. (2001). Mood disorders and suicide. *The Journal of Clinical Psychiatry, 62*(Suppl25), 27–30.

Olesek, K. L., Outcalt, J., Dimaggio, G., Popolo, R., George, S., & Lysaker, P. H. (2016). Cluster B personality disorder traits as a predictor of therapeutic alliance over time in residential treatment for substance use disorders. *The Journal of Nervous and Mental Disease, 204*(10), 736–740. https://doi.org/10.1097/NMD.0000000000000553

Olver, M. E., & Wong, S. C. P. (2009). Therapeutic responses of psychopathic sexual offenders: Treatment attrition, therapeutic change, and long-term recidivism. *Journal of Consulting and Clinical Psychology, 77*(2), 328–336. https://doi.org/10.1037/a0015001

Patrick, C. J., Hicks, B. M., Krueger, R. F., & Lang, A. R. (2005). Relations between psychopathy facets and externalizing in a criminal offender sample. *Journal of Personality Disorders, 19*(4), 339–356. https://doi.org/10.1521/pedi.2005.19.4.339

Pennington, C. R., Cramer, R. J., Miller, H. A., & Anastasi, J. S. (2015). Psychopathy, depression, and anxiety as predictors of suicidal ideation in offenders. *Death Studies, 39*(5), 288–295. https://doi.org/10.1080/07481187.2014.991953

Pham, T. H., & Saloppé, X. (2010). PCL-R psychopathy and its relation to DSM Axis I and II disorders in a sample of male forensic patients in a Belgian security hospital. *International Journal of Forensic Mental Health, 9*(3), 205–214. https://doi.org/10.1080/14999013.2010.517255

Post, R. M., McElroy, S., Kupka, R., Suppes, T., Hellemann, G., Nolen, W., Frye, M., Keck, P., Grunze, H., & Rowe, M. (2018). Axis II personality disorders are linked to an adverse course of Bipolar Disorder. *The Journal of Nervous and Mental Disease, 206*(6), 469–472. https://doi.org/10.1097/nmd.0000000000000819

Price, S. D., Salekin, R. T., Klinger, M. R., & Barker, E. D. (2013). Psychopathy and depression as predictors of psychosocial difficulties in a sample of court evaluated adolescents. *Personality Disorders, Theory, Research, and Treatment, 4*(3), 261–269. https://doi.org/10.1037/per0000011

Rasmussen, K., Storsaeter, O., & Levander, S. (1999). Personality disorders, psychopathy, and crime in a Norwegian prison population. *International Journal of Law and Psychiatry, 22*(1), 91–97. https://doi.org/10.1016/s0160-2527(98)00031-4

Rutherford, M. J., Alterman, A. I., Cacciola, J. S., & McKay, J. R. (1997). Validity of the psychopathy checklist-revised in male methadone patients. *Drug and Alcohol Dependence, 44*(2), 143–149. https://doi.org/10.1016/S0376-8716(96)01329-4

Sakiris, N., & Berle, D. (2019). A systematic review and meta-analysis of the Unified Protocol as a transdiagnostic emotion regulation based intervention. *Clinical Psychology Review, 72*, 101751. https://doi.org/10.1016/j.cpr.2019.101751

Salekin, R. T., Leistico, A.-M. R., Neumann, C. S., DiCicco, T. M., & Duros, R. L. (2004). Psychopathy and comorbidity in a young offender sample: Taking a closer look at psychopathy's potential importance over disruptive behavior disorders. *Journal of Abnormal Psychology, 113*(3), 416–427. https://doi.org/10.1037/0021-843X.113.3.416

Sauer-Zavala, S., Bentley, K. H., & Wilner, J. G. (2015). Transdiagnostic treatment of Borderline Personality Disorder and comorbid disorders: A clinical replication series. *Journal of Personality Disorders, 30*(1), 35–51. https://doi.org/10.1521/pedi_2015_29_179

Sevecke, K., Lehmkuhl, G., & Krischer, M. K. (2009). Examining relations between psychopathology and psychopathy dimensions among adolescent female and male offenders. *European Child & Adolescent Psychiatry, 18*(2), 85–95. https://doi.org/10.1007/s00787-008-0707-7

Sewall, L. A., & Olver, M. E. (2019). Psychopathy and treatment outcome: Results from a sexual violence reduction program. *Personality Disorders, Theory, Research, and Treatment, 10*(1), 59–69. https://doi.org/10.1037/per0000297

Skeem, J., Johansson, P., Andershed, H., Kerr, M., & Louden, J. E. (2007). Two subtypes of psychopathic violent offenders that parallel primary and secondary variants. *Journal of Abnormal Psychology, 116*(2), 395.

Smith, P. N., Selwyn, C. N., Wolford-Clevenger, C., & Mandracchia, J. T. (2013). Psychopathic personality traits, suicide ideation, and suicide attempts in male prison inmates. *Criminal Justice and Behavior, 41*(3), 364–379. https://doi.org/10.1177/0093854813506884

Sram, Z. (2017). The comorbidity of psychopathy and depression: Across different ethnic and sex groups. *The International Journal of Indian Psychology, 4*(3), 2349–3429.

Stadler, C., Manetsch, M., & Vriends, N. (2016). Dialectical behavior therapy approaches with disruptive behavior disorders. *Zeitschrift Fur Kinder- Und Jugendpsychiatrie Und Psychotherapie, 44*(6), 443–454. https://doi.org/10.1024/1422-4917/a000478

Stålenheim, E. G., & Von Knorring, L. (1996). Psychopathy and Axis I and Axis II psychiatric disorders in a forensic psychiatric population in Sweden. *Acta Psychiatrica Scandinavica, 94*(4), 217–223. https://doi.org/10.1111/j.1600-0447.1996.tb09852.x

Stinson, J. D., Becker, J. V., & Tromp, S. (2005). A preliminary study on findings of psychopathy and affective disorders in adult sex offenders. *International Journal of Law and Psychiatry, 28*(6), 637–649. https://doi.org/10.1016/j.ijlp.2004.10.001

Swann, A. C., Lijffijt, M., Lane, S. D., Steinberg, J. L., & Moeller, F. G. (2010). Interactions between bipolar disorder and antisocial personality disorder in trait impulsivity and severity of illness. *Acta Psychiatrica Scandinavica, 121*(6), 453–461. https://doi.org/10.1111/j.1600-0447.2009.01528.x

Swogger, M. T., Conner, K. R., Meldrum, S. C., & Caine, E. D. (2009). Dimensions of psychopathy in relation to suicidal and self-injurious behavior. *Journal of Personality Disorders, 23*(2), 201–210. https://doi.org/10.1521/pedi.2009.23.2.201

Thase, M. E., & Kupfer, D. J. (1996). Recent developments in the pharmacotherapy of mood disorders. *Journal of Consulting and Clinical Psychology, 64*(4), 646–659. https://doi.org/10.1037/0022-006X.64.4.646

Varkovitzky, R. L., Sherrill, A. M., & Reger, G. M. (2017). Effectiveness of the unified protocol for transdiagnostic treatment of emotional disorders among veterans with posttraumatic stress disorder: A pilot study. *Behavior Modification, 42*(2), 210–230. https://doi.org/10.1177/0145445517724539

Vaughn, M. G., Edens, J. F., Howard, M. O., & Smith, S. T. (2009). An investigation of primary and secondary psychopathy in a statewide sample of incarcerated youth. *Youth Violence and Juvenile Justice, 7*(3), 172–188. https://doi.org/10.1177/1541204009333792

Verona, E., Patrick, C. J., & Joiner, T. E. (2001). Psychopathy, antisocial personality, and suicide risk. *Journal of Abnormal Psychology, 110*(3), 462–470. https://doi.org/10.1037/0021-843X.110.3.462

Verona, E., Hicks, B. M., & Patrick, C. J. (2005). Psychopathy and suicidality in female offenders: Mediating influences of personality and abuse. *Journal of Consulting and Clinical Psychology, 73*(6), 1065–1073. https://doi.org/10.1037/0022-006X.73.6.1065

Walton, A., Jeglic, E. L., & Blasko, B. L. (2016). The role of psychopathic traits in the development of the therapeutic alliance among sexual offenders. *Sexual Abuse, 30*(3), 211–229. https://doi.org/10.1177/1079063216637859

Wampold, B. E. (2015). How important are the common factors in psychotherapy? An update. *World Psychiatry, 14*(3), 270–277. https://doi.org/10.1002/wps.20238

Wetterborg, D., Dehlbom, P., Långström, N., Andersson, G., Fruzzetti, A. E., & Enebrink, P. (2018). Dialectical Behavior Therapy for men with Borderline Personality Disorder and antisocial behavior: A clinical trial. *Journal of Personality Disorders*, 1–18. https://doi.org/10.1521/pedi_2018_32_379

Willemsen, J., & Verhaeghe, P. (2012). Psychopathy and internalizing psychopathology. *International Journal of Law and Psychiatry, 35*(4), 269–275. https://doi.org/10.1016/j.ijlp.2012.04.004

Willemsen, J., Vanheule, S., & Verhaeghe, P. (2011). Psychopathy and lifetime experiences of depression. *Criminal Behaviour and Mental Health, 21*(4), 279–294. https://doi.org/10.1002/cbm.812

Wittchen, H. U., Jacobi, F., Rehm, J., Gustavsson, A., Svensson, M., Jönsson, B., Olesen, J., Allgulander, C., Alonso, J., Faravelli, C., Fratiglioni, L., Jennum, P., Lieb, R., Maercker, A., van Os, J., Preisig, M., Salvador-Carulla, L., Simon, R., & Steinhausen, H.-C. (2011). The size and burden of mental disorders and other disorders of the brain in Europe 2010. *European Neuropsychopharmacology, 21*(9), 655–679. https://doi.org/10.1016/j.euroneuro.2011.07.018

Woody, G. E., McLellan, A. T., Luborsky, L., & O'Brien, C. P. (1985). Sociopathy and psychotherapy outcome. *JAMA Psychiatry, 42*(11), 1081–1086. https://doi.org/10.1001/archpsyc.1985.01790340059009

Wozniak, J., Biederman, J., Faraone, S. V., Blier, H., & Monuteaux, M. C. (2001). Heterogeneity of childhood conduct disorder: Further evidence of a subtype of conduct disorder linked to bipolar disorder. *Journal of Affective Disorders, 64*(2), 121–131. https://doi.org/10.1016/S0165-0327(00)00217-2

Zlotnick, C., Kohn, R., Keitner, G., & Della Grotta, S. A. (2000). The relationship between quality of interpersonal relationships and major depressive disorder: Findings from the National Comorbidity Survey. *Journal of Affective Disorders, 59*(3), 205–215. https://doi.org/10.1016/S0165-0327(99)00153-6

Chapter 9
Psychopathy, Trauma, and PTSD Symptoms: Theory and Evidence

Lauren F. Fournier and Edelyn Verona

Abstract This chapter reviews literature on intersections of psychopathy, traumatic experiences, and posttraumatic stress disorder (PTSD), and weighs evidence for putative causal models explaining these relationships. Existing research indicates that experiences of trauma vary with dimension of psychopathic traits, with impulsive-antisocial traits more consistently related to trauma histories, relative to interpersonal-affective traits. There is also evidence that the relationship between interpersonal-affective traits and trauma is more positively related in men than in women, though future work should investigate this possibility. Various models can help explain links between psychopathy and trauma, including those involving gene-environment correlations and interactions, modeling and learning, emotional blunting and instability, and traumatic brain injury (TBI). Though more research is needed, emotional blunting and emotional instability following a traumatic experience, and possibly as a consequence of TBI, are promising potential mechanisms for the development of interpersonal-affective and impulsive-antisocial psychopathic traits, respectively. Treatments targeting emotional dysregulation may be helpful for individuals who exhibit impulsive-antisocial traits and report experiencing trauma, as might assessment for TBI and treatment of post-concussive symptoms. Future work would benefit from investigating emotional blunting and instability as explanatory in the relationships between psychopathy and trauma, and the potential role of TBI and gender in these relationships.

Keywords Psychopathy · Trauma · PTSD · Traumatic brain injury

L. F. Fournier (✉) · E. Verona
University of South Florida, Tampa, FL, USA
e-mail: Lffournier@usf.edu; everona@usf.edu

J. E. Vitale (ed.), *The Complexity of Psychopathy*, Dangerous Behavior in Clinical and Forensic Psychology, https://doi.org/10.1007/978-3-030-83156-1_9

9.1 Introduction

Psychopathy, antisocial personality disorder (ASPD), and associated disinhibited behaviors can co-occur with post-traumatic stress disorder (PTSD) for a number of different reasons and in a number of different ways. For example, PTSD is associated with a marked elevation in risk for substance use (e.g., Krueger et al., 2007; Sartor et al., 2010), suicidality (e.g., Krysinska & Lester, 2010; Verona et al., 2001), and violence (Mills et al., 2006; Collins & Bailey, 1990; Hare & McPherson, 1984). Elevated levels of these behaviors are also observed in and associated with ASPD and some psychopathic traits (Schulz et al., 2016; Trull et al., 2010; Verona et al., 2018). Relatedly, the co-occurrence between lifetime prevalence of PTSD and ASPD in the community is estimated to be between 19% and 21% (Goodwin & Hamilton, 2003; Sareen et al., 2004).

Analysis of the co-occurrence between psychopathy, in particular, and PTSD is complicated by the distinct factors of psychopathy, which are differentially associated with trauma-related constructs (i.e., anxiety; Hicks & Patrick, 2006; Harpur et al., 1989; Hemphill et al., 1994). The current chapter is the first review of associations between PTSD, experiences of trauma, and distinct psychopathic traits, and considers the weight of the evidence of possible explanations for these differential associations. First, we discuss rates of co-occurrence between PTSD, trauma history, and psychopathic traits, especially in detained samples. Second, we highlight how the relationships between psychopathy and trauma may vary depending on the psychopathic traits under study, specifically the impulsive-antisocial and interpersonal-affective features of psychopathy. Third, we discuss the existing evidence for a number of proposed explanations for the reciprocal relationships between psychopathy and trauma, including gene-environment correlations and interactions, vicarious learning, emotional blunting and instability, and brain injury sequelae. Fourth, we briefly explore the extent to which the overlap between psychopathic traits, PTSD, and trauma is relevant in therapy or clinical contexts, especially considering some of the empirical evidence supporting the more viable explanatory models. Finally, we leverage current data and theory to formulate distinct etiological trajectories for co-occurrence of trauma and different psychopathic traits. These trajectories involve differing types of trauma-related emotional dysfunction for differing traits; we propose that emotion dysregulation is central to the development of impulsive-antisocial psychopathic traits, while emotional blunting is central to the development of the interpersonal-affective traits. We conclude broadly that trauma is more consistently linked to the impulsive and antisocial features of psychopathy than the interpersonal-affective features, and that psychopathy and trauma are related through a combination of genetic and environmental influences.

9.2 Definitions and Distinctions

Before discussing the relationships between psychopathy, trauma, and PTSD, it is important to consider how these constructs are defined for the purposes of this chapter. Psychopathy is a constellation of personality traits, including interpersonal manipulativeness, callous affect, impulsivity, and antisocial behavior (Hare, 2003). Psychopathy is not a unitary construct, and much of the literature to date has focused on a two-factor structure of psychopathic traits in which interpersonal and affective features (i.e., interpersonal manipulation, callousness, lack of empathy) comprise one factor (Factor 1) and impulsive lifestyle and antisociality (i.e., irresponsibility, sensation seeking, criminal versatility) comprise another (Factor 2). In this chapter, relationships between distinct psychopathic traits and trauma will be reviewed within the framework of this two-factor structure, as well as some of the sub-facets (e.g., affective).

In terms of trauma, the current review focuses on both traumatic life events (TLEs) and PTSD symptomology in relation to psychopathy traits. PTSD is a diagnosis in the trauma-and-stressor-related disorders section of the DSM-5 (American Psychiatric Association [APA], 2013), the criteria of which include being witness to, or exposed to a traumatic event. Traumatic events include exposure to actual or threatened death, serious injury, or sexual violence, and can be experienced either directly or indirectly, including through direct exposure, witnessing, or learning that a close friend or a relative experienced a trauma. For the diagnosis, an individual must experience intrusive symptoms such as upsetting nightmares or flashbacks to the event, as well as avoidance of reminders of the trauma. Negative changes in mood or thoughts must also be present (e.g., increased negative affect, overly negative thoughts about oneself and the world, and an inability to recall important details of the event), as are trauma-related arousal and reactivity, such as irritability, aggression, hypervigilance, and difficulty sleeping. These symptoms must persist for at least 1 month and cause distress or impairment to an individual's functioning (American Psychiatric Association, 2013). Although some diagnostic criteria for PTSD are trauma-specific (e.g., subsequent nightmares or flashbacks, avoidance of trauma-related reminders), other symptoms include increased risky or aggressive behavior, impairments in functioning, and increased negative affectivity (American Psychiatric Association, 2013), which are also linked to antisociality regardless of trauma history (Fergusson et al., 2005; Jang et al., 2003; Verona et al., 2001).

While a traumatic event is required for a diagnosis of PTSD, experiencing such an event does not necessarily result in PTSD symptomology. The definition of TLEs (events causing threat to one's life or bodily integrity, sudden loss of a loved one, being exposed to a seriously injured, mutilated, or dead body; Green, 1990) in the literature is broader than the definition of a traumatic event necessary for PTSD. It should be noted that there is disagreement in the literature regarding which life events qualify as traumatic and which do not (e.g., Ben-Ezra & Aluf, 2006; Gold et al., 2005; Lancaster et al., 2009). For the purpose of this review, we limit our definition to experiences that tend to overlap with the PTSD criteria for trauma, especially physical or childhood abuse, which are more commonly examined in relation to psychopathy and antisocial behavior (e.g., Cima et al., 2008; Craparo et al., 2013; Forouzan & Nicholls, 2015; Krischer & Sevecke, 2008; Schimmenti et al., 2015).

TLEs do not result solely in psychological distress, as in PTSD; they can result in physical injuries as well, including traumatic brain injury (TBI; Martin et al., 2000; McMillan et al., 2003; Schreiber & Galai-Gat, 1993; Stein & McAllister, 2009). TBIs are defined in the literature as any alteration in brain functioning, including (but not limited to) memory loss, aphasia, and confusion, that is caused by an external force (Menon et al., 2010). They can range from mild to severe, depending on post-injury length of loss of consciousness (from less than 30 min to more than 24 h) and of amnesia (from less than 24 h to 7 days or greater; Carlson et al., 2011; Peterson et al., 2019; Vakil, 2005). A TBI can occur as the result of a number of different events, but in the general population it most commonly occurs following sports injuries, being struck by objects, falls, and vehicle accidents (Peterson et al., 2019).

There is considerable heterogeneity in the TBI literature, however, in that injuries often affect structurally and functionally different areas of the brain, and can result in varying degrees of symptom severity and subsequent behavioral and cognitive changes (Kraus, et al., 2007; Maas et al., 2017), some of which may be relevant to psychopathic traits and some of which may not. For example, TBI damage to ventromedial and dorsolateral frontal regions has been associated with impairments in social cognition, such as theory of mind (see McDonald, 2013, for review), and damage to the dorsolateral prefrontal cortex has also been associated with working memory deficits (Eierud et al., 2014, for review). Structural damage to white matter tracts in connectivity networks has been linked to difficulties with cognitive control processes (Sharp et al., 2014, for review). Thus, neural regions can be involved in a range of different functions, and head trauma can affect a variety of regions and structures in the brain, making this literature complex. There is also the possibility that some of the overlap between features associated with both TBI and impulsive-antisocial psychopathic traits may be related to shared experiences of trauma. For example, a victim of assault may develop an increased sensitivity to threat due to the experience of being attacked, rather than to psychopathic traits or a head injury sustained in the attack. Given these definitions, we now move to discussing the prevalence and overlap between psychopathy, TLEs, PTSD symptomology, and TBI.

9.2.1 Prevalence and Overlap

Potential sources of overlap between PTSD and psychopathic traits are rarely studied, despite the fact that these conditions are both present at relatively high levels in incarcerated and correctional populations. Although the community base rate of psychopathy is estimated to be lower than 1%, around 15–25% of male prisoners in the U.S. score high on psychopathic traits (Hare, 1991). PTSD rates are estimated to be much higher in incarcerated individuals, with as many as 65% meeting criteria for PTSD (Briere et al., 2016; Burton et al., 1994; Cauffman et al., 1998). The relatively high prevalence rates of PTSD among incarcerated populations are likely related to both the increased likelihood of traumatic events associated with a risky or impulsive lifestyle (e.g., Koenen et al., 2005), as well as some overlap between psychopathic traits and the diagnostic criteria of PTSD, as mentioned above. Endorsement of TLEs, more generally, are also remarkably high among incarcerated populations, with upwards of half of incarcerated individuals reporting histories of TLEs (Abram et al., 2007; Erwin et al., 2000; Haugebrook et al., 2010). The prevalence of TLEs has been notably higher among female offender samples, with estimates as high as nearly 80% (Cook et al., 2005; Jordan et al., 1996; Zlotnick, 1997). Research investigating the effects or correlates of trauma is therefore highly important among individuals (and perhaps women especially) with histories of incarceration, a population that is of particular relevance for psychopathy.

TBI resulting from a physical trauma is also present at a relatively high degree among incarcerated populations (25–87% of inmates; Morrell et al., 1998; Slaughter et al., 2003). The presence of TBI following a physical trauma holds potential relevance for psychopathy, as prominent theories of psychopathic personality attribute some of the emotional and behavioral deficits accompanying psychopathy to irregularities in the prefrontal cortex, limbic system, and some other paralimbic structures (e.g., Anderson & Kiehl, 2012). Damage to the prefrontal cortex has been associated with acquired sociopathy, in which sudden changes in personality marked by difficulties in social cognition and social decision-making occur following brain injury (Blair & Cipolotti, 2000; Blumer & Benson, 1975; Damasio, 2000). Recent neuroimaging work has also found psychopathic traits to be associated with structural and functional reductions in prefrontal areas (Anderson & Kiehl, 2012; Kiehl et al., 2001; Yang & Raine, 2009). In regard to the limbic system, both psychopathic traits and TBI have been associated with declines in connectivity between limbic structures and other areas of cortex (Raine et al., 2010; Williamson et al., 2013). It follows that TBI affecting particular neural regions and structures may impact the development or exacerbation of psychopathic dispositions, and thus brain injury can be one pathway by which trauma is linked to development of psychopathic behaviors. At the same time, the resulting manifestation of psychopathy, whether prominent impulsive-antisocial traits or interpersonal-affective features, depends on the mechanisms affected by TBI (e.g., cognitive control vs. emotional dysfunction).

9.3 Multidimensional Nature of Psychopathy and Relationships to Trauma

Relationships between psychopathic traits and PTSD and trauma have focused on psychopathy as both a unitary and a multidimensional construct. Total psychopathy scores have been shown to be both positively related to experiences of TLEs across samples of incarcerated individuals and community members (e.g., Frodi et al.,

2001; Koivisto & Haapasalo, 1996; Patrick et al., 1997; Weiler & Widom, 1996), as well as unrelated to TLEs (Kerig et al., 2012; Marshall & Cooke, 1999; Pham, 2012). The literature relating psychopathy to PTSD symptomology is even more mixed. Whereas results from several studies have indicated that total psychopathy scores are unrelated to PTSD symptoms (Sellbom, 2015; Willemsen et al., 2012), other studies report a positive relationship between PTSD symptoms and overall psychopathy scores (e.g., Blonigen et al., 2012; Sharf et al., 2014; Tatar et al., 2012).

The mixed findings are likely explained by the fact that some aspects of psychopathy overlap with symptoms experienced following TLEs, such as recklessness and aggressive outbursts, while other aspects of psychopathy have been suggested to be protective against or unrelated to internalizing psychopathology, including PTSD (Blonigen et al., 2012; Hicks & Patrick, 2006). In fact, distinct factors of psychopathy show divergent correlates. The impulsive lifestyle and antisocial traits share some features with PTSD (Blonigen et al., 2012; Hare, 2003) and relate to exposure to adverse events (Blonigen et al., 2012; Cima et al., 2008; Forouzan & Nicholls, 2015; Luntz & Widom, 1994; Poythress et al., 2006; Semiz et al., 2007), likely accounting for positive relationships between psychopathy and PTSD. The relationships between PTSD and impulsive-antisocial traits appear to be consistent across different samples. In part, these relationships are in line with theorized developmental trajectories for the impulsive-antisocial traits. That is, TLEs and the difficulties that accompany them are highly implicated in theories on the development of impulsive-antisocial traits, and secondary psychopathy (a variant of psychopathy thought to emerge partly as a result of adverse childhood experiences and more strongly related to negative emotionality, emotional volatility, and the impulsive-antisocial traits; Glenn et al., 2013; Karpman, 1941, 1955; Porter, 1996; Poythress & Skeem, 2006; Poythress et al., 2006; Skeem et al., 2003). Individuals high on impulsive-antisocial psychopathic traits may be more likely to experience TLEs because they engage in impulsive behaviors, often frustrate or anger others, or have inherited such traits from a parent who is in turn more likely to abuse them.

Affective and interpersonal components, in contrast, have shown less consistent relationships with TLEs and PTSD (uncorrelated: Blonigen et al., 2012; Dargis et al., 2016; Forouzan & Nicholls, 2015; Poythress et al., 2006; positively correlated: Graham et al., 2012; Marshall & Cooke, 1999; McBride, 1998; Schimmenti et al., 2015). TLEs and their consequences are not central features in theories of the development of interpersonal-affective traits, or primary psychopathy (the variant of psychopathy historically linked to innate biological deficits in emotional responding; Karpman 1941, 1955; Porter, 1996; Poythress & Skeem, 2006; Schimmenti et al., 2015; Skeem et al., 2003; Willemsen et al., 2012). The interpersonal and affective traits are characterized by blunted affect that may be protective against PTSD symptoms, thus accounting for the lack of correlations in the literature.

In all, there is room for further research examining potential differences in trauma and PTSD histories among individuals high on these psychopathic traits. There is tentative evidence that the mixed literature on interpersonal-affective traits and trauma may be explained by distinct patterns of relationships across gender. Although impulsive-antisocial traits are positively related to TLEs in both men and women, there is more support for a positive relationship between TLEs and interpersonal-affective psychopathic traits in men and boys than in women and girls (Blonigen et al., 2012; Forouzan & Nicholls, 2015; Graham et al., 2012; Krischer & Sevecke, 2008; Schimmenti et al., 2015; Sevecke et al., 2016; Verona et al., 2005; but see Hicks et al., 2010). This may suggest that TLEs relate to *either* greater emotional blunting (interpersonal-affective traits) or greater disinhibition (impulsive-antisocial traits) in men. In women, there is evidence that psychopathy manifests mostly as emotional dysregulation (Sevecke et al., 2016). For example, studies have indicated that symptoms of emotional dysregulation, as expressed in borderline personality disorder (BPD), are associated with psychopathic traits, particularly impulsive-antisocial traits, in women more than men (Hicks et al., 2010; Sprague et al., 2012), and one study found that BPD traits fully accounted for the relationship between impulsive-antisocial psychopathic traits and TLEs in women (Blonigen et al., 2012). It is possible that the mixed results for male samples are simply due to a greater number of studies investigating these effects in men than in women, rather than to gender differences. Few studies on this topic have directly compared the relationship between factors of psychopathy and TLEs in men and women in the same sample, making this an important avenue for future research.

The literature is, in summary, mainly supportive of a positive relationship between impulsive-antisocial psychopathic traits and trauma, but mixed regarding the relationship between interpersonal-affective traits and trauma. Historically, the former have been theoretically linked to trauma, whereas the latter have been theoretically linked to innate expressions of emotional blunting. The relationship between interpersonal-affective traits and trauma may be impacted by additional variables, such as gender. The following sections of this chapter aim to review the evidence (or highlight the lack thereof) in support of proposed models linking psychopathic traits and trauma, and to discuss how support for the theories may vary by the psychopathic traits under study.

9.4 Proposed Models Relating Trauma and Psychopathy

There are a number of potential pathways along which psychopathic traits and trauma may intersect. Below, we critically analyze different explanations for the relationships between psychopathic traits, TLEs and PTSD symptoms, including models respectively highlighting genetic explanations for co-occurrence (e.g., gene-environment correlations), modeling and social learning, emotional dysfunction, and brain injury. Each of these proposed models will be discussed in greater depth, along with support for each as they pertain to different factors of psychopathic traits. As will be discussed, these models are ultimately important for understanding the etiology of psychopathy and have potential implications for the treatment of both psychopathy and trauma-based disorders.

9.4.1 Gene-Environment Correlations

Though the relationship between TLEs and psychopathic traits is often thought of as being linear and causal (with TLEs causing psychopathy), the co-occurrence of TLEs and psychopathic traits may be accounted for in other ways, including gene-environment correlations. For example, one type of TLE (childhood abuse) and psychopathic traits could co-occur because parents who abuse their children carry a genetic predisposition for aggression and impulsivity, which is then transmitted intergenerationally. This passive gene-environment correlation would then result in a spurious correlation between childhood TLE and aggression (DiLalla & Gottesman, 1991; Plomin et al., 1977). According to this explanation, TLEs and psychopathy overlap not because one precedes the other in a causal chain, but because they are both explained by the genetic make-up of parents.

TLEs take an indirect role in the *reactive* gene-environment correlation as well, which posits that children who are born with "difficult" temperaments, including those who may be aggressive or impulsive, are at heightened risk for TLEs because their behaviors can increase frustration and anger in others (Moffitt, 2005; Plomin et al., 1977). Children and adolescents high on psychopathic traits are more likely to get into trouble with the police and at school (McMahon et al., 2010). These problems cause emotional strain and frustration in family members (Arditti et al., 2003), possibly increasing the risk for child abuse directed at these offspring, as parents and caregivers attempt to manage difficult situations. These youths may also be more likely to engage in risk taking behaviors that result in TLEs, PTSD symptoms, and brain injury, though such events can also exacerbate already existing traits. Importantly, passive and reactive gene-environment explanations are not mutually exclusive. For example, a child inheriting a genetic predisposition for aggression from a parent may be more likely to experience TLEs due to aggressive tendencies in that parent (passive), and this risk may also be heightened by the reactions they elicit from the others (reactive).

There have been a number of studies examining gene-environment correlations relating TLEs (particularly childhood abuse) and the development of antisocial behavior. Though these studies focus on antisocial behavior and not psychopathic traits, both antisocial behavior and ASPD are highly related to and overlap considerably with impulsive-antisocial psychopathic traits (Harpur et al., 1989). Previous literature reviews have indicated that antisocial behavior is at least moderately heritable, with genes accounting for approximately 40–50% of the variation (Miles & Carey, 1997; Moffitt, 2005; Rhee & Waldman, 2002); however, some results indicate that heritability or passive gene correlations do not fully account for the effects of TLEs on subsequent antisocial behavior. In a particularly strong example of this, Jaffee et al. (2004) demonstrated in a large longitudinal twin sample that antisocial behavior in parents predicted their likelihood of abusing their children, and that genetic factors accounted for approximately two-thirds of the variance in antisocial behavior in their children, seeming to support passive gene-environment correlation. However, controlling for the genetic relationship between the parent's and child's antisocial behaviors did not eliminate effects of physical maltreatment on childhood antisocial behavior. These results indicate that although antisocial behavior in parents is related to both maltreatment and antisocial behavior in their children, maltreatment exerts compounding influence on offspring antisocial behavior beyond the influence of genetics (Jaffee et al., 2004). Other work utilizing a twin study design has also generally supported a direct effect of childhood trauma on later antisocial behavior (Eaves et al., 2010; Forsman & Långström, 2012; Jonson-Reid et al., 2010), though the causal effect of childhood TLEs has generally been small (see Jaffee et al., 2012 for review). Forsman and Långström (2012) utilized a twin design to investigate the degree to which adult violent offending could be attributed to childhood trauma and genetics, respectively. Their results suggest primary influence of shared genetics and weak causal influence of childhood TLEs in predicting adult violent offending (Forsman & Långström, 2012). Although there is evidence that trauma is causally linked to subsequent antisocial behavior, genetic factors may still account for as much as half of the effect of childhood maltreatment on antisocial behavior, highlighting the importance of both genetics and environment in the development of antisocial behavior (Jaffee et al., 2004).

Research on borderline personality disorder can also be informative about possible genetic and environmental correlates of psychopathy. Previous work has indicated a significant degree of overlap between BPD and impulsive-antisocial psychopathic traits in both women and men (Sprague et al., 2012), and that BPD traits fully account for the relationship between psychopathy and TLEs in women (Blonigen et al., 2012). In contrast to Jaffee et al. (2004), work evaluating gene-environment correlation versus direct exposure explanations for BPD found genetic influences to account for the majority of the relationship between childhood abuse and BPD traits, providing support for a passive or reactive gene-environment relationship instead (Bornovalova et al., 2013). Passive and reactive gene-environment correlations therefore cannot be ruled out in relation to psychopathy, and future research would benefit from considering the relationships between BPD and psychopathic traits in women when examining gene-environment correlations versus direct effects of TLEs on psychopathy.

There is separate evidence in the literature supporting *reactive* gene-environment correlations explaining relationships between trauma and antisocial traits. For example, Ge et al. (1996) found in an adoptive family sample that biological parents' antisocial behaviors were positively related to adoptive parents' antisocial and hostile behaviors toward adopted children, and that this relationship was mediated by children's antisocial behaviors. Additional studies have further supported this, finding that the relationship between prior maltreatment and conduct problems in adolescents could be largely attributed to caregivers' responding to conduct problems with maltreatment (Schulz-Heik et al., 2010). Similar results have been found for children's antisocial behaviors evoking harsh parenting styles (O'Connor et al., 1998), and for callous-unemotional traits predicting parenting practices, including corporal punishment (Hawes et al., 2011). Though these studies support reactive gene-environment correlation as it pertains to the relationship between antisocial behavior and trauma, additional work is needed to understand this relationship in regard to other psychopathic traits (e.g., interpersonal-affective).

Some conclusions can be drawn from these investigations of gene-environment correlations. First, although a propensity to engage in antisocial behavior is often passed down from parents to children, this does not preclude the potentially causal effects of TLEs on antisocial behavior in children, indicating both genes and environment as important in the development of antisocial behavior. Even further, the support for the passive gene-environment correlation model does not exclude the potential for reactive gene-environment correlation, and current work, although limited, is supportive of this model as well. Work on these models is limited in that there is currently very little existing research on gene-environment correlations focusing on psychopathy per se, especially the interpersonal-affective aspects, or the evocative effects of fledgling callous-unemotional traits in children in regard to exposure to traumatic experiences (but see Kimonis et al., 2013). Additional work is needed that includes investigations of the interpersonal-affective features in order to fully evaluate gene-environment correlation explanations of the relationship between psychopathy and trauma.

9.4.2 Gene-Environment Interactions

At another level, psychopathic traits and TLEs may be linked through gene-environment *interactions*, in which the effect that an environmental factor, in this case adverse or traumatic experiences, has on individuals depends upon and interacts with their genotypes (Caspi & Moffitt, 2006). Gene-environment interactions are theorized to be the reason that not all individuals who experience a TLE have the same psychological outcome; only individuals who carry genetic risk who experience a TLE would develop psychopathic traits, for example, while those without genetic risk would not (Gorenstein & Newman, 1980; Meehl, 1962).

Studies of the interactions between specific genes and TLEs have supported the importance of both genetics and environment in the development of antisocial behavior. Prior work has suggested that men with the low-activity allele of the monoamine oxidase A (MAOA-L) gene who are also exposed to childhood maltreatment are at particularly high risk of antisocial behavior (e.g., Caspi et al., 2002; Eme, 2013; Kim-Cohen et al., 2006). Of note, the presence of MAOA-L alone does not predict antisocial behavior—it is only predictive when combined with a history of childhood maltreatment. Other candidate gene studies have likewise shown support for MAOA interactions with other forms of childhood abuse (sexual abuse and emotional abuse/neglect; Derringer et al., 2010; Fergusson et al., 2011) for predicting antisocial behavior. However, these effects have not always replicated. Extreme levels of TLEs have been associated with antisocial behavior regardless of MAOA genotype (Weder et al., 2009), and MAOA-L has been associated with impulsive-antisocial psychopathic traits in adult men, regardless of childhood maltreatment (Haberstick et al., 2005; McDermott et al., 2009; Meyer-Lindenberg et al., 2006; Sadeh et al., 2010).

It is important to note that there are substantial limitations of this work. In general, the candidate gene and gene-environment interaction literature has suffered from poor replicability, likely reflecting a publication bias (Duncan & Keller, 2011; Ficks & Waldman, 2014). Further, although the literature on MAOA gene-environment interactions has been supported by meta-analyses (Byrd & Manuck, 2014; Kim-Cohen et al., 2006), these effects are likely appreciably smaller than reported, as the development of antisocial behavior and psychopathic traits involves numerous genes with very small effects (Holz et al., 2018; Waldman et al., 2018).

Several studies attempting to replicate gene-environment interactions have found null results (Haberstick et al., 2005, 2014; Huizinga et al., 2006; Prichard et al., 2008). While this literature is important to understanding relationships between psychopathy and TLEs, it should be discussed with these considerations in mind.

In sum, there is evidence that traumatic experiences play a role in the development of antisocial traits, which are also heritable, and the genetic and environmental pathways to antisociality are correlated. Thus, studies investigating predictive effects of TLEs on antisocial and psychopathic traits must account for gene effects when drawing conclusions. Work on gene-environment interactions has often demonstrated poor replicability, however. Any specific conclusions at this time should therefore be drawn tentatively.

9.4.3 Modeling and Learning Explanations

Another way in which TLEs and psychopathic traits may co-occur, especially among those genetically predisposed, is through parental modeling or vicarious learning experiences in which children who have experienced TLEs develop aggressive and potentially psychopathic behaviors by observing them in role models (Bandura et al., 1963; Berkowitz, 1993; Parker & Rogers, 1981; Poythress et al., 2006). Here again, genetic and social modeling factors may be additive. For example, an individual may inherit a genetic predisposition for psychopathic traits, live with a biological parent who is more likely to abuse them, and later develop psychopathic traits due to a gene-environment correlation, TLEs, head trauma related to TLEs, and learning by observation of parents high on psychopathic traits. These factors can apply to adult populations and outside the family context as well. Adults predisposed to engage in fighting, substance use, or other risky behaviors are more likely to be exposed to TLEs in associated high-risk environments (i.e. gang membership, combat experience, living in high crime neighborhoods; Panayiotou, 2015; Serin, 1991; Smith & Newman, 1990), and thus observe psychopathic behaviors in others, which reinforces their enactment as useful or adaptive for survival in such environments.

Social learning models relating psychopathy and TLEs are rooted in Bandura's classic work finding that children who observe aggressive behaviors in others are in turn more likely to act aggressively (Bandura, 1973; Bandura et al., 1963). The idea that children model their aggressive behavior after that of role models suggests a possible environmental explanation for the cycle of violence, in which individuals who have been victims are more likely to engage in perpetration themselves (Bandura, 1973; Widom, 1989). There have been a number of studies examining the potentially causal effects of modeling of violence and aggression within laboratory settings, though none has focused on psychopathy. These studies have generally found support for modeling theories, indicating that short-term exposure to antisocial behavior in a role model (i.e., children randomly assigned to view video clips of adults acting aggressively against a doll) is associated with short-term antisocial behavior outcomes (i.e., children act aggressively toward the doll; Bandura et al., 1963; see Ferguson & Savage, 2012 for review). Although these studies provide an important starting point for modeling theories, their effects cannot be assumed to generalize outside of the laboratory and may not be directly relevant to the development of the stable personality traits associated with psychopathy.

Exploration of modeling theories outside of laboratory paradigms has included studies finding that exposure to violence in youth is associated with later antisocial behavior and psychopathic traits (Dargis & Koenigs, 2017; Ferguson et al., 2009; Herrenkohl et al., 2003; Maneta et al., 2017; Patrick et al., 1997; Poythress et al., 2006; Sousa et al., 2011; Weiler & Widom, 1996; White & Widom, 2003; Widom & Maxfield, 1996), although most of these studies have not investigated vicarious learning as a specific mechanism for the TLE-behavior relationship. For example, while one study did find that children's responses when angry modeled those of their parents, with particularly strong effects for boys expressing anger by hitting someone if their fathers also hit someone while angry (Björkqvist, 1997), it is unclear to what extent being witness to these behaviors can be considered a TLE.

Several studies have replicated these effects outside the family context (i.e., witnessing peer victimization, community violence, school violence; Davis et al., 2015; Howard et al., 2012; Kimonis et al., 2008; Schraft et al., 2013; Vogel & Keith, 2015). These studies are especially important because they present in contrast to the gene-environment studies by diminishing the genetic component of the relationship between psychopathy and trauma. Witnessing TLEs outside the biological family therefore provides stronger support for an environmentally-mediated effect of modeling on antisocial and psychopathic traits. However, it is also important to recognize that because these studies have not explored modeling as a specific mechanism linking TLEs and psychopathic traits, other explanations may be equally plausible. It may be that having delinquent peers increases the risk of both witnessing peer victimization and subsequent delinquent behavior (e.g., Toro et al., 2004; Ingoldsby et al., 2006; Monahan et al., 2009), rather than modeling being the link between the two, for example. At the same time, one study using path analysis did find that childhood abuse influenced violent attitudes, which then led to increased involvement with antisocial peers, which then predicted risk for violence (Herrenkohl et al., 2003). These findings suggest that modeling violent attitudes may link abuse and future antisocial behavior, although that was not investigated directly. Witnessing violence (indirect) and being the subject of violence (direct) may have differing impacts on the development of antisocial or psychopathic traits. Although both witnessing and experiencing violence have been linked to later antisociality (Miller et al., 1999; Widom, 1997; Wilson et al., 2009), future research would benefit from exploring these potential differences more fully, as it is currently unclear if modeling is the mechanism through which these relationships develop. In general, the current literature does not offer strong support either for or against modeling/vicarious learning theories connecting TLEs and psychopathy, and more work accounting for potential confounding variables is needed.

9.4.4 Emotional Blunting Theories

Specific theories have been formulated that center the emotional dysfunction sequelae of TLEs to explain the development of psychopathic traits. Porter (1996) proposed that features of psychopathy can emerge out of repeated trauma through which an individual experiences a dissociation between emotion and both cognition and behavior. Dissociation includes depersonalization, derealization, memory recall deficits, and a general feeling of distance from oneself or one's surroundings (Sharpe et al., 2010), and has been identified as a common response following trauma (Halligan et al., 2003; Murray et al., 2002; Vonderlin et al., 2018). Because emotional disconnect is a component of dissociation, some literature suggests it as a possible explanation for the association between trauma and emotional blunting (Porter, 1996; Weiler & Widom, 1996). In other words, empathic responding can be "turned off" over time as the result of repeated abuse or TLEs. Weiler and Widom (1996) suggested that early abuse can result in *desensitization* (becoming emotionally less responsive) to future negative emotional experiences as a defense mechanism, and that this desensitization may extend to a lack of empathy toward others and a lack of emotional responsivity more broadly. Both dissociation and desensitization could account specifically for the development of the interpersonal-affective traits associated with psychopathy.

Support for emotional dissociation models, however, has been notably mixed. This may be due in part to the mixed support for the relationship between interpersonal-affective psychopathic traits and TLEs, in general (e.g., Blonigen et al., 2012; Dargis et al., 2016; Graham et al., 2012; Poythress et al., 2006; Schimmenti et al., 2015). Two key studies testing the proposal that dissociative experiences link interpersonal-affective psychopathic traits and trauma did not support this proposal (Poythress et al., 2006; Tatar et al., 2012). In one study using structural equation modeling, Poythress et al. (2006) did not find that dissociative experiences mediated the relationship between psychopathic traits and trauma (Poythress et al., 2006). Another study even found a negative association between affective psychopathic traits and dissociative experiences (Pham, 2012).

Results have indicated more promise for emotional desensitization (i.e., emotional numbing), rather than dissociative experiences, as a mediator of the TLE-psychopathy relationship. Studies of emotional numbing generally evaluate experiences related to emotional disengagement (e.g., "there are certain emotions that I cannot feel"; Orsillo et al., 2007), whereas studies on dissociation tend to evaluate the disconnect between oneself and the surrounding world more generally (e.g., amnesia for one's behavior, unfamiliarity with surroundings, out-of-body experiences; Bernstein et al., 2001). Several studies find that emotional numbing can explain the relationship between callous-unemotional traits in juveniles and prior victimization (Bennett & Kerig, 2014; Kerig et al., 2012; Kerig & Modrowski, 2018). Reminiscent of the adult literature regarding distinctions between primary and secondary psychopathy variants, the literature on callous-unemotional traits and emotional numbing in youth has also identified two variants: one in which callous-unemotional traits develop in relation to environmental factors such as trauma, likely through emotional numbing, and a second in which these traits are the results of an inherent core affective deficit in an individual and do not appear to be related to trauma to the same degree (Karpman, 1941; Porter, 1996; Skeem et al., 2003). Therefore, although it has yet to be examined directly, TLEs and emotional numbing may be relevant to only a subset of individuals high on psychopathy.

The literature on emotional numbing and dissociation introduces other considerations, especially potential gender differences and relationships to BPD. One study found that TLEs were related to callous-unemotional traits via emotional numbing, and related to BPD symptoms via dissociative experiences (Kerig & Modrowski, 2018). This study also indicated that BPD and dissociation were both significantly more common in maltreated girls compared to maltreated boys, suggesting that there are some gender differences in the effects of victimization on youth traits (Kerig & Modrowski, 2018). Again, this work highlights how gender should be considered when examining different TLE-related outcomes for men and women, with TLEs potentially associated with more emotional dysregulation in girls and more callousness and unempathetic responding in boys. Future work can address these potentially-distinct emotional mechanisms linking TLEs and psychopathic traits in girls versus boys.

9.4.5 Emotional Instability Models

The impulsive-antisocial components of psychopathy may relate to TLEs through emotional dysfunction as well, but in a way that is distinct from that proposed to link TLEs and the interpersonal-affective features of psychopathy. In emotional instability models of psychopathy, TLEs and the negative emotionality that accompanies them may lead to a number of maladaptive coping strategies, other than desensitization, to deal with distress. That is, reactions to TLEs can involve impulsive, aggressive, and antisocial behaviors rooted in emotion dysregulation (Poythress et al., 2006), and these reactions are representative of impulsive-antisocial features of psychopathy. The literature demonstrates that both TLEs and antisocial behavior are linked to abnormalities in emotional processing, particularly a hyperreactivity to and greater engagement with negative emotional stimuli (Kimonis et al., 2012; Tottenham et al., 2010; Verona et al., 2012). Childhood maltreatment, particularly that which occurs earlier in life involving multiple types of maltreatment (i.e., both physical neglect and sexual abuse), has been linked to difficulties in emotion regulation, which are in turn related to externalizing behaviors more broadly (Kim & Cicchetti, 2010). Further, cluster analyses by Dargis and Koenigs (2018) classified psychopathic offenders into subgroups of high and low negative affect, with the high negative affect group reporting significantly greater degrees of childhood maltreatment. Although these studies did not test emotional instability theories directly, the results do suggest that emotion regulation difficulties following TLEs may be related to the development of impulsive-antisocial traits.

Emotional dysregulation is also related to antisocial traits independently of trauma (e.g., Frewen & Lanius, 2006; García-Sancho et al., 2014; Malterer et al., 2008). As one example, Zlotnick (1999) found that ASPD was associated with affective dysregulation, specifically anger modulation difficulties, even after controlling for PTSD symptoms. More definitive evidence is needed showing that emotion dysregulation specifically in response to trauma can lead to impulsive-antisocial traits. Unfortunately, studies examining how TLEs and psychopathy may be related through emotional instability are limited. In one study, Sevecke et al. (2016) found both TLEs and emotion dysregulation to be related to psychopathic traits in youth, but did not investigate whether affective dysregulation mediated the relationship between psychopathy and TLEs.

In sum, the evidence for emotional instability/dysregulation having an effect on or being a mechanism for the relationship between TLEs and impulsive-antisocial traits is limited. This relationship may be explained by the fact that individuals high on psychopathy are at increased risk for both TLEs and emotional dysregulation. It may also be that more nuance is required in these investigations, as negative emotions are complex and multifaceted. Dysregulation of different emotions (i.e., fear, sadness) may link TLEs and psychopathic traits, while others, such as anger, may relate to antisociality or TLEs independently.

9.4.6 Traumatic Brain Injury (TBI) as an Explanatory Variable

Missing from the literature on TLEs and psychopathy is the explanatory role of the physical consequences of traumatic events, in particular head trauma and TBI. This is unfortunate, given that existing research links the sequelae of head trauma with psychopathy-like emotional and cognitive changes. Previous work indicates that TBI is associated with a range of irregularities in emotional functioning relevant to the interpersonal-affective features of psychopathy such as irregular facial mimicry, autonomic responding, and self-reported affective empathy to emotional stimuli, particularly to unpleasant stimuli (de Sousa et al., 2010, 2011, 2012; Saunders et al., 2006). Further, both persons high on psychopathy and persons with TBI show decreased startle potentiation to aversive affective stimuli (Benning et al., 2005; Patrick et al., 1993; Saunders et al., 2006). Thus, across several methodological domains, outcomes for some individuals with TBI reflect deficits in affective empathy and emotional responsivity that are similar to those found in persons high on the interpersonal-affective traits of psychopathy.

Head trauma and TBI also relate to behavioral changes reminiscent of the impulsive-antisocial traits of psychopathy, as individuals with past TBIs have shown increases in aggression, impulsivity, and violence post-injury (Slaughter et al.,

2003; Tate, 1999). TBI is also disproportionately common among criminal offender populations (see Williams et al., 2018, for review), and has been associated with increased risk for multiple arrests, violent offending, and earlier age of offending (Leon-Carrion & Ramos, 2003; Ray & Richardson, 2017; Schwartz, 2021; Williams et al., 2010). Further, TBI has been associated with a number of cognitive deficits, many of which also accompany antisocial behavior. TBI has been associated with impairments in attention and working memory (Bernstein, 2002; Mathias & Wheaton, 2007; McAllister et al., 1999; McDowell et al., 1997), both of which have also been associated with impulsive-antisocial traits of psychopathy (Sadeh & Verona, 2008; Sellbom & Verona, 2007), though the degree and persistence of cognitive impairment associated with TBI appear to vary based on injury severity and location (Dikmen et al., 2009; Ettenhofer & Abeles, 2009; Schretlen & Shapiro, 2003; Segalowitz et al., 2001). There is also some evidence that both TBI and impulsive-antisocial traits are related to the disruption of cognitive processes by negative emotional stimuli and an increased sensitivity to threat, which may result in reactive aggressive behavior (Cale & Lilienfeld, 2006; Mäki-Marttunen et al., 2015; Riley et al., 2004; Verona & Bresin, 2015; Verona et al., 2012).

TBI can act as an exacerbating factor within any of the previously discussed explanatory frameworks and has potential to fit into a chain of events through which TLEs and psychopathy interact. In gene-environment correlations, for example, TBI may occur as a result of an inherited predisposition to impulsive behavior, as such behavior increases the likelihood of injury. Similarly, symptoms following TBI and the care that is sometimes required by others can cause serious strain and frustration, particularly in parents of children with TBIs (Roscigno & Swanson, 2011). Aggression and impulsivity have also been known to follow TBI (Baguley et al., 2006; McHugh & Wood, 2008), and thus may heighten risk for abuse as caretakers try to manage these behaviors. Finally, in line with emotional numbing and instability theories, TBI has been associated with difficulties in emotional expression, recognition, and regulation (Rosenberg et al., 2014; Tate, 1999; van der Horn et al., 2016). Thus, there are several ways in which TBI fits quite well into existing theories positing the relationships between trauma and psychopathy.

Very few studies have explored relationships between TBI and psychopathy, unfortunately, and none have examined whether TBI can explain the development of distinct psychopathic traits. Studies of youth offenders have found significant relationships between psychopathic traits and a history of TBI, but differential relationships with distinct psychopathic traits were not reported (Perron & Howard, 2008; Vaughn et al., 2014). Given the lack of studies, future research should attempt to uncover whether TBI explains any of the relationships reported between psychopathy and certain outcomes (e.g., violent recidivism). These types of investigations are sorely needed to identify the most fruitful targets for rehabilitation and intervention efforts.

Overall, existing literature on TBI and its sequelae suggests that brain injury may show important relationships with psychopathic traits, as the emotional disruption and cognitive changes that sometimes follow TBI can present similarly to those associated with particular facets of psychopathy. Psychopathic traits may also increase a person's risk for TBI through impulsive or externalizing behavior (e.g., increased risk for fighting, motor vehicle accidents, etc.). The ways in which TBI may relate to different dimensions or facets of psychopathic traits has yet to be explored, however, and may be informative in understanding relationships between psychopathic and trauma. Though substantial work is needed in this area, TBI is often tied to TLEs, and may be an important variable in any trauma-related models of psychopathy.

9.5 Treatment Outcomes in Psychopathy and Trauma

The explanatory models above, and some of the evidence supporting them, have implications for appropriate interventions and whether they will be effective in reducing psychopathic behaviors or trauma-based psychopathology. Even without overlapping trauma or PTSD symptoms, increased levels of psychopathic traits are associated with poorer treatment outcomes in both forensic and community populations (e.g., D'Silva et al., 2004; Salekin et al., 2010; Skeem et al., 2002). However, results seem to vary with treatment target. Higher levels of psychopathy have been associated with poorer outcomes in substance use treatment (O'Neill et al., 2003; Richards et al., 2003), whereas the effects of psychopathy on treatment targeting violence reduction are much less certain (Reidy et al., 2013; Skeem et al., 2002). It is unclear whether PTSD and history of TLEs that overlap with psychopathy explain part of the difficulty in treatment course and outcomes observed in psychopathy treatment studies, or vice versa. That is, trauma exposure and PTSD have also been associated with more a more difficult treatment course, including poorer outcomes in substance use treatment, as they are associated with poorer emotion regulation and increased substance use (Ehring & Quack, 2010; Ouimette et al., 1998).

Despite the importance of considering the unique or overlapping roles of TLEs, PTSD, and psychopathy in a treatment context, there has been no direct work on this topic to date. Two potentially relevant studies with military veterans found that antisocial personality is associated with less change in anger during anger management treatment (Marshall et al., 2010) and poorer response to treatment for PTSD (Munley et al., 1994). These studies indicate that antisociality complicates treatment of persons with PTSD, although they do not answer questions about the extent to which overlap across PTSD and antisociality or psychopathy partly accounts for these problematic outcomes. Treatment may not only be more difficult among individuals high on antisocial or psychopathic traits, but the likelihood of seeking treatment may also vary across individuals high on psychopathy, regardless of trauma exposure. In a study that identified primary and secondary variants of high psychopathy (i.e., emotionally stable variant and an aggressive variant, respectively; Hicks et al., 2010), trauma exposure was equally present across both, although the latter was more likely to have received mental health treatment.

Given the potential mechanisms accounting for links between psychopathy and trauma highlighted in the described explanatory models (e.g., emotional numbing), it is likely that targeting trauma symptoms among persons high on psychopathy can help improve rehabilitation, particularly in limiting some of the negative outcomes associated with psychopathy (i.e., impulsivity, reactive aggression). Indeed, a large study of combat veterans indicated that PTSD treatment was associated with a significant decrease in violent behavior across 4 months (Buchanan et al., 2018), and clinically significant reductions of PTSD symptoms following treatment have been associated with decreases in future aggression (Watkins et al., 2018). Though only limited conclusions can be drawn from the existing work, these studies highlight that it is important to assess both trauma exposure and psychopathic traits, as individuals in which the two co-occur are not uncommon and likely need clinical intervention beyond that needed by low-psychopathy individuals with PTSD.

Similar to the lack of treatment studies involving psychopathy and TLEs/PTSD, there is a notable lack of studies examining TBI's effects on treatment of PTSD or of psychopathy (Carlson et al., 2011). This is surprising, given that TBI is highly prevalent among populations that experience both PTSD and psychopathy symptoms. It is possible that interventions that address TBI-related sequalae (e.g., executive functioning, theory of mind) would also help reduce some aspects of psychopathy. For example, work that implements or develops new cognitive rehabilitation technologies for TBI (Chua et al., 2007; see Cicerone et al., 2011 for review) may be extended to the treatment of psychopathy.

In all, work examining how psychopathic traits and trauma intersect in a treatment setting are virtually nonexistent, leaving ample room for future research. The presence of trauma or TBI may be related to a more difficult treatment course, as may the presence of psychopathic traits or antisociality. Future work may consider targeting some of the theoretical explanations proposed above (e.g., emotion dysregulation or modeling) as potential mechanisms of change (or lack thereof) in treatment. Such work may be particularly important in developing therapeutic interventions for persons involved with the criminal justice system, as TLEs, PTSD, TBI, and psychopathy are more common among this population.

9.6 Summary and Conclusions

This review has highlighted several different points at which psychopathy, TLEs, and PTSD intersect. Although this literature is mixed, there are several conclusions that can be drawn. First, there is evidence that facets of psychopathic traits vary in their relation to TLEs, and that this relationship may vary across gender. Impulsive-antisocial traits and behaviors have been consistently related to TLEs and PTSD (Blonigen et al., 2012; Cima et al., 2008; Dargis et al., 2016; Forouzan & Nicholls, 2015; Luntz & Widom, 1994; Poythress et al., 2006; Semiz et al., 2007). The relationship between interpersonal-affective traits and trauma is more variable and potentially more dependent upon other variables. For example, there is more evidence for a positive relationship between these traits and TLEs among men than there is among women (Blonigen et al., 2012; Forouzan & Nicholls, 2015; Graham et al., 2012; Krischer & Sevecke, 2008; Schimmenti et al., 2015; Verona et al., 2005), highlighting the importance of considering gender in future research.

Second, antisociality and TLEs seem related through a combination of genetic and environmental influences, with gene-environment correlations playing a fairly large role. There is evidence to support reactive gene-environment correlations, where antisocial behavior in the child evokes aggressive behavior in parents, potentially leading to TLEs for the child (Ge et al., 1996; Hawes et al., 2011; Schulz-Heik et al., 2010). At the same time, several studies also suggest that TLEs exert some degree of direct causal influence on the development of antisocial behavior (Eaves et al., 2010; Forsam & Langstrom, 2012; Jaffee et al., 2004, 2012; Jonson-Reid et al., 2010; Maas et al., 2008). A different literature implicates gene-environment interactions in the development of impulsive-antisocial psychopathic traits; however, critiques of this area of research (e.g., Duncan & Keller, 2011; Ficks & Waldman, 2014) suggest that conclusions regarding candidate genes should be made cautiously. More research is needed involving genome-wide association studies in very large samples to help delineate potential interactive effects across a large number of genes. Such studies would require very large samples and may be limited in the ability to assess psychopathy with thorough assessments.

9.6.1 Explanatory Models Linking Psychopathy and Trauma

Having established that TLEs likely have at least some impact on the development of psychopathic traits, the mechanisms through which this occurs remain to be determined. There are a number of proposed explanations for this relationship which are not necessarily exclusive of one another. Following the experience of a TLE, modeling, emotional blunting and instability, and TBI could all play a role within a single individual. At present, theories emphasizing emotional blunting hold the most promise for explaining the relationships between psychopathic traits, especially the interpersonal-affective features, and TLEs. Relevant studies indicate that, although high levels of these traits may be more genetically sourced among some individuals, a subset of people high on these traits develop them through emotional blunting following TLEs (Bennett & Kerig, 2014; Kerig et al., 2012; Kerig & Modrowski, 2018). These latter individuals may be most receptive to treatments that address trauma, and such trauma-informed interventions could lead to reductions of callous or antagonistic behaviors among persons showing emotional blunting. TLEs may be less common among the subset of individuals for whom interpersonal-affective psychopathic traits are theorized to be primarily genetically-sourced, even though emotional blunting is still present (Kimonis et al., 2011, 2012; Tatar et al., 2012).

While emotional blunting may be an important factor for understanding the development of interpersonal-affective traits, emotional instability models are promising in regard to linking TLEs and impulsive-antisocial traits. On the one hand, previous work shows that TLEs and antisociality are both related to difficulties in emotion regulation, independent of one another (e.g., Frewen & Lanius, 2006; Garcia-Sancho et al., 2014; Malterer et al., 2008), potentially implicating emotion dysregulation in the development of psychopathic traits following TLEs. On the other hand, it may be the case that emotional instability and TLEs are linked through gene-environment correlations, in which individuals inherit emotional dysregulation from parents who tend to create chaotic and potentially dangerous environments related to their own dysregulation. There is very little direct examination of either possibility. Nonetheless, there is reason to believe that emotional dysregulation may mediate the relationship between TLEs and the impulsive-antisocial features of psychopathy as well. Support for modeling theories finds that children model angry responses of caregivers (Björkqvist, 1997), and thus the antisocial behavior that follows may be a result of modeling maladaptive emotional responses or ineffective emotion regulation strategies, rather than simply modeling the behavior itself. Emotional instability is also implicated in differential manifestations of psychopathic traits in men and women. That is, previous work suggests that psychopathic traits manifest as greater emotional dysregulation in women (Hicks et al., 2010; Sprague et al., 2012), and that BPD traits (many of which reflect emotion dysregulation) mediate the relationship between TLEs and psychopathic traits in women (Blonigen et al., 2012). Emotional instability models may therefore serve a more explanatory role in women than men following TLEs.

9.6.2 Integration of TBI

TBI has been the most understudied mediator of relationships between TLEs and psychopathic traits. The high prevalence of TBI in correctional populations (Morrell et al., 1998; Slaughter et al., 2003) and the similarities between TBI sequelae and correlates of psychopathy (e.g., cognitive deficits, affective irregularities; Bernstein, 2002; Mathias & Wheaton, 2007; McAllister et al., 1999; McDowell et al., 1997; Sadeh & Verona, 2008; Sellbom & Verona, 2007) provide support for TBI as potentially important in the etiology of psychopathy and the relationship between TLEs and psychopathy. The first step to remedy the current gaps in the literature is to determine how strongly TBI predicts different facets of psychopathic traits. After that, specification of this relationship by location and severity of damage, and other potentially important variables (age of injury, lasting symptoms of injury, number of TBIs, etc.) should be pursued.

The next step would then be to determine the extent to which TBI can explain at least some of the relationships between TLEs and psychopathic traits. For example, emotional blunting, such as deficits in empathic responding (de Sousa et al., 2010, 2011, 2012; Saunders et al., 2006), can often result after a TBI. TBI has been also linked to emotion dysregulation that is similar to that found in individuals high on impulsive and antisocial behaviors (Cale & Lilienfeld, 2006; Mäki-Marttunen et al., 2015; Riley et al., 2004; Verona & Bresin, 2015; Verona et al., 2012). Given these putative links, we should consider the ways in which psychological and physical sequalae of trauma may jointly explain the development of psychopathic traits. Because TBIs only occur during a subset of TLEs, in Figs. 9.1a and 9.1b we highlight two potential pathways explaining the relationship between TLEs and psychopathic traits: one with TBI and one without. Among individuals experiencing TLEs that do not involve head injury, psychopathic traits may develop directly as a function of genes, social learning, and/or emotional dysfunction (instability and/or blunting; Fig. 9.1a); whereas in the subset of individuals who experience a TBI as part of a TLE, psychopathic traits may be mediated both through these psychological variables as well as via TBI (see Fig. 9.1b). That is, it is possible that some of the findings linking psychopathic traits with violence, recidivism, or interpersonal

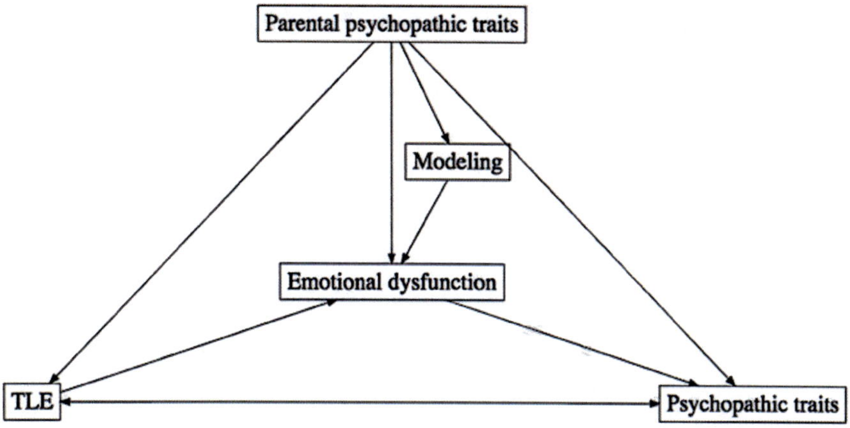

Fig. 9.1a Model of the relationship between trauma and psychopathy without TBI. *TLE* traumatic life event

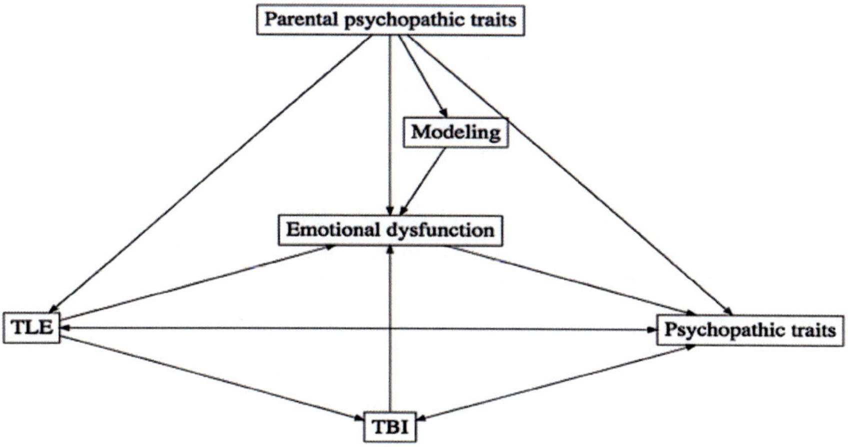

Fig. 9.1b Model of the relationship between trauma and psychopathy with TBI. *TLE* traumatic life event, *TBI* traumatic brain injury

dysfunction are at least partially accounted for by the cognitive and emotional dysfunctions following TBI, and not only by psychological sequelae of trauma or personality dispositions apparent prior to TBI. Future work will be needed to evaluate this model after determining how strongly TBI relates to facets of psychopathic traits.

9.7 Clinical Implications

The current state of this literature as a whole makes drawing conclusions about treatment considerations quite difficult. It seems, however, that antisociality may increase difficulty of treatment for PTSD (Marshall et al., 2010; Munley et al., 1994), but that such treatment may ultimately be successful in decreasing violence and aggression over time (Buchanan et al., 2018; Watkins et al., 2018). Treatments such as Dialectical Behavior Therapy (Linehan, 1993) that target emotional dysregulation may be of particular use among individuals high on the impulsive-antisocial psychopathic traits following a TLE. There currently are no reported studies examining how interpersonal-affective traits of psychopathy may affect or be affected by treatment for PTSD, making this an important avenue for future research. Trauma-informed treatments can be viable approaches, to the extent that emotional blunting accounts for relationships between TLEs and interpersonal-affective traits in a subset of individuals.

Treatment options may vary, however, if the relationship between psychopathy and TLEs is physically mediated by TBI. Some studies have found Cognitive-Behavioral Therapy to be beneficial in reducing post-concussive symptoms (see Al Sayegh et al., 2010, for review), and cognitive rehabilitation techniques beneficial in reducing cognitive deficits such as attention and memory following TBI (see Cicerone et al., 2011, for review). There has also been some preliminary work targeting TBI to reduce inmate risk, and although replication is needed, results are promising, finding that education on adaptive coping for TBI-related deficits limited disciplinary infractions while incarcerated and bettered community integration post-release (Ramos et al., 2018). Importantly, this intervention included working with prison staff to provide better support to inmates with TBIs while incarcerated, a step that may be crucial to outcomes. Of relevance to the proposed models relating TLEs, TBI, and psychopathy, the effects of therapy targeting emotion regulation are not clear and warrant future research.

There is ample room for future work on the relationship between psychopathy and trauma, and such work is important in paving the way for treatment studies. Work investigating emotional blunting and instability theories, TBI, and including tests for gender differences in the relationships between psychopathy and TLEs may be particularly fruitful for future rehabilitation efforts. With time, this work holds promise for limiting the burden of psychopathy and antisocial behavior, through reducing incarceration rates, violent crime, and the distress associated with both PTSD and psychopathy.

References

Abram, K. M., Washburn, J. J., Teplin, L. A., Emanuel, K. M., Romero, E. G., & McClelland, G. M. (2007). Posttraumatic stress disorder and psychiatric comorbidity among detained youths. *Psychiatric Services, 58*(10), 1311–1316.

Al Sayegh, A., Sandford, D., & Carson, A. J. (2010). Psychological approaches to treatment of postconcussion syndrome: A systematic review. *Journal of Neurology, Neurosurgery & Psychiatry, 81*(10), 1128–1134.

American Psychiatric Association. (2013). *Diagnostic and statistical manual of mental disorders* (5th ed.). Author.

Anderson, N. E., & Kiehl, K. A. (2012). The psychopath magnetized: Insights from brain imaging. *Trends in Cognitive Sciences, 16*(1), 52–60.

Arditti, J. A., Lambert-Shute, J., & Joest, K. (2003). Saturday morning at the jail: Implications of incarceration for families and children. *Family Relations, 52*(3), 195–204.

Baguley, I. J., Cooper, J., & Felmingham, K. (2006). Aggressive behavior following traumatic brain injury: How common is common? *The Journal of Head Trauma Rehabilitation, 21*(1), 45–56.

Bandura, A. (1973). *Aggression: A social learning analysis*. Prentice-Hall.

Bandura, A., Ross, D., & Ross, S. A. (1963). Vicarious reinforcement and imitative learning. *The Journal of Abnormal and Social Psychology, 67*(6), 601–607.

Ben-Ezra, M., & Aluf, D. (2006). Traumatic events v. life events: Does it really matter? *The British Journal of Psychiatry, 188*(1), 83–84.

Bennett, D. C., & Kerig, P. K. (2014). Investigating the construct of trauma-related acquired callousness among delinquent youth: Differences in emotion processing. *Journal of Traumatic Stress, 27*(4), 415–422.

Benning, S. D., Patrick, C. J., & Iacono, W. G. (2005). Psychopathy, startle blink modulation, and electrodermal reactivity in twin men. *Psychophysiology, 42*(6), 753–762.

Berkowitz, L. (1993). *Aggression: Its causes, consequences, and control*. Mcgraw-Hill Book Company.

Bernstein, D. M. (2002). Information processing difficulty long after self-reported concussion. *Journal of the International Neuropsychological Society, 8*(5), 673–682.

Bernstein, I. H., Ellason, J. W., Ross, C. A., & Vanderlinden, J. (2001). On the dimensionalities of the Dissociative Experiences Scale (DES) and the Dissociation Questionnaire (DIS-Q). *Journal of Trauma & Dissociation, 2*(3), 101–120.

Björkqvist, K. (1997). Learning aggression from models: From a social learning toward a cognitive theory of modeling. In S. Feshbach & J. Zagrodzka (Eds.), *Aggression* (The plenum series in social/clinical psychology) (pp. 69–81). Springer.

Blair, R. J. R., & Cipolotti, L. (2000). Impaired social response reversal: A case of 'acquired sociopathy'. *Brain, 123*(6), 1122–1141.

Blonigen, D. M., Sullivan, E. A., Hicks, B. M., & Patrick, C. J. (2012). Facets of psychopathy in relation to potentially traumatic events and posttraumatic stress disorder among female prisoners: The mediating role of borderline personality disorder traits. *Personality Disorders, 3*(4), 406–414.

Blumer, D., & Benson, D. F. (1975). Personality changes with frontal and temporal lobe lesions. In D. F. Benson & D. Blumer (Eds.), *Psychiatric aspects of neurological disease* (pp. 151–170). Grune & Stratton.

Bornovalova, M. A., Huibregtse, B. M., Hicks, B. M., Keyes, M., McGue, M., & Iacono, W. (2013). Tests of a direct effect of childhood abuse on adult borderline personality disorder traits: A longitudinal discordant twin design. *Journal of Abnormal Psychology, 122*(1), 180–194.

Briere, J., Agee, E., & Dietrich, A. (2016). Cumulative trauma and current posttraumatic stress disorder status in general population and inmate samples. *Psychological Trauma Theory Research Practice and Policy, 8*(4), 439–446.

Buchanan, A., Stefanovics, E., & Rosenheck, R. A. (2018). Correlates of reduced violent behavior among patients receiving intensive treatment for Posttraumatic Stress Disorder. *Psychiatric Services, 69*(4), 424–430.

Burton, D., Foy, D., Bwanausi, C., Johnson, J., & Moore, L. (1994). The relationship between traumatic exposure, family dysfunction, and post-traumatic stress symptoms in male juvenile offenders. *Journal of Traumatic Stress, 7*(1), 83–93.

Byrd, A. L., & Manuck, S. B. (2014). MAOA, childhood maltreatment and antisocial behavior: Meta-analysis of a gene-environment interaction. *Biological Psychiatry, 75*(1), 9–17.

Cale, E. M., & Lilienfeld, S. O. (2006). Psychopathy factors and risk for aggressive behavior: A test of the "threatened egotism" hypothesis. *Law and Human Behavior, 30*(1), 51–74.

Carlson, K. F., Kehle, S. M., Meis, L. A., Greer, N., MacDonald, R., Rutks, I., Sayer, N. A., Dobscha, S. K., & Wilt, T. J. (2011). Prevalence, assessment, and treatment of mild traumatic brain injury and posttraumatic stress disorder: A systematic review of the evidence. *The Journal of Head Trauma Rehabilitation, 26*(2), 103.

Caspi, A., & Moffitt, T. E. (2006). Gene–environment interactions in psychiatry: Joining forces with neuroscience. *Nature Reviews Neuroscience, 7*(7), 583–590.

Caspi, A., McClay, J., Moffitt, T. E., Mill, J., Martin, J., Craig, I. W., Taylor, A., & Poulton, R. (2002). Role of genotype in the cycle of violence in maltreated children. *Science, 297*(5582), 851–854.

Cauffman, E., Feldman, S., Watherman, J., & Steiner, H. (1998). Posttraumatic stress disorder among female juvenile offenders. *Journal of the American Academy of Child & Adolescent Psychiatry, 37*(11), 1209–1216.

Chua, K. S., Ng, Y. S., Yap, S. G., & Bok, C. W. (2007). A brief review of traumatic brain injury rehabilitation. *Annals of the Academy of Medicine, Singapore, 36*(1), 31.

Cicerone, K. D., Langenbahn, D. M., Braden, C., Malec, J. F., Kalmar, K., Fraas, M., Felicetti, T., Laatsch, L., Harley, J. P., Bergquist, T., Azulay, J., Cantor, J., & Ashman, T. (2011). Evidence-based cognitive rehabilitation: Updated review of the literature from 2003 through 2008. *Archives of Physical Medicine and Rehabilitation, 92*(4), 519–530.

Cima, M., Smeets, T., & Jelicic, M. (2008). Self-reported trauma, cortisol levels, and aggression in psychopathic and non-psychopathic prison inmates. *Biological Psychology, 78*(1), 75–86.

Collins, J. J., & Bailey, S. L. (1990). Traumatic stress disorder and violent behavior. *Journal of Traumatic Stress, 3*(2), 203–220.

Cook, S. L., Smith, S. G., Tusher, C. P., & Raiford, J. (2005). Self-reports of traumatic events in a random sample of incarcerated women. *Women & Criminal Justice, 16*(1–2), 107–126.

Craparo, G., Schimmenti, A., & Caretti, V. (2013). Traumatic experiences in childhood and psychopathy: A study on a sample of violent offenders from Italy. *European Journal of Psychotraumatology, 4*. https://doi.org/10.3402/ejpt.v4i0.21471

D'Silva, K., Duggan, C., & McCarthy, L. (2004). Does treatment really make psychopaths worse? A review of the evidence. *Journal of Personality Disorders, 18*(2), 163–177.

Damasio, A. R. (2000). A neural basis for sociopathy. *Archives of General Psychiatry, 57*(2), 128–129.

Dargis, M., & Koenigs, M. (2017). Witnessing domestic violence during childhood is associated with psychopathic traits in adult male criminal offenders. *Law and Human Behavior, 41*(2), 173–179.

Dargis, M., & Koenigs, M. (2018). Two subtypes of psychopathic criminals differ in negative affect and history of childhood abuse. *Psychological Trauma: Theory, Research, Practice, and Policy, 10*(4), 444.

Dargis, M., Newman, J., & Koenigs, M. (2016). Clarifying the link between childhood abuse history and psychopathic traits in adult criminal offenders. *Personality Disorders, 7*(3), 221–228.

Davis, T., Ammons, C., Dahl, A., & Kliewer, W. (2015). Community violence exposure and callous-unemotional traits in adolescents: Testing parental support as a promotive versus protective factor. *Personality and Individual Differences, 77*, 7–12.

de Sousa, A., McDonald, S., Rushby, J., Li, S., Dimoska, A., & James, C. (2010). Why don't you feel how I feel? Insight into the absence of empathy after severe traumatic brain injury. *Neuropsychologia, 48*(12), 3585–3595.

de Sousa, A., McDonald, S., Rushby, J., Li, S., Dimoska, A., & James, C. (2011). Understanding deficits in empathy after traumatic brain injury: The role of affective responsivity. *Cortex, 47*(5), 526–535.

de Sousa, A., McDonald, S., & Rushby, J. (2012). Changes in emotional empathy, affective responsivity, and behavior following severe traumatic brain injury. *Journal of Clinical and Experimental Neuropsychology, 34*(6), 606–623.

Derringer, J., Krueger, R. F., Irons, D. E., & Iacono, W. G. (2010). Harsh discipline, childhood sexual assault, and MAOA genotype: An investigation of main and interactive effects on diverse clinical externalizing outcomes. *Behavior Genetics, 40*(5), 639–648.

Dikmen, S. S., Corrigan, J. D., Levin, H. S., Machamer, J., Stiers, W., & Weisskopf, M. G. (2009). Cognitive outcome following traumatic brain injury. *The Journal of Head Trauma Rehabilitation, 24*(6), 430–438.

DiLalla, L. F., & Gottesman, I. I. (1991). Biological and genetic contributors to violence: Widom's untold tale. *Psychological Bulletin, 109*(1), 125–129.

Duncan, L. E., & Keller, M. C. (2011). A critical review of the first 10 years of candidate gene-by-environment interaction research in psychiatry. *American Journal of Psychiatry, 168*(10), 1041–1049.

Eaves, L. J., Prom, E. C., & Silberg, J. L. (2010). The mediating effect of parental neglect on adolescent and young adult anti-sociality: A longitudinal study of twins and their parents. *Behavior Genetics, 40*(4), 425–437.

Ehring, T., & Quack, D. (2010). Motion regulation difficulties in trauma survivors: The role of trauma type and PTSD symptom severity. *Behavior Therapy, 41*(4), 587–598.

Eierud, C., Craddock, R. C., Fletcher, S., Aulakh, M., King-Casas, B., Kuehl, D., & LaConte, S. M. (2014). Neuroimaging after mild traumatic brain injury: Review and meta-analysis. *NeuroImage: Clinical, 4*, 283–294.

Eme, R. (2013). MAOA and male antisocial behavior: A review. *Aggression and Violent Behavior, 18*(3), 395–398.

Erwin, B. A., Newman, E., McMackin, R. A., Morrissey, C., & Kaloupek, D. G. (2000). PTSD, malevolent environment, and criminality among criminally involved male adolescents. *Criminal Justice and Behavior, 27*(2), 196–215.

Ettenhofer, M. L., & Abeles, N. (2009). The significance of mild traumatic brain injury to cognition and self-reported symptoms in long-term recovery from injury. *Journal of Clinical and Experimental Neuropsychology, 31*(3), 363–372.

Ferguson, C. J., & Savage, J. (2012). Have recent studies addressed methodological issues raised by five decades of television violence research? A critical review. *Aggression and Violent Behavior, 17*(2), 129–139.

Ferguson, C. J., San Miguel, C., & Hartley, R. D. (2009). A multivariate analysis of youth violence and aggression: The influence of family, peers, depression, and media violence. *The Journal of Pediatrics, 155*(6), 904–908.e3.

Fergusson, D. M., Horwood, L. J., & Ridder, E. M. (2005). Show me the child at seven: The consequences of conduct problems in childhood for psychosocial functioning in adulthood. *Journal of Child Psychology and Psychiatry, 46*(8), 837–849.

Fergusson, D. M., Boden, J. M., Horwood, L. J., Miller, A. L., & Kennedy, M. A. (2011). MAOA, abuse exposure and antisocial behaviour: 30-year longitudinal study. *The British Journal of Psychiatry, 198*(6), 457–463.

Ficks, C. A., & Waldman, I. D. (2014). Candidate genes for aggression and antisocial behavior: A meta-analysis of association studies of the 5HTTLPR and MAOA-uVNTR. *Behavior Genetics, 44*(5), 427–444.

Forouzan, E., & Nicholls, T. L. (2015). Childhood and adolescent characteristics of women with high versus low psychopathy scores: Examining developmental precursors to the malignant personality disorder. *Journal of Criminal Justice, 43*(4), 307–320.

Forsman, M., & Långström, N. (2012). Child maltreatment and adult violent offending: Population-based twin study addressing the 'cycle of violence' hypothesis. *Psychological Medicine, 42*(9), 1977–1983.

Frewen, P. A., & Lanius, R. A. (2006). Toward a psychobiology of posttraumatic self-dysregulation: Reexperiencing, hyperarousal, dissociation, and emotional numbing. *Annals of the New York Academy of Sciences, 1071*(1), 110–124.

Frodi, A., Dernevik, M., Sepa, A., Philipson, J., & Bragesjö, M. (2001). Current attachment representations of incarcerated offenders varying in degree of psychopathy. *Attachment & Human Development, 3*(3), 269–283.

García-Sancho, E., Salguero, J. M., & Fernández-Berrocal, P. (2014). Relationship between emotional intelligence and aggression: A systematic review. *Aggression and Violent Behavior, 19*(5), 584–591.

Ge, X., Conger, R. D., Cadoret, R. J., Neiderhiser, J. M., Yates, W., Troughton, E., & Stewart, M. A. (1996). The developmental interface between nature and nurture: A mutual influence model of child antisocial behavior and parent behaviors. *Developmental Psychology, 32*(4), 574–589.

Glenn, A. L., Johnson, A. K., & Raine, A. (2013). Antisocial personality disorder: A current review. *Current Psychiatry Reports, 15*(12), 427.

Gold, S. D., Marx, B. P., Soler-Baillo, J. M., & Sloan, D. M. (2005). Is life stress more traumatic than traumatic stress? *Journal of Anxiety Disorders, 19*(6), 687–698.

Goodwin, R. D., & Hamilton, S. P. (2003). Lifetime comorbidity of antisocial personality disorder and anxiety disorders among adults in the community. *Psychiatry Research, 117*(2), 159–166.

Gorenstein, E. E., & Newman, J. P. (1980). Disinhibitory psychopathology: A new perspective and a model for research. *Psychological Review, 87*(3), 301–315.

Graham, N., Kimonis, E. R., Wasserman, A. L., & Kline, S. M. (2012). Associations among childhood abuse and psychopathy facets in male sexual offenders. *Personality Disorders, Theory, Research, and Treatment, 3*(1), 66–75.

Green, B. L. (1990). Defining trauma: Terminology and generic stressor dimensions. *Journal of Applied Social Psychology, 20*(20), 1632–1642.

Haberstick, B. C., Lessem, J. M., Hopfer, C. J., Smolen, A., Ehringer, M. A., Timberlake, D., & Hewitt, J. K. (2005). Monoamine oxidase A (MAOA) and antisocial behaviors in the presence of childhood and adolescent maltreatment. *American Journal of Medical Genetics Part B: Neuropsychiatric Genetics, 135B*(1), 59–64.

Haberstick, B. C., Lessem, J. M., Hewitt, J. K., Smolen, A., Hopfer, C. J., Halpern, C. T., Killeya-Jones, L. A., Boardman, J. D., Tabor, J., Siegler, I. C., Williams, R. B., & Mullan Harris, K. (2014). MAOA genotype, childhood maltreatment, and their interaction in the etiology of adult antisocial behaviors. *Biological Psychiatry, 75*(1), 25–30.

Halligan, S. L., Michael, T., Clark, D. M., & Ehlers, A. (2003). Posttraumatic stress disorder following assault: The role of cognitive processing, trauma memory, and appraisals. *Journal of Consulting and Clinical Psychology, 71*(3), 419–431.

Hare, R. D. (1991). *The Hare Psychopathy Checklist-Revised: Manual*. Multi-Health Systems, Incorporated.

Hare, R. D. (2003). *The Hare Psychopathy Checklist—Revised*. Multi-Health Systems, Incorporated.

Hare, R. D., & McPherson, L. M. (1984). Violent and aggressive behavior by criminal psychopaths. *International Journal of Law and Psychiatry, 7*(1), 35–50.

Harpur, T. J., Hare, R. D., & Hakstian, A. R. (1989). Two-factor conceptualization of psychopathy: Construct validity and assessment implications. *Psychological Assessment: A Journal of Consulting and Clinical Psychology, 1*(1), 6–17.

Haugebrook, S., Zgoba, K. M., Maschi, T., Morgen, K., & Brown, D. (2010). Trauma, stress, health, and mental health issues among ethnically diverse older adult prisoners. *Journal of Correctional Health Care, 16*(3), 220–229.

Hawes, D. J., Dadds, M. R., Frost, A. D., & Hasking, P. A. (2011). Do childhood callous-unemotional traits drive change in parenting practices? *Journal of Clinical Child & Adolescent Psychology, 40*(4), 507–518.

Hemphill, J. F., Hart, S. D., Hare, D., & R. (1994). Psychopathy and substance use. *Journal of Personality Disorders, 8*(3), 169–180.

Herrenkohl, T. I., Huang, B., Tajima, E. A., & Whitney, S. D. (2003). Examining the link between child abuse and youth violence: An analysis of mediating mechanisms. *Journal of Interpersonal Violence, 18*(10), 1189–1208.

Hicks, B. M., & Patrick, C. J. (2006). Psychopathy and negative emotionality: Analyses of suppressor effects reveal distinct relations with emotional distress, fearfulness, and anger-hostility. *Journal of Abnormal Psychology, 115*(2), 276.

Hicks, B. M., Vaidyanathan, U., & Patrick, C. J. (2010). Validating female psychopathy subtypes: Differences in personality, antisocial and violent behavior, substance abuse, trauma, and mental health. *Personality Disorders, 1*(1), 38–57.

Holz, N. E., Zohsel, K., Laucht, M., Banaschewski, T., Hohmann, S., & Brandeis, D. (2018). Gene x environment interactions in conduct disorder: Implications for future treatments. *Neuroscience & Biobehavioral Reviews, 91*, 239–258.

Howard, A. L., Kimonis, E. R., Muñoz, L. C., & Frick, P. J. (2012). Violence exposure mediates the relation between callous-unemotional traits and offending patterns in adolescents. *Journal of Abnormal Child Psychology, 40*(8), 1237–1247.

Huizinga, D., Haberstick, B. C., Smolen, A., Menard, S., Young, S. E., Corley, R. P., Stallings, M. C., Grotpeter, J., & Hewitt, J. K. (2006). Childhood maltreatment, subsequent antisocial behavior, and the role of monoamine oxidase A genotype. *Biological Psychiatry, 60*(7), 677–683.

Ingoldsby, E. M., Shaw, D. S., Winslow, E., Schonberg, M., Gilliom, M., & Criss, M. M. (2006). Neighborhood disadvantage, parent–child conflict, neighborhood peer relationships, and early antisocial behavior problem trajectories. *Journal of Abnormal Child Psychology, 34*(3), 293–309.

Jaffee, S. R., Caspi, A., Moffitt, T. E., & Taylor, A. (2004). Physical maltreatment victim to antisocial child: Evidence of an environmentally mediated process. *Journal of Abnormal Psychology, 113*(1), 44–55.

Jaffee, S. R., Strait, L. B., & Odgers, C. L. (2012). From correlates to causes: Can quasi-experimental studies and statistical innovations bring us closer to identifying the causes of antisocial behavior? *Psychological Bulletin, 138*(2), 272.

Jang, K. L., Stein, M. B., Taylor, S., Asmundson, G. J. G., & Livesley, W. J. (2003). Exposure to traumatic events and experiences: Aetiological relationships with personality function. *Psychiatry Research, 120*(1), 61–69.

Jonson-Reid, M., Presnall, N., Drake, B., Fox, L., Bierut, L., Reich, W., Kane, P., Todd, R. D., & Constantino, J. N. (2010). Effects of child maltreatment and inherited liability on antisocial development: An official records study. *Journal of the American Academy of Child & Adolescent Psychiatry, 49*(4), 321–332.

Jordan, B. K., Schlenger, W. E., Fairbank, J. A., & Caddell, J. M. (1996). Prevalence of psychiatric disorders among incarcerated women: II. Convicted felons entering prison. *Archives of General Psychiatry, 53*(6), 513–519.

Karpman, B. (1941). On the need of separating psychopathy into two distinct clinical types: The symptomatic and the idiopathic. *Journal of Criminal Psychopathology, 3*, 112–137.

Karpman, B. (1955). Psychodynamics of child delinquency further contributions: Round table, 1953. *American Journal of Orthopsychiatry, 25*(2), 238.

Kerig, P. K., & Modrowski, C. A. (2018). Testing gender-differentiated models of the mechanisms linking polyvictimization and youth offending: Numbing and callousness versus dissociation and borderline traits. *Journal of Trauma & Dissociation, 19*(3), 347–361.

Kerig, P. K., Bennett, D. C., Thompson, M., & Becker, S. P. (2012). "Nothing really matters": Emotional numbing as a link between trauma exposure and callousness in delinquent youth. *Journal of Traumatic Stress, 25*(3), 272–279.

Kiehl, K. A., Smith, A. M., Hare, R. D., Mendrek, A., Forster, B. B., Brink, J., & Liddle, P. F. (2001). Limbic abnormalities in affective processing by criminal psychopaths as revealed by functional magnetic resonance imaging. *Biological Psychiatry, 50*(9), 677–684.

Kim, J., & Cicchetti, D. (2010). Longitudinal pathways linking child maltreatment, emotion regulation, peer relations, and psychopathology. *Journal of Child Psychology and Psychiatry, 51*(6), 706–716.

Kim-Cohen, J., Caspi, A., Taylor, A., Williams, B., Newcombe, R., Craig, I., & Moffitt, T. (2006). MAOA, maltreatment, and gene–environment interaction predicting children's mental health: New evidence and a meta-analysis. *Molecular Psychiatry, 11*(10), 903.

Kimonis, E. R., Frick, P. J., Munoz, L. C., & Aucoin, K. J. (2008). Callous-unemotional traits and the emotional processing of distress cues in detained boys: Testing the moderating role of aggression, exposure to community violence, and histories of abuse. *Development and Psychopathology, 20*(2), 569–589.

Kimonis, E. R., Skeem, J. L., Cauffman, E., & Dmitrieva, J. (2011). Are secondary variants of juvenile psychopathy more reactively violent and less psychosocially mature than primary variants? *Law and Human Behavior, 35*(5), 381–391.

Kimonis, E. R., Frick, P. J., Cauffman, E., Goldweber, A., & Skeem, J. (2012). Primary and secondary variants of juvenile psychopathy differ in emotional processing. *Development and Psychopathology, 24*(03), 1091–1103.

Kimonis, E. R., Cross, B., Howard, A., & Donoghue, K. (2013). Maternal care, maltreatment and callous-unemotional traits among urban male juvenile offenders. *Journal of Youth and Adolescence, 42*(2), 165–177.

Koenen, K. C., Fu, Q. J., Lyons, M. J., Toomey, R., Goldberg, J., Eisen, S. A., True, W., & Tsuang, M. (2005). Juvenile conduct disorder as a risk factor for trauma exposure and posttraumatic stress disorder. *Journal of Traumatic Stress, 18*(1), 23–32.

Koivisto, H., & Haapasalo, J. (1996). Childhood maltreatment and adulthood psychopathy in light of file-based assessments among mental state examinees. *Studies on Crime & Crime Prevention, 5*(1), 91–104.

Kraus, M. F., Susmaras, T., Caughlin, B. P., Walker, C. J., Sweeney, J. A., & Little, D. M. (2007). White matter integrity and cognition in chronic traumatic brain injury: A diffusion tensor imaging study. *Brain, 130*(10), 2508–2519.

Krischer, M. K., & Sevecke, K. (2008). Early traumatization and psychopathy in female and male juvenile offenders. *International Journal of Law and Psychiatry, 31*(3), 253–262.

Krueger, R. F., Markon, K. E., Patrick, C. J., Benning, S. D., & Kramer, M. D. (2007). Linking antisocial behavior, substance use, and personality: An integrative quantitative model of the adult externalizing spectrum. *Journal of Abnormal Psychology, 116*(4), 645–666.

Krysinska, K., & Lester, D. (2010). Post-traumatic stress disorder and suicide risk: A systematic review. *Archives of Suicide Research, 14*(1), 1–23.

Lancaster, S. L., Melka, S. E., & Rodriguez, B. F. (2009). An examination of the differential effects of the experience of DSM-IV defined traumatic events and life stressors. *Journal of Anxiety Disorders, 23*(5), 711–717.

Leon-Carrion, J., & Ramos, F. J. C. (2003). Blows to the head during development can predispose to violent criminal behaviour: Rehabilitation of consequences of head injury is a measure for crime prevention. *Brain Injury, 17*(3), 207–216.

Linehan, M. M. (1993). *Skills training manual for treating borderline personality disorder*. Guilford Press.

Luntz, B. K., & Widom, C. S. (1994). Antisocial personality disorder in abused and neglected children grown up. *The American Journal of Psychiatry, 151*(5), 670–674.

Maas, C., Herrenkohl, T. I., & Sousa, C. (2008). Review of research on child maltreatment and violence in youth. *Trauma, Violence & Abuse, 9*(1), 56–67.

Maas, A. I. R., Menon, D. K., Adelson, P. D., Andelic, N., Bell, M. J., Belli, A., … Zumbo, F. (2017). Traumatic brain injury: Integrated approaches to improve prevention, clinical care, and research. *The Lancet Neurology, 16*(12), 987–1048.

Mäki-Marttunen, V., Kuusinen, V., Brause, M., Peräkylä, J., Polvivaara, M., dos Santos Ribeiro, R., Öhman, J., & Hartikainen, K. M. (2015). Enhanced attention capture by emotional stimuli in mild traumatic brain injury. *Journal of Neurotrauma, 32*(4), 272–279.

Malterer, M. B., Glass, S. J., & Newman, J. P. (2008). Psychopathy and trait emotional intelligence. *Personality and Individual Differences, 44*(3), 735–745.

Maneta, E. K., White, M., & Mezzacappa, E. (2017). Parent-child aggression, adult-partner violence, and child outcomes: A prospective, population-based study. *Child Abuse & Neglect, 68*, 1–10.

Marshall, L. A., & Cooke, D. J. (1999). The childhood experiences of psychopaths: A retrospective study of familial and societal factors. *Journal of Personality Disorders, 13*(3), 211–225.

Marshall, A. D., Martin, E. K., Warfield, G. A., Doron-Lamarca, S., Niles, B. L., & Taft, C. T. (2010). The impact of antisocial personality characteristics on anger management treatment for veterans with PTSD. *Psychological Trauma Theory Research Practice and Policy, 2*(3), 224–231.

Martin, L., Rosen, L. N., Durand, D. B., Knudson, K. H., & Stretch, R. H. (2000). Psychological and physical health effects of sexual assaults and nonsexual traumas among male and female United States Army soldiers. *Behavioral Medicine, 26*(1), 23–33.

Mathias, J. L., & Wheaton, P. (2007). Changes in attention and information-processing speed following severe traumatic brain injury: A meta-analytic review. *Neuropsychology, 21*(2), 212–223.

McAllister, T. W., Saykin, A. J., Flashman, L. A., Sparling, M. B., Johnson, S. C., Guerin, S. J., Mamourian, A. C., Weaver, J. B., & Yanofsky, N. (1999). Brain activation during working memory 1 month after mild traumatic brain injury: A functional MRI study. *Neurology, 53*(6), 1300–1300.

McBride, M. L. (1998). *Individual and familial risk factors for adolescent psychopathy*. University of British Columbia.

McDermott, R., Tingley, D., Cowden, J., Frazzetto, G., & Johnson, D. D. P. (2009). Monoamine oxidase A gene (MAOA) predicts behavioral aggression following provocation. *Proceedings of the National Academy of Sciences, 106*(7), 2118–2123.

McDonald, S. (2013). Impairments in social cognition following severe traumatic brain injury. *Journal of the International Neuropsychological Society, 19*(3), 231–246.

McDowell, S., Whyte, J., & D'Esposito, M. (1997). Working memory impairments in traumatic brain injury: Evidence from a dual-task paradigm. *Neuropsychologia, 35*(10), 1341–1353.

McHugh, D. L., & Wood, R. L. (2008). Using a temporal discounting paradigm to measure decision-making and impulsivity following traumatic brain injury: A pilot study. *Brain Injury, 22*(9), 715–721.

McMahon, R. J., Witkiewitz, K., & Kotler, J. S. (2010). Predictive validity of callous-unemotional traits measured in early adolescence with respect to multiple antisocial outcomes. *Journal of Abnormal Psychology, 119*(4), 752–763.

McMillan, T. M., Williams, W. H., & Bryant, R. (2003). Post-traumatic stress disorder and traumatic brain injury: A review of causal mechanisms, assessment, and treatment. *Neuropsychological Rehabilitation, 13*(1–2), 149–164.

Meehl, P. E. (1962). Schizotaxia, schizotypy, schizophrenia. *American Psychologist, 17*, 827–838.

Menon, D. K., Schwab, K., Wright, D. W., & Maas, A. I. (2010). Position statement: Definition of traumatic brain injury. *Archives of Physical Medicine and Rehabilitation, 91*(11), 1637–1640.

Meyer-Lindenberg, A., Buckholtz, J. W., Kolachana, B., Hariri, A. R., Pezawas, L., Blasi, G., Wabnitz, A., Honea, R., Verchinski, B., Callicott, J. H., Egan, M., Mattay, V., & Weinberger, D. R. (2006). Neural mechanisms of genetic risk for impulsivity and violence in humans. *Proceedings of the National Academy of Sciences, 103*(16), 6269–6274.

Miles, D. R., & Carey, G. (1997). Genetic and environmental architecture on human aggression. *Journal of Personality and Social Psychology, 72*(1), 207.

Miller, L. S., Wasserman, G. A., Neugebauer, R., Gorman-Smith, D., & Kamboukos, D. (1999). Witnessed community violence and antisocial behavior in high-risk, urban boys. *Journal of Clinical Child Psychology, 28*(1), 2–11.

Mills, K. L., Teesson, M., Ross, J., & Peters, L. (2006). Trauma, PTSD, and substance use disorders: Findings from the Australian National Survey of Mental Health and Well-Being. *American Journal of Psychiatry, 163*(4), 652–658.

Moffitt, T. E. (2005). The new look of behavioral genetics in developmental psychopathology: Gene-environment interplay in antisocial behaviors. *Psychological Bulletin, 131*, 533–554.

Monahan, K. C., Steinberg, L., & Cauffman, E. (2009). Affiliation with antisocial peers, susceptibility to peer influence, and antisocial behavior during the transition to adulthood. *Developmental Psychology, 45*(6), 1520–1530.

Morrell, R. F., Merbitz, C. T., Jain, S., & Jain, S. (1998). Traumatic brain injury in prisoners. *Journal of Offender Rehabilitation, 27*(3–4), 1–8.

Munley, P. H., Bains, D. S., Frazee, J., & Schwartz, L. T. (1994). Inpatient PTSD treatment: A study of pretreatment measures, treatment dropout, and therapist ratings of response to treatment. *Journal of Traumatic Stress, 7*(2), 319–325.

Murray, J., Ehlers, A., & Mayou, R. A. (2002). Dissociation and post-traumatic stress disorder: Two prospective studies of road traffic accident survivors. *British Journal of Psychiatry, 180*(4), 363–368.

O'Neill, M. L., Lidz, V., & Heilbrun, K. (2003). Adolescents with psychopathic characteristics in a substance abusing cohort: Treatment process and outcomes. *Law and Human Behavior, 27*(3), 299–313.

O'Connor, T. G., Deater-Deckard, K., Fulker, D., Rutter, M., & Plomin, R. (1998). Genotype–environment correlations in late childhood and early adolescence: Antisocial behavioral problems and coercive parenting. *Developmental Psychology, 34*(5), 970.

Orsillo, S. M., Theodore-Oklota, C., Luterek, J. A., & Plumb, J. (2007). The development and psychometric evaluation of the emotional reactivity and numbing scale. *The Journal of Nervous and Mental Disease, 195*(10), 830–836.

Ouimette, P. C., Brown, P. J., & Najavits, L. M. (1998). Course and treatment of patients with both substance use and posttraumatic stress disorders. *Addictive Behaviors, 23*(6), 785–795.

Panayiotou, G. (2015). The bold and the fearless among us: Elevated psychopathic traits and levels of anxiety and fear are associated with specific aberrant driving behaviors. *Accident Analysis & Prevention, 79*, 117–125.

Parker, D. R., & Rogers, R. W. (1981). Observation and performance of aggression: Effects of multiple models and frustration. *Personality and Social Psychology Bulletin, 7*(2), 302–308.

Patrick, C. J., Bradley, M. M., & Lang, P. J. (1993). Emotion in the criminal psychopathy: Startle reflex modulation. *Journal of Abnormal Psychology, 102*(1), 82–92.

Patrick, C. J., Zempolich, K. A., & Levenston, G. K. (1997). Emotionality and violent behavior in psychopaths. In A. Raine, P. A. Brennan, D. P. Farrington, & S. A. Mednick (Eds.), *Biosocial bases of violence* (pp. 145–161). Plenum Press.

Perron, B. E., & Howard, M. O. (2008). Prevalence and correlates of traumatic brain injury among delinquent youths. *Criminal Behaviour and Mental Health, 18*(4), 243–255.

Peterson, A. B., Xu, L., Daugherty, J., & Breiding, M. J. (2019). *Surveillance report of traumatic brain injury-related emergency department visits, hospitalizations, and deaths, United States, 2014.*

Pham, T. H. (2012). Psychopathy and traumatic stress. *Journal of Personality Disorders, 26*(2), 213–225.

Plomin, R., DeFries, J. C., & Loehlin, J. C. (1977). Genotype-environment interaction and correlation in the analysis of human behavior. *Psychological Bulletin, 84*(2), 309–322.

Porter, S. (1996). Without conscience or without active conscience? The etiology of psychopathy revisited. *Aggression and Violent Behavior, 1*(2), 179–189.

Poythress, N. G., & Skeem, J. L. (2006). Disaggregating psychopathy. In *Handbook of Psychopathy* (pp. 172–192). The Guilford Press.

Poythress, N. G., Skeem, J. L., & Lilienfeld, S. O. (2006). Associations among early abuse, dissociation, and psychopathy in an offender sample. *Journal of Abnormal Psychology, 115*(2), 288–297.

Prichard, Z., Mackinnon, A., Jorm, A. F., & Easteal, S. (2008). No evidence for interaction between MAOA and childhood adversity for antisocial behavior. *American Journal of Medical Genetics Part B: Neuropsychiatric Genetics, 147*(2), 228–232.

Raine, A., Lee, L., Yang, Y., & Colletti, P. (2010). Neurodevelopmental marker for limbic maldevelopment in antisocial personality disorder and psychopathy. *The British Journal of Psychiatry, 197*(3), 186–192.

Ramos, S. D., Oddy, M., Liddement, J., & Fortescue, D. (2018). Brain injury and offending: The development and field testing of a linkworker intervention. *International Journal of Offender Therapy and Comparative Criminology, 62*(7), 1854–1868.

Ray, B., & Richardson, N. J. (2017). Traumatic brain injury and recidivism among returning inmates. *Criminal Justice and Behavior, 44*(3), 472–486.

Reidy, D. E., Kearns, M. C., & DeGue, S. (2013). Reducing psychopathic violence: A review of the treatment literature. *Aggression and Violent Behavior, 18*(5), 527–538.
Rhee, S. H., & Waldman, I. D. (2002). Genetic and environmental influences on antisocial behavior: A meta-analysis of twin and adoption studies. *Psychological Bulletin, 128*(3), 490–529.
Richards, H. J., Casey, J. O., & Lucente, S. W. (2003). Psychopathy and treatment response in incarcerated female substance abusers. *Criminal Justice and Behavior, 30*(2), 251–276.
Riley, G. A., Brennan, A. J., & Powell, T. (2004). Threat appraisal and avoidance after traumatic brain injury: Why and how often are activities avoided? *Brain Injury, 18*(9), 871–888.
Roscigno, C. I., & Swanson, K. M. (2011). Parents' experiences following children's moderate to severe traumatic brain injury: A clash of cultures. *Qualitative Health Research, 21*(10), 1413–1426.
Rosenberg, H., McDonald, S., Dethier, M., Kessels, R. P., & Westbrook, R. F. (2014). Facial emotion recognition deficits following moderate–severe traumatic brain injury (TBI): Re-examining the valence effect and the role of emotion intensity. *Journal of the International Neuropsychological Society, 20*(10), 994–1003.
Sadeh, N., & Verona, E. (2008). Psychopathic personality traits associated with abnormal selective attention and impaired cognitive control. *Neuropsychology, 22*(5), 669–680.
Sadeh, N., Javdani, S., Jackson, J. J., Reynolds, E. K., Potenza, M. N., Gelernter, J., Lejuez, C. W., & Verona, E. (2010). Serotonin transporter gene associations with psychopathic traits in youth vary as a function of socioeconomic resources. *Journal of Abnormal Psychology, 119*(3), 604–609.
Salekin, R. T., Worley, C., & Grimes, R. D. (2010). Treatment of psychopathy: A review and brief introduction to the mental model approach for psychopathy. *Behavioral Sciences & the Law, 28*(2), 235–266.
Sareen, J., Stein, M. B., Cox, B. J., & Hassard, S. T. (2004). Understanding comorbidity of anxiety disorders with antisocial behavior: Findings from two large community surveys. *The Journal of Nervous and Mental Disease, 192*(3), 178–186.
Sartor, C. E., Mccutcheon, V. V., Pommer, N. E., Nelson, E. C., Duncan, A. E., Waldron, M., Bucholz, K. K., Madden, P. A. F., & Heath, A. C. (2010). Posttraumatic stress disorder and alcohol dependence in young women. *Journal of Studies on Alcohol and Drugs, 71*(6), 810–818.
Saunders, J. C., McDonald, S., & Richardson, R. (2006). Loss of emotional experience after traumatic brain injury: Findings with the startle probe procedure. *Neuropsychology, 20*(2), 224–231.
Schimmenti, A., Di Carlo, G., Passanisi, A., & Caretti, V. (2015). Abuse in childhood and psychopathic traits in a sample of violent offenders. *Psychological Trauma Theory Research Practice and Policy, 7*(4), 340–347.
Schraft, C. V., Kosson, D. S., & McBride, C. K. (2013). Exposure to violence within home and community environments and psychopathic tendencies in detained adolescents. *Criminal Justice and Behavior, 40*(9), 1027–1043.
Schreiber, S., & Galai-Gat, T. (1993). Uncontrolled pain following physical injury as the core-trauma in post-traumatic stress disorder. *Pain, 54*(1), 107–110.
Schretlen, D. J., & Shapiro, A. M. (2003). A quantitative review of the effects of traumatic brain injury on cognitive functioning. *International Review of Psychiatry, 15*(4), 341–349.
Schulz, N., Murphy, B., & Verona, E. (2016). Gender differences in psychopathy links to drug use. *Law and Human Behavior, 40*(2), 159.
Schulz-Heik, R. J., Rhee, S. H., Silvern, L. E., Haberstick, B. C., Hopfer, C., Lessem, J. M., & Hewitt, J. K. (2010). The association between conduct problems and maltreatment: Testing genetic and environmental mediation. *Behavior Genetics, 40*(3), 338–348.
Schwartz, J. A. (2021). A longitudinal assessment of head injuries as a source of acquired neuropsychological deficits and the implications for criminal persistence. *Justice Quarterly, 38*(2), 196–223. https://doi.org/10.1080/07418825.2019.1599044
Segalowitz, S. J., Bernstein, D. M., & Lawson, S. (2001). P300 event-related potential decrements in well-functioning university students with mild head injury. *Brain and Cognition, 45*(3), 342–356.

Sellbom, M. (2015). Elucidating the complex associations between psychopathy and posttraumatic stress disorder from the perspective of trait negative affectivity. *International Journal of Forensic Mental Health, 14*(2), 85–92.

Sellbom, M., & Verona, E. (2007). Neuropsychological correlates of psychopathic traits in a nonincarcerated sample. *Journal of Research in Personality, 41*(2), 276–294.

Semiz, U. B., Basoglu, C., Ebrinc, S., & Cetin, M. (2007). Childhood trauma history and dissociative experiences among Turkish men diagnosed with antisocial personality disorder. *Social Psychiatry and Psychiatric Epidemiology, 42*(11), 865–873.

Serin, R. C. (1991). Psychopathy and violence in criminals. *Journal of Interpersonal Violence, 6*(4), 423–431.

Sevecke, K., Franke, S., Kosson, D., & Krischer, M. (2016). Emotional dysregulation and trauma predicting psychopathy dimensions in female and male juvenile offenders. *Child and Adolescent Psychiatry and Mental Health, 10*(1), 43.

Sharf, A., Kimonis, E. R., & Howard, A. (2014). Negative life events and posttraumatic stress disorder among incarcerated boys with callous-unemotional traits. *Journal of Psychopathology and Behavioral Assessment, 36*(3), 401–414.

Sharp, D. J., Scott, G., & Leech, R. (2014). Network dysfunction after traumatic brain injury. *Nature Reviews Neurology, 10*(3), 156–166.

Sharpe, M., Baldwin, D., & Walker, J. (2010). 17—Neurotic, stress-related and somatoform disorders. In E. C. Johnstone, D. C. Owens, S. M. Lawrie, A. M. McIntosh, & M. Sharpe (Eds.), *Companion to psychiatric studies* (8th ed., pp. 453–491). Elsevier.

Skeem, J. L., Monahan, J., & Mulvey, E. P. (2002). Psychopathy, treatment involvement, and subsequent violence among civil psychiatric patients. *Law and Human Behavior, 26*(6), 577–603.

Skeem, J. L., Poythress, N., Edens, J. F., Lilienfeld, S. O., & Cale, E. M. (2003). Psychopathic personality or personalities? Exploring potential variants of psychopathy and their implications for risk assessment. *Aggression and Violent Behavior, 8*(5), 513–546.

Slaughter, B., Fann, J. R., & Ehde, D. (2003). Traumatic brain injury in a county jail population: Prevalence, neuropsychological functioning and psychiatric disorders. *Brain Injury, 17*(9), 731–741.

Smith, S. S., & Newman, J. P. (1990). Alcohol and drug abuse-dependence disorders in psychopathic and nonpsychopathic criminal offenders. *Journal of Abnormal Psychology, 99*(4), 430.

Sousa, C., Herrenkohl, T. I., Moylan, C. A., Tajima, E. A., Klika, J. B., Herrenkohl, R. C., & Russo, M. J. (2011). Longitudinal study on the effects of child abuse and children's exposure to domestic violence, parent-child attachments, and antisocial behavior in adolescence. *Journal of Interpersonal Violence, 26*(1), 111–136.

Sprague, J., Javdani, S., Sadeh, N., Newman, J. P., & Verona, E. (2012). Borderline personality disorder as a female phenotypic expression of psychopathy? *Personality Disorders, 3*(2), 127–139.

Stein, M. B., & McAllister, T. W. (2009). Exploring the convergence of posttraumatic stress disorder and mild traumatic brain injury. *American Journal of Psychiatry, 166*(7), 768–776.

Tatar, J. R., Cauffman, E., Kimonis, E. R., & Skeem, J. L. (2012). Victimization history and posttraumatic stress: An analysis of psychopathy variants in male juvenile offenders. *Journal of Child & Adolescent Trauma, 5*(2), 102–113.

Tate, R. L. (1999). Executive dysfunction and characterological changes after traumatic brain injury: Two sides of the same coin? *Cortex, 35*(1), 39–55.

Toro, P. A., Urberg, K. A., & Heinze, H. J. (2004). Antisocial behavior and affiliation with deviant peers. *Journal of Clinical Child and Adolescent Psychology, 33*(2), 336–346.

Tottenham, N., Hare, T. A., Quinn, B. T., McCarry, T. W., Nurse, M., Gilhooly, T., Millner, A., Galvan, A., Davidson, M. C., Eigsti, I.-M., Thomas, K. M., Freed, P. J., Booma, E. S., Gunnar, M. R., Altemus, M., Aronson, J., & Thomas, K. M. (2010). Prolonged institutional rearing is associated with atypically large amygdala volume and difficulties in emotion regulation. *Developmental Science, 13*(1), 46–61.

Trull, T. J., Jahng, S., Tomko, R. L., Wood, P. K., & Sher, K. J. (2010). Revised NESARC personality disorder diagnoses: Gender, prevalence, and comorbidity with substance dependence disorders. *Journal of Personality Disorders, 24*(4), 412–426.

Vakil, E. (2005). The effect of moderate to severe traumatic brain injury (TBI) on different aspects of memory: A selective review. *Journal of Clinical and Experimental Neuropsychology, 27*(8), 977–1021.

van der Horn, H. J., Liemburg, E. J., Aleman, A., Spikman, J. M., & van der Naalt, J. (2016). Brain networks subserving emotion regulation and adaptation after mild traumatic brain injury. *Journal of Neurotrauma, 33*(1), 1–9.

Vaughn, M. G., Salas-Wright, C. P., DeLisi, M., & Perron, B. (2014). Correlates of traumatic brain injury among juvenile offenders: A multi-site study. *Criminal Behaviour and Mental Health, 24*(3), 188–203.

Verona, E., & Bresin, K. (2015). Aggression proneness: Transdiagnostic processes involving negative valence and cognitive systems. *International Journal of Psychophysiology, 98*(2), 321–329.

Verona, E., Patrick, C. J., & Joiner, T. E. (2001). Psychopathy, antisocial personality, and suicide risk. *Journal of Abnormal Psychology, 110*(3), 462–470.

Verona, E., Hicks, B. M., & Patrick, C. J. (2005). Psychopathy and suicidality in female offenders: Mediating influences of personality and abuse. *Journal of Consulting and Clinical Psychology, 73*(6), 1065–1073.

Verona, E., Sprague, J., & Sadeh, N. (2012). Inhibitory control and negative emotional processing in psychopathy and antisocial personality disorder. *Journal of Abnormal Psychology, 121*(2), 498–510.

Verona, E., Hoffmann, A., & Edwards, B. (2018). Psychopathic traits and substance use: Co-occurrence and overlapping etiological pathways. In *Routledge international handbook of psychopathy and crime* (pp. 493–507). Routledge.

Vogel, M., & Keith, S. (2015). Vicarious peer victimization and adolescent violence: Unpacking the effects of social learning, general strain, and peer group selection. *Deviant Behavior, 36*(10), 834–852.

Vonderlin, R., Kleindienst, N., Alpers, G. W., Bohus, M., Lyssenko, L., & Schmahl, C. (2018). Dissociation in victims of childhood abuse or neglect: A meta-analytic review. *Psychological Medicine, 48*(15), 2467–2476.

Waldman, I. D., Rhee, S. H., LoParo, D., & Park, Y. (2018). Genetic and environmental influences on psychopathy and antisocial behaivior. In C. J. Patrick (Ed.), *Handbook of psychopathy* (pp. 335–353). The Guilford Press.

Watkins, L. E., Sippel, L. M., Pietrzak, R. H., Hoff, R., & Harpaz-Rotem, I. (2018). Clinically significant change in posttraumatic stress disorder symptoms is associated with lower levels of aggression after residential treatment discharge. *Journal of Traumatic Stress, 31*(2), 265–272.

Weder, N., Yang, B. Z., Douglas-Palumberi, H., Massey, J., Krystal, J. H., Gelernter, J., & Kaufman, J. (2009). MAOA genotype, maltreatment, and aggressive behavior: The changing impact of genotype at varying levels of trauma. *Biological Psychiatry, 65*(5), 417–424.

Weiler, B. L., & Widom, C. S. (1996). Psychopathy and violent behaviour in abused and neglected young adults. *Criminal Behaviour and Mental Health, 6*(3), 253–271.

White, H. R., & Widom, C. S. (2003). Intimate partner violence among abused and neglected children in young adulthood: The mediating effects of early aggression, antisocial personality, hostility and alcohol problems. *Aggressive Behavior, 29*(4), 332–345.

Widom, C. S. (1989). The cycle of violence. *Science, 244*(4901), 160–166.

Widom, C. S. (1997). Child abuse, neglect, and witnessing violence. In *Handbook of antisocial behavior* (pp. 159–170). Wiley.

Widom, C. S., & Maxfield, M. G. (1996). A prospective examination of risk for violence among abused and neglected children. *Annals of the New York Academy of Sciences, 794*(1), 224–237.

Willemsen, J., De Ganck, J., & Verhaeghe, P. (2012). Psychopathy, traumatic exposure, and lifetime posttraumatic stress. *International Journal of Offender Therapy and Comparative Criminology, 56*(4), 505–524.

Williams, W. H., Mewse, A. J., Tonks, J., Mills, S., Burgess, C. N. W., & Cordan, G. (2010). Traumatic brain injury in a prison population: Prevalence and risk for re-offending. *Brain Injury, 24*(10), 1184–1188.

Williams, W. H., Chitsabesan, P., Fazel, S., McMillan, T., Hughes, N., Parsonage, M., & Tonks, J. (2018). Traumatic brain injury: A potential cause of violent crime? *The Lancet Psychiatry, 5*(10), 836–844.

Williamson, J. B., Heilman, K. M., Porges, E., Lamb, D., & Porges, S. W. (2013). A possible mechanism for PTSD symptoms in patients with traumatic brain injury: Central autonomic network disruption. *Frontiers in Neuroengineering, 6*, 13.

Wilson, H. W., Stover, C. S., & Berkowitz, S. J. (2009). The relationship between childhood violence exposure and juvenile antisocial behavior: A meta-analytic review. *Journal of Child Psychology and Psychiatry, 50*(7), 769–779.

Yang, Y., & Raine, A. (2009). Prefrontal structural and functional brain imaging findings in antisocial, violent, and psychopathic individuals: A meta-analysis. *Psychiatry Research: Neuroimaging, 174*(2), 81–88.

Zlotnick, C. (1997). Posttraumatic stress disorder (PTSD), PTSD comorbidity, and childhood abuse among incarcerated women. *The Journal of Nervous and Mental Disease, 185*(12), 761–763.

Zlotnick, C. (1999). Antisocial personality disorder, affect dysregulation and childhood abuse among incarcerated women. *Journal of Personality Disorders, 13*(1), 90–95.

Chapter 10
Psychopathy and Conduct Disorder: Do We Need Additional Specifiers for Adequate Representation?

Andrew P. Bontemps, Blair D. Batky, Beatriz Mendez, and Randall T. Salekin

Abstract Psychopathy is a multicomponent construct that includes interpersonal, affective, lifestyle, and antisocial characteristics (Cleckley, The mask of sanity. Mosby, St. Louis, 1941; Hare, The Hare psychopathy checklist-revised manual. Multi-Health Systems. Tonawanda, New York, 1991). At the child level, there has been a focus on only one component of psychopathy – callous unemotional traits, also referred to as the affective component of psychopathy. However, it has been argued that this focus is too narrow (Salekin, J Child Psychol Psychiatry 58:1180–1200, 2017). The authors of the current chapter review the use of psychopathic traits in the DSM for the diagnosis of CD (and APSD). In addition, the authors review research on the utilization of existing DSM disorders such as ADHD and ODD for the conceptualization of child psychopathy. The authors of this chapter conclude that the field may have inadequate representation of psychopathic personality traits in the DSM for better diagnosing and understanding the various forms of CD. The authors utilize the Proposed Specifiers for Conduct Disorder (PSCD; (Salekin and Hare, Proposed Specifiers for Conduct Disorder (PCSD). Unpublished test, 2016)) as a model to demonstrate how greater representation of psychopathic traits could lead to a better comprehension of CD. The wider conceptualization of child psychopathic traits entails benefits including both a better understanding of the etiology and treatment of youth with various forms of CD.

Keywords Conduct disorder · Psychopathy · PSCD · GM · CU · DI

A. P. Bontemps · B. D. Batky · B. Mendez · R. T. Salekin (✉)
The University of Alabama, Tuscaloosa, AL, USA
e-mail: rsalekin@ua.edu

J. E. Vitale (ed.), *The Complexity of Psychopathy*, Dangerous Behavior in Clinical and Forensic Psychology, https://doi.org/10.1007/978-3-030-83156-1_10

10.1 Introduction

Hervey Cleckley (1941) first described the precursor to modern psychopathic traits in his influential book *The Mask of Sanity.* His rich clinical descriptions drew on his active experience working with an adult inpatient population. Cleckley's ground breaking clinical work led to his seminal list of psychopathic traits, which originally consisted of 21 items (Cleckley, 1941; pp. 338–355). In the second edition of this monograph, Cleckley (1950) narrowed his list to 16 descriptors (pp. 355–356). Subsequent research based on Cleckley's conceptualization subdivided psychopathic traits into categories including interpersonal, affective, lifestyle, and antisocial traits (e.g., Hare, 2003), although Cleckley also alluded to these separate categories. Terminology for the various components of psychopathy has been somewhat dependent on the measurement tool used to assess the traits. For example, the Psychopathy Checklist (PCL-R; Hare, 1991, 2003), one of the first systematic metrics for psychopathy, was originally found to have two factors: Factor 1, which consisted of interpersonal and affective traits (e.g., grandiosity, deceit, low empathy, low guilt, low stress reaction, etc.) and Factor 2, which consisted of impulsive and antisocial traits (e.g., sensation-seeking, risk-taking, social deviance, antisocial behavior) (Harpur et al., 1989).

Later, factor-analytic studies further subdivided the two traditional factors into four distinct facets including interpersonal (facet 1), affective (facet 2), lifestyle (facet 3), and antisocial (facet 4) facets (Hare, 2003). Likewise, researchers have described a multimodal model of psychopathy with the Psychopathic Personality Inventory (PPI; Lilienfeld & Andrews, 1996; Neumann et al., 2008). Specifically, these researchers have shown that the PPI can be subdivided into three trait factors, namely Fearless-Dominance, Self-Centered Impulsivity, and Cold Heartedness. To refer to the categories in a uniform way throughout this chapter, and to be most relevant to the child literature, the model proposed by Salekin (2017) will be used. This model subdivides psychopathic traits into three categories: Grandiose-Manipulative (GM; e.g., manipulation, deceit), Callous Unemotional (CU; e.g., lack of remorse and guilt), and Daring-Impulsive (DI; e.g., risk-taking) traits, plus Conduct Disorder (CD).

Cleckley's work preceded the inception of the first Diagnostic and Statistical Manual of Mental Disorders (DSM-I). Even so, the explicit mention of psychopathy symptoms in diagnostic and statistical manuals has substantially varied. In some diagnostic manuals, there has been a heavy emphasis on personality traits, and in others, there has been an emphasis on behavior. In the most recent diagnostic manuals (e.g., APA, 2000, 2013), the symptoms of psychopathy have tended to be heavily behaviorally-based and incorporated through disorders such as CD and Antisocial Personality Disorder (ASPD). The heavy emphasis on behavioral criteria, as opposed to personality trait criteria, may have occurred for a variety of reasons. First, developers of the diagnostic manuals (i.e., DSM workgroups) may have considered behavioral aspects of psychopathy to best capture the essence (core) of psychopathy (Cloninger, 1978; Robins, 1978; Spitzer et al., 1975). Second, the developers of diagnostic criteria for diagnostic manuals may have viewed the antisocial component of psychopathy to be the most critical component (even if not core) given that it tapped what many believed to be the primary societal concern – antisocial behavior (Robins, 1966). Third, developers of diagnostic criteria for diagnostic manuals may have believed that even if psychopathic personality criteria were not explicitly included in the DSM, other comorbid psychiatric conditions such as ADHD, CD, and ODD, when combined, captured psychopathy and therefore reduced the need for explicit psychopathy criteria (e.g., Lynam, 1996). Although these viewpoints were embraced by some, many researchers believed that the behaviorally-based and comorbidity-based models, alone, omitted many of the important hallmark symptoms of psychopathy.

Recently, the connection between psychopathy, CD, and ASPD has again become more salient due to the addition of the Limited Prosocial Emotions (LPE) specifier to the diagnosis of CD (APA, 2013). The addition of the specifier is believed to capture a subset of youth exhibiting the callous-unemotional component of psychopathy. While considered an advancement in terms of adding psychopathic traits to the nomenclature, Salekin et al. (2018) have questioned whether the inclusion of CU traits alone is sufficient to describe the large variety of youth with conduct problems who are seen in clinics worldwide. Salekin (2017) and colleagues contend that this inclusion of one component of psychopathy offers an incomplete clinical picture and an unsystematic manner with which to incorporate psychopathic traits within the DSM-5 (APA, 2013) and ICD-11 (WHO, 2019). This unsystematic approach raises questions regarding just how psychopathy items should be included in diagnostic and statistical manuals to best help understand CD (and potentially ASPD).

The authors of the current chapter argue that CD and ASPD could benefit from incorporating a more comprehensive psychopathy item set as well as a more systematic manner for the inclusion of psychopathic trait information. The authors suggest that the three dimensions of psychopathy (GM, CU, and DI) outlined in the opening paragraphs may allow for an increasingly clear set of relevant personality characteristics to help describe and explain conduct problems in youth. The authors contend that accounting for the multifaceted nature of psychopathy will be a step forward in reducing the confusion in DSM and ICD manuals and will refine our understanding of the etiology of CD as well as the treatment of youth with CD. Trait-based models will facilitate comprehension of the characterological features that may be driving the behavioral problems. Given this perspective, the authors of the chapter believe that a look back at the DSM's past inclusion of psychopathic traits could be a helpful exercise in examining the comprehensiveness of trait coverage, as well as examining how comorbid conditions may have been used to help explain (understand) psychopathy. The authors further assert that considering the broader inclusion of psychopathic traits and subcomponents could aid in our understanding of the etiology of Conduct Disorder. The authors use a new model for specifying Conduct Disorder, namely the Proposed Specifiers for Conduct Disorder (PSCD), to help the reader contemplate the etiology and eventual treatment of Conduct Disorder. The authors of the chapter believe that closely examining the previously mentioned points of inquiry will help move the field forward with a more optimal and effective use of psychopathic trait criteria to inform CD.

With the aforementioned goals in mind, the aim of this chapter is threefold. First, the authors trace psychopathy's connection to the DSM disorders of CD and ASPD, and the authors evaluate the extent to which the items (and components) of psychopathy are explicitly represented in the successive DSM diagnoses of CD and ASPD. Second, given that some researchers have argued that psychopathy is captured by disorders already present in the DSM (even though they are not termed psychopathy) (Lynam, 1996, 1997; see also Frick, 2021), the authors address whether this conceptualization of comorbid DSM conditions (e.g., ADHD, ODD) is sufficient to forego a more explicit definition of CD and its relationship with psychopathic traits. Finally, the authors discuss the etiology of psychopathy and its connection to CD before drawing specific conclusions regarding how psychopathy's multidimensional nature might be better integrated into the DSM. As mentioned, the authors use the Proposed Specifier for Conduct Disorder scale (Salekin & Hare, 2016) as a framework to discuss how further information on etiology can be garnered by examining the different components of psychopathy in relation to CD. The authors begin with a discussion of how psychopathy has previously been incorporated, in various ways, into successive versions of the DSM.

10.2 Inclusion of Psychopathic Traits and Conduct Problems in the DSM

The DSM, especially after DSM I and DSM II, has typically only included a small to moderate number of psychopathic traits in each successive version of the manual to facilitate the understanding of antisocial characteristics. To provide perspective on this important issue pertaining to item inclusion, the authors examine, through the lens of Cleckley (1941) and Hare (1991), the extent to which various psychopathy items and psychopathy components (i.e., GM, CU, and DI) have been included, and therefore represented, in the DSM over the different versions of the manual. Following this analysis, we draw some brief conclusions pertaining to the manner in which the traits could be more fully incorporated into the formal diagnostic systems.

10.2.1 DSM – I

The first DSM was compiled and distributed in 1952 by the American Psychiatric Association. This first compilation of the manual was an attempt to formalize the classification system of mental disorders in the post-World War II period. Psychopathic traits were incorporated to varying degrees in this earliest version and appear in two separate areas of DSM-I. Disorders with psychopathic traits included the Sociopathic Personality Disorders and the diagnosis of Conduct Disturbance adjustment reaction of childhood. The DSM-I described those with sociopathic personality disturbances (SPDs) as people who have problems conforming "with the prevailing cultural milieu" (APA, 1952, p. 38). Clinicians were advised to first rule-out diagnoses of brain injury and disease, neuroses, or psychoses. The diagnosis of

SPD was from there further divided into three classifications with the Antisocial Reaction class being most relevant to psychopathy. This diagnosis described individuals who were "always in trouble, profiting neither from experience nor punishment," who "demonstrated few or no connections to others," were "emotionally immature or callous," and who "showed little responsibility or judgement" (p. 38). This first version of the DSM had explicit representation of psychopathy, and the representation was equal across the psychopathy components (GM, CU, and DI traits), in addition to including antisocial behavior ("always in trouble").

Conduct Disturbance was an option for diagnosing children, although this diagnosis placed substantially less emphasis on psychopathic traits. Instead, this diagnosis was considered as an adjustment reaction of childhood and was meant to be interpreted as "transient symptomatic reactions of children to some immediate situation or internal emotional conflict" (p. 41). As a result, Conduct Disturbance would have been diagnosed based on antisocial behavior rather than personality traits *per se*.

In sum, there was some representation of psychopathic traits in this first version of the DSM, and the representation was essentially equal across the different dimensions or components of psychopathy, with three (3) GM traits, two (2) CU traits, and two (2) DI traits. Thus, just under half of the Cleckley (1976) items were represented in the adult disorder (this tally includes "always in trouble," which would roughly count under the PSCD CD catgory and maps to Cleckley's item of "inadequately motivated antisocial behavior"). However, none of Cleckley's (1976) or Hare's (1991) criteria were represented in the childhood diagnosis with the exception of the example item of cruelty (see Table 10.1, sections A (adult criteria) and B (child criteria)).

10.2.2 DSM- II

In the second edition of the DSM, psychopathic personality traits were still prevalent. The term Sociopathic Personality Disturbance was no longer used. Instead, the overarching term of Sociopathic Personality Disorders was replaced with Antisocial Personality and was retained under the Personality Disorders section. Those diagnosed with Antisocial Personality were described as being incapable of forming "significant loyalty to other people" and as being "grossly selfish, callous, irresponsible, impulsive, and unable to feel guilt or...learn from experience and punishment" (APA, 1967, p. 43). A new qualifier was added in this version of the DSM requiring that to receive a diagnosis of Antisocial Personality, the individual would need to display more than just "repeated legal or social offenses" (p. 43). This qualifier made it clear that mere antisocial behavior alone was not enough to warrant a diagnosis of Antisocial Personality. Instead, salient personality traits were additionally required for a diagnosis of Antisocial Personality. This stands in stark contrast with the DSM-IV and to some extent the DSM-5 ASPD diagnostic criteria in which the condition can be fully met *without* prominent psychopathic personality traits.

Table 10.1 Level of Use of Psychopathic Traits in the DSM's Antisocial Personality Disorder (APD) and Conduct Disorder (CD) Diagnoses: The Proposed Specifiers for Conduct Disorder (PSCD) scale as a Guide

	PSCD	PSCD	PSCD	PSCD
	GM	CU	DI	CD
Section A **Antisocial Personality Disorder (APD)**				
DSM-I Sociopathic Personality Disturbance (SPD) –Antisocial Reaction	Maintaining no real loyalties to any one person, group, or code Ability to rationalize their behavior so that it appears warranted, reasonable, and justified	Callous Marked emotional immaturity	Hedonistic Lack of judgement Lack of sense of responsibility	Always in trouble
DSM-II Antisocial Personality	Incapable of significant loyalty to individuals, groups, or social values Selfish Blames others or offers plausible rationalizations for their behavior	Callous Unable to feel guilt Unable to learn from experience and punishment	Irresponsible, Impulsive Frustration tolerance low	Not needed ("repeated legal or social offenses is *not* sufficient to justify the diagnosis")
DSM-III Antisocial Personality Disorder (before age 15)	Persistent lying	Lacks remorse	Repeated sexual intercourse in a casual relationship Repeated drunkenness or substance use	Truancy Delinquency Running away from home Vandalism School grades markedly below expectations Chronic violations of rules at home and/or school Initiation of fights

(continued)

Table 10.1 (continued)

	PSCD GM	PSCD CU	PSCD DI	PSCD CD
DSM-III Antisocial Personality Disorder (after age 18)	Disregard for the truth	Lacks remorse	Inability to maintain enduring attachment to a sexual partner Failure to plan ahead, or impulsivity Recklessness	Inability to sustain consistent work behavior Lack of ability to function as a responsible parent Failure to accept social norms with respect to lawful behavior Irritability and aggressiveness: repeated physical fights or assaults; spouse or child beating Failure to honor financial obligations: repeated defaulting on debts, failure to provide child support, failure to support other dependents
DSM-III-R Antisocial Personality Disorder (before 15 years)	Often lied (other than to avoid physical or sexual abuse)			Truant Ran away from home overnight at least twice Initiated physical fights Used a weapon in more than one fight Deliberately destroyed others' property and/or engaged in fire-setting Has stolen with confrontation of a victim Physically cruel to people or animals Forced someone into sexual activity

(continued)

Table 10.1 (continued)

	PSCD GM	PSCD CU	PSCD DI	PSCD CD
DSM-III-R Antisocial Personality Disorder (since age 15)	Repeated lying, use of aliases, or "conning others"	Lacks remorse	Fails to plan ahead, or is impulsive	Is unable to sustain consistent work behavior Fails to conform to social norms with respect to lawful behavior: repeated antisocial acts that are grounds for arrest (e.g., destroying property, harassing others, stealing, pursuing an illegal occupation) Irritable and aggressive Repeatedly fails to honor financial obligations If a parent or guardian one or more of the following: (a) malnutrition of child (b) child's illness resulting from a lack of minimal hygiene (c) failure to obtain medical care for a seriously ill child (d) child's dependence on neighbors or nonresident relatives for food or shelter (e) failure to arrange for a caretaker for young child when parent is away from home Has never sustained monogamous relationship over one year

(continued)

Table 10.1 (continued)

	PSCD GM	PSCD CU	PSCD DI	PSCD CD
DSM-IV, DSM-IV-TR, DSM-5 Antisocial Personality Disorder	Deceitfulness: repeated lying, use of aliases, or conning others for personal profit or pleasure	Lack of remorse	Impulsivity and failure to plan ahead Reckless disregard for safety of self or others	Failure to conform to social norms with respect to lawful behaviors: repeatedly performing acts that are grounds for arrest Irritability and aggressiveness: repeated physical fights or assaults Consistent irresponsibility: repeated failure to sustain consistent work behavior or honor financial obligations
Section B **Conduct Disorder (CD)**				
DSM-I Conduct Disturbance		Cruelty	Use of alcohol	Truancy Stealing Destructiveness Sexual offenses
DSM-II Unsocialized Aggressive Reaction of Childhood (UARC)	Lying [Vengefulness] [Hostile teasing]			Overt/covert hostile disobedience Physical and verbal aggressiveness Destructiveness Temper tantrums Solitary stealing Hostile teasing
DSM-II Group Delinquent Reaction of Childhood (GDRC)				Steal Skip school Stay out late at night Shoplifting Sexual delinquency

(continued)

Table 10.1 (continued)

	PSCD GM	PSCD CU	PSCD DI	PSCD CD
DSM-III Conduct Disorder Aggressive Undersocialized		Failure to establish normal degree of affection, empathy, bond with others		Thefts outside the home involving confrontation with the victim Physical violence against persons or property (vandalism, rape, breaking and entering, etc.)
DSM-III Conduct Disorder Non-Aggressive Undersocialized	Persistent, serious lying Blame externalization Being out for personal gain	Failure to establish normal degree of affection, empathy, bond with others		Violations of a variety of important rules at home or school Repeated running away from home overnight Stealing not confronting a victim
DSM-III-R Conduct Disorder	Often lies			Stolen with/without confrontation of a victim Run away from home overnight Deliberately engaged in fire-setting Truant from school Broken in to someone else's house, building, or car Deliberately destroyed others property Used a weapon in more than one fight Initiates physical fights Physically cruel to people or animals Forced someone into sexual activity with him or her

(continued)

Table 10.1 (continued)

	PSCD	PSCD	PSCD	PSCD
	GM	CU	DI	CD
DSM-IV, DSM-IV-TR, DSM-5	Lies to obtain goods or favors or to avoid obligations	Lack of remorse or guilt (DSM-5 LPE specifier) Callous – Lack of empathy (DSM-5 LPE specifier) Unconcerned about performance (DSM-5 LPE specifier) Shallow or deficient affect (DSM-5 LPE specifier)		Bullies, threatens, or intimidates others Initiates physical fights Used a weapon that can cause serious physical harm to others Stolen with/without confronting a victim Deliberately engaged in fire-setting Deliberately destroyed others' property Broken into someone else's house, building, or car Stays out at night despite parental prohibition Run away from home overnight Physically cruel to people or animals Forced someone into sexual activity Truant

Note. *GM* grandiose manipulative traits, *CU* callous unemotional traits, *DI* Daring impulsive traits, *CD* Conduct Disorder. Some of the items did not fit neatly into one category. For instance, in the DSM-I, the authors of this chapter put the item "cruelty" under CU traits for Conduct Disturbance, but the item could also be considered a GM trait. Similalrly, for the DSM-II, the authors placed "failure to learn from punishment" under CU traits, but this item could also be placed under DI traits. For the DSM-II Conduct disturbance, the authors placed "vengefulness" and "hostile teasing" in brackets under GM, however, technically, they are only indirectly related to Cleckley (1976) or Hare (1991) criteria and thus are not counted as items that map to either scholar.

At the child-level, the two diagnoses could be given including Unsocialized Aggressive Reaction in Childhood (UARC) and Group Delinquent Reaction in Childhood (GDRC). These diagnoses were divided between behavior that originated within the individual (i.e., internally- or personally-motivated antisocial behavior) and behavior that occurred as a result of group membership (i.e., externally-motivated antisocial behavior). The UARC described children who were either overtly or covertly hostile, aggressive, or destructive toward others (APA, 1967). They were also described as disobedient, quarrelsome, vengeful, and destructive. It also specified that the diagnosis should be differentiated from Antisocial

Personality. The GDRC diagnosis described individuals who had joined a "delinquent peer group" (p. 51) and had participated in various antisocial acts with the group, such as stealing or truancy (APA, 1967).

In sum, as in DSM-I, the DSM-II explicitly mentioned psychopathic personality traits for the adult condition and showed roughly equal dispersion of psychopathic traits with two (2) GM traits, two (2) CU traits, and three (3) DI traits —roughly half of Cleckley's criteria. Notably, as reported, the DSM-II makes the point that antisocial behavior is not sufficient on its own for a diagnosis of Antisocial Personality. Some hallmark psychopathic traits were needed for the diagnosis. As with DSM-I, few psychopathic personality traits were included in the childhood disorder of Unsocialized Aggressive Reaction of Childhood (UARC) or Group Delinquent Reaction of Childhood (GDRC). However, UARC did include lying, hostile teasing of other children, and vengefulness that might be considered GM traits, but lying is the only GM trait that connects directly with Cleckley (1976) and Hare (2003) (see Table 10.1, sections A and B).

10.2.3 DSM–III and DSM–III–R

In the DSM-III (APA, 1980), *Conduct Disorder* was formally introduced, replacing the term conduct disturbance. Compared to earlier editions, the DSM-III and DSM-III-R (APA, 1987) diagnoses for ASPD and CD became more specific in their descriptions of the symptoms of each disorder, as well as the number of symptoms required for individuals to receive a diagnosis. ASPD required 3 of 15 symptoms to meet diagnostic criteria for this disorder. Included among these 15 symptoms were three explicit psychopathic traits including, "lying," "inability for enduring attachment to others," and "inability to sustain consistent work." At the same time, the DSM-III dropped some of the previously required psychopathic trait-level items included in the DSM-II diagnosis (i.e., "lack of remorse," "callousness," or "inability to learn from punishment") (APA, 1980). However, the DSM-III-R reintroduced one of the previous cornerstones of psychopathy from the DSM, namely "lack of remorse."

With regard to CD, the DSM-III and DSM-III-R differed substantially in their recognition of a larger number of explicit psychopathic personality traits. The DSM-III featured a number of psychopathic traits, including interpersonal or affective traits for CD criteria (APA, 1980, 1987). This may be surprising as some consider the DSM-5's addition of LPE to CD to be the first time this inclusion of psychopathic traits has occurred, but we see in the DSM-III that psychopathic traits were included for CD. In the DSM-III, four types of CD were specified. Children with CD were differentiated between those who had the capability to form social ties (i.e. socialized types) and those who did not (i.e. undersocialized types; APA, 1980). Children with the undersocialized type were described as failing to develop normal "affection, empathy, or bond[s]" (APA, 1980, p. 48) with others, regardless of the social groups to which the individual belonged. The socialized type, by comparison, could form social ties and experience empathy but rarely did so outside of their preferred group. Aggressive and nonaggressive types were also differentiated based on the presence or absence of physical violence against others (APA, 1980). "Lying" was retained as a key symptom but only in the undersocialized- and socialized- nonaggressive categories. It was not included in the socialized-and undersocialized- aggressive categories.

In the DSM-III-R, the diagnosis of CD was simplified from four types to one syndrome. Although generally considered one category, CD could be further specified. For instance, DSM-III-R CD could be specified as mild, moderate, and severe, as well as with three "types" that included group, solitary, and undifferentiated (APA, 1987). Both versions included "lying" as a criterion, but in the DSM-III-R, lying was included in the broader set of thirteen items. The DSM-III-R, however, removed emotional callousness symptoms, such as "failure to establish a normal degree of affection, empathy, or bond with others" (APA, 1987, p. 48), thereby removing a large portion of affective psychopathic traits (similar to CU traits). Thus, under the DSM-III, individuals were likely able to be assessed for elevated affective psychopathic traits, whereas this was not the case with the DSM-III-R. Both versions did include a sole GM trait, namely "lying." There were few DI traits in the DSM-III or DSM-III-R, although some characteristics could be indicative of daring traits, such as "fire-setting" and "running away."

Taken together, the DSM-III included several psychopathic personality traits in its criteria for ASPD, including "irresponsibility," "inability to form enduring attachment," and "lying." This DSM-III version therefore offers some representation of psychopathic traits, but the vast majority of items for a diagnosis of ASPD appear to be behavioral. The DSM-III-R retained the items of "irresponsibility," "inability to form enduring attachment," and "lying," and added "lack of remorse." Thus, the representation of psychopathy is considered low with one (1) GM trait, one or two (1–2) CU traits, and one (1) DI trait. However, as previously mentioned, the remaining behavioral items are generally related to irresponsibility (e.g., "poor parental practices").

With regard to CD in childhood, the DSM-III actually contained quite a few GM and CU traits. This version included "lying," "blame externalization," and "being out for personal gain" (3 GM traits). Also, the section on "failure to establish a normal degree of affection, empathy, or bond with others" included an additional three (3) CU items, such as "lack of remorse/guilt," "unconcern for others," and "short, limited friendships" (APA, 1987). Thus, childhood disorders in this version of the DSM had substantial psychopathic personality trait representation, although some of the terminology (undersocialized and socialized) was confusing. Furthermore, clinicians had to consider some of the criteria that reflected pathological characteristics, such as "lying," in combination with those that reflected positive characteristics (to be reversed), such as "feels guilt" and "extends him/herself to others when nothing to gain," which also generated some confusion. Nonetheless, this version of the DSM included roughly 4 of the 16 Cleckley criteria at the adult level, and 7 of the 16 criteria at the child level (see Table 10.1 sections A and B).

10.2.4 DSM–IV and DSM–IV–TR

The DSM-IV and DSM-IV-TR reincorporated several of the core psychopathic personality traits listed by Cleckley and explicitly noted that ASPD is akin to psychopathy. The diagnosis also maintained ASPD's direct connection to CD as evidenced by the criterion that there must be signs of CD prior to age 15 (APA, 1994). With regard to the traits closely tied to those of Cleckley's (1964) prototypical psychopath, the DSM-IV continued to include "lying," "lack of remorse," "impulsivity," and "irresponsibility," in addition to the previously included symptoms of aggressiveness and law-breaking (APA, 1994). Thus, there was representation of all three components of psychopathy, plus antisocial conduct. However, as the current diagnosis only requires three of seven criteria, an individual might qualify for the diagnosis of ASPD without exhibiting any of the individual psychopathic traits. Research has shown that this can, and does, lead to confusion when attempting to measure and disentangle what many argue are different personality-based syndromes (e.g. Crego & Widiger, 2015; Hare, 1996; Lilienfeld, 1994; Rogers, 1995). Furthermore, the description for ASPD in the DSM-5 states that ASPD has been previously called psychopathy, which, according to some, may inappropriately equate the two conditions (APA, 2013; see also Ogloff, 2006).

For CD, between DSM-III-R and DSM-IV, the specifier for solitary or group type was eliminated in favor of a specifier asking the clinician to note whether the individual's behavior began during childhood or adolescence. The DSM-IV grouped the CD symptoms into categories including "Aggression to people and animals," "Destruction of property," "Deceitfulness or theft," and "Serious violations of rules" (APA, 1994). The diagnosis of CD also required that the behavior caused clinically significant impairment (APA, 1994). Although the diagnoses of CD and ASPD remained linked through their criteria, the diagnosis of CD did not follow the changes made to the diagnosis of ASPD regarding the inclusion of personality traits in addition to observable behavior (APA, 1994). Rather, the criteria for CD in DSM-IV were more behaviorally- based relative to those in DSM-III and DSM-III-R (APA, 1980, 1987, 1994).

In sum, the DSM-IV and DSM-IV-TR diagnoses included several psychopathic personality traits but also remained highly behavioral. At the adult level, there was representation of several psychopathic personality traits, including one (1) GM trait (deceitfulness), one (1) CU trait (lack of remorse), and three (3) DI traits (reckless disregard, impulsivity, and irresponsible). For individuals diagnosed with CD, the characteristics were predominantly behavioral, with psychopathic traits limited to a single GM trait (i.e., lying). Thus, it might be expected for individuals with CD to have elevated scores in GM traits due to potential lying and manipulation of others, but explicit CU and DI traits were not included in DSM-IV (APA, 1994). Considering only three out of fifteen of the CD criteria need to be met to receive a diagnosis of CD, many individuals with a diagnosis of CD may not exhibit any psychopathic traits at all (APA, 1994). Overall, the explicit representation of psychopathic traits in this version of the DSM was low at the adult level (3/16 traits), and extremely low at the child level (1/16 traits) (see Table 10.1, sections A and B).

10.2.5 DSM-5

The most recent DSM, the DSM-5 (APA, 2013), included several psychopathic personality traits for a diagnosis of ASPD. These included "deceitfulness," "lack of remorse," "reckless disregard," "impulsivity," and "irresponsibility." While the Section II criteria for ASPD largely did not change between DSM-IV-TR and DSM-5, Section III of the DSM-5 included additional psychopathic traits for ASPD. In addition, the DSM-5 brought back some of the affective traits for CD that were evident in the DSM-III. Specifically, affective traits were reintroduced to the diagnosis of CD in the form of the limited prosocial emotion (LPE) specifier (APA, 2013). With the specifier, clinicians were asked to determine whether an individual has shown a pattern of at least two of four characteristics over a period of 12 months: lack of remorse or guilt, callous lack of empathy, unconcerned about performance, and shallow or deficient affect (APA, 2013). By adding personality traits, the CD diagnosis more closely relates to the ASPD criteria of lack of remorse and consistent irresponsibility (APA, 1994). Although the addition of the LPE specifier likely represents an advancement in specifying CD subtypes, it only brings an element of the original Cleckley (1964) psychopathic personality to the diagnosis of CD, and, as we have noted previously, much more could be done to further specify CD (Salekin et al., 2018).

In sum, the adult diagnosis of ASPD includes "deceitfulness" (lying), "lack of remorse," "impulsivity," "recklessness" and "irresponsibility," as well as "antisocial conduct." Therefore, there is some representation of the psychopathic personality items for each component of psychopathy with one (1) GM item, one (1) CU item, and three (3) DI items. These items reflect certain Cleckley (1964) criteria, such as "lack of remorse and shame" and "general poverty in major affective reactions." At the child level, the addition of the LPE specifier allows for the inclusion of additional CU traits, which brings CD closer to adult ASPD. However, as previously noted, the representation at the adult level is low, and the current definition of CD does not adequately represent GM and DI traits (see Table 10.1, sections A and B).

10.2.6 Summary and Integration

The various versions of the DSM, while inclusive of psychopathic traits through the diagnostic criteria associated with ASPD and CD, have yet to develop systematic models that allow for the wider inclusion of psychopathic traits and their relation to antisocial behavior and conduct problems. Perhaps the best attempt to include a wide representation of psychopathic traits was the DSM-III CD criteria set (i.e., aggressive vs. nonaggressive and socialized vs. unsocialized; APA, 1980). This version of CD included GM traits, CU traits, and DI traits. However, the terminology was confusing, and the hallmark symptom of "lying" was only included in the nonaggressive subtypes and could not be utilized with the aggressive subtypes. The DSM-5 also includes a larger number of psychopathic personality traits for both ASPD and CD although the various psychopathy components are not equally represented (APA, 2013). Moreover, the relevance of some of the DSM-5 LPE specifier items have been questioned (Lahey, 2014). This section, which provided a look back at the previous DSMs, makes clear that the wider conceptualization of psychopathic traits to specify CD and ASPD has not been met. We argue that the partial inclusion of psychopathic personality traits may lead to problems with diagnosis, developing accurate etiological models, and creating efficacious treatment programs (Lahey, 2014; Salekin, 2017).

10.3 Psychopathy and DSM Comorbidity: Is there a Need for the Addition of Psychopathy Criteria if we already have ADHD, CD, and ODD?

An argument for excluding psychopathy criteria sets in the DSM has been the proposition that psychopathy is already captured by existing DSM conditions such as ADHD, CD, and ODD. That is, each condition, or a combination of the conditions, *is* psychopathy, even though the conditions are not termed psychopathy (Lynam, 1996, 1997; Smith & Hung, 2012; see Frick, 2021 for updated version of the argument). In this section, we cover several arguments pertaining to the manner in which DSM "comorbidity" has been considered to account for or conceptualize psychopathy. Specifically, we examine the comorbid subtype position (i.e., "fledgling psychopath" hypothesis), the ADHD mediation model, and the CD mediation model. In addition, some scholars hold the belief that other DSM disorders (or features of disorders) such as Oppositional Defiant Disorder (ODD) in combination with CD might also sufficiently explain psychopathy. We cover these proposed comorbidity models below and discuss whether they offer a compelling rationale for foregoing or limiting the inclusion of explicit psychopathic trait criteria in the DSM and ICD diagnostic manuals.

10.3.1 Fledgling Psychopath Model

Lynam (1996, 1997) previously argued that psychopathy is likely already captured in the DSM by the diagnoses of ADHD and CD. In his seminal paper, which referred to the "fledgling psychopath," Lynam (1996) highlighted how childhood psychopathy can be understood in terms of existing DSM disorders (e.g., ADHD, CD; Lynam, 1996). In his work examining the development of psychopathy, Lynam (1996, 1997) described the construct of the fledgling psychopath as encompassing youth who are high in conduct problems, inattention, hyperactivity, and impulsivity (Sevecke & Kosson, 2010; Smith & Hung, 2012). In line with the central thesis of the fledgling psychopath construct, subsequent work has found that higher rates of psychopathic traits tend to emerge in youth exhibiting both ADHD and CD symptoms (e.g., Barry et al., 2000; DeLisi et al., 2014). Retrospective research with psychopathic adults further supports the construct, with offenders in one study endorsing significant difficulties with attention, hyperactivity, impulsivity, and conduct problems during childhood relative to their non-psychopathic counterparts (Johansson et al., 2005). Other work, however, has yielded inconsistent findings, showing that ADHD symptoms are only implicated in psychopathy through their association with conduct problems (Abramowitz et al., 2004; Colledge & Blair, 2001; Hoong et al., 2006; Sevecke et al., 2009). This suggests that the role of ADHD in psychopathy may be fully explained by ADHD's comorbidity with CD.

Component-level analyses have been comparatively more mixed (Becker et al., 2013; Michonski & Sharp, 2010). For example, Becker et al. (2013) found that conduct problems and ADHD symptoms did not interact to predict GM traits, although results revealed a marginal interaction of conduct problems and ADHD symptoms in predicting CU traits. By contrast, Michonski and Sharp (2010) did not find evidence of such relationships. In sum, there is a lack of consistent evidence regarding the fledgling psychopath hypothesis, calling into question the impact of features like inattention and hyperactivity relative to conduct problems in the development of psychopathy (Smith & Hung, 2012). Of note, it has further been argued that the fledgling psychopath model of childhood psychopathy places much less emphasis on GM (i.e., interpersonal) and CU (i.e., affective) traits in favor of a focus on DI traits (i.e., impulsivity) (Pardini & Loeber, 2007), despite the former components being integral to the psychopathy construct.

10.3.2 Conduct Problem Mediation Model

A second model for understanding comorbidity in relation to psychopathy has been referred to as "conduct problem-mediation." This model proposes that it is conduct problems alone that have an influence on psychopathy. In this model, ADHD's link to psychopathy and criminality is based on hyperactive children's increased risk to manifest conduct problems, which in turn puts them at risk for the development of psychopathic traits and serious antisocial behavior (Smith & Hung, 2012). Nevertheless, it should be noted that even youth *without* ADHD who end up with conduct problems could also be on a path to eventual psychopathy. Earlier work has provided some support for conduct problems independently contributing to the emergence of psychopathic traits (Babinski et al., 1999; Taylor et al., 1996). This conduct problem mediation model may also stem from the work of Robins (1966), who suggested that behavioral traits of "sociopathy" more reliably assess psychopathic personality. However, the asymmetric relations between psychopathy, ASPD and CD indicate that not all children with CD have co-occurring psychopathic traits. There has been little research at the component level to support the conduct problem mediation hypothesis.

10.3.3 ADHD Mediation Model

A third proposal is the ADHD mediation model, where theorists argue that the symptoms of ADHD contribute to the development of psychopathy and serious antisocial behavior. Proponents of this model suggest that ADHD can operate as an individual risk factor for the development of psychopathy (Smith & Hung, 2012). In part, this hypothesis stems from behavioral genetics research and the notion that the mechanisms of ADHD ("always on the go – like a motor") may lead to psychopathy via sensation-seeking. There is some support for ADHD contributing separately to the development of psychopathic traits and/or serious offending long associated with psychopathy (Babinski et al., 1999; Taylor et al., 1996). However, other research has supplied only limited support for the ADHD mediation model. Some work has primarily identified a relationship between ADHD and DI traits or ADHD and conduct problems (Colledge & Blair, 2001; Frick et al., 2000; Mathias et al., 2007; Piatigorsky & Hinshaw, 2004; Salekin, 2017).

At the component level, research has suggested that the connection between ADHD and psychopathy may be dependent on the type of ADHD (e.g., Hyperactive v. Inattentive) as well as potentially the component of psychopathy being investigated. For instance, Daring Impulsive (DI) traits may be particularly relevant (Smith & Hung, 2012), although, even research using finer distinctions is not well replicated nor compelling (e.g. Colledge & Blair, 2001; Frick et al., 2000; Haas et al., 2011; Mathias et al., 2007; Nigg, 2006). Thus, the evidence is limited for this ADHD mediation model hypothesis for explaining psychopthy.

Nonetheless, the literature demonstrates that the disorders of ADHD and CD do tend to co-occur to some extent (Angold et al., 1999; Barkley, 2006; Bendiksen et al., 2017; Biederman et al., 1991; Connor et al., 2010; Di Trani et al., 2013; Faraone et al., 1998; Fowler et al., 2009; Jensen & Steinhausen, 2015; Kosson et al., 2002; Rowe et al., 2002; Rowe et al., 2010a, b; Willcutt et al., 2012). Moreover, children with comorbid conditions can exhibit more problems than children with a single psychiatric condition (DeLisi et al., 2011; Kaplan & Cornell, 2004; Loeber et al., 1995; Lynam, 1996; Odgers et al., 2008; Piatigorsky & Hinshaw, 2004; Sevecke & Kosson, 2010). With that being said, comorbidity between ADHD and CD with psychopathic traits may largely stem from the overlap between the impulsivity dimension of psychopathy and the Hyperactivity/Impulsivity component of ADHD, indicating that impulsivity and/or conduct problems may drive their relationship.

10.3.4 ODD Temperament Model

A fourth model is the ODD temperament model, whereby the temperament of psychopathy is already captured within the DSM through the ODD diagnosis. Early stepping-stone models considered ODD to be a lead in to CD, and subsequently to ASPD (Loeber, 1991). Loeber (1991) outlined a three-pathway model for explaining serious juvenile delinquency. This model delineated the pathways of conflict with authority, overt antisocial behavior, and covert antisocial behavior. Authority conflict, or oppositionality, was the first problem on the pathway to subsequent difficulties including conduct problems and the eventual development of ASPD. Similarly, Lahey and Waldman (2012) claimed that oppositionality might constitute a temperament-based risk factor for CD and later serious delinquency. Specifically, they believed that three temperaments (one being "oppositionality") combined to explain the most serious forms of juvenile delinquency and potentially psychopathy. While these ODD temperament models have mostly been applied to help explain serious juvenile offending, some have been more specifically connected to psychopathy.

Stringaris and Goodman (2009), as well as Burke (2009), showed that ODD could be divided into three dimensions including "irritable" (e.g. angry, resentful), "headstrong" (e.g. blame-externalization, argumentative), and "hurtful" (e.g. spitefulness) facets (Burke, 2009; Burke et al., 2014; Lavigne et al., 2015; Stringaris & Goodman, 2009). Cross-sectional and longitudinal studies have demonstrated that the irritability facet of ODD yielded a strong relationship with internalizing symptoms associated with anxiety and depression, but not with CD (Barker & Salekin, 2012; Burke et al., 2010; Stringaris et al., 2009; Stringaris & Goodman, 2009). By contrast, the headstrong factor has been related to mild CD but not severe CD. Notably, the spiteful dimension has been linked to more severe CD and even psychopathic traits (Stringaris & Goodman, 2009), suggesting that the dimensions of ODD may co-occur with different forms of psychopathology (see also Burke, 2012; Ezpeleta, et al., 2012; Rowe et al., 2010a, b; Stringaris et al., 2012; Whelan et al., 2013). While the ODD temperament line of study is interesting, the component that is most relevant to psychopathy appears to be a single item (hurtful or spiteful) and subsequent research has increasingly shown that this "dimension" more often than not folds into the headstrong (oppositional) dimension.

Notably, the DSM-III did not conceptualize youth with ODD as developing later antisocial personality. Instead, youth with ODD were expected to develop passive-aggressive personality disorder in adulthood, with the DSM-III stating that "some children with Oppositional Disorder as adults may have a disorder meeting the criteria for Passive Aggressive Personality Disorder" (APA, 1980, p. 305). It is not clear what role ODD will have in our understanding of psychopathy in the long-term, as it was originally intended to be a downward extension of Passive-Aggressive Personality Disorder, a diagnosis excluded from the current edition of the DSM. The work of Stringaris and Goodman (2009) and Burke et al. (2010) suggests only one item might be related specifically to the concept of psychopathy. These single items may be worth further investigation, although we believe, given the low level of item coverage, they are unlikely to prove a sufficient measure of psychopathy. ODD in childhood may simply extend to ODD-like symptoms in adulthood.

10.3.5 Summary and Integration

Existing DSM disorders have be hypothesized to explain (capture) psychopathy. However, these indirect methods are likely to be less effective than straightforwardly targeting the symptoms of psychopathy and anchoring those symptoms to the conceptualizations of Cleckley (1976) and Hare (2003). The fledgling psychopath hypothesis, although compelling, has not been well supported by subsequent research especially when accounting for GM and CU traits. This also appears to be the case for the conduct problem and the ADHD mediation models. While examining the comorbidity of CD and psychopathy allows for greater understanding of the interconnections between the conditions, there are also conceptual reasons to surmise that ADHD, ODD, and CD on their own do not comprise the totality of the symptoms of psychopathy, nor do they accurately predict the condition. Given the lack of evidence that these comorbid disorders capture, or designate, psychopathy, we contend that more fully representing relevant psychopathy symptoms will improve the overall precision in the DSM and ICD diagnoses of CD. Moreover, their inclusion will facilitate our understanding of the etiology and treatment of the condition. With this in mind, we turn to etiological models for psychopathy and CD.

10.4 Psychopathic Traits and the Etiology of Conduct Disorder

Psychopathy is a broad construct underpinned by multiple dimensions along with conduct problems (Salekin, 2017). Quay (1965) developed one of the first etiological theories regarding psychopathy, basing its development on a low-arousal model. Effectively, Quay (1965) argued that underlying psychopathy manifested in sensation-seeking (i.e., modern DI traits), leading to what were subsequently described as the behavioral characteristics of psychopathy. He later adapted this model to include environmental impacts as they pertain to the ways in which psychopathy's expression may be influenced by factors such as parenting practices (Quay, 1965, 1972). This model, as noted, might be akin to explaining psychopathy through a sensation-seeking model for youth who have a high level of behavioral activity. As research has increasingly turned from sensation-seeking-based explanations to examining affective traits in youth (CU traits), researchers have attempted to explain the etiology of psychopathy via primarily affective models.

Specifically, Frick and colleagues (Frick & Viding, 2009; Frick & White, 2008) adopted Lykken's (1957) low-fear model and have argued that children high in CU traits appear to have lower temperamental fear and lower emotional reactivity, particularly to negative emotional stimuli. Lykken (1957) suggested that those higher in psychopathic traits generally experience reduced anxiety and it was also believed that children might experience lower levels of anxiety. Later research has indicated that abnormally low levels of certain emotional experiences such as guilt, empathy, and fear may lead to antisocial behavior. Individuals higher in psychopathic traits may not learn to inhibit antisocial acts since they may not feel emotional distress from engaging in these behaviors (e.g. Frick & Viding, 2009; Frick & White, 2008). This model has been used to suggest that those with psychopathic traits appear to be less sensitive to punishment, further preventing these children from developing prosocial empathy and guilt. Finally, research suggests that CU traits have a strong genetic component, and environmental influences such as parenting styles may not be as influential in the development of CU traits (Frick, 2012). However, this model also represents a somewhat narrow view of the etiology for psychopathy as it overlooks other trait dimensions central to the construct.

Thus, despite some important theoretical efforts to determine the etiology of psychopathy, we contend that it might be more informative to consider the multifaceted nature of psychopathy and potentially manifold etiological mechanisms. Such an approach for understanding the etiology of psychopathy necessitates examining in detail the broader construct of psychopathy as well as its underpinning dimensions. In our view, this methodology would glean additional critical information regarding the processes of psychopathy. As proposed in Salekin (2017), we suggest that this should be done by using measures with a wide representation of psychopathic traits and their relation to Conduct Disorder. In this regard, Salekin and Hare (2016) developed the Proposed Specifiers for Conduct Disorder (PSCD) to advance research on the causal mechanisms of psychopathy. As previously noted, the PSCD has four subsets of items that can be used to investigate the graded nature of psychopathy and CD and the distinct correlates that are related to each dimension (López Romero et al., 2019; Luo et al., 2020). In Table 10.2, we provide the items for the PSCD which has now been validated in several studies (e.g., López Romero et al., 2019; Luo et al., 2020; Muratori et al., 2021; Ribeiro da Silva et al, 2022).

Overall, there has been increasing interest in determining whether psychopathic traits *beyond* CU traits may be informative in understanding etiological pathways to CD or in designating subtypes of the disorder (e.g. Frogner et al., 2018; Salekin, 2016; Salekin, et al. 2018). Increasing evidence suggests that other dimensions (e.g. GM and DI traits) may be valuable in understanding CD and potentially even designating subtypes. For instance, there is evidence that children who display elevated CU traits as well as psychopathic traits involving deceitfulness, grandiosity, and sensation-seeking (i.e. GM and DI traits) have more severe and persistent conduct problems than children displaying high levels of CU traits alone (e.g., Frogner et al., 2018). A combination of varied psychopathic traits rather than CU traits alone may therefore help to account for the etiology, maintenance, and severity of conduct problems over time. Additionally, using the multidimensional psychopathy construct may allow for more stable prediction of CD severity compared to using just CU traits (e.g., Colins et al., 2018).

Other studies suggest that considering the interactions between different psychopathy subdimensions is also important for understanding conduct problems (Fanti et al., 2018; Somma et al., 2018). In particular, grandiosity and narcissism may be especially useful to examine in conjunction with CU traits. Indeed, GM traits appear to predict problematic behavior among youth independently of CU traits (Jezior et al., 2016). This research suggests that youth high in GM traits may engage in aggressive behavior in order to defend positive self-views and may be more willing to exploit others for personal gain (Washburn et al., 2004). Moreover, some studies indicate that GM and CU traits appear to act synergistically to lead to higher levels of conduct problems (Fanti et al., 2018; Somma et al., 2018). Fanti et al. (2018) found that the association between CU traits and conduct problems was significantly stronger when high levels of GM traits were also present. Youth high in CU traits alone may have little motivation to engage in prosocial behavior, but youth who are high in GM and CU traits may be particularly motivated to engage in

Table 10.2 The Proposed Specifiers for Conduct Disorder (PSCD; Salekin & Hare, 2016)

GM traits	CU traits	DI traits	CD traits
I can turn on the charm in any situation	I don't waste time thinking about how I may have hurt others	I am daring	I have stolen things
I am a very important person	I can turn and walk away from someone who is hurt	I like a lot of change and/or adventure	I have engaged in physical aggression against animals or people
I am very good at most things I do	When people are happy or upset I don't seem to care	I get a thrill out of doing risky things	I have destroyed property
Lying is easy for me	I like it when others are afraid of me	I feel like I need a lot of stimulation	I break (violate) a lot of rules
I take advantage of others	Some people consider me to be a mean person	I like to live in the moment	I started breaking rules before the age of 10
I am a natural story teller	I rarely feel guilt or remorse	Some people think I am reckless	I can be argumentative and defiant (ODD)

Note. There are 2 items included on the PSCD that can be optionally tallied for the CD scale. These include the early starter specifier ("I started breaking rules before the age of 10") and one ODD item ("I can be argumentative and defiant")

antisocial acts to advance their own self-interest while disregarding others' needs (Fanti et al., 2018). Fanti et al. (2018) demonstrated that youth who are elevated on GM traits, CU traits, and DI traits appear to be the most problematic, and adding disinhibition to a combination of high GM and high CU traits seems to further exacerbate conduct problems (Fanti et al., 2018). GM and DI also appear to combine to predict worse outcomes in some studies, even though impulsivity is a consistent risk factor for conduct problems throughout adolescence (e.g., Mann et al., 2018). Further research on the broader construct of psychopathy in youth may be helpful in discerning the specific etiological processes that underlie each subdimension and whether additional specifiers of CD should be considered to account for the unique variance explained by GM and DI traits (Frogner, et al., 2018). Additional studies are emerging to suggest that psychopathy dimensions add value to our understanding of CD (see Breaux et al., 2019).

Finally, what the LPE specifier adds to the diagnosis of CD has been debated in the literature (e.g., Colins et al., 2020; Déry et al., 2019; Edens et al., 2017; Frick & Myers, 2017; Lahey, 2014; Salekin et al., 2018). As noted above, there have been studies suggesting that the LPE specifier in the DSM-5 designates a more severe and psychopathic presentation of CD (Pardini et al., 2012; Pechorro et al., 2015). However, there are also arguments that the LPE specifier may not designate a stable subgroup of individuals with CD and that children high and low in CU traits may not have significantly different behavioral outcomes (Lahey, 2014; Sakai et al., 2016). More specifically, Lahey (2014) argues that more research is needed on the diagnostic validity and utility of CU traits and on whether using a more parsimonious construct, such as CD severity, would be more useful in designating subtypes. Also, Sakai et al. (2016) demonstrated that the specifier was highly unreliable and did not designate the worst CD cases (see also Déry et al., 2019). More research on the LPE specifier may be warranted, to determine if item content could be improved

(Colins et al., 2020; Edens et al., 2017). Lahey (2014) reviewed work demonstrating that there is heterogeneity within CU traits themselves and that unemotionality has a relatively low correlation with being callous or uncaring. In light of these findings, assessment content and method for CU may require further study and potential refinement. Fortunately, research is starting to examine psychopathy content, and to test models incorporating broader psychopathy against single componenet models.

10.5 Conclusion

Historically, psychopathic traits have been connected to DSM CD and APSD diagnoses. However, this connection has often lacked clarity, coherence, and completeness, including in the most recent DSM-5 (APA, 2013). This chapter reviewed the diagnoses for CD and ASPD across versions of the DSM to better comprehend the extent to which psychopathic traits have been included as DSM criteria. In sum, there have been shifts in the extent to which psychopathic personality traits have been incorporated into diagnostic statistical manuals' criteria for disorders marked by antisocial behavior. The authors contend that the psychopathy dimensions of GM, CU, and DI may be particularly useful in better understanding the CD condition. It is unlikely that comorbid conditions (i.e., ADHD and ODD) will adequately explain the full spectrum of psychopathic personality traits on their own. Instead, utilizing comorbid conditions could lead to misdiagnoses, misprediction, and generally further blur the clinical picture. Considering the wider psychopathic condition and its subdimensions will be necessary to fully understand the etiological pathways to CD. The authors of the present chapter suggest that the three dimensions of psychopathy might clarify some of these difficulties with respect to specifying CD and perhaps ASPD, allowing for an increasingly clear and broad set of psychopathic traits to play a role in explaining conduct problems in youth. The authors believe accounting for the multifaceted psychopathy construct would be a step forward in refining our understanding of the etiology as well as the treatment of youth with CD across the globe.

References

Abramowitz, C. S., Kosson, D. S., & Seidenberg, M. (2004). The relationship between childhood attention deficit hyperactivity disorder and conduct problems and adult psychopathy in male inmates. *Personality and Individual Differences, 36*(5), 1031–1047.

American Psychiatric Association. (1952). *Diagnostic and statistical manual of mental disorders*. Author.

American Psychiatric Association. (1967). *Diagnostic and statistical manual of mental disorders* (2nd ed.). Author.

American Psychiatric Association. (1980). *Diagnostic and statistical manual of mental disorders* (3rd ed.). Author.

American Psychiatric Association. (1987). *Diagnostic and statistical manual of mental disorders* (3rd ed., rev.). Author.

American Psychiatric Association. (1994). *Diagnostic and statistical manual of mental disorders* (4th ed., text rev.). Author.

American Psychiatric Association. (2000). *Diagnostic and statistical manual of mental disorders: DSM-IV-TR*. Washington, DC: Author.

American Psychiatric Association. (2013). *Diagnostic and statistical manual of mental disorders* (5th ed.). Author.

Angold, A., Costello, E. J., & Erkanli, A. (1999). Comorbidity. *The Journal of Child Psychology and Psychiatry and Allied Disciplines, 40*(1), 57–87.

Babinski, L. M., Hartsough, C. S., & Lambert, N. M. (1999). Childhood conduct problems, hyperactivity-impulsivity, and inattention as predictors of adult criminal activity. *The Journal of Child Psychology and Psychiatry and Allied Disciplines, 40*(3), 347–355.

Barker, E. D., & Salekin, R. T. (2012). Irritable oppositional defiance and callous unemotional traits: Is the association partially explained by peer victimization? *Journal of Child Psychology and Psychiatry, 53*(11), 1167–1175.

Barkley, R. A. (2006). *Attention-deficit hyperactivity disorder: A handbook for diagnosis and treatment* (3rd ed.). Guilford.

Barry, C. T., Frick, P. J., DeShazo, T. M., McCoy, M., Ellis, M., & Loney, B. R. (2000). The importance of callous–unemotional traits for extending the concept of psychopathy to children. *Journal of Abnormal Psychology, 109*(2), 335–340.

Becker, S. P., Luebbe, A. M., Fite, P. J., Greening, L., & Stoppelbein, L. (2013). Oppositional defiant disorder symptoms in relation to psychopathic traits and aggression among psychiatrically hospitalized children: ADHD symptoms as a potential moderator. *Aggressive Behavior, 39*(3), 201–211.

Bendiksen, B., Svensson, E., Aase, H., Reichborn-Kjennerud, T., Friis, S., Myhre, A. M., & Zeiner, P. (2017). Co-occurrence of ODD and CD in preschool children with symptoms of ADHD. *Journal of Attention Disorders, 21*(9), 741–752.

Biederman, J., Newcorn, J., & Sprich, S. (1991). Comorbidity of attention deficit hyperactivity disorder. *American Journal of Psychiatry, 148*(5), 564–577.

Breaux, R., Babinski, D. E., Willoughby, M. T., Haas, S. M., Coles, E. K., Pelham, W. E., ... Waschbusch, D. A. (2019). Examining psychopathic traits in children using the child psychopathy scale–revised. *Journal of Abnormal Child Psychology*, 1–13.

Burke, J. D. (2009). The relationship between conduct disorder and oppositional defiant disorder and their continuity with antisocial behaviors: Evidence from longitudinal clinical studies. In *Externalizing disorders of childhood: Refining the research agenda for DSM-V*. American Psychiatric Association.

Burke, J. D. (2012). An affective dimension within oppositional defiant disorder symptoms among boys: Personality and psychopathology outcomes into early adulthood. *Journal of Child Psychology and Psychiatry, 53*(11), 1176–1183.

Burke, J. D., Hipwell, A. E., & Loeber, R. (2010). Dimensions of oppositional defiant disorder as predictors of depression and conduct disorder in preadolescent girls. *Journal of the American Academy of Child & Adolescent Psychiatry, 49*(5), 484–492.

Burke, J. D., Boylan, K., Rowe, R., Duku, E., Stepp, S. D., Hipwell, A. E., & Waldman, I. D. (2014). Identifying the irritability dimension of ODD: Application of a modified bifactor model across five large community samples of children. *Journal of Abnormal Psychology, 123*(4), 841.

Cleckley, H. (1941). *The mask of sanity: An attempt to reinterpret the so-called psychopathic personality*. Mosby.

Cleckley, H. (1950). *The mask of sanity An attempt to clarify some issues about the so-called psychopathic personality* (2nd ed.). Mosby.

Cleckley, H. (1964). *The mask of sanity: An attempt to clarify some issues about the so-called psychopathic personality*. Ravenio Books.

Cleckley, H. (1976). *The mask of sanity* (5th ed.). Mosby.

Cloninger, C. R. (1978). The antisocial personality. *Hospital Practice, 13*(8), 97–106.

Colins, O. F., Andershed, H., Salekin, R. T., & Fanti, K. A. (2018). Comparing different approaches for subtyping children with conduct problems: Callous-unemotional traits only versus the multidimensional psychopathy construct. *Journal of Psychopathology and Behavioral Assessment, 40*(1), 6–15.

Colins, O. F., van Damme, L., Hendriks, A. M., & Georgiou, G. (2020). The DSM-5 with limited prosocial emotions specifier for conduct disorder: A systematic review. *Journal of Psychopathology and Behavioral Assessment, 42*(2), 248–258.

Colledge, E., & Blair, R. J. R. (2001). The relationship in children between the inattention and impulsivity components of attention deficit and hyperactivity disorder and psychopathic tendencies. *Personality and Individual Differences, 30*(7), 1175–1187.

Connor, D. F., Steeber, J., & McBurnett, K. (2010). A review of attention-deficit/hyperactivity disorder complicated by symptoms of oppositional defiant disorder or conduct disorder. *Journal of Developmental & Behavioral Pediatrics, 31*(5), 427–440.

Crego, C., & Widiger, T. A. (2015). Psychopathy and the DSM. *Journal of Personality, 83*(6), 665–677.

Déry M., Bégin V., Toupin J., & Temcheff C. (2019). Clinical utility of the limited prosocial emotions specifier in the childhood-onset subtype of conduct cisorder. *Canadian Journal of Psychiatry, 64*(12), 838-845. https://doi.org/10.1177/0706743719885469.

DeLisi, M., Vaughn, M., Beaver, K. M., Wexler, J., Barth, A. E., & Fletcher, J. M. (2011). Fledgling psychopathy in the classroom: ADHD subtypes, psychopathy, and reading comprehension in a community sample of adolescents. *Youth Violence and Juvenile Justice, 9*(1), 43–58.

DeLisi, M., Dansby, T., Peters, D. J., Vaughn, M. G., Shook, J. J., & Hochstetler, A. (2014). Fledgling psychopathic features and pathological delinquency: New evidence. *American Journal of Criminal Justice, 39*(3), 411–424.

Di Trani, M., Di Roma, F., Scatena, M. C., & Donfrancesco, R. (2013). Severity of symptomatology and subtypes in ADHD children with comorbid oppositional defiant and conduct disorders. *International Journal on Disability and Human Development, 12*(3), 283–287.

Edens, J. F., Mowle, E. N., Clark, J. W., & Magyar, M. S. (2017). "A psychopath by any other name?": Juror perceptions of the DSM-5 "limited prosocial emotions" specifier. *Journal of Personality Disorders, 31*(1), 90–109.

Ezpeleta, L., Granero, R., de la Osa, N., Penelo, E., & Domènech, J. M. (2012). Dimensions of oppositional defiant disorder in 3-year-old preschoolers. *Journal of Child Psychology and Psychiatry, 53*(11), 1128–1138.

Fanti, K. A., Kyranides, M. N., Lordos, A., Colins, O. F., & Andershed, H. (2018). Unique and interactive associations of callous-unemotional traits, impulsivity and grandiosity with child and adolescent conduct disorder symptoms. *Journal of Psychopathology and Behavioral Assessment, 40*(1), 40–49.

Faraone, S. V., Biederman, J., Weber, W., & Russell, R. L. (1998). Psychiatric, neuropsychological, and psychosocial features of DSM-IV subtypes of attention-deficit/hyperactivity disorder: Results from a clinically referred sample. *Journal of the American Academy of Child & Adolescent Psychiatry, 37*(2), 185–193.

Fowler, T., Langley, K., Rice, F., Whittinger, N., Ross, K., van Goozen, S., Owen, M. J., O'Donovan, M. C., van den Bree, M. B. M., & Thapar, A. (2009). Psychopathy traits in adolescents with childhood attention-deficit hyperactivity disorder. *The British Journal of Psychiatry, 194*(1), 62–67.

Frick, P. J. (2012). Developmental pathways to conduct disorder: Implications for future directions in research, assessment, and treatment. *Journal of Clinical Child & Adolescent Psychology, 41*(3), 378–389.

Frick, P. J. (2021). Editorial: Testing the validity of the limited prosocial emotions specifier. *Journal of the American Academy of Child and Adolescent Psychiatry, 60*(8), 952–954. https://doi.org/10.1016/j.jaac.2020.12.020

Frick, P. J., & Myers, T. D. (2017). Conduct disorder and callous-unemotional traits. *The Wiley Handbook of Disruptive and Impulse-Control Disorders*, 37–54.

Frick, P. J., & Viding, E. (2009). Antisocial behavior from a developmental psychopathology perspective. *Development and Psychopathology, 21*(4), 1111–1131.

Frick, P. J., & White, S. F. (2008). Research review: The importance of callous-unemotional traits for developmental models of aggressive and antisocial behavior. *Journal of Child Psychology and Psychiatry, 49*(4), 359–375.

Frick, P. J., Bodin, S. D., & Barry, C. T. (2000). Psychopathic traits and conduct problems in community and clinic-referred samples of children: Further development of the psychopathy screening device. *Psychological Assessment, 12*(4), 382.

Frogner, L., Andershed, A. K., & Andershed, H. (2018). Psychopathic personality works better than CU traits for predicting fearlessness and ADHD symptoms among children with conduct problems. *Journal of Psychopathology and Behavioral Assessment, 40*(1), 26–39.

Haas, S. M., Waschbusch, D. A., Pelham, W. E., King, S., Andrade, B. F., & Carrey, N. J. (2011). Treatment response in CP/ADHD children with callous/unemotional traits. *Journal of Abnormal Child Psychology, 39*(4), 541–552.

Hare, R. D. (1991). *The Hare psychopathy checklist-revised manual. Multi-health systems.* Tonawanda.

Hare, R. D. (1996). Psychopathy and antisocial personality disorder: A case of diagnostic confusion. *Psychiatric Times, 13*(2), 39–40.

Hare, R. D. (2003). *Manual for the Hare psychopathy checklist-revised* (2nd ed.). Multi-Health Systems.

Harpur, T. J., Hare, R. D., & Hakstian, A. R. (1989). Two-factor conceptualization of psychopathy: Construct validity and assessment implications. *Psychological Assessment: A Journal of Consulting and Clinical Psychology, 1*(1), 6–17.

Hoong, W., Houghton, S., & Chapman, E. (2006). Relationships between attention deficit/hyperactivity disorder, conduct disorder, psychopathy, and aggression: The fledgling psychopath hypothesis. *Trends in Attention Deficit Hyperactivity Disorder Research, 99.*

Jensen, C. M., & Steinhausen, H. C. (2015). Comorbid mental disorders in children and adolescents with attention-deficit/hyperactivity disorder in a large nationwide study. *ADHD Attention Deficit and Hyperactivity Disorders, 7*(1), 27–38.

Jezior, K. L., McKenzie, M. E., & Lee, S. S. (2016). Narcissism and callous-unemotional traits prospectively predict child conduct problems. *Journal of Clinical Child and Adolescent Psychology, 45*(5), 579–590.

Johansson, P., Kerr, M., & Andershed, H. (2005). Linking adult psychopathy with childhood hyperactivity-impulsivity-attention problems and conduct problems through retrospective self-reports. *Journal of Personality Disorders, 19*(1), 94–101.

Kaplan, S. G., & Cornell, D. G. (2004). Psychopathy and ADHD in adolescent male offenders. *Youth Violence and Juvenile Justice, 2*(2), 148–160.

Kosson, D. S., Cyterski, T. D., Steuerwald, B. L., Neumann, C. S., & Walker-Matthews, S. (2002). The reliability and validity of the psychopathy checklist: Youth version (PCL: YV) in nonincarcerated adolescent males. *Psychological Assessment, 14*(1), 97–109.

Lahey, B. B. (2014). What we need to know about callous-unemotional traits: Comment on Frick, Ray, Thornton, and Kahn (2014). *Psychological Bulletin, 140*, 58–63.

Lahey, B. B., & Waldman, I. D. (2012). Annual research review: Phenotypic and causal structure of conduct disorder in the broader context of prevalent forms of psychopathology. *Journal of Child Psychology and Psychiatry, 53*(5), 536–557.

Lavigne, J. V., Bryant, F. B., Hopkins, J., & Gouze, K. R. (2015). Dimensions of oppositional defiant disorder in young children: Model comparisons, gender and longitudinal invariance. *Journal of Abnormal Child Psychology, 43*(3), 423–439. https://doi.org/10.1007/s10802-014-9919-0

Lilienfeld, S. O. (1994). Conceptual problems in the assessment of psychopathy. *Clinical Psychology Review, 14*(1), 17–38.

Lilienfeld, S. O., & Andrews, B. P. (1996). Development and preliminary validation of a self-report measure of psychopathic personality traits in noncriminal population. *Journal of Personality Assessment, 66*(3), 488–524.

Loeber, R. (1991). Antisocial behavior: More enduring than changeable? *Journal of the American Academy of Child & Adolescent Psychiatry, 30*(3), 393–397.

Loeber, R., Green, S. M., Keenan, K., & Lahey, B. B. (1995). Which boys will fare worse? Early predictors of the onset of conduct disorder in a six-year longitudinal study. *Journal of the American Academy of Child & Adolescent Psychiatry, 34*(4), 499–509.

López-Romero, L., Romero, E., Colins, O. F., Andershed, H., Hare, R. D., & Salekin, R. T. (2019). Proposed specifiers for conduct disorder (PSCD): Preliminary validation of the parent version in a Spanish sample of preschoolers. *Psychological Assessment, 31*(11), 1357–1367.

Luo, J., Wang, M.-C., Neumann, C. S., Hare, R. D., & Salekin, R. T. (2020, August). Factor structure and construct validity of the proposed specifier for conduct disorder (PSCD) scale in Chinese adolescents. *Assessment.* https://doi.org/10.1177/1073191120949914

Lykken, D. T. (1957). A study of anxiety in the sociopathic personality. *Journal of Abnormal and Social Psychology, 55*(1), 6–10.

Lynam, D. R. (1996). Early identification of chronic offenders: Who is the fledgling psychopath? *Psychological Bulletin, 120*(2), 209–234.

Lynam, D. R. (1997). Pursuing the psychopath: Capturing the fledgling psychopath in a nomological net. *Journal of Abnormal Psychology, 106*(3), 425.

Mann, F. D., Paul, S. L., Tackett, J. L., Tucker-Drob, E. M., & Harden, K. P. (2018). Personality risk for antisocial behavior: Testing the intersections between callous–unemotional traits, sensation seeking, and impulse control in adolescence. *Development and Psychopathology, 30*(1), 267–282.

Mathias, C. W., Furr, R. M., Daniel, S. S., Marsh, D. M., Shannon, E. E., & Dougherty, D. M. (2007). The relationship of inattentiveness, hyperactivity, and psychopathy among adolescents. *Personality and Individual Differences, 43*(6), 1333–1343.

Michonski, J. D., & Sharp, C. (2010). Revisiting Lynam's notion of the "fledgling psychopath": Are HIA-CP children truly psychopathic-like? *Child and Adolescent Psychiatry and Mental Health, 4*(1), 24.

Muratori, P., Buonanno, C., Gallani, A., Grossi, G., Levantini, V., Milone, A., Pisano, S., Salekin, R. T., Sesso, G., Masi, G., & Nocentini, A. (2021). Validation of the Proposed Specifiers for Conduct Disorder (PSCD) scale in a sample of Italian students. *Children, 8*, 1020. https://doi.org/10.3390/children81111020.

Neumann, C. S., Malterer, M. B., & Newman, J. P. (2008). Factor structure of the psychopathic personality inventory (PPI): Findings from a large incarcerated sample. *Psychological Assessment, 20*(2), 169–174.

Nigg, J. T. (2006). Temperament and developmental psychopathology. *Journal of Child Psychology and Psychiatry, 47*(3–4), 395–422.

Odgers, C. L., Moffitt, T. E., Broadbent, J. M., Dickson, N., Hancox, R. J., Harrington, H., … Caspi, A. (2008). Female and male antisocial trajectories: From childhood origins to adult outcomes. *Development and Psychopathology, 20*(2), 673–716.

Ogloff, J. R. P. (2006). Psychopathy/antisocial personality disorder conundrum. *Australian and New Zealand Journal of Psychiatry, 40*(6–7), 519–528.

Pardini, D. A., & Loeber, R. (2007). Interpersonal and affective features of psychopathy in children and adolescents: Advancing a developmental perspective introduction to special section. *Journal of Clinical Child and Adolescent Psychology, 36*(3), 269–275.

Pardini, D., Stepp, S., Hipwell, A., Stouthamer-Loeber, M., & Loeber, R. (2012). The clinical utility of the proposed DSM-5 callous-unemotional subtype of conduct disorder in young girls. *Journal of the American Academy of Child & Adolescent Psychiatry, 51*(1), 62–73.

Pechorro, P., Jiménez, L., Hidalgo, V., & Nunes, C. (2015). The DSM-5 limited prosocial emotions subtype of conduct disorder in incarcerated male and female juvenile delinquents. *International Journal of Law and Psychiatry, 39*, 77–82.

Piatigorsky, A., & Hinshaw, S. P. (2004). Psychopathic traits in boys with and without attention-deficit/hyperactivity disorder: Concurrent and longitudinal correlates. *Journal of Abnormal Child Psychology, 32*(5), 535–550.

Quay, H. C. (1965). Psychopathic personality as pathological stimulation-seeking. *American Journal of Psychiatry, 122*(2), 180–183.

Quay, H. C. (1972). Patterns of aggression, withdrawal, and immaturity. In H. C. Quay & J. S. Werry (Eds.), *Psychopathological disorders of childhood*. Wiley.

Robins, L. N. (1966). *Deviant children grown up: A sociological and psychiatric study of the psychopathic personality*. Williams & Wilkins.

Robins, L. N. (1978). Sturdy childhood predictors of adult antisocial behavior: Replications from longitudinal studies. *Psychological Medicine, 8*(4), 611–622.

Ribeiro da Silva, D., Sousa, R., Rijo, D., Mendez, B., Tsang, S., & Salekin, R. T. (2022). Proposed Specifiers for Conduct Disorder (PSCD): Factor structure and validation of the self-report version in community and forensic samples of Portuguese youth. *Assessment*. https://doi.org/10.1177/10731911211044534.

Rogers, R. (1995). *Diagnostic and structured interviewing*. PAR.

Rowe, R., Maughan, B., Pickles, A., Costello, E. J., & Angold, A. (2002). The relationship between DSM-IV oppositional defiant disorder and conduct disorder: Findings from the Great Smoky Mountains study. *Journal of Child Psychology and Psychiatry, 43*(3), 365–373.

Rowe, R., Costello, E. J., Angold, A., Copeland, W. E., & Maughan, B. (2010a). Developmental pathways in oppositional defiant disorder and conduct disorder. *Journal of Abnormal Psychology, 119*(4), 726.

Rowe, R., Maughan, B., Moran, P., Ford, T., Briskman, J., & Goodman, R. (2010b). The role of callous and unemotional traits in the diagnosis of conduct disorder. *Journal of Child Psychology and Psychiatry, 51*(6), 688–695.

Sakai, J. T., Mikulich-Gilbertson, S. K., Young, S. E., Rhee, S. H., McWilliams, S. K., Dunn, R., … Hopfer, C. J. (2016). Adolescent male conduct-disordered patients in substance use disorder treatment: Examining the "limited prosocial emotions" specifier. *Journal of Child and Adolescent Substance Abuse, 25*(6), 613–625.

Salekin, R. T. (2017). Research review: What do we know about psychopathic traits in children? *Journal of Child Psychology and Psychiatry, 58*(11), 1180–1200.

Salekin, R. T. (2016). Pychopathy in childhood: Why should we care about grandiose-manipulative and daringimpulsive traits? *British Journal of Psychiatry, 209*(3), 189–191. https://doi.org/10.1192/bjp.bp.115.179051.

Salekin, R. T., & Hare, R. D. (2016). *Proposed specifiers for conduct disorder (PCSD)*. Unpublished test.

Salekin, R. T., Andershed, H., Batky, B. D., & Bontemps, A. P. (2018). Are callous unemotional (CU) traits enough? *Journal of Psychopathology and Behavioral Assessment, 40*(1), 1–5.

Sevecke, K., & Kosson, D. S. (2010). Relationships of child and adolescent psychopathy to other forms of psychopathology. In R. T. Salekin & D. R. Lynam (Eds.), *Handbook of child and adolescent psychopathy* (pp. 284–314). The Guilford Press.

Sevecke, K., Kosson, D. S., & Krischer, M. K. (2009). The relationship between attention deficit hyperactivity disorder, conduct disorder, and psychopathy in adolescent male and female detainees. *Behavioral Sciences & the Law, 27*(4), 577–598.

Smith, C. S., & Hung, L. C. (2012). The relative influence of conduct problems and attention-deficit hyperactivity disorder in the development of adolescent psychopathy. *Aggression and Violent Behavior, 17*(6), 575–580. https://doi.org/10.1016/j.avb.2012.08.003

Somma, A., Andershed, H., Borroni, S., Salekin, R. T., & Fossati, A. (2018). Psychopathic personality traits in relation to self-report delinquency in adolescence: Should we mind about interaction effects? *Journal of Psychopathology and Behavioral Assessment, 40*(1), 69–78.

Spitzer, R. L., Endicott, J., & Robins, E. (1975). Clinical criteria for psychiatric diagnosis and DSM-III. *The American Journal of Psychiatry, 132*(11), 1187–1192.

Stringaris, A., & Goodman, R. (2009). Three dimensions of oppositionality in youth. *Journal of Child Psychology and Psychiatry, 50*(3), 216–223.

Stringaris, A., Cohen, P., Pine, D. S., & Leibenluft, E. (2009). Adult outcomes of youth irritability: A 20-year prospective community-based study. *American Journal of Psychiatry, 166*(9), 1048–1054.

Stringaris, A., Zavos, H., Leibenluft, E., Maughan, B., & Eley, T. C. (2012). Adolescent irritability: Phenotypic associations and genetic links with depressed mood. *American Journal of Psychiatry, 169*(1), 47–54.

Taylor, E., Chadwick, O., Heptinstall, E., & Danckaerts, M. (1996). Hyperactivity and conduct problems as risk factors for adolescent development. *Journal of the American Academy of Child & Adolescent Psychiatry, 35*(9), 1213–1226.

Washburn, J. J., McMahon, S. D., King, C. A., Reinecke, M. A., & Silver, C. (2004). Narcissistic features in young adolescents: Relations to aggression and internalizing symptoms. *Journal of Youth and Adolescence, 33*(3), 247–260.

Whelan, Y. M., Stringaris, A., Maughan, B., & Barker, E. D. (2013). Developmental continuity of oppositional defiant disorder subdimensions at ages 8, 10, and 13 years and their distinct psychiatric outcomes at age 16 years. *Journal of the American Academy of Child & Adolescent Psychiatry, 52*(9), 961–969.

World Health Organization (2019). *International Statistical Classification of Diseases and Related Health Problems (11th ed.)*. World Health Organization.

Willcutt, E. G., Nigg, J. T., Pennington, B. F., Solanto, M. V., Rohde, L. A., Tannock, R., … Lahey, B. B. (2012). Validity of DSM-IV attention deficit/hyperactivity disorder symptom dimensions and subtypes. *Journal of Abnormal Psychology, 121*(4), 991–1010.

Chapter 11
Psychopathy and Substance Use Disorders

Grace M. Brennan, Allison M. Stuppy-Sullivan, and Arielle R. Baskin-Sommers

Abstract The association between substance use disorders (SUDs) and antisocial behavior is one of the most reliable and important themes in the SUDs literature. Among individuals who engage in antisocial behavior, individuals with psychopathy are at significantly higher risk for SUDs (the term "substance" is used throughout this chapter to include alcohol and drugs). In this chapter, we will detail the existing empirical evidence highlighting the link between psychopathy and SUDs, with special consideration for the varied presentations of psychopathy based on the way the construct is measured and the type of sample used in each study. We also briefly discuss potential mechanisms that may reinforce this link between psychopathy and SUDs. Finally, we close with evidence-based considerations and recommendations for assessing and treating SUDs in individuals with psychopathy. Specifying patterns of associations between psychopathy and SUDs has important clinical and legal implications.

Keywords Psychopathy · Substance use disorders (SUDs) · Substance use · Factor 2 · Assessment · Treatment

11.1 Links Between Psychopathy and Substance Use Disorders

The association between substance use disorders (SUDs) and antisocial behavior is one of the most reliable and important themes in the SUDs literature (Compton et al., 2005; Grant et al., 2004). Among individuals who engage in antisocial behavior, individuals with psychopathy are at significantly higher risk for diverse SUDs (the term "substance" is used in a broad sense throughout this chapter to include alcohol and drugs). Even among incarcerated individuals (who already exhibit

G. M. Brennan · A. M. Stuppy-Sullivan · A. R. Baskin-Sommers (✉)
Yale University, New Haven, CT, USA
e-mail: arielle.baskin-sommers@yale.edu

J. E. Vitale (ed.), *The Complexity of Psychopathy*, Dangerous Behavior in Clinical and Forensic Psychology, https://doi.org/10.1007/978-3-030-83156-1_11

elevated rates of SUDs compared to individuals in the general population; Fazel et al., 2006), individuals with psychopathy can be up to five times more likely to have a lifetime SUD diagnosis (Smith & Newman, 1990). Rates among individuals with psychopathy are as high as 92.9% for alcohol use disorder and 73.5% for drug use disorder (Smith & Newman, 1990); for comparison, in the general, population, lifetime prevalence rates for and alcohol use disorder and drug use disorder are 30.3% (Hasin et al., 2007) and 10.3% (Compton et al., 2007), respectively. These staggeringly high rates underscore the interconnected relationship between psychopathy and SUDs. The overarching goal of the present chapter is to describe the existing literature linking psychopathy and SUDs, and to provide evidence-based recommendations for assessment and treatment of individuals with co-morbid psychopathy and SUDs.

Psychopathy is a debilitating form of personality disorder characterized by a constellation of traits, including manipulativeness, lack of empathy, impulsivity, and chronic antisociality (Gretton et al., 2004; Hare & McPherson, 1984; Kruh et al., 2005; Murrie et al., 2004; Salekin et al., 1996; Serin & Amos, 1995). Psychopathy affects approximately 1% of the general population and approximately 15% to 25% of incarcerated offenders (Hare, 2003; Kiehl & Hoffman, 2011). In adults, the gold-standard assessment of psychopathy is Hare's Psychopathy Checklist-Revised (PCL-R; Hare, 2003), an interview-based measure of the interpersonal/affective (Factor 1) and impulsive/antisocial (Factor 2) traits characteristic of this personality pathology (Hare et al., 1990; Harpur et al., 1989; see Table 11.1 for items and examples). Using this measure, psychopathy is construed as a unitary construct (i.e., total score) that can be subdivided into component traits (e.g., Factors). More recent factor analyses indicate that three- (Cooke & Michie, 2001) and four-facet (Hare & Neumann, 2005; Neumann et al., 2012) solutions also can subdivide the traits associated with psychopathy. For example, in the four-facet model, the two Factors can each be further subdivided into two component facets. Under Factor 1, the component facets are known as the interpersonal facet (Facet 1) and the affective facet (Facet 2). Under Factor 2, the component facets are known as the impulsive facet (Facet 3) and the antisocial facet (Facet 4) (in addition to Table 11.1, see Sect. 11.1.2 below for more information regarding the traits that make up each Factor and facet).

In youth, psychopathy is expressed through a combination of interpersonal, callous-unemotional (CU; affective), and impulsive/antisocial (e.g., conduct problems) traits. In incarcerated and community samples of youth, the prevalence of psychopathy is on average between 9–25% depending on the instruments (e.g., Psychopathy Checklist: Youth Version [PCL:YV; Forth et al., 2003]; Youth Psychopathic Traits Inventory [YPI; Andershed et al., 2002]) and cut-off scores used to distinguish psychopathic and non-psychopathic youth, the types of institutions/settings, and the composition (e.g., males and females) of the samples (Kosson et al., 2002; Lynam et al., 2007; Salekin et al., 2004). Additionally, in the most recent update to the Diagnostic and Statistical Manual of Mental Disorders, Version 5 (DSM-5; American Psychiatric Association, 2013) a specifier was added to conduct disorder (CD): CD with limited prosocial emotions (i.e., CU). Youth with this

Table 11.1 List of diagnostic criteria for psychopathy according to the psychopathy checklist—revised

PCL-R items	Examples
Factor 1	
Facet 1: Interpersonal facet	
Glibness/superficial charm	Telling stories that place oneself in an unreasonably positive light; charming others in an insincere manner
Grandiose sense of self-worth	Displaying an attitude that one is superior to others
Pathological lying	Using an alias to evade detection by police
Conning/manipulative	Committing identity fraud; using blackmail to control others
Facet 2: Affective facet	
Lack of remorse or guilt	Regarding oneself as the true victim of one's crime; repeated engagement in the same criminal act
Shallow affect	Failing to experience a normal range of emotions (e.g., experiencing only anger); lacking sustained expression of any emotion
Callous/lack of empathy	Expressing an attitude that victims of crimes get what they deserve; failing to intuit the emotions of others
Failure to accept responsibility	Attributing blame for one's misdeeds to society or to others; minimizing the impact of one's own behavior
Factor 2	
Facet 3: Impulsive facet	
Need for stimulation/ proneness to boredom	Experimenting with a range of different substances; experiencing excessive boredom with the routine of everyday life
Parasitic lifestyle	Living with someone without contributing to paying bills
Lack of realistic long-term goals	Expressing intentions to pursue a career in an area in which one has no knowledge
Impulsivity	Moving without having a plan for where one will live or work
Irresponsibility	Failing to pay child support, bills, and loan repayments; drunk driving
Facet 4: Antisocial facet	
Poor behavioral controls	Engaging in many physical fights (e.g., 20+); showing more aggression when under the influence of substances
Early behavior problems	Using weapons to threaten or harm others before the age of 13; abusing alcohol or sniffing glue before the age of 13
Juvenile delinquency	Committing grand theft auto before the age of 18
Revocation of conditional release	Receiving a new criminal charge while on probation or parole; submitting a dirty urine screen while on parole
Criminal versatility	Committing a wide range of different crime types (e.g., drug charges, assault, disorderly conduct, theft, etc.)
Other items	
Promiscuous sexual behavior	Having sex with a large number (e.g., 20+) of different partners
Many short-term marital relationships	Co-habitating with several different (e.g., 3+) partners over the course of the lifetime

CD specifier display the callous use of others, a lack of remorse or guilt, and an absence of empathy. Youth falling into this category represent approximately 32–46.1% of those with CD (Herpers et al., 2012) and represent a group who are at particularly high risk for meeting criteria for psychopathy in adulthood (Frick, 2009).

Although psychopathy is often discussed as a unitary construct, there is a long tradition of distinguishing psychopathic subtypes in both adults and youth. A leading classification scheme involves categorizing individuals as having either primary or secondary psychopathy (Karpman, 1941; Kimonis et al., 2011; Skeem et al., 2007). Primary psychopathy is associated with a lack of anxiety and is presumed to be a consequence of some intrinsic deficit that hampers self-regulation and normal adjustment. Secondary psychopathy is associated with comparable levels of

Table 11.2 Lists of diagnostic criteria for DSM-5 substance use disorder (current criteria), and DSM-IV substance use disorder (previous criteria)

DSM-5 substance use disorder criteria (2 or more of the following for any level of diagnosis)	DSM-IV substance use disorder criteria
Craving or a strong desire or urge to use the substance (newly added)	
	Abuse criteria (1 or more of the following in the absence of a dependence diagnosis):
	Recurrent substance-related legal problems (removed in DSM-5)
Recurrent substance use in situations where it is physically hazardous	Recurrent substance use in situations where it is physically hazardous
Recurrent use resulting in a failure to fulfill major role obligations at work, school, or home	Recurrent use resulting in a failure to fulfill major role obligations at work, school, or home
Continued use despite having persistent or recurrent interpersonal problems caused or exacerbated by the effects of the substance	Continued use despite having persistent or recurrent interpersonal problems caused or exacerbated by the effects of the substance
	Dependence criteria (3 or more of the following):
Substance is taken in larger amounts or over a longer period than was intended	Substance is taken in larger amounts or over a longer period than was intended
Persistent desire or unsuccessful efforts to cut down or control use	Persistent desire or unsuccessful efforts to cut down or control use
Great deal of time spent in activities necessary to obtain the substance, use it, or recover from its effects	Great deal of time spent in activities necessary to obtain the substance, use it, or recover from its effects
Important social, occupational, or recreational activities are given up or reduced because of use	Important social, occupational, or recreational activities are given up or reduced because of use
Continued use despite knowledge of having a persistent or recurrent physical or psychological problem that is likely to have been caused or exacerbated by use	Continued use despite knowledge of having a persistent or recurrent physical or psychological problem that is likely to have been caused or exacerbated by use
Tolerance	Tolerance
Withdrawal	Withdrawal

antisocial behavior, but is thought to stem from social disadvantage, child maltreatment, excessive neurotic anxiety, and/or other forms of psychopathology. Taken together, across gender, stages of development, and subtype, psychopathy is associated with disruptions in interpersonal, emotional, and behavioral functioning.

As noted above, psychopathy and SUDs are commonly comorbid. This high rate of comorbidity is probably not surprising, since individuals with SUDs often have higher rates of impulsivity and aggression. In recent years, the operationalization of SUDs using the Diagnostic and Statistical Manual for Mental Disorders (American Psychiatric Association, 2013) has shifted. In 2000, under the DSM-IV (American Psychiatric Association, 2000) SUDs were diagnosed as either "substance abuse" or "substance dependence." Substance abuse was associated with four diagnostic criteria, and substance dependence was associated with a separate set of seven diagnostic criteria (see Table 11.2). In 2013, there was a substantial overhaul of the diagnostic scheme, such that SUDs are now rated on a continuum of severity, from mild to moderate to severe levels. If thresholds are met for 2–3 criteria, an individual is diagnosed with a mild SUD; if thresholds are met for 4–5 criteria, an individual is diagnosed with a moderate SUD; and if thresholds are met for 6 or more criteria, an individual is diagnosed with a severe SUD.[1] Moreover, the "legal problems due to substance use" criterion was removed and a criterion for "craving" was added in the DSM-5.

In addition to formal diagnostic criteria, there are other important substance use-related factors to consider. First are factors that quantify substance use and specify the nature of substance use. The *quantity of substances used* (often operationalized as the frequency of substance use over a given time period, or a total amount calculated by multiplying the quantity of substance used per occasion by the frequency of use) relates to substance-related problems (though is not synonymous with problems). *Age at initiation of* substance use is a predictor of long-term impairments, such that individuals who begin using substances at an earlier age are more likely to experience more severe problems across multiple life domains (Brook et al., 2002), including substance-related violence, injuries, intoxicated driving, and absenteeism from school or work (Gruber et al., 1996). Substance use *versatility* (the number of different substances used) relates to a higher likelihood of exposure to particularly risky substances (e.g., opioids) and indicates a potentially more severe course of substance use (Moss et al., 2014). Second, there are factors that characterize the extent to which substance use causes problems. One of the most commonly assessed factors is the *severity of substance misuse.* This factor represents a more dimensional measure of substance-related problems compared to categorical diagnoses, and can potentially capture more information about the degree to which substance use is interfering in an individual's life (e.g., evaluated using measures such as the Michigan Alcohol Screening Test [Selzer, 1971] or the Drug Abuse Screening Test [Skinner, 1982]). Third, and finally, there are factors that capture subjective aspects

[1] Given the recency of the DSM-5, no studies to date examined how psychopathy relates to DSM-5 diagnoses.

of substance use, including *motives for using substances*. Research indicates that individuals use substances for a range of different reasons (e.g., to experience positive feelings, to cope with stress or negative emotions, to facilitate social interactions). Specific motives, particularly using substances to cope with stress or negative emotions, tend to be associated with more frequent and more problematic substance use (Cooper, 1994; Hyman & Sinha, 2009). In sum, quantity of substance use, age at initiation of substance use, substance use versatility, severity of substance-related problems, and substance use motives are important factors to consider when examining patterns of substance misuse.

In the sections that follow, we will review the empirical evidence linking psychopathy and SUDs. In this review, we pay special consideration to the varied presentations of psychopathy based on the way the construct is measured and the type of sample (e.g., based on gender, age, etc.) used in each study. Specifying patterns of associations between psychopathy and SUDs is important for a variety of reasons that carry both clinical and legal implications. A better understanding of this association is needed not only because substance misuse is harmful on its own, but also because there is evidence that substance use and misuse can exacerbate the dangerous and destructive behaviors that characterize psychopathy (e.g., aggression; Birkley et al., 2013).

11.1.1 Patterns of Associations Between Psychopathy and SUDs

Across a wide range of sample types (i.e., correctional, epidemiological, community, clinical), psychopathy as a unitary construct is associated with higher rates of SUD diagnoses (Rice & Harris, 1995; Smith & Newman, 1990), particularly for illicit drugs compared to alcohol (Coid et al., 2009a; Hemphill et al., 1994). Moreover, psychopathy is consistently associated with more frequent and extensive use of substances (Cope et al., 2014; Sylvers et al., 2011), earlier initiation of substance use (Brennan, Stuppy-Sullivan, et al., 2017b; Vincent et al., 2003) and age of onset of substance abuse (Gustavson et al., 2007), and greater substance use versatility (Hemphill et al., 1994; Lynam et al., 1999). In terms of motives for using substances, psychopathy total scores are not consistently related to specific motives, especially after controlling for frequency of substance use (Salatino et al., 2018). Taken together, psychopathy is clearly associated with higher rates of SUDs, heavier use of a variety of substances, as well as a more chronic and severe course of substance-related problems; however, psychopathy is not associated with specific substance use motives.

Both clinical observations and empirical investigations have uncovered differences in how SUDs manifest in individuals with psychopathy, in comparison to both non-psychopathic individuals with SUDs as well as individuals with different antisocial pathologies. In his seminal writings, Cleckley (1941) wrote that substance use in individuals with psychopathy follows a presentation that is distinct from that of other individuals who chronically use substances and engage in antisocial behavior. For example, Cleckley (1941) commented that alcohol does not drive the behavior of individuals with psychopathy, but rather acts as a catalyst that spurs the expression of already existing tendencies. The alcohol use of an individual with psychopathy also does not seem to stem from strong affective urges or motivations to avoid withdrawal. This is in contrast to the substance use of the "neurotic drinker" who uses due to specific motivations to feel good or better, and a desire to continue using substances in order to avoid withdrawal (Cleckley, 1941). Consistent with these observations, compared to other antisocial individuals (who do not share the interpersonal/affective features of psychopathy), individuals with psychopathy tend to initiate substance use at a younger age but have less severe SUDs (Brennan, Stuppy-Sullivan, et al., 2017b). These differences highlight the importance of considering psychopathy as an influence on the expressed symptomatology of SUDs, as well as the importance of differentiating individuals with psychopathy from individuals with other antisocial pathologies.

11.1.2 Patterns of Associations Between Psychopathy Factors/Facets and SUDs

Some researchers advocate for parsing the unitary construct of psychopathy into its component Factors. This type of work has led to conclusions that the interpersonal/affective traits (Factor 1) are the core personality traits of psychopathy, while the impulsive/antisocial traits (Factor 2) reflect behavioral dysregulation and criminality more broadly (Patrick, 2007). Whereas an individual with high levels of interpersonal/affective traits may present as a smooth-talking manipulator who exploits others in a calculated manner and does not feel remorse for their actions, an individual with high levels of impulsive/antisocial traits may present as an emotionally dysregulated risk-taker who lacks the self-control to inhibit their aggressive and criminal behavior. The two Factors show distinct associations with external correlates. For example, Factor 2 (i.e., impulsive/antisocial) traits are associated with depressive symptoms and suicide attempts, whereas Factor 1 (i.e., interpersonal/affective) traits are not (Hunt et al., 2015; Verona et al., 2001). Consistent with this general dissociation, the associations between these psychopathy Factors and SUDs also appear to diverge.

Both Factor 1 and Factor 2 relate to higher levels of substance use (Kramer et al., 2017; Miller et al., 2011). However, Factor 2 (i.e., impulsive/antisocial) traits are generally more strongly associated with substance use-related problems. For example, higher Factor 2 scores relate to a greater number of SUD diagnoses (Brennan et al., 2017b; Hemphill et al., 1994). Additionally, inmates with higher levels of Factor 2 traits report an earlier age of initiation of use across a variety of substances (Brennan et al., 2017b; Smith & Newman, 1990), and Factor 2 is more strongly associated with SUD symptoms (Hart et al., 1991; Hart & Hare, 1989; Reardon et al., 2002; Smith & Newman, 1990).

Although many studies fail to detect an association between the interpersonal/affective (i.e., Factor 1) traits and SUD symptoms and diagnoses (Hart & Hare, 1989; Korponay et al., 2017; Smith & Newman, 1990), results are somewhat inconsistent. On the one hand, some studies found evidence of positive associations between the interpersonal/affective traits and substance-related problems for specific drugs such as cocaine. For example, Denomme et al. (2018) report that a cocaine-dependent group of offenders had higher levels of Factor 1 traits (as well as Factor 2 traits) compared to a non-dependent group of offenders. Walsh et al. (2007) found that Factor 1 was positively associated with cocaine dependence symptoms among European Americans. On the other hand, some studies found negative associations between Factor 1 traits and substance-related problems (e.g., Schulz et al., 2015).[2]

Beyond diagnoses and the nature of substance use, there is evidence that the reasons underlying substance use in individuals with higher interpersonal/affective (i.e., Factor 1) versus impulsive/antisocial (i.e., Factor 2) traits may be different. The impulsive/antisocial (Factor 2) traits appear to relate more consistently to specific motives for using substances. For example, Reardon et al. (2002) found significant associations between Factor 2 and all drinking motives assessed (i.e., motives pertaining to enhancement of positive mood, coping with negative emotions, and socializing with others), but no associations between Factor 1 and drinking motives in a sample of male inmates. In another study of previously incarcerated offenders, Salatino et al. (2018) found that both Factor 1 and Factor 2 traits were associated with motives to enhance positive mood and socialize with others. However, after controlling for frequency of use, only the relationship between Factor 2 and enhancement motives (i.e., aiming to enhance positive mood) for drinking remained, while Factor 1 was again unrelated to drinking motives (Salatino et al., 2018).

Overall, across metrics of substance use and misuse, individuals with higher levels of impulsive/antisocial (i.e., Factor 2) traits appear to have the highest risk for chronic and severe SUDs. Moreover, the repeated presence of negative associations between the interpersonal/affective (i.e., Factor 1) traits and indicators of SUDs raises the question of whether interpersonal/affective traits are protective against

[2] It is worth noting that differences in statistical approaches across studies may account for some of the inconsistent findings for the associations between Factor 1 and substance use-related factors. When examining associations between psychopathy Factors and substance use variables, in some studies researchers enter the Factor scores simultaneously into a statistical analysis, while in other studies researchers enter the Factor scores separately. These two techniques allow researchers to answer two different questions: entering psychopathy Factor scores simultaneously allows researchers to examine the contributions of the *unique* variance of each Factor (removing variance shared between the Factors), whereas entering Factor scores separately allows researchers to examine the *independent* associations of each Factor (without removing shared variance) with substance use. When researchers examine unique variance of the two factors, Factor 1 is more likely to show negative associations with substance use-related factors; however, when researchers examine independent associations of each factor, Factor 1 typically shows no associations with substance use-related factors (see Lynam et al., 2006 for a review of the hazards of examining unique variance associated with psychopathy factors).

SUDs. For example, Reardon et al. (2002) found that although levels of alcohol *use* were similarly elevated among two groups of inmates showing divergent profiles of psychopathic traits (i.e., inmates with high Factor 1 and high Factor 2 traits, and inmates with high Factor 2 but low Factor 1 traits), the high-Factor-1/high-Factor-2 inmates demonstrated less severe alcohol problems compared to the low-Factor-1/high-Factor-2 inmates. In contrast to these findings, Hunt et al. (2015) directly tested the question of whether interpersonal/affective traits confer protection against SUDs by means of moderation analyses, and found no evidence of protective effects of Factor 1 against SUDs. More research is needed to reconcile these findings and identify at what levels (if any) interpersonal/affective traits may exert protective effects.

At the level of psychopathy facets, there is evidence that each of the four facets may contribute to substance-related factors, although findings generally point to stronger positive associations for impulsive/antisocial-related facets compared to interpersonal/affective-related facets. Both the Facet 3 (impulsive) and Facet 4 (antisocial) are robustly and consistently associated with a greater likelihood of SUD diagnoses across a range of substance categories (Coid et al., 2009a; Coid et al., 2009b). Facet 1 (interpersonal) and Facet 2 (affective), however, are only associated with a greater likelihood of use and problems for a circumscribed range of substances (e.g., cocaine; Coid et al., 2009a, b). Other work suggests that it may be the interpersonal (compared to affective) traits that contribute more strongly to substance-related problems within Factor 1; conversely, the impulsive (compared to antisocial) traits may contribute more strongly to substance-related problems within Factor 2. For example, in the study by Walsh et al. (2007) the *positive* association between Factor 1 and cocaine dependence symptoms appeared to be driven by Facet 2 (interpersonal facet), while the *negative* association between Factor 1 and marijuana dependence symptoms appeared to be driven by Facet 1 (affective facet). Furthermore, in this same study, for cannabis and opioids, Facet 3 (impulsive facet) was more strongly associated with number of dependence symptoms than was Facet 4 (antisocial facet). Taken together, consistent with findings at the Factor level, the Factor 2-related facets (i.e., impulsive and antisocial traits) are more clearly implicated in substance use and misuse.

11.1.3 Patterns of Associations Between Psychopathy Subtype and SUDs

Psychopathy is related to low interpersonal emotions and flagrant disregard for personal welfare and the welfare of others. However, psychopathy can manifest in different ways, with primary and secondary subtypes relating to somewhat divergent personality profiles and external correlates. For example, whereas primary psychopathy is associated with deliberateness and emotional stability, secondary psychopathy is associated with poor impulse control and emotional reactivity (Hicks et al., 2004, 2010). Accordingly, although psychopathy subtypes are not interchangeable with PCL-R factor scores, primary psychopathy is more strongly associated with the core personality traits of psychopathy (i.e., the interpersonal/affective traits of Factor 1), while secondary psychopathy is more strongly associated with the disinhibited behavior of psychopathy (i.e., the impulsive/antisocial traits of Factor 2; Hicks et al., 2012). Moreover, individuals with secondary psychopathy tend to be more angry, aggressive, and prone to violence (Blackburn & Lee-Evans, 1985; Hicks et al., 2004; Kimonis et al., 2011). Primary and secondary subtypes of psychopathy are related to the expression of SUDs in psychopathy as well.

Multiple studies indicate that secondary psychopathy is more strongly associated with substance misuse. For example, research has demonstrated elevated substance use and substance-related problems in individuals classified as having secondary psychopathy (Hicks et al., 2004; Magyar et al., 2011). Moreover, Skeem et al. (2007) examined substance use-related factors across a wide range of substances, and reported that individuals characterized as displaying secondary psychopathy showed a pattern of more severe substance-related pathology for a variety of substances. Therefore, although primary and secondary psychopathy are described as similar constructs that emerge for different reasons, there is mounting evidence that these two subtypes might represent distinguishable pathologies that meaningfully relate to important clinical outcomes (e.g., violence, substance misuse).

11.1.4 Patterns of Associations Between Psychopathy Across Developmental Stages and SUDs

Psychopathy is associated with earlier substance use initiation. For that reason, youth with elevated psychopathic traits warrant heightened attention as a group at high risk for proceeding along a trajectory of serious, chronic substance misuse. Moreover, some evidence suggests that substance use early in life can place individuals on a trajectory of heightened psychopathic traits (Hawes et al., 2015), thereby further increasing their risk of persistent criminality and violence. Therefore, it is crucial to examine early developmental stages and understand the factors leading to the onset and maintenance of substance use and SUDs.

Generally, similar patterns of associations between substance use and psychopathic traits are found among youth and adults. In terms of SUDs, adolescents with higher levels of psychopathic traits exhibit higher rates of SUDs (Cauffman et al., 2009) and more symptoms of alcohol and drug misuse (Hemphälä & Tengström, 2010; Hillege et al., 2010; Mailloux et al., 1997; Salekin et al., 2004). Harvey et al. (1996) compared adolescent psychiatric patients who abused only one substance (alcohol) with those who abused multiple substances, and reported that the latter group exhibited higher psychopathy scores, implicating psychopathy as a risk factor for abuse of multiple substances. Substance abuse is so strongly linked with psychopathic traits in adolescence that Murrie and Cornell (2000) found that a substance abuse proneness measure correctly classified 79% of adolescents as either high-psychopathy or low-psychopathy, outperforming the various other indices tested.

Levels of psychopathic traits in adolescents also impacts substance use broadly and the nature of use. Adolescents with higher levels of psychopathic traits are more likely to use alcohol, marijuana, and other substances (Dembo et al., 2007). Additionally, adolescents with higher levels of psychopathic initiate use earlier (Corrado et al., 2004; Mailloux et al., 1997). Moreover, adolescents with higher levels of psychopathic traits show greater substance use versatility (Mailloux et al., 1997).

When examining the associations between the Factor scores and substance use among adolescents, patterns of use are largely consistent with findings in adults. Paralleling findings in adults, the impulsive/antisocial (i.e., Factor 2) traits are generally more strongly related to substance use-related factors than the interpersonal/affective (i.e., Factor 1) traits in adolescents. In terms of age at initiation of substance use, while Corrado et al. (2004) found that higher PCL:YV Factor 2 (but not Factor 1) scores were negatively associated with age at initiation of drug use, Mailloux et al. (1997) found that *both* Factor 1 and Factor 2 (also measured using the PCL:YV) were negatively associated with age at initiation of drug use. Furthermore, with respect to substance-related problems, studies consistently identify positive associations between the impulsive/antisocial (Factor 2) traits and SUD symptoms, while evidence is slightly less consistent for positive associations between the interpersonal/affective (Factor 1) traits and SUD symptoms (Gillen et al., 2016; Hillege et al., 2010). Finally, similar to findings in adults, Factor 2 (but not Factor 1) is related to coping motives for substance use in adolescents (Gillen et al., 2016).

The distinction between primary and secondary psychopathy appears similar in regard to the associations with SUDs in adolescents as in adults. Kimonis et al. (2012), using multiple substance-related outcome measures, found that adolescents exhibiting a secondary psychopathy profile had a higher likelihood of meeting criteria for a SUD and reported a higher likelihood of using substances while incarcerated. However, there is mixed evidence regarding the association between primary/secondary psychopathy and other substance-related outcomes in adolescents. Some studies of adolescents found that secondary psychopathy was associated with more frequent use (Kimonis et al., 2012; Vaughn et al., 2009), while a more recent study found that primary and secondary psychopathy were associated with similar baseline levels and rates of increase in alcohol and marijuana use (Waller & Hicks, 2019). Taken together, these findings suggest that even though adolescents who fit profiles of primary versus secondary psychopathy may exhibit similar rates of substance use (at least for certain substance categories such as marijuana), it is the adolescents who fit the profile of the secondary subtype who exhibit higher rates of SUDs and related problems.

Longitudinal investigations of links between psychopathic traits and SUDs represent valuable approaches for identifying developmental trajectories and risk factors associated with the co-occurrence of psychopathy and SUDs. Several longitudinal studies have identified contributions of psychopathy as a unitary construct, as well as the Factors, to substance use outcomes measured at a later timepoint. In terms of psychopathy as a unitary construct, Loney et al. (2007) assessed a sample of male adolescents and found that psychopathy predicted greater nicotine and cannabis (but not alcohol) dependence symptoms at 6-year follow-up. Of note, there is evidence that conceptualizing psychopathy as a unitary construct by considering all four facets of psychopathy (i.e., interpersonal, affective, impulsive, and antisocial traits) provides the most power for predicting future substance use. Specifically, Andershed et al. (2018) grouped adolescents into six mutually exclusive categories based on whether they displayed high or low levels of each psychopathy facet. The adolescents who displayed elevated levels of all four facets were more likely than any other group to exhibit persistently elevated substance use over the following 3 years.

In terms of the psychopathy Factors, consistent with cross-sectional findings, the impulsive/antisocial (i.e., Factor 2) traits are generally a stronger predictor than the interpersonal/affective (i.e., Factor 1) traits of substance-related outcomes, including alcohol and marijuana dependence symptoms (Charalampous et al., 2019; Loney et al., 2007) and drug problems (Vize et al., 2016). However, there is evidence that it is not just the impulsive/antisocial (Factor 2) traits that are important in predicting substance use outcomes; the interpersonal/affective (Factor 1) traits appear to predict some substance-related outcomes as well. Wymbs et al. (2012) assessed CD and CU traits and found that sixth-grade CU traits (akin to Factor 1 traits in adults) uniquely predicted ninth-grade substance use and substance-related problems for both alcohol and marijuana. In another study of adolescents, Baskin-Sommers et al. (2015a, b) reported that a stable trajectory of high CU traits predicted greater substance use versatility in adulthood. Finally, fearless dominance (a construct purportedly analogous to Factor 1, though see critiques by Lynam & Miller, 2012) in youth predicted the presence of alcohol problems (but not drug problems) in adulthood (Vize et al., 2016). Taken together, although findings in adolescents and adults might suggest that the impulsive/antisocial (Factor 2) traits are the driver of the psychopathy-SUD link, it is important to consider all aspects of the unitary psychopathy construct (including the interpersonal/affective traits of Factor 1) to identify youth at highest risk of chronic substance misuse.

Additionally, some recent evidence suggests that it is not only the case that psychopathy predicts substance use outcomes at later timepoints; there also are bidirectional, reciprocal effects of psychopathic traits and substance use. For example, two studies identified prospective associations between alcohol use and the level of psychopathic traits measured at later timepoints. In a sample of adolescents, Charalampous et al. (2019) reported that alcohol dependence symptoms predicted interpersonal psychopathy traits at a later timepoint. In a sample of young justice-involved males, Hawes et al. (2015) used a within-individual approach to examine associations between alcohol use and psychopathic traits over time. They found that increases in alcohol use were associated with increases in subsequent levels of psychopathic traits. More specifically, when an individual engaged in alcohol use that exceeded their normal amount of alcohol consumption (given their overall trajectory), they displayed subsequent increases in psychopathic traits, relative to their average levels of these traits. Thus, it is becoming increasingly clear that substance use can impact the development of psychopathic traits.

11.1.5 Patterns of Associations Between Gender Expressions of Psychopathy and SUDs

Gender is important to consider in the expression of psychopathy. Although the vast majority of psychopathy research has focused on males, the body of research on female psychopathy has grown substantially in recent years (see Verona & Vitale, 2018 for a review). Depending on the specific study, the prevalence rates of psychopathy found among females is lower compared to males (e.g., 9–30% prevalence in females versus 15–25% in males; Nicholls et al., 2005), and females tend to exhibit lower mean levels of psychopathic traits (Salekin et al., 1997). Moreover, although standard assessments (e.g., PCL measures) appear to be acceptable for use in females (Bolt et al., 2004), psychopathy scores on these measures are less predictive of general and violent recidivism in females compared to males (Edens et al., 2007; Odgers et al., 2005; Vincent et al., 2008). Furthermore, consistent with evidence that psychopathy is more strongly related to anxiety and negative emotionality in females compared to males (Vitale et al., 2002), psychopathy in females bears a greater phenotypic resemblance to borderline personality disorder (characterized by pervasive emotional dysregulation and unstable interpersonal relationships) than psychopathy in males (Sprague et al., 2012). Given that psychopathy can manifest differently in females compared to males, it is important to examine potential gender differences in psychopathy's association with substance use-related factors.

The few studies that examined substance use and SUDs as they relate to psychopathy in women indicate that psychopathic traits in women show similar patterns of association with substance use (Miller et al., 2011), substance-related problems (Schulz et al., 2015), and substance use motives (Kennealy et al., 2007) as psychopathic traits in men. Specifically, studies using all-female or mixed-gender samples provide robust evidence that women (similar to men) show impulsive/antisocial (Factor 2)-specific associations with more SUD diagnoses, heavier use of a wide variety of substances, younger age at initiation of illicit drug use, greater substance use versatility, and more SUD symptoms (Kennealy et al., 2007; Rutherford et al., 1996; Schulz et al., 2015; Sellbom et al., 2017). Similar to findings in males, there is some evidence of associations between Factor 1 traits and substance use indices for a circumscribed range of substances (e.g., frequency of opioid use), with evidence for Facet 1 (interpersonal facet) driving this association (Kennealy et al., 2007). Additionally, mirroring findings in males, Factor 2 traits are positively associated with multiple drinking motives (i.e., motives related to facilitating social interactions, coping with negative emotions, and enhancing positive feelings), while Factor 1 traits are unrelated to these motives (Kennealy et al., 2007). Finally, research confirms that secondary psychopathy in women is associated with greater substance use and problems (Hicks et al., 2010).

Studies that used mixed-gender samples and directly compared men and women yield some evidence that gender moderates the associations between psychopathy and substance-related factors. Schulz et al. (2015), who used a sample of community members with drug use problems and histories of incarceration, found that

Factor 2 was more strongly related to illicit drug use in women compared to men, while Factor 1 was more strongly associated with a later age at initiation of drug use in women compared to men. Moreover, in adults there is evidence that Factor 1 is related to substance use in men but not women (Miller et al., 2011). These findings suggest that, to a greater extent in women compared to men, the impulsive/antisocial (i.e., Factor 2) traits exert promotive effects on substance use, whereas the interpersonal/affective (i.e., Factor 1) traits exert protective effects (Schulz et al., 2015). However, Sellbom et al. (2017) failed to find moderating effects of gender across four samples drawn from forensic, correctional, and university settings. More research is needed to clarify whether gender consistently influences the link between psychopathy factors and SUDs, but there is some evidence to suggest that the interpersonal/affective (Factor 1) traits may relate more to SUDs in males compared to females.

When examining gender differences in youth, Hemphälä and Tengström (2010) found evidence that, while Factor 2 (i.e., impulsive/antisocial) traits were positively associated with SUD symptoms (for both alcohol and other drugs) in both males and females in a substance-abusing adolescent sample, it was only among males that Factor 1 (i.e., interpersonal/affective) traits were positively associated with SUD symptoms. Hillege et al. (2010) demonstrated that CU traits (which represent Factor 1 traits) were positively associated with scores on a measure of problematic alcohol use in males but not females. Finally, Wymbs et al. (2012), using a longitudinal design, demonstrated a stronger prospective association between CU traits and substance use outcomes measured at a later timepoint for boys compared to girls. Overall, in combination with the adult data, consideration of the level of affective traits (Facet 2), specifically, as an earlier risk factor (and not just a correlate) for chronic and severe substance use may be particularly important in males compared to females. By contrast, the aspects of psychopathy driving substance use and misuse in females appear to be the impulsive/antisocial (i.e., Factor 2) traits or secondary psychopathy. This association could be consistent with the observation that women with psychopathy tend to exhibit greater emotional dysregulation and impulsivity than what is typically seen in men with psychopathy.

11.2 Mechanisms That Increase Risk for SUDs in Psychopathy

There is clear evidence for a strong association between psychopathy and SUDs. Both cross-sectional and longitudinal studies show that psychopathy increases risk for SUDs, and there is some evidence that SUDs elevate risk for psychopathic traits. In this section, we will explore different levels of analysis to highlight potential reasons underlying the high rates of comorbidity and particular expressions of SUDs in psychopathy. We will review research on personality characteristics, cognitive-affective features, and neural functioning as three levels of analysis particularly important for understanding the association between SUDs and psychopathy.

With respect to personality, there appear to be certain personality characteristics that most strongly contribute to the high rates of overlap between psychopathy and SUDs. In particular, both impulsivity (Hopley & Brunelle, 2012) and sensation seeking (Rutherford et al., 1996) play key roles in driving the behaviors observed in psychopathy and SUDs. As a personality characteristic, impulsivity is considered a tendency to act without planning or consideration, whereas sensation seeking is the tendency to pursue novel or exciting experiences. Notably, both of these personality characteristics conceptually overlap with traits of psychopathy, namely those within the impulsive facet. The association between the impulsive facet and substance misuse (Walsh et al., 2007) might reflect a shared expression of these personality characteristics that increase the severity of SUDs in psychopathy. Moreover, specific subtypes of psychopathy may express these characteristics to a greater extent. For example, alcohol and marijuana use appears to be driven by higher impulsivity (e.g., doing things without thinking, general self-control) for individuals with secondary psychopathy but not primary psychopathy (Waller & Hicks, 2019). Taken together, at the level of personality characteristics, impulsivity and sensation-seeking might be two characteristics that relate to elevated SUDs in psychopathy and/or specific psychopathy subtypes. It is important to note, though, that these characteristics are common across several antisocial expressions (e.g., antisocial personality disorder, general trait externalizing) and should not be considered a specific predictor of psychopathy or related substance use.

At the level of cognitive-affective features, experimental research associates psychopathy with an aberrant expression of interpersonal emotions and an exaggerated fixation on information relevant to immediate goals (Baskin-Sommers & Newman, 2012). As a result of these dysfunctions, individuals with psychopathy tend to adopt a myopic perspective, such that they are particularly adept at focusing directly on an immediate goal, but fail to integrate important contextual cues, such as emotion or cues signaling the consequences of their behavior. This dysfunction may allow individuals with psychopathy to experiment with substances when they are available, but simultaneously interfere with their ability to process, reflect upon, and respond to the negative consequences of their substance use. Thus, individuals with psychopathy may initiate substance use, try a wide variety of substances in a premeditated fashion, and continue use (in spite of problems) because they do not integrate information related to the consequences of their use (Brennan et al., 2017a).

Finally, some studies have examined neural functioning in response to substance-related cues in psychopathy. One functional magnetic resonance imaging (fMRI) study found that adults with psychopathy displayed blunted neural responses to drug cues in craving-related brain regions (e.g., prefrontal cortex and amygdala; Cope et al., 2014), a finding that was replicated in a sample of adolescents (Vincent et al., 2018). Similarly, another fMRI study found that a longer history of substance use was associated with greater neural reactivity to drug-related cues in cocaine-dependent offenders with low levels of psychopathic traits, but not in cocaine-dependent offenders with high levels of psychopathic traits (Denomme et al., 2018). These findings suggest that although individuals with psychopathy can engage in excessive and problematic substance use, they show unique patterns of neural reactivity to substance-related reward cues. Whereas substance-abusing populations generally tend to exhibit neural hyperreactivity to substance-related cues, individuals with psychopathy fail to exhibit this pattern and show *blunted* neural reactivity. One interpretation of this pattern is that, rather than being driven by intense and affectively laden urges to use substances when exposed to substance cues, the substance use of psychopathic individuals may be more purposeful and dissociated from affective processes.

11.3 Assessment Considerations

Throughout the chapter thus far, we highlight the largely consistent findings associating psychopathy to SUDs. However, some issues related to the assessment of psychopathy and SUDs were apparent in the above review. Namely, what measures were used in research and what constructs were measured in each study seemed to impact the pattern of findings. In the following sections, we will discuss important considerations for the assessment of psychopathy and substance use.

11.3.1 Assessing Psychopathy

There are many areas to consider when assessing people for SUDs, including their pattern of use, routes of administration, and biopsychosocial history. In this section, we will highlight two important considerations for assessing psychopathy in individuals with excessive substance use or SUDs. First, it is crucial to consider the specific characteristics of the sample or individual client. Second, it is crucial to consider the availability of collateral information (e.g., institutional records; family member's report).

There are several well-validated measures of psychopathy. In correctional populations, as noted above, the PCL-R is the gold standard measure of psychopathy. While the PCL-R appears to be a reliable and valid measure of psychopathy and its Factor structure has been well-replicated (Alterman et al., 1993; Rutherford et al., 1996), interpretations of PCL-R Factor scores should be made with caution in non-incarcerated SUD patients, based on evidence that the two-factor structure may not generalize to these individuals (McDermott et al., 2000). More specifically, instead of a two-factor structure, McDermott et al. (2000) found that a unitary model of psychopathy (i.e., psychopathy total score) provided the best fit within a substance-dependent sample. The main implication of this finding for assessing psychopathy is that, when using the PCL-R with individuals who present primarily as SUD patients, it may be more useful to base clinical formulations and recommendations on a consideration of the more parsimonious total PCL-R score, rather than on separate consideration of the two factor scores. However, one way to tap distinct expressions of unitary psychopathy would be to evaluate the primary and secondary psychopathy subtypes using measures of trait anxiety (e.g., State-Trait Anxiety Inventory Trait Scale; Spielberger et al., 1983) or negative emotionality (Multidimensional Personality Questionnaire—Brief; Patrick et al., 2002). Consideration of these subtypes might provide clues into the nature of substance use and misuse for individuals expressing different psychopathy subtypes, despite both subtypes displaying high psychopathic phenotypes.

When collateral information is unavailable or when time or resources (e.g., for assessment or training staff) are limited, another possibility for assessing psychopathy in individuals with SUDs is to use a validated self-report measure of psychopathic traits. For adults, well-validated self-report measures across several types of samples (e.g., community, incarcerated, college students) are the Self-Report Psychopathy Scale (SRP; Paulhus et al., 2017) and the Psychopathic Personality Index (PPI; Lilienfeld & Widows, 2005). For adolescents, validated self-report measures include the Youth Psychopathic Traits Inventory (YPI; Andershed et al., 2002) and the self-report version of the Antisocial Process Screening Device (APSD; Frick & Hare, 2001).[3] Although total scores on all of these measures generally show expected positive relationships with substance use and misuse (e.g., Neal & Sellbom, 2012; Poythress et al., 2006), there is important variability among measures that should be taken into consideration when deciding how to assess psychopathic traits.

For example, in terms of adult measures, the PPI may not be the most useful measure for clinical risk assessment or SUD treatment purposes. Findings indicate that PPI Factor 1 (i.e., fearless dominance) generally exhibits negative correlations with substance-related factors (Hunt et al., 2015) and appears to index traits that are more adaptive and more protective (e.g., against SUDs) than Factor 1 scores derived from other measures (Miller & Lynam, 2012). In terms of youth measures, findings indicate that the YPI appears to be poorly suited for indexing liability for SUDs; thus, like the PPI, the YPI may be an inappropriate choice for assessing psychopathic traits when the practical purpose is clinical risk assessment or treatment. Two separate longitudinal studies (Colins et al., 2015; Vaughn et al., 2008) that used the YPI to assess psychopathy failed to replicate previous findings of a prospective association between psychopathic traits and substance use outcomes later in life. This may be related to the fact that the YPI is based on a three-factor model and thus omits items indexing antisocial aspects of psychopathy, which are known to relate strongly to substance misuse (Coid et al., 2009a). In sum, self-report measures can provide efficient and low-cost means of assessing psychopathy, but the suitability of each measure for the goal at hand should be carefully considered.

[3] The Inventory of Callous-Unemotional Traits (ICU; Kimonis et al., 2008) is a validated measure of the affective traits of psychopathy for children, adolescents, and young adults, but based on evidence for the importance of all four psychopathy facets in predicting substance-related outcomes, the ICU should not be used as a stand-alone psychopathy measure; instead, if the ICU is used, another measure indexing the remaining psychopathic traits (i.e., interpersonal, impulsive, and antisocial) should be used alongside it.

11.3.2 Assessing SUDs

The assessment of SUDs in individuals with psychopathy involves special considerations based on evidence that unique personality and SUD profiles characterize psychopathy. In this section, we will highlight three areas for evaluators to consider in their assessments. First, an evaluator should take into account an individual's level of insight. Second, it is important for an evaluator to consider the expression and nature of substance use and SUDs within psychopathy. Finally, evaluators should reflect on an individual's motivations for using substances.

When assessing SUDs in individuals with elevated psychopathic traits, clinicians must remain aware of the tendency among individuals with psychopathy to lack insight into the effects of their behavior on others and to minimize problems in general. The implications of these tendencies are that clinicians must ask targeted, specific questions that rely as little as possible on the patient's subjective interpretation of the effects of their substance use. For example, when administering the SCID-5 for SUDs, after posing the question, "Did your use of alcohol ever cause problems with other people?" the clinician should ask targeted follow-up questions based on their knowledge of the individual's life history and relationships. Examples of targeted follow-up questions are: "Did your girlfriend ever complain that she did not like the way you acted when you drank alcohol?" or "Did your parents ever threaten to kick you out of the house because of your alcohol use?" These follow-up questions are not only more specific than the broad question of interpersonal problems (and thus more likely to cue recall of relevant experiences); they also frame the questions in a way that does not require the individual to make a value judgment about whether their substance use was problematic, but instead prompt the individual to relate whether an event occurred.

SUDs are diagnosed at a high rate among individuals with psychopathy. However, for individuals with psychopathy, the symptom profile of SUDs maybe expressed in a different way than in those without psychopathy. Evidence shows that individuals with psychopathy who meet criteria for SUDs may be less likely to experience symptoms of craving and withdrawal compared to individuals without psychopathy who meet criteria for SUDs (Cleckley, 1941; Cope et al., 2014). Thus, it is important for clinicians to recognize that the absence of craving and/or withdrawal experienced by a SUD patient with psychopathy should not necessarily indicate that the patient has less SUD-related impairment.

The nature of substance use in individuals with psychopathy is likely to differ from that in individuals without psychopathy. Cleckley (1941) noted, "[a] major point about the psychopath and his relation to alcohol can be found in the shocking, fantastic, uninviting, or relatively inexplicable behavior which emerges when he drinks—sometimes when he drinks only a little." (p. 365). In particular, it is useful to differentiate between substance use and substance-related problems. Although heavier or more frequent substance use is related to more severe problems, these two aspects of an individual's experience do not exhibit a one-to-one correspondence. For example, someone may drink alcohol daily and experience a similar (or lesser) degree of alcohol-related problems compared to an individual who drinks alcohol heavily twice per week. In these cases, more frequent use (i.e., daily use) does not translate into more alcohol-related problems. This may be a self-evident point, but it is highlighted here because many research studies combine these categories into a composite variable or do not specify which category they are measuring. This issue not only limits the ability to draw more fine-grained conclusions about the associations between psychopathy and substance-related factors, but also reduces the likelihood of capturing the full substance-related experience of individuals with psychopathy. Taken together, it is useful to consider separately several aspects of substance use and related problems.

Finally, substance use motives are an important mediating factor in the association between psychopathy and severity of substance-related pathology, particularly for individuals with high levels of impulsive/antisocial (i.e., Factor 2) traits. A comprehensive assessment of SUDs in individuals would benefit from inclusion of a measure of substance use motives (e.g., the Drinking Motives Questionnaire Revised; Cooper, 1994; Risky, Impulsive, Self-Destructive Behavior Questionnaire; Sadeh & Baskin-Sommers, 2016) to enhance understanding of the function(s) of substance use for a given individual and to inform treatment planning. Conversely, a different approach may be warranted for individuals whose interpersonal/affective (i.e., Factor 1) traits dominate the clinical picture. Although the literature suggests that substance use motives (as traditionally assessed) do not appear to explain the substance use behavior of individuals with higher levels of interpersonal/affective traits, there are some important caveats to bear in mind. It is possible that the more common and traditionally assessed substance use motives (e.g., coping) simply do not fit the experience of individuals with high interpersonal/affective traits, and that alternative, yet-to-be-identified motives better explain these individuals' substance use. It also is possible that the more traditionally assessed motives do apply to individuals with higher interpersonal/affective traits, but that these individuals lack insight into their own motives, perhaps in part owing to their affective deficits (Patrick, 2007). These two possibilities suggest that it is important not to rely completely on pre-existing measures of substance use motives, to ask open-ended questions about the individual's motives that may identify motives not captured by existing measures, to conduct functional analyses of substance use behavior, and to discuss the insights generated in a collaborative manner with the individual. Together, these strategies will allow for greater progress toward gaining insight and uncovering candidate motives and/or functions of substance use in individuals with psychopathy.

11.4 Clinical Interventions

Drug-related problems exact an enormous cost on society. Offenders account for over $107 billion of the $181 billion annual cost of drug abuse in the United States (National Institute on Drug Abuse, 2006). Therefore, the development of more efficacious and cost-effective interventions for offenders with SUDs is a necessity from both a public health and cost-benefit perspective. Moreover, there are special considerations when working with individuals with psychopathy in a clinical context.

Traditional psychotherapy approaches for psychopathy focus on changing the general personality structure of individuals with psychopathy through lengthy courses of talk therapy. This is in contrast to a leading model of offender treatment, the risk-need-responsivity (RNR) model (Bonta & Andrews, 2007), which promotes the idea that treatment of high-risk offenders (e.g., offenders with psychopathy) should focus on modifying specific risk factors (e.g., substance misuse) known to contribute to engagement in criminal and violent behavior. Consistent with the RNR model, modern treatment approaches suggest that more targeted strategies for reducing harmful substance use behaviors can be beneficial.

For example, recent work has evaluated interventions that target substance use in individuals with elevated psychopathic traits using motivational interviewing (MI) approaches. MI is a therapeutic technique that aims to build intrinsic motivation to change by guiding clients to explore and resolve ambivalence. It emphasizes the client's autonomy by framing change as something that is completely up to the client, and it manages resistance by highlighting how the client could benefit from reducing problematic behaviors. Research demonstrates that it is generally effective for reducing substance use among both adults (Smedslund et al., 2011) and adolescents (Jensen et al., 2011). Yet, evidence for the effectiveness of this treatment for individuals with psychopathy and SUDs is mixed. Salekin et al. (2012) found that a 12-session treatment program that included MI techniques was effective at reducing CU traits and improving behavior. By contrast, Swogger et al. (2016) found that individuals with high levels of Factor 1 (i.e., interpersonal/affective) traits had worse substance use outcomes following brief MI. It is well-documented that individuals with psychopathy are less likely to present for treatment voluntarily (Durbeej et al., 2014; Swogger et al., 2016), and thus exhibit lower levels of motivation to change. To increase treatment engagement among individuals with high levels of interpersonal/affective traits, clinicians may focus on maximizing self-relevance within the MI context. For example, during an MI intervention, the clinician might highlight the ways in which reducing substance use can benefit the client in terms of enhancing their status, increasing their earnings, achieving their own personal goals, and attaining freedom. However, more research is needed to examine the impact of length of intervention and at what stage of development the intervention might be most effective (e.g., in youth versus adults).

As another example of a targeted intervention approach, recent work has evaluated cognitive remediation interventions that target the psychopathy-specific cognitive-affective mechanisms that are thought to drive harmful substance use. Baskin-Sommers et al. (2015a, b) developed and tested a computerized training package for adult offenders with psychopathy and SUDs. The training package was designed specifically to remediate the key cognitive-affective dysfunctions that characterize psychopathy; namely, to enhance integration of contextual cues, particularly emotion. Results demonstrated that individuals who completed the targeted training package (consisting of six weekly sessions) demonstrated improved cognitive-affective functioning, both on trained tasks as well as more general (non-trained) cognitive-affective tasks. An aspect of the study design worth noting was that offenders were divided into two groups: a psychopathy group and an externalizing group. Using a 2 × 2 crossover design, offenders characterized as psychopathic or as externalizing were randomly assigned to one of two computerized training packages. In contrast with the psychopathy training package, the externalizing package was designed to ameliorate cognitive-affective dysfunctions associated with externalizing; namely, to improve inhibitory control and enhance the regulation of affect. As with the psychopathy group, only those from the externalizing group that received the etiology-matched training improved on trained and non-trained tasks indexing externalizing-specific dysfunctions. Moreover, there was evidence of iatrogenic effects of training if externalizing individuals received training that did not target their underlying etiology. These findings highlight the utility of cognitive remediation as a strategy for intervening on SUDs in psychopathy and emphasize the importance of targeting the specific mechanisms associated with subtypes of antisocial offenders.

The recommendations to consider MI and cognitive remediation are just two examples of treatment approaches that follow from understanding the psychopathic presentation and how that relates to substance use. However, the heterogeneity among individuals with psychopathy has important implications for tailoring SUD interventions to address each individual's characteristics, needs, and motivations (Gudonis et al., 2009). Considering the presentation and underlying motivations of a secondary psychopathy or female psychopathy presentation might indicate a focus on emotional aspects of behavior (e.g., Dialectical Behavior Therapy; Dimeff & Linehan, 2008). Regardless of the specific approach, across therapeutic interventions, it is necessary to identify and target the underlying mechanisms that drive behavior within the individual.

11.5 Conclusions

This chapter reviewed psychopathy's robust associations with a variety of substance use-related indices, including heightened diagnosis risk, greater substance use, greater substance use versatility, earlier substance use initiation, and more severe substance-related problems. The impulsive/antisocial traits of psychopathy (i.e., Factor 2) are the main driver of these effects. When the impulsive facet (Facet 3) and the antisocial facet (Facet 4) are examined, the impulsive facet, which includes traits such as impulsivity and need for stimulation/proneness to boredom, appears more strongly associated with substance use and substance-related problems. However, longitudinal studies provide evidence that the unitary psychopathy construct (i.e., traits across *both* interpersonal/affective [i.e., Factor 1] and impulsive/antisocial traits) predict trajectories of chronic and elevated substance use and substance-related pathology. While interpersonal/affective traits are not consistently associated with substance use motives, impulsive/antisocial traits show associations with emotion-based motives for substance use, including coping with negative emotions and enhancing positive emotions. Mirroring effects for psychopathy factors, secondary psychopathy is associated with more severe substance-related pathology compared to primary psychopathy. Overall, it is clear that psychopathy is related to substance use, but there is important nuance when characterizing this relationship.

Future research should focus on building knowledge in several key domains. First, more research is needed to characterize patterns of associations between psychopathy and the DSM-5 SUD symptoms and diagnoses. Second, future research efforts should aim to assess different substance-related indices (e.g., frequency of use, severity of substance-related problems) separately to build a more in-depth understanding of the associations between psychopathy and substance use. Finally, and most importantly, more rigorous controlled treatment studies are needed to evaluate treatments for SUDs in psychopathy and build more effective treatments for dissemination among individuals with psychopathy. One crucial question as it relates to the treatment of SUDs in psychopathy is whether treating SUDs can lead to improvements in terms of other outcomes (e.g., lowered recidivism, decreased aggression) in individuals with psychopathy. Although this question has not been directly tested, research suggests that SUDs exacerbate the dangerous behavior of individuals with psychopathy and thus represent a worthy target for intervention. Targeted interventions designed to match the distinctive personality characteristics, cognitive-affective features, and neural functions of individuals with psychopathy have shown promise thus far, and continued efforts along these lines can lead to further progress in reducing the dangerousness of psychopathy.

References

Alterman, A. I., Cacciola, J. S., & Rutherford, M. J. (1993). Reliability of the revised psychopathy checklist in substance abuse patients. *Psychological Assessment, 5*(4), 442–448. https://doi.org/10.1037/1040-3590.5.4.442

American Psychiatric Association. (2000). *Diagnostic and statistical manual of mental disorders (DSM-IV-TR)*. American Psychiatric Publishing.

American Psychiatric Association. (2013). *Diagnostic and statistical manual of mental disorders (DSM-5)*. American Psychiatric Publishing.

Andershed, H. A., Kerr, M., Stattin, H., & Levander, S. (2002). Psychopathic traits in non-referred youths: A new assessment tool. In E. Blaauw & L. Sheridan (Eds.), *Psychopaths: Current international perspectives* (pp. 131–158). Elsevier.

Andershed, H. A., Colins, O. F., Salekin, R. T., Lordos, A., Kyranides, M. N., & Fanti, K. A. (2018). Callous-unemotional traits only versus the multidimensional psychopathy construct as predictors of various antisocial outcomes during early adolescence. *Journal of Psychopathology and Behavioral Assessment, 40*(1), 16–25. https://doi.org/10.1007/s10862-018-9659-5

Baskin-Sommers, A., & Newman, J. P. (2012). Cognition-emotion interactions in psychopathy: Implications for theory and practice. In *Psychopathy and law: A practitioner's guide* (1st ed., pp. 79–97). Wiley.

Baskin-Sommers, A., Curtin, J. J., & Newman, J. P. (2015a). Altering the cognitive-affective dysfunctions of psychopathic and externalizing offender subtypes with cognitive remediation. *Clinical Psychological Science, 3*(1), 45–57. https://doi.org/10.1177/2167702614560744

Baskin-Sommers, A., Waller, R., Fish, A. M., & Hyde, L. W. (2015b). Callous-unemotional traits trajectories interact with earlier conduct problems and executive control to predict violence and substance use among high risk male adolescents. *Journal of Abnormal Child Psychology, 43*(8), 1529–1541. https://doi.org/10.1007/s10802-015-0041-8

Birkley, E. L., Giancola, P. R., & Lance, C. E. (2013). Psychopathy and the prediction of alcohol-related physical aggression: The roles of impulsive antisociality and fearless dominance. *Drug and Alcohol Dependence, 128*(1–2), 58–63. https://doi.org/10.1016/j.drugalcdep.2012.08.011

Blackburn, R., & Lee-Evans, J. M. (1985). Reactions of primary and secondary psychopaths to anger-evoking situations. *British Journal of Clinical Psychology, 24*(2), 93–100. https://doi.org/10.1111/j.2044-8260.1985.tb01319.x

Bolt, D. M., Hare, R. D., Vitale, J. E., & Newman, J. P. (2004). A multigroup item response theory analysis of the psychopathy checklist–revised. *Psychological Assessment, 16*(2), 155–168. https://doi.org/10.1037/1040-3590.16.2.155

Bonta, J., & Andrews, D. A. (2007). Risk-need-responsivity model for offender assessment and rehabilitation. *Rehabilitation, 6*(1), 1–22.

Brennan, G. M., Hyde, L. W., & Baskin-Sommers, A. R. (2017a). Antisocial pathways associated with substance use disorders: Characterizing etiological underpinnings and implications for treatment. *Current Opinion in Behavioral Sciences, 13*, 124–129.

Brennan, G. M., Stuppy-Sullivan, A. M., Brazil, I. A., & Baskin-Sommers, A. R. (2017b). Differentiating patterns of substance misuse by subtypes of antisocial traits in male offenders. *The Journal of Forensic Psychiatry & Psychology, 28*(3), 341–356. https://doi.org/10.1080/14789949.2017.1280072

Brook, D. W., Brook, J. S., Zhang, C., Cohen, P., & Whiteman, M. (2002). Drug use and the risk of major depressive disorder, alcohol dependence, and substance use disorders. *Archives of General Psychiatry, 59*(11), 1039–1044.

Cauffman, E., Kimonis, E. R., Dmitrieva, J., & Monahan, K. C. (2009). A multimethod assessment of juvenile psychopathy: Comparing the predictive utility of the PCL:YV, YPI, and NEO PRI. *Psychological Assessment, 21*(4), 528–542. https://doi.org/10.1037/a0017367

Charalampous, K., Stavrinides, P., Georgiou, S., & Giasemidou, P. (2019). Is there a psychopathic element in adolescent drinking? A longitudinal study. *European Journal of Developmental Psychology, 16*(1), 47–65. https://doi.org/10.1080/17405629.2017.1334547

Cleckley, H. (1941). *The mask of sanity*. Mosby.

Coid, J., Yang, M., Ullrich, S., Roberts, A., & Hare, R. D. (2009a). Prevalence and correlates of psychopathic traits in the household population of Great Britain. *International Journal of Law & Psychiatry, 32*(2), 65–73. https://doi.org/10.1016/j.ijlp.2009.01.002

Coid, J., Yang, M., Ullrich, S., Roberts, A., Moran, P., Bebbington, P., et al. (2009b). Psychopathy among prisoners in England and Wales. *International Journal of Law and Psychiatry, 32*(3), 134–141. https://doi.org/10.1016/j.ijlp.2009.02.008

Colins, O. F., Andershed, H., & Pardini, D. A. (2015). Psychopathic traits as predictors of future criminality, intimate partner aggression, and substance use in young adult men. *Law and Human Behavior, 39*(6), 547–558. https://doi.org/10.1037/lhb0000148

Compton, W. M., Conway, K. P., Stinson, F. S., Colliver, J. D., & Grant, B. F. (2005). Prevalence, correlates, and comorbidity of DSM-IV antisocial personality syndromes and alcohol and specific drug use disorders in the United States: Results from the National Epidemiologic Survey on Alcohol and Related Conditions. *The Journal of Clinical Psychiatry, 66*(6), 677–685.

Compton, W. M., Thomas, Y. F., Stinson, F. S., & Grant, B. F. (2007). Prevalence, correlates, disability, and comorbidity of DSM-IV drug abuse and dependence in the United States: Results from the National Epidemiologic Survey on Alcohol and Related Conditions. *Archives of General Psychiatry, 64*(5), 566–576. https://doi.org/10.1001/archpsyc.64.5.566

Cooke, D. J., & Michie, C. (2001). Refining the construct of psychopathy: Towards a hierarchical model. *Psychological Assessment, 13*(2), 171–188.

Cooper, M. L. (1994). Motivations for alcohol use among adolescents: Development and validation of a four-factor model. *Psychological Assessment, 6*(2), 117–128. https://doi.org/10.1037/1040-3590.6.2.117

Cope, L. M., Vincent, G. M., Jobelius, J. L., Nyalakanti, P. K., Calhoun, V. D., & Kiehl, K. A. (2014). Psychopathic traits modulate brain responses to drug cues in incarcerated offenders. *Frontiers in Human Neuroscience, 8*, 87. Retrieved from https://doi.org/10.3389/fnhum.2014.00087

Corrado, R. R., Vincent, G. M., Hart, S. D., & Cohen, I. M. (2004). Predictive validity of the psychopathy checklist: Youth version for general and violent recidivism. *Behavioral Sciences & the Law, 22*(1), 5–22. https://doi.org/10.1002/bsl.574

Dembo, R., Jainchill, N., Turner, C., Fong, C., Farkas, S., & Childs, K. (2007). Levels of psychopathy and its correlates: A study of incarcerated youths in three states. *Behavioral Sciences & the Law, 25*(5), 717–738. https://doi.org/10.1002/bsl.784

Denomme, W. J., Simard, I., & Shane, M. S. (2018). Neuroimaging metrics of drug and food processing in cocaine-dependence, as a function of psychopathic traits and substance use severity. *Frontiers in Human Neuroscience, 12*(350). https://doi.org/10.3389/fnhum.2018.00350

Dimeff, L. A., & Linehan, M. M. (2008). Dialectical behavior therapy for substance abusers. *Addiction Science & Clinical Practice, 4*(2), 39–47.

Durbeej, N., Palmstierna, T., Berman, A. H., Kristiansson, M., & Gumpert, C. H. (2014). Offenders with mental health problems and problematic substance use: Affective psychopathic personality traits as potential barriers to participation in substance abuse interventions. *Journal of Substance Abuse Treatment, 46*(5), 574–583. https://doi.org/10.1016/j.jsat.2014.01.002

Edens, J. F., Campbell, J. S., & Weir, J. M. (2007). Youth psychopathy and criminal recidivism: A meta-analysis of the psychopathy checklist measures. *Law and Human Behavior, 31*(1), 53–75. https://doi.org/10.1007/s10979-006-9019-y

Fazel, S., Bains, P., & Doll, H. (2006). Substance abuse and dependence in prisoners: A systematic review. *Addiction, 101*(2), 181–191. https://doi.org/10.1111/j.1360-0443.2006.01316.x

Forth, A. E., Kosson, D. S., & Hare, R. D. (2003). *The Hare psychopathy checklist: Youth version*. Multi-Health Systems.

Frick, P. J. (2009). Extending the construct of psychopathy to youth: Implications for understanding, diagnosing, and treating antisocial children and adolescents. *The Canadian Journal of Psychiatry, 54*(12), 803–812.

Frick, P. J., & Hare, R. D. (2001). *The antisocial process screening device*. Multi-Health Systems.

Gillen, C. T. A., Barry, C. T., & Bater, L. R. (2016). Anxiety symptoms and coping motives: Examining a potential path to substance use-related problems in adolescents with psychopathic traits. *Substance Use & Misuse, 51*(14), 1920–1929. https://doi.org/10.1080/10826084.2016.1201510

Grant, B. F., Hasin, D. S., Stinson, F. S., Dawson, D. A., Chou, S. P., Ruan, W. J., et al. (2004). Prevalence, correlates, and disability of personality disorders in the United States: Results from the National Epidemiologic Survey on alcohol and related conditions. *Journal of Clinical Psychiatry, 65*(7), 948–958. https://doi.org/10.1001/archpsyc.64.5.566

Gretton, H. M., Hare, R. D., & Catchpole, R. E. (2004). Psychopathy and offending from adolescence to adulthood: A 10-year follow-up. *Journal of Consulting and Clinical Psychology, 72*(4), 636–645. https://doi.org/10.1037/0022-006x.72.4.636

Gruber, E., DiClemente, R. J., Anderson, M. M., & Lodico, M. (1996). Early drinking onset and its association with alcohol use and problem behavior in late adolescence. *Preventive Medicine, 25*(3), 293–300. https://doi.org/10.1006/pmed.1996.0059

Gudonis, L. C., Derefinko, K., & Giancola, P. R. (2009). The treatment of substance misuse in psychopathic individuals: Why heterogeneity matters. *Substance Use & Misuse, 44*(9–10), 1415–1433. https://doi.org/10.1080/10826080902961625

Gustavson, C., Ståhlberg, O., Sjödin, A.-K., Forsman, A., Nilsson, T., & Anckarsäter, H. (2007). Age at onset of substance abuse: A crucial covariate of psychopathic traits and aggression in adult offenders. *Psychiatry Research, 153*(2), 195–198. https://doi.org/10.1016/j.psychres.2006.12.020

Hare, R. D. (2003). *Manual for the revised psychopathy checklist* (2nd ed.). Multi-Health Systems.

Hare, R. D., & McPherson, L. M. (1984). Violent and aggressive behavior by criminal psychopaths. *International Journal of Law & Psychiatry, 7*(1), 35–50. https://doi.org/10.1016/0160-2527(84)90005-0

Hare, R. D., & Neumann, C. S. (2005). Structural models of psychopathy. *Current Psychiatry Reports, 7*(1), 57–64.

Hare, R. D., Harpur, T. J., Hakstian, A. R., Forth, A. E., Hart, S. D., & Newman, J. P. (1990). The revised psychopathy checklist: Reliability and factor structure. *Psychological Assessment: A Journal of Consulting and Clinical Psychology, 2*(3), 338–341. https://doi.org/10.1037/1040-3590.2.3.338

Harpur, T. J., Hare, R. D., & Hakstian, A. R. (1989). Two-factor conceptualization of psychopathy: Construct validity and assessment implications. *Psychological Assessment, 1*, 6–17. https://doi.org/10.1037/1040-3590.1.1.6

Hart, S. D., & Hare, R. D. (1989). Discriminant validity of the psychopathy checklist in a forensic psychiatric population. *Psychological Assessment, 1*(3), 211–218. https://doi.org/10.1037/1040-3590.1.3.211

Hart, S. D., Forth, A. E., & Hare, R. D. (1991). The MCMI-II and psychopathy. *Journal of Personality Disorders, 5*(4), 318–327. https://doi.org/10.1521/pedi.1991.5.4.318

Harvey, P. D., Stokes, J. L., Lord, J., & Pogge, D. L. (1996). Neurocognitive and personality assessment of adolescent substance abusers: A multidimensional approach. *Assessment, 3*(3), 241–253. https://doi.org/10.1177/107319119600300305

Hasin, D. S., Stinson, F. S., Ogburn, E., & Grant, B. F. (2007). Prevalence, correlates, disability, and comorbidity of DSM-IV alcohol abuse and dependence in the United States: Results from the National Epidemiologic Survey on Alcohol and Related Conditions. *Archives of General Psychiatry, 64*(7), 830–842. https://doi.org/10.1001/archpsyc.64.7.830

Hawes, S. W., Crane, C. A., Henderson, C. E., Mulvey, E. P., Schubert, C. A., & Pardini, D. A. (2015). Codevelopment of psychopathic features and alcohol use during emerging adulthood: Disaggregating between- and within-person change. *Journal of Abnormal Psychology, 124*(3), 729–739. https://doi.org/10.1037/abn0000075

Hemphälä, M., & Tengström, A. (2010). Associations between psychopathic traits and mental disorders among adolescents with substance use problems. *British Journal of Clinical Psychology, 49*(1), 109–122. https://doi.org/10.1348/014466509x439216

Hemphill, J. F., Hart, S. D., & Hare, R. (1994). Psychopathy and substance use. *Journal of Personality Disorders, 8*(3), 169–180. https://doi.org/10.1521/pedi.1994.8.3.169

Herpers, P. C., Rommelse, N. N., Bons, D. M., Buitelaar, J. K., & Scheepers, F. E. (2012). Callous–unemotional traits as a cross-disorders construct. *Social Psychiatry and Psychiatric Epidemiology, 47*(12), 2045–2064.

Hicks, B. M., Markon, K. E., Patrick, C. J., Krueger, R. F., & Newman, J. P. (2004). Identifying psychopathy subtypes on the basis of personality structure. *Psychological Assessment, 16*(3), 276–288. https://doi.org/10.1037/1040-3590.16.3.276

Hicks, B. M., Vaidyanathan, U., & Patrick, C. J. (2010). Validating female psychopathy subtypes: Differences in personality, antisocial and violent behavior, substance abuse, trauma, and mental health. *Personality Disorders: Theory, Research, and Treatment, 1*(1), 38–57. https://doi.org/10.1037/a0018135

Hicks, B. M., Carlson, M. D., Blonigen, D. M., Patrick, C. J., Iacono, W. G., & Mcgue, M. (2012). Psychopathic personality traits and environmental contexts: Differential correlates, gender differences, and genetic mediation. *Personality Disorders: Theory, Research, and Treatment, 3*(3), 209–227. https://doi.org/10.1037/a0025084

Hillege, S., Das, J., & de Ruiter, C. (2010). The youth psychopathic traits inventory: Psychometric properties and its relation to substance use and interpersonal style in a Dutch sample of non-referred adolescents. *Journal of Adolescence, 33*(1), 83–91. https://doi.org/10.1016/j.adolescence.2009.05.006

Hopley, A. A., & Brunelle, C. (2012). Personality mediators of psychopathy and substance dependence in male offenders. *Addictive Behaviors, 37*(8), 947–955. https://doi.org/10.1016/j.addbeh.2012.03.031

Hunt, E., Bornovalova, M. A., Kimonis, E. R., Lilienfeld, S. O., & Poythress, N. G. (2015). Psychopathy factor interactions and co-occurring psychopathology: Does measurement approach matter? *Psychological Assessment, 27*(2), 583–595. https://doi.org/10.1037/pas0000055

Hyman, S. M., & Sinha, R. (2009). Stress-related factors in cannabis use and misuse: Implications for prevention and treatment. *Journal of Substance Abuse Treatment, 36*(4), 400–413. https://doi.org/10.1016/j.jsat.2008.08.005

Jensen, C. D., Cushing, C. C., Aylward, B. S., Craig, J. T., Sorell, D. M., & Steele, R. G. (2011). Effectiveness of motivational interviewing interventions for adolescent substance use behavior change: A meta-analytic review. *Journal of Consulting and Clinical Psychology, 79*(4), 433–440. https://doi.org/10.1037/a0023992

Karpman, B. (1941). On the need of separating psychopathy into two distinct clinical types: The symptomatic and the idiopathic. *Journal of Criminology and Psychopathology, 3*, 112–137.

Kennealy, P. J., Hicks, B. M., & Patrick, C. J. (2007). Validity of factors of the psychopathy checklist—Revised in female prisoners: Discriminant relations with antisocial behavior, substance abuse, and personality. *Assessment, 14*(4), 323–340. https://doi.org/10.1177/1073191107305882

Kiehl, K. A., & Hoffman, M. B. (2011). The criminal psychopath: History, neuroscience, treatment, and economics. *Jurimetrics, 51*, 355–397.

Kimonis, E. R., Frick, P. J., Skeem, J. L., Marsee, M. A., Cruise, K., Munoz, L. C., et al. (2008). Assessing callous–unemotional traits in adolescent offenders: Validation of the inventory of callous–unemotional traits. *International Journal of Law and Psychiatry, 31*(3), 241–252. https://doi.org/10.1016/j.ijlp.2008.04.002

Kimonis, E. R., Skeem, J. L., Cauffman, E., & Dmitrieva, J. (2011). Are secondary variants of juvenile psychopathy more reactively violent and less psychosocially mature than primary variants? *Law and Human Behavior, 35*(5), 381–391. https://doi.org/10.1007/s10979-010-9243-3

Kimonis, E. R., Tatar, J. R., & Cauffman, E. (2012). Substance-related disorders among juvenile offenders: What role do psychopathic traits play? *Psychology of Addictive Behaviors, 26*(2), 212–225. https://doi.org/10.1037/a0028047

Korponay, C., Pujara, M., Deming, P., Philippi, C., Decety, J., Kosson, D. S., et al. (2017). Impulsive-antisocial psychopathic traits linked to increased volume and functional connectivity within prefrontal cortex. *Social Cognitive and Affective Neuroscience, 12*, 1169–1178.

Kosson, D. S., Cyterski, T. D., Steuerwald, B. L., Neumann, C. S., & Walker-Matthews, S. (2002). The reliability and validity of the psychopathy checklist: Youth version (PCL: YV) in nonincarcerated adolescent males. *Psychological Assessment, 14*(1), 97.

Kramer, M. P., Stevenson, B. L., & Dvorak, R. D. (2017). Primary psychopathy and alcohol pathology in college students: The role of protective behavioral strategies. *The American Journal of Drug and Alcohol Abuse, 43*(6), 719–726. https://doi.org/10.1080/00952990.2016.1278222

Kruh, I. P., Frick, P. J., & Clements, C. B. (2005). Historical and personality correlates to the violence patterns of juveniles tried as adults. *Criminal Justice and Behavior, 32*(1), 69–96. https://doi.org/10.1177/0093854804270629

Lilienfeld, S. O., & Widows, M. R. (2005). *Psychopathic personality inventory-revised: Professional manual*. Psychological Assessment Resources.

Loney, B. R., Taylor, J., Butler, M. A., & Iacono, W. G. (2007). Adolescent psychopathy features: 6-year temporal stability and the prediction of externalizing symptoms during the transition to adulthood. *Aggressive Behavior, 33*(3), 242–252. https://doi.org/10.1002/ab.20184

Lynam, D. R., Whiteside, S., & Jones, S. (1999). Self-reported psychopathy: A validation study. *Journal of Personality Assessment, 73*(1), 110–132.

Lynam, D. R., Hoyle, R. H., & Newman, J. P. (2006). The perils of partialling: Cautionary tales from aggression and psychopathy. *Assessment, 13*(3), 328–341. https://doi.org/10.1177/1073191106290562

Lynam, D. R., Caspi, A., Moffitt, T. E., Loeber, R., & Stouthamer-Loeber, M. (2007). Longitudinal evidence that psychopathy scores in early adolescence predict adult psychopathy. *Journal of Abnormal Psychology, 116*(1), 155–165. https://doi.org/10.1037/0021-843X.116.1.155

Lynam, D. R., & Miller, J. D. (2012). Fearless dominance and psychopathy: A response to Lilienfeld et al. *Personality Disorders: Theory, Research, and Treatment, 3*(3), 341–353.

Magyar, M. S., Edens, J. F., Lilienfeld, S. O., Douglas, K. S., & Poythress, N. G., Jr. (2011). Examining the relationship among substance abuse, negative emotionality and impulsivity across subtypes of antisocial and psychopathic substance abusers. *Journal of Criminal Justice, 39*(3), 232–237. https://doi.org/10.1016/j.jcrimjus.2011.02.013

Mailloux, D. L., Forth, A. E., & Kroner, D. G. (1997). Psychopathy and substance use in adolescent male offenders. *Psychological Reports, 81*(2), 529–530.

McDermott, P. A., Alterman, A. I., Cacciola, J. S., Rutherford, M. J., Newman, J. P., & Mulholland, E. M. (2000). Generality of psychopathy checklist—Revised factors over prisoners and substance-dependent patients. *Journal of Consulting and Clinical Psychology, 68*(1), 181–186. https://doi.org/10.1037/0022-006X.68.1.181

Miller, J. D., & Lynam, D. R. (2012). An examination of the psychopathic personality inventory's nomological network: A meta-analytic review. *Personality Disorders: Theory, Research, and Treatment, 3*(3), 305–326. https://doi.org/10.1037/a0024567

Miller, J. D., Watts, A., & Jones, S. E. (2011). Does psychopathy manifest divergent relations with components of its nomological network depending on gender? *Personality and Individual Differences, 50*(5), 564–569. https://doi.org/10.1016/j.paid.2010.11.028

Moss, H. B., Chen, C. M., & Yi, H.-Y. (2014). Early adolescent patterns of alcohol, cigarettes, and marijuana polysubstance use and young adult substance use outcomes in a nationally representative sample. *Drug and Alcohol Dependence, 136*, 51–62. https://doi.org/10.1016/j.drugalcdep.2013.12.011

Murrie, D. C., & Cornell, D. G. (2000). The Millon adolescent clinical inventory and psychopathy. *Journal of Personality Assessment, 75*(1), 110–125. https://doi.org/10.1207/S15327752JPA7501_8

Murrie, D. C., Cornell, D. G., Kaplan, S., McConville, D., & Levy-Elkon, A. (2004). Psychopathy scores and violence among juvenile offenders: A multi-measure study. *Behavioral Sciences & the Law, 22*(1), 49–67. https://doi.org/10.1002/bsl.573

National Institute on Drug Abuse. (2006). *Drug addiction treatment in the criminal justice system.* Retrieved from https://www.drugabuse.gov/related-topics/criminal-justice/drug-addiction-treatment-in-criminal-justice-system

Neal, T. M. S., & Sellbom, M. (2012). Examining the factor structure of the Hare self-report psychopathy scale. *Journal of Personality Assessment, 94*(3), 244–253. https://doi.org/10.1080/00223891.2011.648294

Neumann, C. S., Schmitt, D. S., Carter, R., Embley, I., & Hare, R. D. (2012). Psychopathic traits in females and males across the globe. *Behavioral Sciences & the Law, 30*(5), 557–574. https://doi.org/10.1002/bsl.2038

Nicholls, T. L., Ogloff, J. R., Brink, J., & Spidel, A. (2005). Psychopathy in women: A review of its clinical usefulness for assessing risk for aggression and criminality. *Behavioral Sciences & the Law, 23*(6), 779–802. https://doi.org/10.1002/bsl.678

Odgers, C. L., Reppucci, N. D., & Moretti, M. M. (2005). Nipping psychopathy in the bud: An examination of the convergent, predictive, and theoretical utility of the PCL-YV among adolescent girls. *Behavioral Sciences & the Law, 23*(6), 743–763. https://doi.org/10.1002/bsl.664

Patrick, C. J. (2007). Getting to the heart of psychopathy. In H. Herve & J. C. Yuille (Eds.), *The psychopath: Theory, research, and social implications* (pp. 207–252). Erlbaum.

Patrick, C. J., Curtin, J. J., & Tellegen, A. (2002). Development and validation of a brief form of the multidimensional personality questionnaire. *Psychological Assessment, 14*(2), 150–163. https://doi.org/10.1037//1040-3590.14.2.150

Paulhus, D. L., Neumann, C. S., & Hare, R. D. (2017). *Manual for the self-report psychopathy scale*. Multi-Health Systems.

Poythress, N. G., Dembo, R., Wareham, J., & Greenbaum, P. E. (2006). Construct validity of the youth psychopathic traits inventory (YPI) and the antisocial process screening device (APSD) with justice-involved adolescents. *Criminal Justice and Behavior, 33*(1), 26–55. https://doi.org/10.1177/0093854805282518

Reardon, M. L., Lang, A. R., & Patrick, C. J. (2002). An evaluation of relations among antisocial behavior, psychopathic traits, and alcohol problems in incarcerated men. *Alcoholism: Clinical and Experimental Research, 26*(8), 1188–1197. https://doi.org/10.1111/j.1530-0277.2002.tb02655.x

Rice, M. E., & Harris, G. T. (1995). Psychopathy, schizophrenia, alcohol abuse, and violent recidivism. *International Journal of Law and Psychiatry, 18*(3), 333–342. https://doi.org/10.1016/0160-2527(95)00015-A

Rutherford, M. J., Cacciola, J. S., Alterman, A. I., & McKay, J. R. (1996). Reliability and validity of the revised psychopathy checklist in women methadone patients. *Assessment, 3*(2), 145–156. https://doi.org/10.1177/107319119600300206

Sadeh, N., & Baskin-Sommers, A. (2016). Risky, impulsive, and self-destructive behavior questionnaire (RISQ): A validation study. *Assessment, 24*, 1080–1094. https://doi.org/10.1177/1073191116640356

Salatino, A. C., Tangney, J. P., Stuewig, J. B., & Chrosniak, L. D. (2018). Are borderline personality symptoms and psychopathy differentially related to drinking motives of former jail inmates? *Journal of Personality Disorders*, 1–16. https://doi.org/10.1521/pedi_2018_32_377

Salekin, R. T., Rogers, R., & Sewell, K. W. (1996). A review and meta-analysis of the psychopathy checklist and psychopathy checklist-revised: Predictive validity of dangerousness. *Clinical Psychology: Science and Practice, 3*(3), 203–215.

Salekin, R. T., Rogers, R., & Sewell, K. W. (1997). Construct validity of psychopathy in a female offender sample: A multitrait-multimethod evaluation. *Journal of Abnormal Psychology, 106*(4), 576–585.

Salekin, R. T., Leistico, A.-M. R., Neumann, C. S., & DiCicco, T. M. (2004). Psychopathy and comorbidity in a young offender sample: Taking a closer look at psychopathy's potential importance over disruptive behavior disorders. *Journal of Abnormal Psychology, 113*(3), 416–427. https://doi.org/10.1037/0021-843X.113.3.416

Salekin, R. T., Tippey, J. G., & Allen, A. D. (2012). Treatment of conduct problem youth with interpersonal callous traits using mental models: Measurement of risk and change. *Behavioral Sciences & the Law, 30*(4), 470–486.

Schulz, N., Murphy, B., & Verona, E. (2015). Gender differences in psychopathy links to drug use. *Law and Human Behavior*. https://doi.org/10.1037/lhb0000165

Sellbom, M., Donnelly, K. M., Rock, R. C., Phillips, T. R., & Ben-Porath, Y. S. (2017). Examining gender as moderating the association between psychopathy and substance abuse. *Psychology, Crime & Law, 23*(4), 376–390. https://doi.org/10.1080/1068316X.2016.1258466

Selzer, M. L. (1971). The Michigan alcoholism screening test: The quest for a new diagnostic instrument. *The American Journal of Psychiatry, 127*(12), 1653–1658. https://doi.org/10.1176/ajp.127.12.1653

Serin, R. C., & Amos, N. L. (1995). The role of psychopathy in the assessment of dangerousness. *International Journal of Law and Psychiatry, 18*(2), 231–238.

Skeem, J. L., Johansson, P., Andershed, H., Kerr, M., & Louden, J. E. (2007). Two subtypes of psychopathic violent offenders that parallel primary and secondary variants. *Journal of Abnormal Psychology, 116*(2), 395–409. https://doi.org/10.1037/0021-843X.116.2.395

Skinner, H. A. (1982). The drug abuse screening test. *Addictive Behaviors, 7*(4), 363–371. https://doi.org/10.1016/0306-4603(82)90005-3

Smedslund, G., Berg, R. C., Hammerstrom, K. T., Steiro, A., Leiknes, K. A., Dahl, H. M., et al. (2011). Motivational interviewing for substance abuse. *Cochrane Database of Systematic Reviews*, (5), Cd008063. https://doi.org/10.1002/14651858.CD008063.pub2

Smith, S. S., & Newman, J. P. (1990). Alcohol and drug abuse-dependence disorders in psychopathic and nonpsychopathic criminal offenders. *Journal of Abnormal Psychology, 99*(4), 430–439. https://doi.org/10.1037/0021-843X.99.4.430

Spielberger, C. D., Gorsuch, R. L., Lushene, R., Vagg, P. R., & Jacobs, G. A. (1983). *Manual for the state-trait anxiety inventory STAI (form Y)*. Consulting Psychologists Press.

Sprague, J., Javdani, S., Sadeh, N., Newman, J. P., & Verona, E. (2012). Borderline personality disorder as a female phenotypic expression of psychopathy? *Personality Disorders: Theory, Research, and Treatment, 3*(2), 127–139. https://doi.org/10.1037/a0024134

Swogger, M. T., Conner, K. R., Caine, E. D., Trabold, N., Parkhurst, M. N., Prothero, L. M., et al. (2016). A test of core psychopathic traits as a moderator of the efficacy of a brief motivational intervention for substance-using offenders. *Journal of Consulting and Clinical Psychology, 84*(3), 248.

Sylvers, P., Landfield, K. E., & Lilienfeld, S. O. (2011). Heavy episodic drinking in college students: Associations with features of psychopathy and antisocial personality disorder. *Journal of American College Health, 59*(5), 367–372. https://doi.org/10.1080/07448481.2010.511363

Vaughn, M. G., Newhill, C. E., DeLisi, M., Beaver, K. M., & Howard, M. O. (2008). An investigation of psychopathic features among delinquent girls: Violence, theft, and drug abuse. *Youth Violence and Juvenile Justice, 6*(3), 240–255. https://doi.org/10.1177/1541204007312298

Vaughn, M. G., Edens, J. F., Howard, M. O., & Smith, S. T. (2009). An investigation of primary and secondary psychopathy in a statewide sample of incarcerated youth. *Youth Violence and Juvenile Justice, 7*(3), 172–188. https://doi.org/10.1177/1541204009333792

Verona, E., & Vitale, J. (2018). Psychopathy in women: Assessment, manifestations, and etiology. In C. J. Patrick (Ed.), *Handbook of psychopathy* (2nd ed.). Guilford.

Verona, E., Patrick, C. J., & Joiner, T. E. (2001). Psychopathy, antisocial personality, and suicide risk. *Journal of Abnormal Psychology, 110*(3), 462–470.

Vincent, G. M., Vitacco, M. J., Grisso, T., & Corrado, R. R. (2003). Subtypes of adolescent offenders: Affective traits and antisocial behavior patterns. *Behavioral Sciences & the Law, 21*(6), 695–712. https://doi.org/10.1002/bsl.556

Vincent, G. M., Odgers, C. L., McCormick, A. V., & Corrado, R. R. (2008). The PCL: YV and recidivism in male and female juveniles: A follow-up into young adulthood. *International Journal of Law and Psychiatry, 31*(3), 287–296. https://doi.org/10.1016/j.ijlp.2008.04.012

Vincent, G. M., Cope, L. M., King, J., Nyalakanti, P., & Kiehl, K. A. (2018). Callous-unemotional traits modulate brain drug craving response in high-risk young offenders. *Journal of Abnormal Child Psychology, 46*(5), 993–1009. https://doi.org/10.1007/s10802-017-0364-8

Vitale, J. E., Smith, S. S., Brinkley, C. A., & Newman, J. P. (2002). The reliability and validity of the psychopathy checklist-revised in a sample of female offenders. *Criminal Justice and Behavior, 29*(2), 202–231.

Vize, C. E., Lynam, D. R., Lamkin, J., Miller, J. D., & Pardini, D. (2016). Identifying essential features of juvenile psychopathy in the prediction of later antisocial behavior: Is there an additive, synergistic, or curvilinear role for fearless dominance? *Clinical Psychological Science, 4*(3), 572–590. https://doi.org/10.1177/2167702615622384

Waller, R., & Hicks, B. M. (2019). Trajectories of alcohol and marijuana use among primary versus secondary psychopathy variants within an adjudicated adolescent male sample. *Personality Disorders: Theory, Research, and Treatment, 10*, 87–96. https://doi.org/10.1037/per0000303

Walsh, Z., Allen, L. C., & Kosson, D. S. (2007). Beyond social deviance: Substance use disorders and the dimensions of psychopathy. *Journal of Personality Disorders, 21*(3), 273–288. https://doi.org/10.1521/pedi.2007.21.3.273

Wymbs, B. T., McCarty, C. A., King, K. M., McCauley, E., Vander Stoep, A., Baer, J. S., et al. (2012). Callous-unemotional traits as unique prospective risk factors for substance use in early adolescent boys and girls. *Journal of Abnormal Child Psychology, 40*(7), 1099–1110. https://doi.org/10.1007/s10802-012-9628-5

Chapter 12
Psychopathy and Personality Disorders

Cristina Crego

Abstract Everybody, including those individuals with psychological problems, has their own unique personality, that is, their characteristic manner of thinking, feeling, behaving, and relating to others (John et al., Handbook of personality: theory and research, 3rd edn. Guilford, 2008). Some people are typically introverted, quiet, and withdrawn, whereas others are more extraverted, active, and outgoing. Some individuals are consistently anxious, self-conscious, and apprehensive, whereas others are routinely relaxed, self-assured and unconcerned. Personality traits are integral to each person's sense of self, as they involve what people value, how they think and feel about things, what they like to do, and what they are like most every day throughout much of their lives. For some people, these personality traits will be maladaptive to the point that they would constitute a personality disorder. A personality disorder (PD) is defined in the Diagnostic and Statistical Manual of Mental Disorders-5 (DSM-5) as "an enduring pattern of inner experience and behavior that deviates markedly from the expectations of the individual's culture, is pervasive and inflexible, has an onset in adolescence or early adulthood, is stable over time, and leads to distress or impairment" (APA, Diagnostic and statistical manual of mental disorders, 5th edn. Author, 2013, p. 645).

Keywords Psychopathy · Diagnosis · Assessment · Personality disorder · DSM-5

12.1 Introduction

Everybody, including those individuals with psychological problems, has their own unique personality, that is, their characteristic manner of thinking, feeling, behaving, and relating to others (John et al., 2008). Some people are typically introverted, quiet, and withdrawn, whereas others are more extraverted, active, and outgoing. Some individuals are consistently anxious, self-conscious, and apprehensive,

C. Crego (✉)
Longwood University, Farmville, VA, USA
e-mail: cregocm@longwood.edu

J. E. Vitale (ed.), *The Complexity of Psychopathy*, Dangerous Behavior in Clinical and Forensic Psychology, https://doi.org/10.1007/978-3-030-83156-1_12

whereas others are routinely relaxed, self-assured and unconcerned. Personality traits are integral to each person's sense of self, as they involve what people value, how they think and feel about things, what they like to do, and what they are like most every day throughout much of their lives. For some people, these personality traits will be maladaptive to the point that they would constitute a personality disorder. A personality disorder (PD) is defined in the Diagnostic and Statistical Manual of Mental Disorders-5 (DSM-5) as "an enduring pattern of inner experience and behavior that deviates markedly from the expectations of the individual's culture, is pervasive and inflexible, has an onset in adolescence or early adulthood, is stable over time, and leads to distress or impairment" (APA, 2013, p. 645).

It is estimated that 10–15% of the general population would meet criteria for one of the 10 DSM-5 personality disorders (Torgersen, 2012) and the prevalence of personality disorders within clinical settings is estimated to be well above 50% (Zimmerman & Mattia, 2001). For example, as many as 60% of inpatients within some clinical settings are diagnosed with borderline personality disorder (APA, 2013). However, the prevalence of personality disorders is generally underestimated in clinical practice, due to a lack of time to provide sufficiently systematic or comprehensive evaluations of personality functioning (Miller et al., 2012) and perhaps due as well to a reluctance to diagnose personality disorders because insurance companies may consider them to be untreatable (Zimmerman & Mattia, 1999). Personality disorders are among the most difficult of disorders to treat because they involve well-established behaviors that can be integral to a client's self-image (Millon, 2011).

12.2 Diagnostic Criteria for Personality Disorder

Broadly speaking, the DSM-5 (APA, 2013) lists six requirements for the diagnosis of a personality disorder (see Table 12.1).

However, each respective personality disorder also has its own specific criteria. For example, the diagnostic criteria for Antisocial Personality Disorder (ASPD) states that these individuals must demonstrate "disregard for and violation of other's rights since age 15, as indicated by one of seven sub features: Failure to obey laws and norms by engaging in behavior which results in criminal arrest, or would warrant criminal arrest, lying, deception, and manipulation, for profit or self-amusement, impulsive behavior, irritability and aggression, manifested as frequently assaults others, or engages in fighting, blatantly disregards safety of self and others, a pattern of irresponsibility and lack of remorse for actions" (APA, 2013, p. 659). Further, ASPD also requires that individuals were diagnosed with conduct disorder prior to the age of 15.

It is notable that ASPD has been included within every edition of the DSM. One might even characterize ASPD as the prototypic personality disorder, as the term "psychopath" originally referred to all cases of personality disorder (Schneider, 1923). Although the DSM-5 ASPD label is sometimes still used interchangeably

Table 12.1 Criteria for the diagnosis of personality disorder (APA, 2013, pp. 646–647)

A. An enduring pattern of inner experience and behavior the deviates markedly from the expectations of the individual's culture. This pattern is manifested in two (or more) of the following areas: 1. Cognition (i.e., ways of perceiving and interpreting self, other people and events) 2. Affectivity (i.e., the range, intensity, liability, and appropriateness of emotional response) 3. Interpersonal functioning 4. Impulse control
B. The enduring pattern is inflexible and pervasive across a broad range of personal and social situations.
C. The enduring pattern leads to clinically significant distress or impairment in social, occupational, or other important areas of functioning.
D. The pattern is stable and of long duration, and its onset can be traced back at least to adolescence or early adulthood. E. The enduring pattern is not better accounted for as a manifestation or consequence of another mental disorder.
F. The enduring pattern is not due to the direct physiological effects of a substance (e.g., a drug abuse, a medication) or a general medical condition (e.g., head trauma).

with the alternative label of "psychopathy" (Crego & Widiger, 2015) and there are important overlaps between ASPD and psychopathy that will be noted throughout this text, nonetheless, ASPD and psychopathy do not overlap perfectly. There are important differences in the symptoms, trajectory, and correlates that have led many to argue that the syndromes should be kept distinct (e.g., Lykken, 2018; Ogloff et al., 2016).

The diagnostic criteria for ASPD in the DSM has a rich empirical history. However, by the time of DSM-5, there was considerably more research concerning psychopathy than ASPD. Similarly, whereas in the last century there were texts devoted to ASPD (e.g., Stoff et al., 1997), in this century, the texts have focused increasingly on psychopathy (e.g., Patrick, 2006). Blashfield and Intoccia (2000) conducted a literature review concerning the APA personality disorders and concluded that, while ASPD has a substantial body of literature, over the last 30 years, new research in this area has been limited. If they had included psychopathy within their search, they would have likely concluded that the research was more truly alive and well, as much of the research concerning this personality disorder had shifted to studies of psychopathy.

In developing the DSM-5, it appeared to be the intention to shift the diagnosis of ASPD toward Hare and/or Cleckley's conceptualization of psychopathy. This was explicitly evident in the proposal to change the name from "antisocial" to "antisocial/psychopathic" (Skodol, 2010). What resulted, however, was not consistent with this intention. As noted above, the final diagnostic criteria for ASPD in the DSM-5 do not go beyond the DSM-IV criterion set to represent additional traits of Hare/Cleckley psychopathy. This outcome was part of a larger debate surrounding the conceptualization of personality disorder, more generally.

12.3 The DSM-5 Personality Disorder Proposals

Prior to DSM-III, mental disorder diagnosis was notoriously unreliable, as it was based on clinicians providing an impressionistic matching of what they knew about a patient (on the basis of unstructured assessments) to a narrative paragraph description of a prototypic case. No specific or explicit guidelines were provided as to which features were necessary or even how many to consider (Spitzer et al., 1980). Spitzer and Fleiss (1974) reviewed nine major studies of inter-rater diagnostic reliability and found that kappa values for the diagnosis of a personality disorder ranged from a low of .11 to .56, with a mean of only .29. DSM-II (APA, 1968) was blamed for much of this poor reliability, along with idiosyncratic clinical interviewing (Spitzer et al., 1978). A significant shift occurred with the publication of DSM-III, when specific and explicit criterion sets were developed (APA, 1980). This movement towards more specific diagnosis was spearheaded by Feighner et al. (1972), who developed specific and explicit criterion sets for 14 mental disorders. As expressed more recently by Kendler et al. (2010), "the renewed interest in diagnostic reliability in the early 1970s-substantially influenced by the Feighner criteria-proved to be a critical corrective and was instrumental in the renaissance of psychiatric research witnessed in the subsequent decades" (p. 141).

By the time of DSM-IV (APA, 1994), even with these advances in diagnosis, there was considerable criticism of the APA categorical model of personality disorder classification (Clark, 2007; Widiger & Trull, 2007). These criticisms included an excessive diagnostic co-occurrence, arbitrary and inconsistent diagnostic boundaries, insufficient coverage, and the use of a single diagnostic term to describe a heterogeneous constellation of maladaptive personality traits. For example, in DSM–IV–TR, any five of nine optional criteria were required for the diagnosis of Borderline Personality Disorder (BPD; APA, 2000). As a result, there were 256 different combinations of criteria from which it was possible to receive the same diagnosis of BPD (Ellis et al., 2009) and it was even possible for two individuals to meet the DSM–IV–TR criteria for BPD yet have only one diagnostic feature in common. In light of the limitations of the APA categorical model, and in an attempt to address these issues, Widiger and Simonsen (2005) proposed that PDs be conceptualized dimensionally, rather than categorically.

When the development of DSM-5 began, authors from the Personality and Personality Disorders Work Group (PPDWG) acknowledged these limitations and that personality disorder conceptualization was under construction. At the outset, the Chair and Vice Chair of DSM-5 indicated that the primary contribution of DSM-5 would be a shift toward a dimensional model of classification (e.g., Regier, 2008; Regier et al., 2010). The Nomenclature Work Group of a DSM-5 research planning conference, charged with addressing fundamental assumptions of the diagnostic system, concluded that it would be "important that consideration be given to advantages and disadvantages of basing part or all of DSM-V on dimensions rather than categories" (Rounsaville et al., 2002, p. 12). They suggested that a dimensional model be developed in particular for the personality disorders, and it was suggested that, in the event that a dimensional model performed well and was satisfactory to clinicians, it might be beneficial to investigate dimensional methodologies in different spaces (Rounsaville et al., 2002). A subsequent DSM-5 research planning conference was devoted to documenting the empirical support for this shift in the personality disorders section (Widiger & Simonsen, 2005). This was followed by a third DSM-5 research planning conference that was devoted to proposals to shift the entire manual to a dimensional model, including the personality disorders (Krueger et al., 2008).

The final proposal by the Personality and Personality Disorders Work Group (PPDWG) included a "level of functioning" that considered separately self and interpersonal functioning, as well as a 5-domain, 25-maladaptive trait model that could be used by itself to describe a patient, but was also part of newly proposed diagnostic criterion sets for the traditional personality disorder categories (Krueger et al., 2011). The five broad domains were negative affectivity, detachment, psychoticism, antagonism, and disinhibition.

Under this proposal, the diagnostic criteria for ASPD consisted of four deficits in self and interpersonal functioning and seven maladaptive personality traits (APA, 2011). The seven traits were: manipulativeness, deceitfulness, callousness, and hostility from the domain of antagonism, and irresponsibility, impulsivity, and risk-taking from the domain of disinhibition. In terms of the ASPD/psychopathy question, there were (initially) no traits from negative affectivity or detachment, which would align ASPD more closely to psychopathy. Instead, this initial list of traits aligned very well with the DSM-IV criterion set for ASPD (Lynam & Vachon, 2012). For example, missing from the description were traits included within the widely used Psychopathy Checklist-Revised (PCL-R; Hare, 2003) that were also not included within DSM-IV, such as arrogance, glib charm, lack of empathy, and shallow affect (Hare, 2003; Widiger et al., 1996). While "grandiosity" is included within the dimensional trait model (APA, 2013), and aligns closely with PCL-R grandiose sense of self-worth (Hare, 2003), it was not included within the dimensional trait description of ASPD, nor even within the eventually added psychopathy specifier.

Rather than emphasize the PCL-R criteria for psychopathy, the authors of the DSM-5 ASPD model referred instead to a new model of psychopathy, developed concurrently with DSM-5: the triarchic model of psychopathy, assessed via the Triarchic Psychopathy Measure (TriPM; Patrick et al., 2009). This model identifies three constructs considered to be essential to the understanding of psychopathy: boldness, meanness, and disinhibition. TriPM Boldness relates closely with the fearless-dominance factor of the Psychopathic Personality Inventory-Revised (PPI-R; Lilienfeld & Widows, 2005), as well as the emotional stability factor of the Elemental Psychopathy Assessment (EPA; Lynam et al., 2011).

As a result, after the final posting on the DSM-5 website, further revisions were made to the proposed criterion set for ASPD. More specifically, three additional traits were provided as potential specifiers for psychopathy: low anxiousness, low social withdrawal, and high attention-seeking (APA, 2013). These traits were said to represent TriPM boldness and/or PPI-R fearless-dominance: "High attention-seeking and low withdrawal capture the social potency (assertive/dominant) component of psychopathy, whereas low anxiousness captures the stress immunity (emotional stability/resilience) component" (APA, 2013, p. 765).

The final proposal set forth by the PPDWG was approved by the DSM-5 Task Force, but rejected by a DSM-5 scientific oversight committee and the APA Board of Trustees. The rationale for this rejection is unclear, although it is likely due to the magnitude of the proposed changes, vocal opposition to them, and the inadequate documentation of their empirical support (Skodol et al., 2013; Widiger, 2013). There is a considerable body of research to support the dimensional trait proposal, but a criticism of the PPDWG literature review was that it was confined largely to the studies authored by work group members (Blashfield & Reynolds, 2012), failing to cite a considerable body of additional research (Widiger et al., 2012b). For example, it was important for the proposal to be something that clinicians found useful (Rounsaville et al., 2002) and there have been a number of studies documenting empirically that clinicians prefer the dimensional trait model over the existing diagnostic categories (e.g., Glover et al., 2012; Lowe & Widiger, 2009; Samuel & Widiger, 2006). However, this research was not included within the PPDWG literature review (APA, 2012). Included instead were two studies that suggested a lack of support by clinicians for such a shift (i.e., Rottman et al., 2009; Spitzer et al., 2008). In any case, it was clear that there was considerable opposition to the proposal by well-known and well-regarded PD clinicians (e.g., Gunderson, 2010a; Shedler et al., 2010).

In the end, DSM-5 (APA, 2013) still includes 10 personality disorders. These diagnoses and their criterion sets are identical to those included in the prior editions, DSM-IV-TR (APA, 2000) and DSM-IV (1994). Nonetheless, the dimensional trait proposal is included within Section III of DSM-5, for emerging models and measures (APA, 2013). Further, the introduction to DSM-5 explicitly acknowledges the failure of the categorical model: "the once plausible goal of identifying homogeneous populations for treatment and research resulted in narrow diagnostic categories that did not capture clinical reality, symptom heterogeneity within disorders, and significant sharing of symptoms across multiple disorders" (APA, 2013, p. 12). It is further asserted that dimensional approaches will "supersede current categorical approaches in coming years" (p. 13).

Even with the opposition to the DSM-5 proposal, the 11th edition of the World Health Organization's (WHO) International Classification of Diseases (ICD-11) proposed an even more radical shift in PD classification involving, among other things, a dimension trait approach. This is notable because once ICD-11 is officially implemented, the clinicians in all member countries of the WHO will be shifting to this new model of personality disorder. Each member country of the WHO is obligated to use the ICD-11 or at least use a nomenclature that is in compliance with and/or is not fundamentally inconsistent with ICD-11 (First et al., 2015; Frances et al., 1995). Thus, the continued use of the DSM–5 personality disorder diagnostic categories (e.g., antisocial, borderline, narcissistic) could be said to be fundamentally inconsistent with the ICD-11 and with the practice of psychiatry throughout the rest of the world.

The ICD-11 proposal represented a paradigm shift in how personality disorder is conceptualized, moving away from the ICD-10 categorical syndromes to a dimensional trait classification (Krueger, 2016; Tyrer, 2014). The ICD-11 proposal sought to replace all of the ICD-10 personality disorder categories with a general personality disorder severity rating and a five-domain dimensional trait model (Tyrer et al., 2015). The five trait domains were negative affectivity, detachment, disinhibition, anankastia (i.e., compulsivity), and dissocial (i.e., antagonism). This proposal for ICD-11 did meet with some objections (e.g., Bateman, 2011; Gunderson & Zanarini, 2011), but not to the point that it was completely derailed. The final version of the proposal revised the severity rating to include some of the self- and interpersonal-functioning components from DSM-5, and added to the five-domain trait model a borderline domain (which is essentially equivalent to DSM-5 BPD).

This last addition makes sense given the status of BPD in the field. BPD is of substantial clinical interest (Gunderson, 2010b; Gunderson & Zanarini, 2011) and any national or international conference on personality disorders is dominated largely by presentations concerning BPD. BPD is also the only personality disorder category for which an empirically validated treatment protocol has been developed (APA, 2001). Clinicians were understandably concerned that the lack of an explicit reference to this syndrome within the ICD-11 would be problematic to its continued research and clinical funding and its inclusion would appear to be a reasonable compromise (Tyrer et al., 2019).

The ICD-11 revision was made official in 2019, and all member countries of the WHO will likely begin using this new classification of personality disorder by 2022. Each member of the WHO is obligated to use a nomenclature that closely conforms or is in compliance with the ICD and is not fundamentally inconsistent (First et al., 2015). Continuing to use the DSM-5 Section II (APA, 2013) personality disorder diagnostic categories (e.g., paranoid, schizoid, antisocial, histrionic, dependent, and narcissistic), would be fundamentally inconsistent with the ICD-11 and with the practice of psychiatry throughout the rest of the world. Thus, a change to the DSM-5 conceptualization is likely to occur shortly following the release of ICD-11.

12.4 Five-Factor Model of Personality Disorder

If changes to the DSM-5 conceptualization occur in an attempt to increase consistency between itself and the ICD-11, then PDs will be conceptualized from a dimensional trait model perspective across the globe. In fact, the dimensional trait models of both DSM-5 and ICD-11 are coordinated with the Five Factor Model (FFM) of general personality structure (Widiger & Costa, 2013), which is the predominant model of general personality structure (John et al., 2008). Thus, an understanding of the FFM and its application to personality disorder is useful in understanding how a trait model might apply in a diagnostic system.

The FFM was developed empirically, through the study of the trait terms within the language. Language can be understood as a sedimentary deposit of the observations of persons over the thousands of years of the language's development and transformation. The assumption is that the most important domains of personality functioning would be those with the greatest number of terms to describe and differentiate their various manifestations and nuances, and the structure of personality would be evident in the empirical relationship among the trait terms (Goldberg, 1993). Such lexical analyses of languages have typically identified five fundamental dimensions of personality: neuroticism (or negative affectivity) versus emotional stability, introversion versus extraversion, closedness versus openness to experience, antagonism versus agreeableness, and conscientiousness (constraint) versus disinhibition. Each of the five broad domains of the FFM can be differentiated further in terms of underlying facets. For example, the facets of antagonism versus agreeableness include suspiciousness versus trusting gullibility, callous tough-mindedness versus tender-mindedness, confidence and arrogance versus modesty and meekness, exploitation versus altruism and sacrifice, oppositionalism and aggression versus compliance, and deception and manipulation versus straightforwardness and honesty (Costa & McCrae, 1992).

Empirical support for the FFM is substantial (McCrae & Costa, 2003; Widiger, 2017), including multivariate behavior genetics (Jarnecke & South, 2017), childhood antecedents (Caspi et al., 2005; Mervielde et al., 2005), temporal stability across the life span (Roberts & DelVecchio, 2000), and cross-cultural validity (Allik & Realo, 2017). The FFM has also been shown across a vast empirical literature to be useful in predicting a substantial number of important life outcomes, both positive and negative (Ozer & Benet-Martinez, 2006). Importantly, given the debates surrounding the use of dimensional models for the DSM-5, Skodol et al. (2005) have noted that "similar construct validity has been more elusive to attain with the current [DSM-5] personality disorder categories" (p. 1923). This suggests that there are greater benefits to modeling personality pathology after the extensively validated FFM rather than attempting to develop a model for personality pathology that, while based on and similar to the FFM, lacks the same evidence of validity.

The FFM is robust in its coverage of abnormal as well as normal personality functioning. A substantial body of research now indicates that the FFM successfully accounts for the symptoms and traits of the DSM-5 and ICD-11 personality disorders (Oltmanns & Widiger, 2018a; Samuel & Widiger, 2008; Widiger et al., 2013). The FFM not only demonstrates construct validity, but also includes all of the maladaptive traits within the DSM-5 Section III and ICD-11 maladaptive trait models. As stated in DSM-5, the "five broad domains [of the DSM-5 trait model] are maladaptive variants of the five domains of the extensively validated and replicated personality model known as the 'Big Five,' or the Five Factor Model of personality" (APA, 2013, p. 773). Similarly, as expressed by the authors of the ICD-11 trait model, "Negative Affective [aligns] with neuroticism, Detachment with low extraversion, Dissocial with low agreeableness, Disinhibited with low conscientiousness and Anankastic with high conscientiousness" (Mulder et al., 2016, p. 85).

Each of the DSM-5 personality disorder syndromes are also readily understood as maladaptive and/or extreme variants of the FFM domains and facets (Lynam & Widiger, 2001; Samuel & Widiger, 2004) and existing measures of the FFM can in fact be used to provide valid assessments for most of the DSM-5 personality disorders (Miller, 2012). For example, DSM-5 obsessive-compulsive personality disorder (OCPD) is primarily a disorder of maladaptively extreme conscientiousness, including the FFM facets of deliberation (OCPD rumination), self-discipline, achievement-striving (OCDP workaholism), dutifulness (OCPD over conscientiousness, scrupulousness about matters of ethics and morality), order (OCPD preoccupation with details), and competence (OCPD perfectionism). The FFM description also goes beyond the DSM-IV-TR diagnostic criteria by including high anxiousness, low impulsiveness, low excitement-seeking, and closed mindedness to feelings, values, ideas, and actions (Samuel et al., 2012). In addition, measures to assess the DSM-5 personality disorders from the perspective of the FFM, such as the Five-Factor Borderline Inventory (Mullins-Sweatt et al., 2012) have also been developed (Widiger et al., 2012a).

Empirical support for the integration of the DSM-IV-TR (and DSM-5) personality nomenclature with the FFM is summarized by Widiger et al. (2012a, b). Overall, there are a number of advantages of an FFM of personality disorder (Widiger & Trull, 2007). The dimensional trait model addresses the many fundamental limitations of the categorical system (e.g., heterogeneity within diagnoses, inadequate coverage, lack of consistent diagnostic thresholds, and excessive diagnostic co-occurrence). It provides a description of abnormal personality functioning within the same model and language used to describe general personality structure, allowing for a more comprehensive system that would enable clinicians to identify personality strengths as well as deficits. It also transfers to the psychiatric nomenclature a wealth of knowledge concerning the origins, development, universality, and stability of personality structure (Widiger & Trull, 2007). Finally, it represents a significant step toward a rapprochement and integration of psychiatry with psychology.

The personality traits associated with psychopathy can also be captured by the FFM general personality structure (Lynam & Widiger, 2007; Widiger & Lynam, 1998). Due to psychopathy surpassing ASPD in its empirical interest, a FFM measure of ASPD was never developed. Alternatively, Miller et al. (2001) surveyed psychopathy researchers, asking them to describe a prototypic psychopath in terms of the 30 facets of the FFM on a 1 to 5 point scale (1 = extremely low, 5 = extremely high). The description included all of the traits of antagonism (e.g., exploitation, callousness, arrogance, aggression, and manipulation), along with traits of extraversion (excitement-seeking, assertiveness, and boldness), low neuroticism (lack of anxiousness and glib charm), high neuroticism (angry hostility and impulsivity), and low conscientiousness (rashness, immorality, disinhibition, and irresponsibility). In other words, the researchers considered the prototypic psychopath to be bold (i.e., high in assertiveness and excitement-seeking) and fearless (low in anxiousness and vulnerability). The Miller et al. (2001) description also characterized the prototypic psychopath as being high in competence, but Miller et al. (2001) suggested this might have been perceived competence rather than actual competence.

12.5 Personality Disorder Clinical Assessment Considerations and Techniques

There are a number of techniques available for the assessment of DSM-IV-TR (now DSM-5) PDs. These include interviews (unstructured or semi-structured), self-reports, and informant-reports. Covered herein will be interviews and self-reports. Also covered will be approaches to the assessment of DSM-5 Section III PDs.

12.5.1 *Interviews: Unstructured*

Not surprisingly, the most common method for eliciting information regarding PD symptoms in clinical practice is the use of an unstructured clinical interview. An unstructured clinical interview is one in which clinicians use their own personal and idiosyncratic questions (and order) to guide assessment (Westen, 1997). These interviews will vary both across and within clinicians; that is, no two clinicians will use the same unstructured interview and the same clinician may not ask the same questions or use the same order with each patient. Clinicians often prefer this methodology, as it is perceived as providing greater flexibility and spontaneity while taking less time; these features are often believed to result in an interview that is more likely to generate good clinical rapport (Westen, 1997).

12.5.2 *Interviews: Semi-structured*

The most commonly used assessment methodology in PD research to study the etiology, pathology, prevalence, and treatment of PD is a semi-structured interview. Fully structured interviews have been confined largely to studies concerning epidemiology wherein a large number of participants are interviewed via the phone and/or by lay interviewers (e.g. Trull et al., 2010). Semi-structured interviews provide specific questions that must be asked of each patient; in addition, questions are included that allow for the assessment of each symptom. This approach ensures the systematic and comprehensive assessment of all symptoms for each PD and thus allows the rater to apply the DSM diagnostic guidelines in a consistent manner.

Semi-structured interviews differ from fully structured interviews in that they provide the assessor with some latitude regarding follow-up queries and encourage the rater to use clinical judgment based on observations to make each rating, rather than relying solely on the patients' answers. For instance, the Structured Clinical Interview for DSM-IV-TR Axis II PDs (SCID-II; First et al., 1997), a popular semi-structured interview of DSM-IV-TR PDs, encourages raters to consider behavior manifested during the interview when rating whether a patient tends to show "arrogant, haughty behaviors or attitudes" (a symptom of narcissistic PD), in addition to asking an explicit question about this symptom (i.e., "Do you find that there are very few people that are worth your time and attention?"; p. 28).

There are five semi-structured interviews that were designed to assess all official DSM-IV-TR/DSM-5 PDs. These interviews include: (1) Diagnostic Interview for DSM-IV Personality Disorders (DIPD-IV; Zanarini et al., 1987, 1996); (2) International Personality Disorder Examination (IPDE; Loranger, 1999); (3) Personality Disorder Interview-IV (PDI-IV; Widiger et al., 1995); (4) Structured Clinical Interview for DSM-IV Axis II Personality Disorders (SCID-II; First & Gibbon, 2004); and (5) Structured Interview for DSM-IV Personality Disorders (SIDP-IV; Pfohl et al., 1997). Although these interviews all have the same aim, they differ in important ways, including the number of questions used (range: SCID-II: 303 questions to IPDE: 537), provision of a detailed manual (e.g., PDI-IV: yes; DIPD-IV: no), organization of questions by PD (e.g., SCID-II) or content area (e.g., close relations; work; SIDP-IV) or both (PDI-IV), and empirical support (i.e., SCID-II, SIDP-IV, and IPDE have been used the most frequently). An additional difference is that the SCID-II has a self-report screening instrument that can be used before the interview to identify the PDs that warrant closer attention.

In addition to the five comprehensive semi-structured interviews of DSM-IV-TR/DSM-5 PDs, there are also interviews aimed at assessing only one specific PD such as borderline (e.g., Revised Diagnostic Interview for Borderlines [DIB-R]; Zanarini et al., 1989) and narcissistic (e.g., Diagnostic Interview for Narcissism [DIN]; Gunderson et al., 1990)—although neither of these interviews were designed to be perfectly in-line with their respective DSM-IV-TR/DSM-5 counterparts. These semi-structured interviews provide a great deal of information regarding their respective constructs but take considerable time given their relatively specific yield (i.e., one PD).

12.5.3 Self-Reports

There are a number of self-report inventories that can be used for the assessment of DSM PDs. Self-report measures of PD have several advantages and disadvantages. On the positive side, self-report measures are efficient in terms of time and cost (e.g., clinician does not have to be involved), are fully structured and thus involve no idiosyncrasies from one administration to the next, can include validity scales to assess for invalid responding, and can be used in conjunction with semi-structured interviews as screening devices. The disadvantages of this approach include the tendencies of individuals to over-endorse PD symptoms on these self-report instruments (which can lead to a high rate of false-positives), the small to moderate convergence with informant and interview ratings, and the necessity for the patient to have some degree of insight into his/her cognitions, emotions, and behaviors as they relate to the PDs. Some suggest that self-report inventories be used to identify potential PD elevations that warrant follow-up with all or portions of a respective semi-structured interview (e.g., Widiger & Samuel, 2005).

Table 12.2 Self Report Instruments for the Assessment of DSM-IV-TR/DSM-5 Personality Disorders

Title of Assessment Instrument	Acronym	Citation
Assessment of DSM-IV Personality Disorders	ADP-IV	Schotte et al. (1998)
Coolidge Axis II Inventory	CATI	Coolidge and Merwin (1992)
Millon Clinical Multiaxial Inventory—III	MCMI-III	Millon et al. (1997)
Minnesota Multiphasic Personality Inventory-2 DSM-IV PD scales	MMPI-2 PDs	Hathaway et al. (1989), Morey et al. (1985), Colligan et al. (1994) and Somwaru and Ben-Porath (1995)
Multi-source Assessment of Personality Pathology	MAPP	Oltmanns and Turkheimer (2006)
NEO Personality Inventory—Revised PD	NEO PI-R	Costa and McCrae (1992)
Five Factor Model Personality Disorder scales	FFMPD	Bagby and Widiger (2018) and Widiger et al. (2012a, b)
Personality Diagnostic Questionnaire-4	PDQ-4+	Hyler (1994)
OMNI Personality Inventory	OMNI	Loranger (2001)
Schedule for Nonadaptive and Adaptive Personality	SNAP	Simms and Clark (2006)
Structured Clinical Interview for DSM-IV PDs: Personality Questionnaire	SCID-II P/Q	First et al. (1997)
Wisconsin Personality Disorders Inventory	WISPI	Klein et al. (1993)

There are at least 12 self-report assessment inventories that can be used to assess all of the DSM-IV-TR/DSM-5 PDs (Table 12.2), although some utilize the symptoms as described in DSM-III-R to do so (e.g., Coolidge Axis II Inventory [CATI]; Coolidge & Merwin, 1992). Of these self-report inventories, the ones that are the most straightforward, specific, and directly coordinated with the DSM are the PDQ-4, SCID-II PQ, CATI, ADP-IV, and MAPP. Like the DSM itself, these measures are atheoretical and simply assess each DSM-IV-TR PD criterion (DSM-III-R in the case of the CATI) using one or more questions for each. There are also a number of self-report inventories to assess individual personality disorders, such as the Narcissistic Personality Inventory (Raskin & Terry, 1988), and the Personality Assessment Inventory (PAI; Morey & Hopwood, 2006). Particular interest in psychopathy (versus ASPD more generally) has led to the development of a number of alternative self-report measures specifically for psychopathy, including the TriPM (Patrick et al., 2009) and PPI-R (Lilienfeld & Widows, 2005). A review of these is beyond the scope of this chapter but there are reviews published elsewhere (e.g., see Lilienfeld & Fowler, 2006, for a more comprehensive review of self-report measures of psychopathy).

Several other self-report inventories can provide DSM-IV-TR PD scores as part of a broader inventory; these measures include the SNAP, MMPI-2 PD scales, OMNI, PAI (for DSM-III-R antisocial and borderline PDs only), and FFM PD similarity and count scores from the NEO PI-R. These five inventories can provide scores on the DSM PDs but require completion of a broader inventory to accomplish this feat (e.g. MMPI-2: 567 items; SNAP: 375; NEO PI-R: 240). The NEO PI-R (Costa & McCrae, 1992) is a 240-item, self-report measure of general personality traits as conceptualized by the Five Factor Model. The measure assesses the five broad domains that are consistent with the domains that are likely to be included within the DSM-5 dimensional trait model (i.e., neuroticism, extraversion, openness, agreeableness, and conscientiousness) as well as 30 narrower facets. This dimensional measure of general personality functioning can be used to generate FFM PD scores in the form of both similarity scores and counts that closely parallel the proposed diagnostic criterion sets for DSM-5. Both of these mechanisms are based on a quantitative prototype matching methodology. The FFM PD prototypes can be based on researchers' ratings (Lynam & Widiger, 2001), clinicians' ratings (Samuel & Widiger, 2004), and meta-analytic results (Miller et al., 2008; Samuel & Widiger, 2008). The majority of the extant literature (e.g., Miller et al., 2004; Trull et al., 2003), however, has been based on the researchers' ratings (Lynam & Widiger, 2001) in which individuals who had published on a given DSM-IV-TR PD rated a prototypical individual with that PD on the 30 narrow facets of the FFM.

As discussed earlier, a series of Five-Factor Model Personality Disorder (FFMPD) scales have also been developed (Bagby & Widiger, 2018; Widiger et al., 2012a, b). Each was constructed by first identifying which facets of the NEO Personality Inventory-Revised (NEO PI-R) trait model for FFM appeared to be most relevant for a respective personality disorder. The facet selections were based on researchers' FFM descriptions of each personality disorder (Lynam & Widiger, 2001), clinicians' descriptions (Samuel & Widiger, 2004), and FFM-personality disorder research (Samuel & Widiger, 2008). Scales were constructed to assess the maladaptive variants of each facet that were specific to each personality disorder. This effort resulted in seven scales assessing maladaptive variants of conscientiousness (e.g., Workaholism, Perfectionism, and Ruminative Deliberation), five for maladaptive agreeableness (e.g., Gullibility, Subservience, and Timorousness), nine for maladaptive extraversion (e.g., Exhibitionism, Thrill-Seeking, and Authoritative), six for maladaptive openness (e.g., Aberrant Ideas and Odd and Eccentric), and even four for low neuroticism (e.g., Indifference and Invulnerability). All of the initial validation studies provided empirical support for their convergent (and discriminant) validity with the respective pole of the FFM domain, and these relationships have been cross-validated in subsequent studies (Bagby & Widiger, 2018).

12.5.4 Assessment of DSM-5 Section III Personality Disorders: Level of Personality Functioning

DSM-5 includes an assessment of level of functioning that considers separately self and interpersonal functioning. For self-functioning, ratings take into account (1) *identity integration* (i.e., regulation of self-states; coherence of sense of time and personal history; ability to experience a unique self and to identify clear boundaries between self and others; capacity for self-reflection), (2) *integrity of self-concept* (i.e., regulation of self-esteem and self-respect, sense of autonomous agency; accuracy of self-appraisal; quality of self-representation [e.g., degrees of complexity, differentiation, and integration]), and (3) *self-directedness* (i.e., establishment of internal standards for one's behavior; coherence and meaningfulness of both short-term and life goals). For interpersonal functioning, ratings take into account (1) *empathy* (i.e., ability to mentalize [create an accurate model of another's thoughts and emotions]; capacity for appreciating others' experiences; attention to range of others' perspectives; understanding of social causality), (2) *intimacy and cooperativeness* (i.e., depth and duration of connection with others; tolerance and desire for closeness; reciprocity of regard and support and its reflection in interpersonal/social behavior), and (3) *complexity and integration of representations of others* (i.e., cohesiveness, complexity and integration of mental representations of others; use of other-representations to regulate self). To facilitate this assessment, narrative descriptions are provided for each of five levels of self and interpersonal functioning (APA, 2013). In addition, self-report scales for their assessment have also been developed (Bender et al., 2011).

12.5.5 Assessment of DSM-5 Section III Personality Disorders: Personality Trait Profile

DSM-5 also includes a dimensional trait model consisting of five broad domains (i.e., negative affectivity, detachment, antagonism, disinhibition, and peculiarity or psychoticism) that are underlaid by 25 specific facets. Each of these traits are rated on a four-point scale ranging from 0 (very little or not at all descriptive) to 3 (extremely descriptive). These 25 traits form the other component of the DSM-5 diagnostic criteria for each personality disorder type being retained (APA, 2013). For example, the traits of withdrawal, intimacy avoidance, anhedonia, and anxiousness would be used for the diagnosis of avoidant personality disorder. The primary assessment technique and measure used to assess the DSM-5 trait model is the Personality Inventory for DSM-5 (PID-5; Krueger et al., 2011). The PID-5 is the official self-report measure of the dimensional trait model included in Section III of DSM-5 for emerging measures and models (APA, 2013). A considerable body of research has rapidly accumulated concerning the validity of the PID-5 (Krueger & Markon, 2014). This 25-trait model can also be assessed using clinician ratings via the DSM-5 Clinicians' Personality Trait Rating Form (i.e., Clinicians' PTRF).

Progress has occurred over the past 25 years with respect to the assessment of personality disorders. Much of this progress can be attributed to the increased attention given to PDs by their placement on a separate axis of the DSM, as well as the development of specific and explicit criterion sets. The fact that so many alternative semi-structured interviews and self-report inventories exist is a testament to strong clinical and research interest in these constructs. However, this also highlights the lack of consensus and certainty over how these constructs should be assessed. Nevertheless, the stage has been set for major changes in how PDs are assessed and diagnosed beginning with the DSM-5 and into the future, and it will be of particular importance for future research to address whether these upcoming changes result in improvement in their assessments.

12.6 Comorbidity

The term "comorbidity" refers to the co-occurrence of independent disorders, each with presumably its own separate etiology, pathology, and treatment implications (Feinstein, 1970). Diagnostic comorbidity is important in part because it is such a pervasive phenomenon; it is a rare psychiatric patient who meets diagnostic criteria for just one disorder (Widiger & Clark, 2000). Diagnostic comorbidity is also important because it is evident that the etiology, course, treatment, and outcome of a disorder are influenced heavily by the presence of comorbid conditions. Finally, comorbidity is important because the nature and extent of its occurrence are problematic to the conceptualization of mental disorders as distinct clinical conditions (Lilienfeld et al., 1994; Widiger & Clark, 2000). As expressed by the primary authors of DSM-5, "Epidemiologic and clinical studies have shown extremely high rates of comorbidities among the disorders, undermining the hypothesis that the syndromes represent distinct etiologies" (Kupfer et al., 2002, p. xviii). Diagnostic co-occurrence can reflect the co-occurrence of independent conditions, overlapping diagnostic criterion sets, or the presence of a common, underlying pathology. Comorbidity is a particularly challenging issue for personality disorders.

A number of studies have explored the comorbidity and covariation of psychopathy with the personality disorders included within recent editions of the DSM; psychopathy has been consistently reported to covary with ASPD and narcissistic personality disorder, as well as to some degree with BPD. In the following sections, the overlap between psychopathy and ASPD and these syndromes' comorbidity with other DSM personality disorders, substance use disorders, and criminal behavior will be considered.

12.6.1 Psychopathy, Antisocial Personality Disorder, and Externalizing Problems

As described earlier, the DSM-5 defines ASPD as a pervasive pattern of disregard for and violation of the rights of others (APA, 2013). Its primary diagnostic criteria include deceitfulness, impulsivity, recklessness, aggressiveness, irresponsibility, criminal activity, and indifference to the mistreatment of others. DSM-5 ASPD overlaps substantially with PCL-R psychopathy. The primary differences are the inclusion of glib charm, arrogance, lack of empathy, and shallow affect within the PCL-R, and the requirement within DSM-5 for the evidence of conduct disorder within childhood (Crego & Widiger. 2015). More recent formulations of psychopathy have extended its description to include such traits as fearlessness (Malterer et al., 2010), boldness (Patrick et al., 2009), dominance, and invulnerability (Lynam et al., 2011).

There has been a considerable body of research on the diagnostic co-occurrence of psychopathy with ASPD. This research has generally suggested that most cases of psychopathy diagnosed within prison or other forensic settings would meet the DSM-IV-TR (APA, 2000) criteria for ASPD (which were carried forward into DSM-5), but only about half of the cases of ASPD would meet criteria for psychopathy (Hare, 2003; Hare & Neumann, 2008). There are certainly notable differences between psychopathy, as diagnosed with the PCL-R (Hare, 2003) and the DSM (APA, 1980, 2000) ASPD criterion sets (e.g., Crego & Widiger, 2015; Hare & Neumann, 2008; Rogers et al., 2000; Widiger et al., 1996). The source of the differences between these diagnostic conceptions can be traced to the origins of the DSM and their development.

Despite the differences in ASPD and psychopathy criteria, externalizing behavior problems are a feature of both psychopathy and ASPD. For example, ASPD includes such traits as disinhibition and antagonism (Kotov et al., 2017; Kruefer & Markon, 2014), as well as aggressiveness, criminal acts, impulsivity, irritability, recklessness, and irresponsibility (APA, 2013). Similarly, the PCL-R (Hare, 2003) criteria include impulsivity, irresponsibility, criminal versatility, and juvenile delinquency. Both ASPD and psychopathy also often co-occur with other externalizing disorders, including substance use disorders (Crego & Widiger, 2015). Given this overlap, it is not surprising that psychopathy and ASPD have similar associations to a range of variables, including Narcissistic Personality Disorder and substance use disorder.

12.6.2 Psychopathy, ASPD, and Narcissistic Personality Disorder

Narcissistic personality disorder (NPD) involves a pervasive pattern of grandiosity (in fantasy or behavior), need for admiration or adulation, and lack of empathy (APA, 2013). Its primary diagnostic criteria include a grandiose sense of self-importance; preoccupation with success, power, brilliance, or beauty; a belief that one is special and can only be understood by high status individuals; a demand for excessive admiration; a strong sense of entitlement; an exploitation of others; lack of empathy; and arrogance. There is a substantial body of research on narcissism (Miller et al., 2010; Pincus & Lukowitsky, 2010), although, surprisingly, NPD was actually slated for deletion from DSM-5 (Skodol, 2012).

NPD was first included within the APA diagnostic manual in DSM-III (APA, 1980). Its inclusion "was suggested by an increasing psychoanalytic literature and by the isolation of narcissism as a personality factor in a variety of psychological studies" (Frances, 1980, p. 1053). However, it has not been included in the World Health Organization's (WHO) International Classification of Diseases (ICD-10; WHO, 1992), despite its presence in the DSM since 1980, as it has been perceived internationally as largely an American concept. There has been some concern that the DSM-5 criterion set may place too much emphasis on a grandiose narcissism, which can be associated with success in work and career, and fails to adequately recognize a vulnerable narcissism indicated by a need for admiration, self-devaluation, and feelings of vulnerability, humiliation, or rage in response to criticism or rebuke (Miller et al., 2010; Pincus & Lukowitsky, 2010). It is suggested that narcissistic persons fluctuate between states of grandiosity and vulnerability (Oltmanns & Widiger, 2018b), and when in the latter state will not appear at all arrogant, grandiose, or conceited.

Narcissism has a theoretical and clinical literature that is independent of psychopathy. Nevertheless, there have long been cross-references within both literatures (Widiger & Crego, 2018). For example, psychodynamic views of narcissism suggest that many features of psychopathy are apparent within narcissistic persons (Kernberg, 1998). Antisocial and psychopathic tendencies are sometimes conceptualized as being on a continuum with narcissism, with both involving a motivation to dominate, humiliate, and manipulate others. Consistent with this, Kernberg (1970), a narcissism theorist, suggested that "the antisocial personality may be considered a subgroup of the narcissistic personality" (p. 51), whereas psychopathy theorists Hart and Hare (1998) suggested that "psychopathy can be viewed as a higher-order construct with two distinct, albeit related facets, one of which is very similar to the clinical concept of narcissism" (p. 429).

Some of the features of NPD are explicitly suggestive of psychopathy, notably a grandiose sense of self-importance and arrogant, haughty behaviors (akin to psychopathic arrogant self-appraisal), lack of empathy, and interpersonal exploitation. In light of these shared features, it has even been intimated that NPD is closer to Cleckley's (1941) conception of psychopathy than is ASPD (Hare et al., 1991; Harpur et al., 2002). Psychopathy's association with narcissism is also captured by the "dark triad" model, which encompasses the personality traits of narcissism, Machiavellianism, and psychopathy (Paulhus & Williams, 2002). Consistent with the comorbidity found between NPD and psychopathy, although all three dark triad traits are conceptually distinct, empirical evidence shows them to be overlapping; they are all also associated with a callous-manipulative interpersonal style (Jones & Paulhus, 2010).

When the DSM-IV (APA, 1994) was being developed, some consideration was given to including additional features of PCL-R psychopathy to the ASPD criteria, in particular glib charm, arrogance, and lack of empathy (Widiger & Corbitt, 1995). However, a significant concern with this proposal was that these features were also central to the diagnosis of NPD and that their inclusion would have markedly increased the diagnostic co-occurrence of ASPD with NPD. The authors of the NPD criterion set (Gunderson et al., 1991) considered the antisocial and narcissistic personality disorders to be qualitatively distinct conditions and argued that revisions should help differentiate between the disorders rather than further increase their overlap. The final decision for DSM-IV was to acknowledge that glib charm, arrogance, and lack of empathy are included within other conceptualizations of ASPD and that their inclusion within the criterion set would likely increase the validity of the assessment of ASPD within prison and other forensic settings (APA, 1994).

This debate served to highlight just how much psychopathy arches across these two disorders (ASPD and NPD) and also illustrates some of the key features that they have in common (i.e. glib charm, arrogance, and lack of empathy). Further, the tension between this overlap on one hand and the need to address one of the issues inherent to PDs (excessive diagnostic comorbidity) and to limit the conceptualization of ASPD so that it remains distinct from NPD on the other emphasizes how challenging it is to bring the conceptualization of ASPD closer to psychopathy.

12.6.3 Psychopathy, ASPD, and Borderline Personality Disorder

Borderline Personality Disorder (BPD) was a new addition to DSM-III (APA, 1980; Spitzer et al., 1979). However, it has since become the single most frequently diagnosed (Gunderson, 2001) and studied (Blashfield & Intoccia, 2000) personality disorder and it is the only personality disorder syndrome being retained within the ICD-11. BPD also has rich empirical support ranging from the development of well-validated self-report inventories to treatment interventions (Mullins-Sweatt et al., 2012).

BPD is a pervasive pattern of impulsivity and instability in interpersonal relationships, affect, and self-image (APA, 2013). Its primary diagnostic criteria include frantic efforts to avoid abandonment, unstable and intense relationships, impulsivity (e.g., substance abuse, binge eating, or sexual promiscuity), recurrent suicidal thoughts and gestures, self-mutilation, and episodes of rage and anger.

Much like NPD, BPD has a theoretical and clinical literature that is independent of psychopathy. Like ASPD, BPD is comorbid with a number of DSM mental disorders and problem behaviors including mood disorders, substance use disorder, and externalizing problems such as criminality (Eaton et al., 2011; Grant et al., 2008). This co-occurrence likely reflects shared risk factors (Torgersen, 2012). Comorbidity between ASPD, psychopathy, and BPD has been documented and is found to be associated with a broad spectrum of antisocial outcomes beginning with childhood conduct disorder and continuing to violence in adulthood, drug/alcohol dependence, and cognitive disturbance (Freestone et al., 2012)

12.6.4 Psychopathy, ASPD, and Substance Use Disorders

The comorbidity of substance use disorder with both ASPD and psychopathy is substantial (Widiger & Crego, 2018). These are externalizing disorders that are characterized in large part by disinhibitory, reckless, and indulgent behavior

(Krueger et al., 2002). Alcohol and/or drug use are even included within the diagnostic criteria for ASPD and/or psychopathy. For example, driving while intoxicated is listed as a potential indicator of the "reckless disregard" criterion for ASPD, and one of Cleckley's (1941, 1976) criteria for psychopathy was "fantastic and uninviting behavior with drink." Many other behaviors that would count toward a diagnosis of ASPD and/or psychopathy—such as thefts, deception, conning, poor work history, and recklessness—could be due, at least in part, to a history of dyscontrolled drug usage. In the development of DSM-III, DSM-III-R, and DSM-IV, it was suggested that an exclusion criterion be added to ASPD to disallow the diagnosis when the behaviors involved substance usage (Widiger & Corbitt, 1995). However, this exclusion criterion has never been added because the differentiation between ASPD and substance dependence is facilitated by the requirement for evidence of conduct disorder in childhood. The presence of conduct disorder prior to the age of 15 will often date the onset of ASPD prior to the onset of a substance-related disorder, making it unlikely that the adult antisocial acts involving substance-related behaviors are secondary to an adult substance-related disorder. The PCL-R includes two similar diagnostic criteria (i.e., early behavior problems and juvenile delinquency), but, in contrast to DSM-5 ASPD, the PCL-R does not require the childhood antecedents to be evident for the diagnosis of psychopathy (Hare, 2003).

Differentiation between ASPD and substance use disorder is more complicated if the onset and course of the substance usage are congruent with the onset and course of the ASPD behaviors. However, if both have been evident prior to the age of 15 and persist thereafter into adulthood, it may then be clinically meaningless to differentiate them. Both disorders would likely be present. Persons with ASPD can develop a substance use disorder, and a substance use disorder can contribute to the development of ASPD (Widiger & Crego, 2018). In such cases, it might be useful to recognize that both warrant recognition and treatment.

12.7 Criminal Behavior

The relationship of criminality to psychopathy warrants particular consideration, as the extent to which psychopathy should be diagnosed on the basis of criminal and/or antisocial behavior has been hotly debated (Hare & Neumann, 2008, 2010; Skeem & Cooke, 2010). A longstanding criticism of the DSM-III through DSM-IV is that the ASPD criterion sets placed too much emphasis on criminal behavior. Hare (1986), for example, suggested that DSM-III ASPD was unable to identify psychopathic persons who lacked a criminal history because it purportedly relied heavily on criminal behavior for its diagnosis: "DSM-III has difficulty in identifying individuals who fit the classic picture of psychopathy but who manage to avoid early or formal contact with the criminal justice system" (Hare, 1986, p. 21). This charge is somewhat ironic, as Skeem and Cooke (2010) eventually suggested that the PCL-R suffers from the same limitation by placing too much emphasis on criminal history for its diagnosis: "The two-factor model [of the PCL-R] poorly identifies this 'great majority of psychopaths' who escape contact with the legal system or simply express their psychopathic tendencies in a manner that does not conflict with the law" (Skeem & Cooke, 2010, p. 435).

The criticism of DSM-III was perhaps overstated given that most of the DSM-III diagnostic criteria made no explicit reference to criminal activity (referring instead to poor work history, irresponsible parenting, relationship infidelity, aggression, lack of planning, and financial irresponsibility). On the other hand, it was certainly true that the DSM-III and DSM-III-R ASPD criterion sets identified considerably more persons with ASPD within prison settings than would be identified as psychopathic using the PCL-R (Hare, 2003; Hare et al., 2012).

As suggested from the DSM-IV ASPD field trial (Widiger et al., 1996), criminal behavior is not a particularly useful indicator of psychopathy within prison or forensic settings, the primary settings for the majority of PCL-R research. The reason is rather clear, in that criminal behavior is universal within a prison population. In contrast, within routine clinical settings, adult criminal behavior is more specific to –and therefore may be a more useful indicator of—persons who are psychopathic. The DSM-IV (now DSM-5) diagnostic criteria for ASPD were presented in a descending order of diagnostic value (Gunderson, 1998) and adult criminal behavior is listed first because it is the most useful criterion within general clinical settings (Widiger & Corbitt, 1995).

Criminal behavior, and violent criminal behavior, in particular, has been closely associated with psychopathy (Hart, 1998, p. 355; cf. Skeem & Cooke, 2010). Psychopathy is a diagnostic concept that was developed in part to help understand and explain criminal behavior (Hare & Neumann, 2008) and many studies have indicated that psychopathy as defined by the PCL-R has been successful in identifying a particularly callous, dangerous, and remorseless subset of criminals who repeatedly engage in particularly heinous, brutal, and exploitative acts (Hare et al., 2012).

As noted by Patrick (2006), "without exception, all the individuals represented in [Cleckley's] case histories engage in repeated violations of the law-including truancy, vandalism, theft, fraud, forgery, fire-setting, drunkenness and disorderly conduct, assault, reckless driving, drug offences, prostitution, and escape" (p. 608). As expressed by Cleckley (1976), "not only is the psychopath undependable, but also in more active ways he cheats, deserts, annoys, brawls, fails, and lies without any apparent compunction" (p. 343). In sum, "there is no question that Cleckley considered persistent antisocial deviance to be characteristic of psychopaths" (Patrick, 2006, p. 608).

However, it is also worth noting though that very few of Cleckley's psychopaths were cruel, angry, hostile, callous, aggressive, or even just mean (Crego & Widiger, 2016). They were exploitative, duplicitous, dishonest, unempathic, insincere, and manipulative, but not in any particularly vicious or brutal manner. None of Cleckley's psychopaths committed murder or rape, let alone serial murder or serial rape (Patrick, 2006). These are not the psychopaths that are typically portrayed in the media or clinical literature, such as Clyde Barrow, Ted Bundy, Kenneth Bianchi, or Henry Hill, who committed many severe crimes of violence (Lilienfeld & Arkowitz,

2007; Widiger & Crego, 2018). This is not to suggest that a serial murder, such as Ted Bundy (Samuel & Widiger, 2007), is not accurately described as being psychopathic, but that the cruel, heinous, depraved, and barbarous acts of such persons are not evident in the psychopaths of Cleckley (Crego & Widiger, 2016; Skeem et al., 2011). Their antisocial acts were, for the most part, petty, if not even pointless. The Cleckley psychopaths were not persons pursuing a productive criminal career, having successfully worked their way up in organized crime. Their antisocial acts were said by Cleckley to be "inadequately motivated;" that is, often with no apparent benefit or value. The Cleckley psychopath with the highest score on inadequately motivated antisocial behavior was Tom, who "wandered more or less aimlessly, sometimes shooting at a [farmer's] chickens, setting fire to a rural privy … or perhaps loitering about a cigar store or a poolroom, reading the comics, throwing rocks at squirrels in a park, perpetuating small thefts or swindles" (Cleckley, 1955, p. 91).

Although it is not difficult to imagine a psychopathic person without a criminal record or even a criminal history, it is perhaps difficult to imagine a psychopathic person not having a history infused with unethical, predatory, and other disreputable acts. Skeem and Cooke (2010) made a distinction between criminal and antisocial behavior, noting that "Criminal" behavior is sanctioned by the legal system, whereas "antisocial" behavior is more inclusive, involving "behavior that defeats the interests of the social order" (p. 435). "Snakes in suits" (i.e., psychopathic persons in business, law or other white-collar professions; Babiak & Hare, 2006) may not in fact break many laws, but they will significantly bend, massage, and work the rules to an unfair, self-serving advantage. Although Skeem and Cooke (2010) were quite critical of including criminal behavior within an assessment of psychopathy, they did feel that "some antisocial behavior seems inherent to the interpersonal and affective core of psychopathy (e.g., noncriminal manipulative behavior)" (p. 435). Indeed, it is difficult to imagine a person being exploitative, callous, selfish, unremorseful, egocentric, deceitful, and manipulative but not engaging in any significant unethical and/or antisocial behavior (Hare & Neumann, 2008).

12.8 Clinical Interventions

Treating personality disorders can be challenging. PDs are relatively unique because they are often "ego-syntonic," that is, most persons are largely comfortable with their selves, and with their characteristic manner of behaving, feeling, and relating to others. As a result, persons rarely seek treatment for their antisocial, narcissistic, histrionic, paranoid, and/or schizoid personality disorder. Further, persons typically lack insight into the maladaptivity of their personality.

One clear exception is BPD (and, perhaps, also avoidant personality disorder). Neuroticism is the domain of general personality structure that concerns inherent feelings of emotional pain and suffering, including feelings of distress, anxiety, depression, self-consciousness, helplessness, and vulnerability. Persons who have very high elevations on neuroticism (i.e., persons with borderline personality disorder) experience life as one of pain and suffering, and they will seek treatment to alleviate this severe emotional distress. Persons with avoidant personality may also seek treatment for their high levels of neuroticism (anxiousness and self-consciousness) and introversion (social isolation). In contrast, narcissistic persons will rarely seek treatment to reduce their arrogance; paranoid persons rarely seek treatment to reduce their feelings of suspiciousness; and antisocial persons rarely (or at least willfully) seek treatment to reduce their disposition for criminality, aggression, and irresponsibility.

Nevertheless, maladaptive personality traits will be evident in many individuals seeking treatment for other mental disorders, such as anxiety, mood, and substance use. Many of the persons with a substance use disorder will have antisocial personality traits; many of the persons with mood disorder will have borderline personality traits. As stated earlier in this chapter, the prevalence of personality disorders within clinical settings is estimated to be well above 50% (Torgersen, 2012) and as many as 60% of inpatients within some clinical settings are diagnosed with borderline personality disorder (APA, 2000). Antisocial personality disorder may be diagnosed in as many as 50% of inmates within a correctional setting (Hare et al., 2012). It is estimated that 10–15% of the general population meets criteria for at least one of the 10 DSM-IV-TR personality disorders (Torgersen, 2012), and quite a few more individuals are likely to have maladaptive personality traits not covered by one of the 10 DSM-IV-TR diagnoses.

The presence of a personality disorder will often have an impact on the treatment of other mental disorders, typically inhibiting or impairing responsivity. Antisocial persons will tend to be irresponsible and negligent; borderline persons can form intensely manipulative attachments to their therapists; paranoid patients will be unduly suspicious and accusatory; narcissistic patients can be dismissive and denigrating; and dependent patients can become overly attached to and feel helpless without their therapists.

It is a misnomer though to suggest that personality disorders cannot themselves be treated. Personality disorders are among the most difficult of disorders to treat because they involve well-established behaviors that can be integral to a client's self-image (Millon, 2011). Nevertheless, much has been written on the treatment of personality disorder (e.g., Beck et al., 1990; Gunderson & Gabbard, 2000) and there is empirical support for clinically and socially meaningful changes in response to psychosocial and pharmacologic treatments (Perry & Bond, 2000). The development of an ideal or fully healthy personality structure is unlikely to occur through the course of treatment, but given the considerable social, public health, and personal costs associated with some of the personality disorders, such as ASPD and BPD, even moderate adjustments in personality functioning can represent quite significant and meaningful change. Space limitations prohibit detailed clinical coverage of all 10 DSM-5 personality disorders. Therefore, discussed herein are some treatment considerations for the three personality disorders for which there has been the most research and which are the most closely associated with psychopathy: antisocial, narcissistic, and borderline.

12.8.1 Antisocial Personality Disorder

ASPD is considered to be the among most difficult personality disorders to treat (Gunderson & Gabbard, 2000; Hare et al., 2012). Individuals with ASPD, especially those who would also meet criteria for psychopathy, can be seductively charming and may declare a commitment to change, but they often lack sufficient motivation. Their declarations of desire to change might even be dishonest. They will also fail to appreciate the future costs associated with antisocial acts (e.g., imprisonment and lack of meaningful interpersonal relationships), and may stay in treatment only as required by an external source, such as a parole. Residential programs that provide a carefully controlled environment with high levels of structure and supervision, combined with peer confrontation, have been recommended (Gunderson & Gabbard, 2000). However, it is unknown what benefits may be sustained after the ASPD individual leaves this environment.

During inpatient treatment, individuals with ASPD may manipulate and exploit staff and fellow patients. Studies have indicated that outpatient therapy is not likely to be successful, although the extent to which persons with ASPD are entirely unresponsive to treatment may have been somewhat exaggerated (Salekin, 2002). Rather than attempt to develop a sense of conscience in these individuals, therapeutic techniques should perhaps be focused on rational and utilitarian arguments against repeating past mistakes. These approaches would focus on the tangible, material value of prosocial behavior (Young et al., 2003).

12.8.2 Narcissistic Personality Disorder

People rarely seek treatment for their narcissism. Although some narcissistic persons seeking treatment for a growing sense of discontent and futility with their lives (Ronningstam, 2005), more typically, individuals with NPD enter treatment seeking assistance for another problem, such as substance abuse (secondary to career stress), mood disorder (secondary to career setback), or even something quite specific, such as test anxiety. Once an individual with NPD is in treatment, he or she will have difficulty perceiving the relationship as collaborative and will likely attempt to dominate, impress or devalue the therapist. They can idealize their therapists (to affirm that the therapist is indeed of sufficient status or quality to be treating them) but they may also devalue the therapist to affirm to themselves a sense of superiority. How the therapist might best to respond is often unclear, as the establishment and maintenance of rapport will be an immediate and ongoing issue. At times, it may be preferable to accept the praise or criticism, whereas at other times it may be preferable to confront and discuss the motivation for the devaluation (or the idealization). Therapists must be careful not to become embroiled within intellectual conflicts and competitions with these clients. Narcissistic persons can be acutely aware of the self-esteem conflicts of their therapist, and it is best for the therapist to model a comfortable indifference to losing disputes or conflicts.

12.8.3 Borderline Personality Disorder

The APA (2001) has published practice guidelines for the psychotherapeutic and pharmacologic treatment of persons with BPD. Because borderline patients can present with significant suicide risk, a thorough evaluation of the potential for suicidal ideation and activity should have the initial priority (Hooley et al., 2012). In contrast to most other personality disorders, manualized and empirically-validated treatment protocols have been developed for BPD (APA, 2001). These include Mentalization Based Therapy (MBT; Bateman & Fonagy, 2012), which uses structured techniques to help persons with BPD to "mentalize", or stand outside their feelings and more accurately observe the feelings within themselves and others, and Dialectical Behavior Therapy (DBT; Linehan & Schmidt, 1995; Lynch et al., 2007; Lynch & Cuper, 2012), which is a form of cognitive-behavior therapy that draws on principles from Zen Buddhism, dialectical philosophy, and behavioral science.

DBT is the most common form of cognitive-behavioral for BPD. The treatment has four components: individual therapy, group skills training, telephone coaching, and a therapist consultation team, and will typically last a full year (Lynch & Cuper, 2012). As such, it is a relatively expensive form of treatment, but research has indicated that its benefits far outweighs its costs, both financially and socially. The dialectical component of DBT was derived largely from Zen Buddhist principles of overcoming suffering through acceptance (Linehan, 1993). Mastery of conflict is achieved in part through no longer struggling or fighting adversity; pain is overcome when it is accepted as an inevitable, fundamental part of life. This principle is taught in part through the meditative technique of mindfulness, in which one attempts to empty one's mind of all thoughts, but accepts whenever and wherever the mind naturally travels. DBT initially focuses on reducing self-harm and para-suicidal behaviors that are disruptive to treatment. Contracts may be implemented, wherein time with the therapist is limited secondary to treatment disruptive behavior. This can even go so far as to include suspension of treatment secondary to suicidal behavior. After mastery of treatment disruptive behavior, DBT teaches coping skills focused on emotional control and interpersonal relatedness. Individuals in DBT attend regular sessions with an individual therapist and discuss problems in applying the new skills. These sessions are augmented with a didactic skills-training group.

Clients with BPD form relationships with therapists that are similar to their other significant relationships; that is, the therapeutic relationship can often be tremendously unstable, intense, and volatile. Ongoing consultation with colleagues is recommended to address potential negative reactions toward the client (e.g., distancing, rejecting, or abandoning the patient in response to feelings of anger or frustration) as well as positive reactions (e.g., fantasies of being the therapist who in fact rescues or cures the patient, or romantic, sexual feelings in response to a seductive patient). Sessions should emphasize the building of a strong therapeutic alliance, monitoring self-destructive and suicidal behaviors, validation of suffering and abusive experience (but also helping the client take responsibility for actions), promotion of self-reflection rather than impulsive action, and setting limits on self-destructive behavior

(Gunderson, 2001). The tendency of borderline patients to engage in "splitting" (polarization of an emotional response) should also be carefully monitored and addressed (e.g., devaluation of prior therapists, coupled with idealization of current therapist).

In light of the impact that DBT has had in the area of treatment for BPD, it is unclear why specific and explicit treatment manuals have not been developed for other personality disorders. This may reflect a regrettable assumption that personality disorders are unresponsive to treatment. It may also reflect the complexity of their treatment. As noted earlier, each DSM-IV-TR disorder is a heterogeneous constellation of maladaptive personality traits. In fact, a person can meet diagnostic criteria for the antisocial, borderline, schizoid, schizotypal, narcissistic, and avoidant personality disorders and yet have only one diagnostic criterion in common. In addition, patients meeting diagnostic criteria for one personality disorder will often meet diagnostic criteria for another. This degree of diagnostic overlap and heterogeneity of membership hinders tremendously efforts to identity a specific etiology, pathology, or treatment for any particular personality disorder as there is so much variation within any group of patients sharing the same diagnosis (Smith & Zapolski, 2009).

Of course, this diagnostic overlap and complexity did not prevent researchers and clinicians from developing DBT and MBT. A further reason for the weak progress in treatment development is that, as noted earlier, persons rarely seek treatment for their personality disorder. This can make it difficult to obtain a sufficiently large group of persons with (for instance) narcissistic or obsessive-compulsive disorder to participate in a treatment outcome study, one receiving the manualized treatment protocol, the other receiving treatment-as-usual.

12.9 Conclusions

Maladaptive personality traits will often impair or impede the treatment of other mental disorders and therefore should be a focus of clinical assessment and treatment. Section III of DSM-5, for emerging models and measures, and the ICD-11 include domain trait models that are closely aligned, both conceptually and empirically, with the five-factor model of general personality structure. The FFM and these dimensional maladaptive trait models offer a compelling alternative to the categorical diagnosis of personality disorders provided in Section II of DSM-5. Advantages of understanding personality disorders in terms of these dimensional trait models include the provision of more specific descriptions of individual patients (including adaptive as well as maladaptive personality functioning), the avoidance of arbitrary categorical distinctions, and the ability to bring to bear the extensive amount of research on the heritability, temperament, development, and course of general personality functioning of the FFM to an understanding of personality disorders.

Consistent with this maladaptive trait approach, psychopathy is a personality syndrome consisting of a constellation of maladaptive (and perhaps adaptive) personality traits. The core traits are antagonistic (i.e., callousness, exploitativeness, manipulativeness, deceitfulness, lack of empathy, and aggression), coupled with traits of low conscientiousness (laxness, irresponsibility, and rashness), high extraversion (assertiveness, boldness, and excitement-seeking), high neuroticism (angry hostility), and low neuroticism (fearlessness and glib charm). Psychopathy may indeed represent a dangerous combination of traits. However, although psychopathic persons pose a considerable threat to others, they are also harmful to themselves, as their lives are replete with loss, impairment, and failure, including imprisonment and at times even death. Psychopathy, particularly the externalizing aspects of this disorder, relates highly to other personality disorders, including ASPD, NPD, and BPD, as well as other problem behaviors. The complexity of the relationship between these disorders and the problematic behaviors that accompany them highlight the importance of continuing to investigate the best assessment and treatment approaches. A maladaptive trait approach is likely to offer benefits above and beyond categorical approaches to achieving these goals.

References

Allik, J., & Realo, A. (2017). Universal and specific in the five factor model. In T. A. Widiger (Ed.), *The Oxford handbook of the five factor model* (pp. 173–190). Oxford University Press.

American Psychiatric Association. (1968). *Diagnostic and statistical manual of mental disorders* (2nd ed.). Author.

American Psychiatric Association. (1980). *Diagnostic and statistical manual of mental disorders* (3rd ed.). Author.

American Psychiatric Association. (1994). *Diagnostic and statistical manual of mental disorders* (4th ed.). Author.

American Psychiatric Association. (2000). *Diagnostic and statistical manual of mental disorders* (4th ed., text revision). Author.

American Psychiatric Association. (2001). *Practice guidelines for the treatment of patients with borderline personality disorder*. American Psychiatric Association.

American Psychiatric Association. (2011, June). *T 04 Antisocial personality disorder (dissocial personality disorder)*. Retrieved from http://web.archive.org/web/20110726005003/http://www.dsm5.org/ProposedRevisions/Pages/proposedrevision.aspx?rid=16

American Psychiatric Association. (2012, May, 1). *Rationale for the proposed changes to the personality disorders classification in DSM-5*. Retrieved from http://www.dsm5.org/ProposedRevision/Pages/PersonalityDisorders.aspx

American Psychiatric Association. (2013). *Diagnostic and statistical manual of mental disorders* (5th ed.). Author.

Babiak, P., & Hare, R. D. (2006). *Snakes in suits: When psychopaths go to work*. Regan Books/Harper Collins Publishers.

Bagby, R. M., & Widiger, T. A. (2018). Five factor model personality disorder scales: An introduction to a special section on assessment of maladaptive variants of the five factor model. *Psychological Assessment, 30*, 1–9.

Bateman, A. W. (2011). Throwing the baby out with the bathwater? *Personality and Mental Health, 5*, 274–280.

Bateman, A. W., & Fonagy, P. (2012). Mentalization-based treatment of borderline personality disorder. In T. A. Widiger (Ed.), *The Oxford handbook of personality disorders* (pp. 767–784). Oxford University Press.

Beck, A. T., Freeman, A., & Associates. (1990). *Cognitive therapy of personality disorders*. Guilford Press.

Bender, D., Morey, L., & Skodol, A. E. (2011). Toward a model for assessing level of personality functioning in *DSM–5*, Part I: A review of theory and methods. *Journal of Personality Assessment, 93*, 332–346.

Blashfield, R. K., & Intoccia, V. (2000). Growth of the literature on the topic of personality disorders. *American Journal of Psychiatry, 157*, 472–473.

Blashfield, R. K., & Reynolds, S. M. (2012). An invisible college view of the DSM-5 personality disorder classification. *Journal of Personality Disorders, 26*, 821–829.

Caspi, A., Roberts, B. W., & Shiner, R. L. (2005). Personality development: Stability and change. *Annual Review of Psychology, 56*, 453–484.

Clark, L. A. (2007). Assessment and diagnosis of personality disorder: Perennial issues and an emerging reconceptualization. *Annual Review of Psychology, 57*, 277–257.

Cleckley, H. (1941). *The mask of sanity*. Mosby.

Cleckley, H. (1955). *The mask of sanity* (3rd ed.). Mosby.

Cleckley, H. (1976). *The mask of sanity* (5th ed.). Mosby.

Colligan, R. C., Morey, L. C., & Offord, K. P. (1994). MMPI/MMPI-2 personality disorder scales. Contemporary norms for adults and adolescents. *Journal of Clinical Psychology, 50*, 168–200.

Coolidge, F. L., & Merwin, M. M. (1992). Reliability and validity of the Coolidge Axis II Inventory: A new inventory for the assessment of personality disorders. *Journal of Personality Assessment, 59*, 223–238.

Costa, P. T., Jr., & McCrae, R. R. (1992). *Revised NEO Personality Inventory (NEO-PI-R) and NEO Five Factor Inventory (NEO-FFI) professional manual*. Psychological Assessment Resources.

Crego, C., & Widiger, T. A. (2015). Psychopathy and the DSM. *Journal of Personality, 83*, 665–677.

Crego, C., & Widiger, T. A. (2016). Cleckley's psychopaths: Revisited. *Journal of Abnormal Psychology, 125*, 75–87.

Eaton, N. R., Krueger, R. F., Keyes, K. M., Skodol, A. E., Markon, K. E., Grant, B. F., & Hasin, D. S. (2011). Borderline personality disorder co-morbidity: Relationship to the internalizing-externalizing structure of common mental disorders. *Psychological Medicine, 41*, 1041–1050.

Ellis, A., Abrams, M., & Abrams, L. D. (2009). *Personality theories: Critical perspectives*. Sage Publications Inc.

Feighner, J. P., Robins, E., Guze, S. B., Woodruff, R. A., Winokur, G., & Munoz, R. (1972). Diagnostic criteria for use in psychiatric research. *Archives of General Psychiatry, 26*, 57–63.

Feinstein, A. R. (1970). The pre-therapeutic classification of co-morbidity in chronic disease. *Journal of Chronic Diseases, 23*, 455–468.

First, M. B., & Gibbon, M. (2004). The Structured Clinical Interview for DSM-IV Axis I Disorders (SCID-I) and the Structured Clinical Interview for DSM-IV Axis II Disorders (SCID-II). In M.J. Hilsenroth, D.L. Segal, & M. Hersen (Eds.). *Comprehensive handbook of psychological assessment, Volume 2. Personality assessment* (pp. 134–143). : Wiley.

First, M. B., Gibbon, M., Spitzer, R. L., Williams, J. B. W., & Benjamin, L. S. (1997). *Structured Clinical Interview for DSM-IV Axis II Personality Disorders (SCID-II)*. American Psychiatric Press.

First, M. B., Reed, G. M., Hyman, S. E., & Saxena, S. (2015). The development of the ICD-11 clinical descriptions and diagnostic guidelines for mental and behavioural disorders. *World Psychiatry, 14*, 82–90.

Frances, A. J. (1980). The DSM-III personality disorders section: A commentary. *American Journal of Psychiatry, 137*, 1050–1054.

Frances, A. J., First, M. B., & Pincus, H. A. (1995). *DSM–IV guidebook*. American Psychiatric Press.

Freestone, M., Taylor, C., Milsom, S., Mikton, C., Ullrich, S., Phillips, O., & Coid, J. (2012). Assessments and admissions during the first 6 years of a UK medium secure DSPD service. *Criminal Behaviour and Mental Health, 22*, 91–107.

Glover, N., Crego, C., & Widiger, T. A. (2012). The clinical utility of the five-factor model of personality disorder. *Personality Disorders, Theory, Research, and Treatment, 3*, 176–184.

Goldberg, L. R. (1993). The structure of phenotypic personality traits. *American Psychologist, 48*, 26–34.

Grant, B. F., Chou, S. P., Goldstein, R. B., Huang, B., Stinson, F. S., Saha, T. D., Smith, S. M., Dawson, D. A., Pulay, A. J., Pickering, R. P., & Ruan, J. (2008). Prevalence, correlates, disability, and comorbidity of *DSM-IV* borderline personality disorder: Results from the Wave 2 National Epidemiologic Survey on Alcohol and Related Conditions. *Journal of Clinical Psychiatry, 69*, 533–545.

Gunderson, J. G. (1998). DSM-IV personality disorders: Final overview. In T. A. Widiger, A. Frances, H. A. Pincus, R. Ross, M. B. First, W. Davis, & M. Kline (Eds.), *DSM-IV sourcebook* (Vol. 4, pp. 1123–1140). American Psychiatric Association.

Gunderson, J. G. (2001). *Borderline personality disorder: A clinical guide*. American Psychiatric Press.

Gunderson, J. G. (2010a). Commentary on "Personality traits and the classification of mental disorders: Toward a more complete integration in DSM-5 and an empirical model of psychopathology". *Personality Disorders, Theory, Research, and Treatment, 1*, 119–122.

Gunderson, J. G. (2010b). Revising the borderline diagnosis for DSM-V: An alternative proposal. *Journal of Personality Disorders, 24*, 694–708.

Gunderson, J. G., & Gabbard, G. O. (Eds.). (2000). *Psychotherapy for personality disorders*. American Psychiatric Press.

Gunderson, J. G., & Zanarini, M. C. (2011). Deceptively simple—Or radical shift? *Personality and Mental Health, 5*, 260–262.

Gunderson, J. G., Ronningstam, E., & Bodkin, A. (1990). The diagnostic interview for narcissistic patients. *American Journal of Psychiatry, 47*, 676–680.

Gunderson, J. G., Ronningstam, E., & Smith, L. (1991). Narcissistic personality disorder: A review of data on DSM-III-R descriptions. *Journal of Personality Disorders, 5*, 167–177.

Hare, R. D. (1986). Twenty years experience with the Cleckley psychopath. In W. H. Reid, D. Dorr, J. I. Walker, & J. W. Bonner III (Eds.), *Unmasking the psychopath* (pp. 3–27). W.W. Norton.

Hare, R. D. (2003). *Hare Psychopathy Checklist Revised (PCL-R). Technical manual*. Multi-Health Systems.

Hare, R. D., & Neumann, C. S. (2008). Psychopathy as a clinical and empirical construct. *Annual Review of Clinical Psychology, 4*, 217–246.

Hare, R. D., & Neumann, C. S. (2010). The role of antisociality in the psychopathy construct: Comment on Skeem and Cooke (2010). *Psychological Assessment, 22*, 446–454.

Hare, R. D., Hart, S. D., & Harpur, T. J. (1991). Psychopathy and the DSM-IV criteria for antisocial personality disorder. *Journal of Abnormal Psychology, 100*, 391–398.

Hare, R. D., Neumann, C. S., & Widiger, T. A. (2012). Psychopathy. In T. A. Widiger (Ed.), *Oxford handbook of personality disorder* (pp. 478–504). Oxford University Press.

Harpur, T. J., Hart, S. D., & Hare, R. D. (2002). Personality of the psychopath. In P. T. Costa & T. A. Widiger (Eds.), *Personality disorders and the five factor model of personality* (2nd ed., pp. 299–324). American Psychological Association.

Hart, S. D. (1998). Psychopathy and risk for violence. In D. J. Cooke, A. E. Forth, & R. D. Hare (Eds.), *Psychopathy: Theory, research, and implications for society* (pp. 355–373). Kluwer.

Hart, S. D., & Hare, R. D. (1998). Association between psychopathy and narcissism: Theoretical reviews and empirical evidence. In E. F. Ronningstam (Ed.), *Disorders of narcissism: Diagnostic, clinical, and empirical implications* (pp. 415–436). American Psychiatric Press.

Hathaway, S. R., McKinley, J. C., Butcher, J. N., Dahlstrom, W. G., Graham, J. R., & Tellegen, A. (1989). *Minnesota multiphasic personality inventory test booklet*. Regents of the University of Minnesota.

Hooley, J. M., Cole, S. H., & Gironde, S. (2012). Borderline personality disorder. In T. A. Widiger (Ed.), *The Oxford handbook of personality disorders* (pp. 409–436). Oxford University Press.

Hyler, S. E. (1994). *Personality Diagnostic Questionnaire-4 (PDQ-4)*. Unpublished test. New York State Psychiatric Institute.

Jarnecke, A. M., & South, S. C. (2017). Behavior and molecular genetics of the five factor model. In T. A. Widiger (Ed.), *The Oxford handbook of the five factor model* (pp. 301–318). Oxford University Press.

John, O. R., Robins, R. W., & Pervin, L. A. (Eds.). (2008). *Handbook of personality: Theory and research* (3rd ed.). Guilford.

Jones, D. N., & Paulhus, D. L. (2010). Differentiating the dark triad within the interpersonal circumplex. In L. M. Horowitz & S. N. Strack (Eds.), *Handbook of interpersonal theory and research* (pp. 249–267). Guilford.

Kendler, K., Munoz, R. A., & Murphy, G. (2010). The development of the Feighner criteria: A historical perspective. *American Journal of Psychiatry, 167*, 134–142.

Kernberg, O. F. (1970). Factors in the treatment of narcissistic personalities. *Journal of the American Psychoanalytic Association, 18*, 51–85.

Kernberg, O. F. (1998). Pathological narcissism and narcissistic personality disorder: Theoretical background and diagnostic classification. In E. F. Ronningstam (Ed.), *Disorders of narcissism: Diagnostic, clinical, and empirical implications* (pp. 29–52). American Psychiatric Press.

Klein, M. H., Benjamin, L. S., Rosenfeld, R., Treece, C., Husted, J., & Greist, J. H. (1993). The Wisconsin Personality Disorders Inventory: I. Development, reliability, and validity. *Journal of Personality Disorders, 7*, 285–303.

Kotov, R., Krueger, R. F., Watson, D., Achenbach, T. M., Althoff, R. R., Bagby, M., … Zimmerman, M. (2017). The Hierarchical Taxonomy of Psychopathology: A dimensional alternative to traditional nosologies. *Journal of Abnormal Psychology, 126*, 454–477.

Krueger, R. F. (2016). The future is now: Personality disorder and the ICD-11. *Personality and Mental Health, 10*, 118–119.

Krueger, R. F., & Markon, K. E. (2014). The role of the DSM-5 personality trait model in moving toward a quantitative and empirically based approach to classifying personality and psychopathology. *Annual Review of Clinical Psychology, 10*, 477–501.

Krueger, R. F., Hicks, B. M., Patrick, C. J., Carlson, S. R., Iacono, W. G., & McGue, M. (2002). Etiologic connections among substance dependence, antisocial behavior, and personality: Modeling the externalizing spectrum. *Journal of Abnormal Psychology, 111*, 411–424.

Krueger, R. F., Skodol, A. E., Livesley, W. J., Shrout, P. E., & Huang, Y. (2008). Synthesizing dimensional and categorical approaches to personality disorders: Refining the research agenda for DSM-IV Axis II. In J. E. Helzer, H. C. Kraemer, R. F. Krueger, H.-U. Wittchen, P. J. Sirovatka, & D. A. Regier (Eds.), *Dimensional approaches to diagnostic classification: Refining the research agenda for DSM-V* (pp. 85–100). American Psychiatric Association.

Krueger, R. F., Eaton, N. R., Clark, L. A., Watson, D., Markon, K. E., Derringer, J., Skodol, A., & Livesley, W. J. (2011). Deriving an empirical structure of personality pathology for DSM-5. *Journal of Personality Disorders, 25*, 170–191.

Kupfer, D. J., First, M. B., & Regier, D. A. (2002). Introduction. In D. J. Kupfer, M. B. First, & D. A. Regier (Eds.), *A research agenda for DSM-V* (pp. xv–xxiii). American Psychiatric Association.

Lilienfeld, S. O., & Arkowitz, H. (2007). What "psychopath" means. *Scientific American Mind, 18*, 80–81.

Lilienfeld, S. O., & Fowler, K. (2006). The self-report assessment of psychopathy: Problems, pitfalls, and promises. In C. J. Patrick (Ed.), *Handbook of psychopathy* (pp. 107–132). Guilford Press.

Lilienfeld, S. O., & Widows, M. R. (2005). *Psychopathic Personality Inventory—Revised professional manual*. Psychological Assessment Resources, Inc.

Lilienfeld, S. O., Waldman, I. D., & Israel, A. C. (1994). A critical examination of the use of the term "comorbidity" in psychopathology research. *Clinical Psychology: Science and Practice, 1*, 71–83.

Linehan, M. M. (1993). *Cognitive-behavioral treatment of borderline personality disorder*. Guilford Press.

Linehan, M. M., & Schmidt, H., III. (1995). The dialectics of effective treatment of borderline personality disorder. In W. T. O'Honohue & L. Krasner (Eds.), *Theories of behavior therapy: Exploring behavior change* (pp. 553–584). American Psychological Association.

Loranger, A. W. (1999). *International Personality Disorder Examination (IPDE)*. Psychological Assessment Resources.

Loranger, A. W. (2001). *OMNI Personality inventories. Professional manual*. Psychological Assessment Resources.

Lowe, J. R., & Widiger, T. A. (2009). Clinicians' judgments of clinical utility: A comparison of the DSM-IV with dimensional models of personality disorder. *Journal of Personality Disorders, 23*, 211–229.

Lykken, D. T. (2018). Psychopathy, sociopathy, and antisocial personality disorder. In C. J. Patrick (Ed.), *Handbook of psychopathy* (2nd ed., pp. 22–38). The Guilford Press.

Lynam, D. R., & Vachon, D. D. (2012). Antisocial personality disorder in DSM-5: Missteps and missed opportunities. *Personality Disorders, Theory, Research, and Treatment, 3*, 483–495.

Lynam, D. R., & Widiger, T. A. (2001). Using the five factor model to represent the DSM-IV personality disorders: An expert consensus approach. *Journal of Abnormal Psychology, 110*, 401–412.

Lynam, D. R., & Widiger, T. A. (2007). Using a general model of personality to identify the basic elements of psychopathy. *Journal of Personality Disorders, 21*, 160–178.

Lynam, D. R., Gaughan, E. T., Miller, J. D., Miller, D. J., Mullins-Sweatt, S., & Widiger, T. A. (2011). Assessing the basic traits associated with psychopathy: Development and validation of the Elemental Psychopathy Assessment. *Psychological Assessment, 23*, 108–124.

Lynch, T. R., & Cuper, P. F. (2012). Dialectical behavior therapy of borderline and other personality disorders. In T. A. Widiger (Ed.), *The Oxford handbook of personality disorders* (pp. 785–793). Oxford University Press.

Lynch, T. R., Trost, W. T., Salsman, N., & Linehan, M. M. (2007). Dialectical behavior therapy for borderline personality disorder. *Annual Review of Clinical Psychology, 3*, 181–206.

Malterer, M. B., Lilienfeld, S. O., Neumann, C. S., & Newman, J. P. (2010). Concurrent validity of the Psychopathic Personality Inventory with offender and community samples. *Assessment, 17*, 3–15.

McCrae, R. R., & Costa, P. T. (2003). *Personality in adulthood: A five-factor theory perspective* (2nd ed.). Guilford.

Mervielde, I., De Clercq, B., De Fruyt, F., & Van Leeuwen, K. (2005). Temperament, personality and developmental psychopathology as childhood antecedents of personality disorders. *Journal of Personality Disorders, 19*, 171–201.

Miller, J. D. (2012). Five-factor model personality disorder prototypes: A review of their development, validity, and comparison with alternative approaches. *Journal of Personality, 80*, 1565–1591.

Miller, J. D., Lyman, D. R., Widiger, T. A., & Leukefeld, C. (2001). Personality disorders as extreme variants of common personality dimensions: Can the Five Factor Model adequately represent psychopathy? *Journal of Personality, 69*, 253–276.

Miller, J. D., Reynolds, S. K., & Pilkonis, P. A. (2004). The validity of the five-factor model prototypes for personality disorders in two clinical samples. *Psychological Assessment, 16*, 310–322.

Miller, J. D., Lynam, D. R., Pham-Scottez, A., De Clercq, B., Rolland, J. P., & De Fruyt, F. (2008). Using the Five-Factor Model of personality to score the DSM-IV personality disorders. *Annales Médico Psychologiques, 166*, 418–426.

Miller, J. D., Widiger, T. A., & Campbell, W. K. (2010). Narcissistic personality disorder and the DSM-V. *Journal of Abnormal Psychology, 119*, 640–649.

Miller, J. D., Few, L. R., & Widiger, T. A. (2012). Assessment of personality disorders and related traits: Bridging DSM-IV-TR and DSM-5. In T. A. Widiger (Ed.), *Oxford handbook of personality disorder* (pp. 108–140). Oxford University Press.

Millon, T. (2011). *Disorders of personality: Introducing a DSM/ICD spectrum from normal to abnormal* (3rd ed.). Wiley.

Millon, T., Millon, C., & Davis, R. (1997). *MCMI-III manual* (2nd ed.). National Computer Systems.

Morey, L. C., & Hopwood, C. J. (2006). The Personality Assessment Inventory and the measurement of normal and abnormal personality constructs. In S. Strack (Ed.), *Differentiating normal and abnormal personality* (2nd ed., pp. 451–471). Springer.

Morey, L. C., Waugh, M. H., & Blashfield, R. K. (1985). MMPI scales for DSM-III personality disorders: Their derivation and correlates. *Journal of Personality Assessment, 49*, 245–251.

Mulder, R. T., Horwood, J., Tyrer, P., Carter, J., & Joyce, P. R. (2016). Validating the proposed ICD-11 domains. *Personality and Mental Health, 10*, 84–95.

Mullins-Sweatt, S. N., Edmundson, M., Sauer-Zavala, S. E., Lynam, D. R., Miller, J. D., & Widiger, T. A. (2012). Five-factor measure of borderline personality traits. *Journal of Personality Assessment, 94*, 475–487.

Ogloff, J. R. P., Campbell, R. E., & Shepherd, S. M. (2016). Disentangling psychopathy from antisocial personality disorder: An Australian analysis. *Journal of Forensic Psychology Research and Practice, 16*, 198–215.

Oltmanns, T. F., & Turkheimer, E. (2006). Perceptions of self and others regarding pathological personality traits. In R. F. Krueger & J. L. Tackett (Eds.), *Personality and psychopathology* (pp. 71–111). Guilford.

Oltmanns, J. R., & Widiger, T. A. (2018a). A self-report measure for the ICD-11 dimensional trait model proposal: The Personality Inventory for ICD-11. *Psychological Assessment, 30*, 154–169.

Oltmanns, J. R., & Widiger, T. A. (2018b). Assessment of fluctuation between grandiose and vulnerable narcissism: Development and initial validation of the FLUX scales. *Psychological Assessment, 30*, 1612–1624.

Ozer, D. J., & Benet-Martinez, V. (2006). Personality and the prediction of consequential outcomes. *Annual Review of Psychology, 57*, 401–421.

Patrick, C. J. (2006). Back to the future: Cleckley as a guide to the next generation of psychopathy research. In C. J. Patrick (Ed.), *Handbook of psychopathy* (pp. 605–617). Guilford.

Patrick, C. J., Fowles, D. C., & Krueger, R. F. (2009). Triarchic conceptualization of psychopathy: Developmental origins of disinhibition, boldness, and meanness. *Development and Psychopathology, 21*, 913–938.

Paulhus, D. L., & Williams, K. M. (2002). The Dark Triad of personality: Narcissism, achiavellianism, and psychopathy. *Journal of Research in Personality, 36*, 556–563.

Perry, J. C., & Bond, M. (2000). Empirical studies of psychotherapy for personality disorders. In J. Gunderson & G. Gabbard (Eds.), *Psychotherapy for personality disorders* (pp. 1–31). American Psychiatric Press.

Pfohl, B., Blum, N., & Zimmerman, M. (1997). *Structured interview for DSM-IV personality*. American Psychiatric Press.

Pincus, A. L., & Lukowitsky, M. R. (2010). Pathological narcissism and narcissistic personality disorder. *Annual Review of Clinical Psychology, 6*, 421–446.

Raskin, R., & Terry, H. (1988). A principal-components analysis of the Narcissistic Personality Inventory and further evidence of its construct validity. *Journal of Personality and Social Psychology, 54*, 890–902.

Regier, D. A. (2008). Forward: Dimensional approaches to psychiatric classification. In J. E. Helzer, H. C. Kraemer, R. F. Krueger, H.-U. Wittchen, P. J. Sirovatka, & D. A. Regier (Eds.), *Dimensional approaches to diagnostic classification: Refining the research agenda for DSM-V* (pp. xvii–xxiii). American Psychiatric Association.

Regier, D. A., Narrow, W. E., Kuhl, E. A., & Kupfer, D. J. (2010). The conceptual development of DSM-V. *American Journal of Psychiatry, 166*, 645–655.

Roberts, B. W., & DelVecchio, W. F. (2000). The rank-order consistency of personality traits from childhood to old age: A quantitative review of longitudinal studies. *Psychological Bulletin, 126*, 3–25.

Rogers, R., Salekin, R. T., Sewell, K. W., & Cruise, K. R. (2000). Protoypical analysis of antisocial personality disorder: A study of inmate samples. *Criminal Justice and Behavior, 27*(2), 234–255.

Ronningstam, E. (2005). Narcissistic personality disorder: A review. In M. Maj, H. S. Akiskal, J. E. Mezzich, & A. Okasha (Eds.), *Personality disorders* (pp. 278–327). John Wiley & Sons.

Rottman, B. M., Ahn, W. K., Sanislow, C. A., & Kim, N. S. (2009). Can clinicians recognize DSM-IV personality disorders from five-factor model descriptions of patient cases? *American Journal of Psychiatry, 196*, 356–374.

Rounsaville, B. J., Alarcon, R. D., Andrews, G., Jackson, J. S., Kendell, R. E., Kendler, K. S., & Kirmayer, L. J. (2002). Toward DSM-V: Basic nomenclature issues. In D. J. Kupfer, M. B. First, & D. A. Regier (Eds.), *A research agenda for DSM-V* (pp. 1–30). American Psychiatric Press.

Salekin, R. T. (2002). Psychopathy and therapeutic pessimism: Clinical lore or clinical reality? *Clinical Psychology Review, 22*, 79–112.

Samuel, D. B., & Widiger, T. A. (2004). Clinicians' personality descriptions of prototypic personality disorders. *Journal of Personality Disorders, 18*, 286–308.

Samuel, D. B., & Widiger, T. A. (2006). Clinicians' judgments of clinical utility: A comparison of the DSM-IV and five factor models. *Journal of Abnormal Psychology, 115*, 298–308.

Samuel, D. B., & Widiger, T. A. (2007). Describing Ted Bundy's personality and working toward DSM-V. *Independent Practitioner, 27*, 20–22.

Samuel, D. B., & Widiger, T. A. (2008). A meta-analytic review of the relationships between the five-factor model and DSM-IV-TR personality disorders: A facet level analysis. *Clinical Psychology Review, 28*, 1326–1342.

Samuel, D. B., Riddell, A. D. B., Lynam, D. R., Miller, J. D., & Widiger, T. A. (2012). A five-factor measure of obsessive-compulsive personality traits. *Journal of Personality Assessment, 94*, 456–465.

Schneider, K. (1923). *Psychopathic personalities*. Charles. C. Thomas.

Schotte, C. K. W., De Doncker, D., Vankerckhoven, C., Vertommen, H., & Cosyns, P. (1998). Self-report assessment of the DSM-IV personality disorders. Measurement of trait and distress characteristics: The ADP-IV. *Psychological Medicine, 28*, 1179–1188.

Shedler, J., Beck, A., Fonagy, P., Gabbard, G. O., Gunderson, J. G., Kernberg, O., Michels, R., & Westen, D. (2010). Personality disorders in DSM-5. *American Journal of Psychiatry, 167*, 1027–1028.

Simms, L. J., & Clark, L. A. (2006). The Schedule for Nonadaptive and Adaptive Personality (SNAP): A dimensional measure of traits relevant to personality and personality pathology. In S. Strack (Ed.), *Differentiating normal and abnormal personality* (2nd ed., pp. 431–449). Springer.

Skeem, J. L., & Cooke, D. J. (2010). Is criminal behavior a central component of psychopathy? Conceptual directions for resolving the debate. *Psychological Assessment, 22*, 433–445.

Skeem, J. L., Polaschek, D. L., Patrick, C. J., & Lilienfeld, S. O. (2011). Psychopathic personality bridging the gap between scientific evidence and public policy. *Psychological Science in the Public Interest, 12*, 95–162.

Skodol, A. E. (2010, February 10). *Rationale for proposing five specific personality types*. Retrieved from http://www.dsm5.org/ProposedRevisions/Pages/RationaleforProposingFiveSpecificPersonalityDisorderTypes.aspx

Skodol, A. E. (2012). Personality disorders in DSM-5. *Annual Review of Clinical Psychology, 8*, 317–344.

Skodol, A. E., Oldham, J. M., Bender, D. S., Dyck, I. R., Stout, R. L., Morey, L. C., Shea, M. T., Zanarini, M. C., Sanislow, C. A., Grilo, C. M., McGlashan, T. H., & Gunderson, J. G. (2005). Dimensional representations of DSM-IV personality disorders: Relationships to functional impairment. *American Journal of Psychiatry, 162*, 1919–1925.

Skodol, A. E., Morey, L. C., Bender, D. S., & Oldham, J. M. (2013). The ironic fate of the personality disorders in DSM-5. *Personality Disorders, Theory, Research, and Treatment, 4*, 342–349.

Smith, G. G., & Zapolski, T. C. B. (2009). Construct validation of personality measures. In J. N. Butcher (Ed.), *Oxford handbook of personality assessment* (pp. 81–98). Oxford University Press.

Somwaru, D. P., & Ben-Porath, Y. S. (1995). *Development and reliability of MMPI-2 based personality disorder scales*. Paper presented at the 30th Annual Workshop and Symposium on Recent Developments in Use of the MMPI-2 & MMPI-A. St. Petersburg Beach, Florida.

Spitzer, R. L., & Fleiss, J. L. (1974). A re-analysis of the reliability of psychiatric diagnosis. *British Journal of Psychiatry, 125*, 341–347.

Spitzer, R. L., Endicott, J., & Robins, E. (1978). Research diagnostic criteria: Rationale and reliability. *Archives of General Psychiatry, 35*, 773–782.

Spitzer, R. L., Endicott, J., & Gibbon, M. (1979). Crossing the border into borderline personality and borderline schizophrenia. *Archives of General Psychiatry, 36*, 17–24.

Spitzer, R. L., Williams, J. B. W., & Skodol, A. E. (1980). DSM-III: The major achievements and an overview. *American Journal of Psychiatry, 137*, 151–164.

Spitzer, R. L., First, M. B., Shedler, J., Westen, D., & Skodol, A. (2008). Clinical utility of five dimensional systems for personality diagnosis. *Journal of Nervous and Mental Disease, 196*, 356–374.

Stoff, D. M., Breiling, J., & Maser, J. D. (Eds.). (1997). *Handbook of antisocial behavior*. Wiley.

Torgersen, S. (2012). Epidemiology. In T. A. Widiger (Ed.), *The Oxford handbook of personality disorders* (pp. 186–205). Oxford University Press.

Trull, T. J., Widiger, T. A., Lynam, D. R., & Costa, P. T. (2003). Borderline personality disorder from the perspective of general personality functioning. *Journal of Abnormal Psychology, 112*, 193–202.

Trull, T. J., Jahng, S., Tohmko, R. L., Wood, P. K., & Sher, K. J. (2010). Revised NESARC personality disorder diagnoses: Gender, prevalence, and comorbidity with substance-dependence disorders. *Journal of Personality Disorders, 24*, 412–426.

Tyrer, P. (2014). Time to choose – DSM-5, ICD-11, or both? *Archives of Psychiatry and Psychotherapy, 3*, 5–8.

Tyrer, P., Reed, G. M., & Crawford, M. J. (2015). Classification, assessment, prevalence, and effect of personality disorder. *Lancet, 385*, 717–726.

Tyrer, P., Mulder, R., Kim, Y.-R., & Crawford, M. J. (2019). The development of the ICD-11 classification of personality disorders: An amalgam of science, pragmatism and politics. *Annual Review of Clinical Psychology, 15*, 481–502.

Westen, D. (1997). Divergences between clinical and research methods for assessing personality disorders: Implications for research and evolution of Axis II. *American Journal of Psychiatry, 154*, 895–903.

Widiger, T. A. (2013). DSM-5 personality disorders: A postmortem and future look. *Personality Disorders, Theory, Research, and Treatment, 4*, 382–387.

Widiger, T. A. (Ed.). (2017). *The Oxford handbook of the five-factor model*. Oxford University Press.

Widiger, T. A., & Clark, L. A. (2000). Toward DSM-V and the classification of psychopathology. *Psychological Bulletin, 126*, 946–963.

Widiger, T. A., & Corbitt, E. M. (1995). Antisocial personality disorder in DSM-IV. In W. J. Livesley (Ed.), *The DSM-IV personality disorders* (pp. 103–126). Guilford Press.

Widiger, T. A., & Costa, P. T. (Eds.). (2013). *Personality disorders and the five-factor model of personality*. American Psychological Association.

Widiger, T. A., & Crego, C. (2018). Psychopathy and DSM-5 psychopathology. In C. J. Patrick (Ed.), *Handbook of psychopathy* (2nd ed., pp. 281–298). Guilford Press.

Widiger, T. A., & Lynam, D. R. (1998). Psychopathy from the perspective of the five-factor model of personality. In T. Millon, E. Simonsen, M. Birket-Smith, & R. D. Davis (Eds.), *Psychopathy: Antisocial, criminal, and violent behaviors* (pp. 171–187). Guilford.

Widiger, T. A., & Samuel, D. B. (2005). Evidence based assessment of personality disorders. *Psychological Assessment, 17*, 278–287.

Widiger, T. A., & Simonsen, E. (2005). The American Psychiatric Association's research agenda for the DSM-V. *Journal of Personality Disorders, 19*, 103–109.

Widiger, T. A., & Trull, T. J. (2007). Plate tectonics in the classification of personality disorder: Shifting to a dimensional model. *American Psychologist, 62*, 71–83.

Widiger, T. A., Mangine, S., Corbitt, E. M., Ellis, C. G., & Thomas, G. V. (1995). *Personality Disorder Interview-IV: A semistructured interview for the assessment of personality disorders. Professional manual*. Psychological Assessment Resources.

Widiger, T. A., Cadoret, R., Hare, R., Robins, L., Rutherford, M., Zanarini, M., Alterman, A., Apple, M., Corbitt, E., Forth, A., Hart, S., Kultermann, J., Woody, G., & Frances, A. (1996). DSM-IV antisocial personality disorder field trial. *Journal of Abnormal Psychology, 105*, 3–16.

Widiger, T. A., Lynam, D. R., Miller, J. D., & Oltmanns, T. F. (2012a). Measures to assess maladaptive variants of the five-factor model. *Journal of Personality Assessment, 94*, 450–455.

Widiger, T. A., Samuel, D. B., Mullins-Sweat, S., Gore, W. L., & Crego, C. (2012b). Integrating normal and abnormal personality structure: The five-factor model. In T. A. Widiger (Ed.), *The Oxford handbook of personality disorders* (pp. 82–107). Oxford University Press.

Widiger, T. A., Costa, P. T., Gore, W. L., & Crego, C. (2013). Five factor model personality disorder research. In T. A. Widiger & P. T. Costa (Eds.), *Personality disorders and the five-factor model of personality* (3rd ed., pp. 75–100). American Psychological Association.

World Health Organization. (1992). *The ICD-10 classification of mental and behavioural disorders: Clinical descriptions and diagnostic guidelines*. World Health Organization.

Young, J. E., Klosko, J. S., & Weishaar, M. E. (2003). *Schema therapy: A practitioner's guide*. Guilford Press.

Zanarini, M. C., Frankenburg, F. R., Chauncey, D. L., & Gunderson, J. G. (1987). The Diagnostic Interview for Personality Disorders: Interrater and test-retest reliability. *Comprehensive Psychiatry, 28*, 467–480.

Zanarini, M. C., Gunderson, J. G., Frankenburg, F. R., & Chauncey, D. L. (1989). The Revised Diagnostic Interview for Borderlines: Discriminating BPD from other Axis II disorders. *Journal of Personality Disorders, 3*, 10–18.

Zanarini, M. C., Frankenburg, F. R., Sickel, A. E., & Yong, L. (1996). *The diagnostic interview for DSM-IV personality disorders (DIPD-IV)*. McLean Hospital.

Zimmerman, M., & Mattia, J. I. (1999). Differences between clinical and research practices in diagnosing borderline personality disorder. *American Journal of Psychiatry, 156*, 1570–1574.

Zimmerman, M., & Mattia, J. I. (2001). The Psychiatric Diagnostic Screening Questionnaire: Development, reliability and validity. *Comprehensive Psychiatry, 42*, 175–189.

Chapter 13
Forensic Rehabilitation Perspectives: Applying a Two-Component Framework to Interventions for Adults with Psychopathy

Julie Blais, Natasha S. Maltais, and Andrew E. Brankley

Abstract Individuals with psychopathic traits commit a disproportionate amount of crime (Coid J, Yang M, Soc Psychiatry Psychiatr Epidemiol 46:473–480, 2011; Kiehl KA, Hoffman MB, Jurimetrics J 51:355–397, 2011), are more violent than offenders without psychopathic traits (Lynam DR, J Abnorm Psychol 106:425–438, 1997; Porter S, Birt A, Boer DP, Law Hum Behav 25:647–661, 2001), and are estimated to cost the criminal justice system billions of dollars each year (Kiehl KA, Hoffman MB, Jurimetrics J 51:355–397, 2011). Treating psychopathic individuals and reducing their impact on society is therefore of utmost importance. This chapter begins by reviewing the operationalization and measurement of the construct of psychopathy in order to give context to the focus of intervention and the mechanisms for change. Next is a review of attempts to change the core personality traits of psychopathy (i.e., lack of empathy, deceitfulness) followed by a discussion of methodological issues and challenges with this approach to contextualize the source of therapeutic pessimism. This chapter also reviews treatment approaches that focus on behavioral changes which provide a more promising model of intervention. Although psychopathy is a challenging issue to address in treatment, there is now sufficient evidence to support the notion that individuals higher in psychopathy are not immune to making positive lifestyle and behavioral changes.

Keywords Psychopathy · Evidence-based treatment · Responsivity · Two-component model · Desistance · Good lives model · Management

---

J. Blais (✉)
Dalhousie University, Halifax, NS, Canada
e-mail: julie.blais@dal.ca

N. S. Maltais
Carleton University, Ottawa, ON, Canada

A. E. Brankley
Kurt Freund Phallometric Lab & Sexual Behaviours Clinic, Toronto, ON, Canada

J. E. Vitale (ed.), *The Complexity of Psychopathy*, Dangerous Behavior in Clinical and Forensic Psychology, https://doi.org/10.1007/978-3-030-83156-1_13

13.1 Introduction

Psychopathy can be conceptualized as a constellation of personality traits and behaviors that describe an individual who is antagonistic, manipulative, callous, erratic, and impulsive (Hare, 2003; Neumann et al., 2007). Although people with psychopathic traits represent 1% of the general population (e.g., Coid et al., 2009) and approximately 20–25% of the prison population (Hare, 2003), they exert a substantial cost to society. Individuals with psychopathic traits commit a disproportionate amount of crime (Coid & Yang, 2011; Kiehl & Hoffman, 2011), are more violent than offenders without psychopathic traits (Lynam, 1997; Porter et al., 2001), and are estimated to cost the criminal justice system billions of dollars each year (Kiehl & Hoffman, 2011). Overall, psychopathy can be viewed as a serious and pervasive public health concern (Reidy et al., 2015). Treating psychopathic individuals and reducing their impact on society is therefore of utmost importance.

This chapter begins by reviewing the operationalization and measurement of the construct of psychopathy in order to give context to the focus of intervention and the mechanisms for change. Next is a review of attempts to change the core personality traits of psychopathy (i.e., lack of empathy, deceitfulness) followed by a discussion of methodological issues and challenges with this approach to contextualize the source of therapeutic pessimism. This chapter also reviews treatment approaches that focus on behavioral changes which provide a more promising model of intervention. Although psychopathy is a challenging issue to address in treatment, there is now sufficient evidence to support the notion that individuals higher in psychopathy are not immune to making positive lifestyle and behavioral changes.

13.2 A Treatment Target with Distinct, Interrelated Features

In this chapter we adopt the operationalization of psychopathy put forth by the Psychopathy Checklist-Revised (PCL-R; Hare, 2003). The PCL-R is a construct rating scale comprised of 20 items scored between 1 (absent) and 2 (present) with total scores ranging from 0 to 40 (see Hare et al. (2017) for a detailed review). Several surveys have demonstrated that the PCL-R is the most common tool used in forensic and clinical settings (e.g., Hurducas et al., 2014; Neal & Grisso, 2014). PCL-R scores are also strong predictors of future violent and general recidivism (e.g., Leistico et al., 2008), both reactive and instrumental violence (Blais et al., 2014), institutional misconducts (Guy et al., 2005), sexual offending (Hawes et al., 2013), and failure on conditional release (Hart et al., 1988). As a result, the PCL-R is sometimes considered the "gold standard" of psychopathy measures (e.g., Acheson, 2005; Cooke & Michie, 2001).

Although the PCL-R model of psychopathy is traditionally conceptualized as a categorical phenomenon (i.e., "non-psychopaths" vs. "psychopaths"), examinations of the latent structure of the PCL-R support a dimensional interpretation (e.g., Guay et al., 2007). In other words, variations on PCL-R scores denote incremental differences in the level of expressed psychopathy. Although several factor structures have been proposed for the PCL-R, there is now ample support for the four-facet model consisting of the Interpersonal, Affective, Lifestyle, and Antisocial facets (Hare & Neumann, 2008; Neumann et al., 2007). These four facets can also be collapsed to represent the more traditional two-factor model of psychopathy (Hare, 1991) with Factor 1 representing the affective and interpersonal aspects and Factor 2 the lifestyle and antisocial aspects.

Factor 1 and Factor 2 show independent, even divergent, associations with important treatment-relevant constructs. For example, Wallace et al. (2009) found that Factor 1 was uniquely related to less reactivity in the region of the brain associated with the Behavioral Inhibition System (BIS; Gray & McNaughton, 2000) while Factor 2 was related to increased reactivity of the Behavioral Activation System (BAS). These results indicate that individuals with higher Factor 1 scores (sometimes referred to as Primary Psychopathy; Lykken, 1995) may be uniquely difficult to treat given their lower levels of anxiety and decreased sensitivity to behavioral consequences (i.e., low BIS). Those with higher Factor 2 scores, or Secondary Psychopathy, may, in turn, be more amenable to treatment given associations between high BAS and reward-seeking behaviors and positive emotional states (Newman et al., 2005; Wallace et al., 2009).

Further evidence for the distinct role of Factor 1 and 2 can be found by examining brain abnormalities that feature prominently in etiological models of psychopathy (see Yang and Raine (2017) for a detailed review). Whereas deficiencies in the prefrontal cortex (associated with more impulsive, aggressive behavior) have been equally related to total, Factor 1, and Factor 2 scores (Yang et al., 2005), deficiencies in the amygdala (associated with reduced ability to process emotional stimuli; Müller et al., 2003) have shown stronger associations with the affective and interpersonal features of psychopathy (Factor 1) as opposed to the impulsive and behavioral features (Factor 2; de Oliveira-Souza et al., 2008; Yang et al., 2009). Glenn et al. (2010) further found that Factor 1 traits/behaviors were related to increased volume of the striatum, which is involved in the initiation and persistence of reward-seeking behaviors and poor decision-making. Taken together, although very few studies have examined differential associations between psychopathy factors and structural differences in specific brain regions, the evidence that does exist suggests that Factor 1 traits/behaviors would be particularly problematic in treatment settings aimed at changing outcomes through rewards and punishments.

13.3 No Reliable Means to Change the Core Psychopathy Traits (Factor 1)

The original description of our modern conception of psychopathy (i.e., Cleckley, 1976) included the belief that treatment for these individuals would be pointless. This description also placed the affective and interpersonal components, now found under Factor 1, as the defining features of psychopathy. Therefore, treatment pessimism was likely tied to the belief that personality traits such as glibness, grandiosity, pathological lying, shallow affect, and lack of remorse represent relatively enduring and stable ways of interacting with the world. Certainly, there is ample evidence for the stability of personality traits across the lifespan (e.g., Caspi et al., 2005; Caspi & Silva, 1995). In addition, based on the neuropsychological research summarized above, clinicians may doubt the success of treatment when clients continue to show superficial, if any, regard for the consequences of their behavior.

The question then becomes, can personality traits be changed through appropriate treatment interventions? A recent meta-analysis by Roberts et al. (2017) examined the extent to which personality traits, conceptualized by the Big Five model, could be changed through intervention across 207 studies. The authors considered several intervention types (e.g., cognitive-behavioral, pharmacological) and a number of different presenting problems (e.g., depression, anxiety, personality disorder, etc.). Overall, treatment interventions were related to changes in personality traits both in the short-term and over longer follow-up periods. People with personality disorders made the most change of any presenting problem. While these results are promising, to date, no well-designed treatment studies exist that specifically target psychopathic personality traits.

A single study by Baskin-Sommers et al. (2015) provides preliminary evidence for the possibility of changing cognitive-emotional impairments related to psychopathic traits (e.g., blunted affect, enhanced goal-directed behavior; Baskin-Sommers et al., 2013). Participants ($N = 141$) were assessed with the PCL-R and placed into two groups before completing a six-week computer training program. The "externalizing" group included participants who scored a 12 or greater on Factor 2, but below the median on Factor 1. The "psychopathy" group included participants who scored a 12 or greater on Factor 2 and above the median on Factor 1. Half of each group was matched to complete programs focused on their specific affective deficits (i.e., attention to context for the "psychopathy" group and affective cognitive control for the "externalizing" group) and the other half received the opposite group's program. Participants who received congruent programs exhibited improved performance on the trained tasks and tasks that were not included in their training. Participants who completed the programs that were unrelated to their deficits did not show similar improvements (Baskin-Sommers et al., 2015). Although a promising study, further research is required to establish if such training translates to outside behavioral change and whether this change can be retained for a meaningful period of time.

Personality is developmental, meaning that changes in personality are not solely explained by neurobiological features, but also by experiences and relationships (Caspi, 1998; Caspi et al., 2005). Although Roberts et al. (2017) demonstrated that personality traits do in fact reliably change in treatment, especially amongst those who have chronic problematic traits, the current gap is in our understanding and application of these general findings to the treatment of psychopathic personality traits specifically. Although there is some preliminary evidence that changes in Factor 1 could be possible (Baskin-Sommers et al., 2015), the proposed treatment program (i.e., cognitive-affective retraining program) is not currently widely accepted or implemented in the treatment of personality disorders. Until further research is conducted, it would be unwise to pursue Factor 1 as a legitimate treatment target. Given this conclusion, it is necessary to move beyond changing psychopathic traits specifically, and to instead focus on changing problematic behavioral outcomes, mainly criminal offending.

13.4 Offender Rehabilitation

Historically, the debate concerning effective offender rehabilitation has shifted from a "nothing works" perspective made popular by Martinson's reviews in the 1970s (e.g., Martinson, 1974), to a more optimistic, yet cautious, view in the 1990s based on Lipsey's meta-analytic work (Lipsey, 1992, 1995), to a general acceptance today that offenders can be treated when provided with appropriate rehabilitation programs (see Andrews and Bonta (2010) for a detailed review). Offenders with psychopathic traits, however, present a unique challenge for treatment providers given their low treatment motivation, their antagonistic interpersonal style, and high rates of treatment dropout (Olver, 2016). In this section, we place psychopathy within three well-established correctional paradigms, namely Risk, Need, and Responsivity (RNR; Andrews & Bonta, 2010; Andrews et al., 2006), the Good Lives Model (Ward, 2002; Ward & Brown, 2004), and desistance (Porporino, 2010; Ward & Laws, 2010). While the focus is on describing how psychopathy can be adapted within each of these paradigms, we also provide cautions and limitations that should be considered when dealing with individuals with psychopathic traits.

We have also organized our discussion around two important considerations. First, as previously summarized, psychopathy is a multi-dimensional construct. While total scores are most often used when making risk-relevant decisions in the criminal justice system (e.g., preventative detention hearings; Blais & Forth, 2014), relying on total scores within treatment programs is not advisable because of the differential associations between psychopathy factor scores and relevant treatment outcomes (e.g., Factor 1 is more strongly related to problematic treatment behaviors; Olver & Wong, 2011). The incorporation of psychopathy within correctional paradigms therefore requires a consideration of Factor 1 and Factor 2, separately. Second, it is important to specify that the outcome of interest for correctional treatment programs is not the same as that of treatment programs designed for specific psychological or personality disorders. While treatment programs designed for specific disorders target aspects of that disorder with the goal of improving general and social functioning (e.g., improving emotional stability, decreasing self-injurious behaviors; McMain et al., 2009), the ultimate goal of correctional treatment programs is a reduction in the risk of reoffending.

13.4.1 The Risk, Need, and Responsivity (RNR) Model

One of the greatest developments in corrections research has been the creation and validation of the Risk, Need, and Responsivity (RNR) model outlining effective correctional practice (Andrews & Bonta, 2010; Bonta & Andrews, 2017). The RNR model draws on a general personality (individual factors) and cognitive social learning (changing modes of thinking and behavior) theory to identify who should be subjected to correctional treatment (Risk), what should be targeted within that treatment (Need), and how treatment should be delivered (Responsivity; Bonta & Andrews, 2017). To provide a brief review, the risk principle states that rehabilitation will be most successful when the intensity of the treatment is matched with the risk level posed by the individual. Here, the highest 'dose' of treatment (often determined by the number of hours spent within the program) would be provided to the highest risk individual as determined by a structured and validated risk assessment scale (Andrews & Bonta, 1994, 2010). The risk principle therefore assumes that offender risk can be reliably determined prior to the initiation of a correctional program (Andrews et al., 1990).

The need principle identifies what should be targeted within the intervention program, namely criminogenic needs. Criminogenic needs are dynamic factors that, when appropriately targeted, would result in reductions in reoffending (Andrews et al., 1990). Within the RNR model, important dynamic factors are found within the "Central Eight" risk factors (with the exception of criminal history which would not be considered a true dynamic factor as it can only increase with time; Bonta & Andrews, 2017). The dynamic factors within the "Central Eight" are: antisocial personality pattern (e.g., impulsive, aggressive, callous), antisocial cognition (e.g., negative attitudes towards the criminal justice system), antisocial associates (e.g., disproportionate association with antisocial peers), family/marital circumstances (e.g., quality of interpersonal relationships), school/work (e.g., quality of relationships within these settings), leisure/recreation (e.g., lack of engagement in prosocial activities), and substance abuse (Andrews & Bonta, 2010).

The RNR model also defines factors that are considered non-criminogenic needs. These are factors that are similarly dynamic in that they can be changed over time; however, such changes would not be associated with changes in risk for reoffending (Andrews & Dowden, 2007). Non-criminogenic needs should not be the primary focus of treatment interventions and instead, should be treated as potential treatment barriers. Non-criminogenic needs include many of the treatment targets for programs aimed at specific personality disorders such as personal distress, emotional regulation, and dealing with experiences of early trauma (e.g., Clarkin et al., 2016). Further examples of non-criminogenic needs include self-esteem, internalizing problems such as depression or anxiety, empathy, and denial (Hanson et al., 2009).

The responsivity principle encompasses two components. The general responsivity principle identifies cognitive social learning strategies as the most effective way to change behavior emphasizing both the relationship (i.e., establishing an appropriate prosocial connection with the client) and structural (i.e., modeling and reinforcement of prosocial goals) aspects of treatment (Andrews & Bonta, 2010). Specific responsivity identifies factors that will either help or hinder the rehabilitation process. Such factors must be considered to maximize an individual's ability to benefit from rehabilitation efforts (Andrews & Bonta, 2010). For example, individual characteristics that should be considered include treatment motivation, individual differences in personality, age, gender, and culture (Bonta & Andrews, 2017). It is under the specific responsivity principle that non-criminogenic needs can be targeted in order to enhance treatment motivation and reduce barriers to full participation.

While the RNR principles are considered core components of the RNR model, Andrews and Bonta (2010) have further outlined additional overarching, clinical, and organizational principles. Overarching principles include: (a) respect for persons and the delivery of an ethical and just treatment program, (b) the importance of basing treatment on sound psychological theory, and (c) the ultimate goal of reducing crime can occur both within and outside the justice system. The most important additional clinical principle outlines that multiple treatment needs should be targeted to maximize treatment benefit (breadth). Finally, organizational goals further outline that community-based programs are preferred over institutional programs, that staff must maintain high-quality relationships with clients while modeling appropriate prosocial behavior, and that appropriate oversight is required to ensure treatment integrity in adhering to RNR principles (Andrews & Bonta, 2010).

The RNR model has helped guide the creation of validated risk assessment scales and has provided an abundance of literature on effective correctional practices (e.g., Andrews & Dowden, 2007; Dowden & Andrews, 2000; Hanson et al., 2009; see Andrews and Bonta (2010) for further review). There also appears to be an incremental effect of RNR principles with treatment programs showing greater reductions in recidivism with the increase in the number of RNR principles that are adhered to (Dowden & Andrews, 1999, 2000; Hanson et al., 2009). Several meta-analyses have demonstrated that treatment programs based on the RNR model are effective for reducing recidivism among violent offenders (Dowden & Andrews, 2000), sexual offenders (Hanson et al., 2009), female offenders (Dowden & Andrews, 1999) and youth offenders (Koehler et al., 2014).

13.4.2 *The RNR Model and Psychopathy*

Risk The risk principle outlines that the level or intensity of correctional programming should match the risk level of the client. In applying this principle to individuals with psychopathic traits, it is therefore important to review the literature on the relationship between psychopathy and risk. There have been several meta-analytic examinations of this relationship (e.g., Kennealy et al., 2010; Leistico et al., 2008; Salekin et al., 1996; Walters, 2003a, b). The general finding is that psychopathy (most often measured by the PCL-R) is moderately and significantly related to general and violent recidivism. The results for sexual recidivism are somewhat mixed with some studies showing weak correlations between psychopathy and sexual recidivism (e.g., Gretton et al., 2001), and others demonstrating a stronger effect (e.g., Hanson & Morton-Bourgon, 2009) with evidence of an interaction between psychopathy and sexual deviance (increased risk when high psychopathy scores are combined with the presence of sexual deviancy; Hawes et al., 2013).

The relationship between psychopathy and risk also appears to depend on the factor of psychopathy under consideration. Factor 2, or the behavioral manifestations of psychopathy (i.e., impulsivity, poor behavioral controls, criminal history), has consistently produced stronger relationships to risk outcomes compared to Factor 1 (i.e., glibness, shallow affect, lack of remorse; Kennealy et al., 2010; Leistico et al., 2008). That is not to say, however, that Factor 1 is irrelevant to risk. In fact, Factor 1 has shown equivalent relationships to Factor 2 when examining specific outcomes such as reactive and instrumental aggression (Blais et al., 2014), inpatient aggression (Langton et al., 2011), and domestic violence (Swogger et al., 2007).

Overall, there is consistent evidence for a moderate relationship between psychopathy and risk for general and violent recidivism and a somewhat weaker association with sexual recidivism. As such, in applying the risk principle, individuals scoring higher on psychopathy would need more intensive rehabilitative programming. As a demonstration of the risk principle, Mailloux et al. (2003) examined risk factors among a group of 337 sexual offenders placed within either low, moderate, or high treatment intensity groups. There was a clear incremental effect of PCL-R scores with those in the high intensity group having significantly higher scores compared to the moderate group, who in turn had significantly higher scores than the low intensity group. That is not to say, however, that the absence of psychopathic traits would result in an individual being categorized as low risk, and therefore in need of less treatment. As outlined in the Central Eight risk/need factors, there are many other criminogenic needs that should be considered when classifying the risk of the client.

Need Applying the need principle to individuals with psychopathic traits is interesting as psychopathy is itself encompassed within the criminogenic need of antisocial personality pattern (APP). However, not all of the psychopathy traits and behaviors are related to APP. As outlined by Andrews and Bonta (2010), the conceptualization of APP within the lens of psychopathy facets emphasizes history of antisocial behavior, weak self-control, and poor problem solving, essentially analogous to the Lifestyle and Antisocial facets of the PCL-R. Less important to the conception of APP are the affective and interpersonal aspects of psychopathy such as glibness, conning/manipulation, and shallow affect. Factor 2 traits are therefore more appropriate treatment targets compared to Factor 1 traits.

In applying the need principle, we can also consider differences in the type and severity of criminogenic needs among psychopathic and non-psychopathic offenders. The actual types of criminogenic needs experienced by both groups are not expected to be very different. Wong and Burt (2007) used the Violence Risk Scale (VRS; Wong & Gordon, 2006) to compare the criminogenic needs profiles of a group of psychopathic offenders who had recidivated violently to a group of psychopathic offenders who had not. Overall, those who did not recidivate were older at release, had less lengthy criminal histories, fewer violent incidents within institutions, were less aggressive, and had better community supports. These results provide support for the benefit of applying the needs principle to the treatment of psychopathic offenders in that psychopathic individuals with fewer criminogenic needs were less likely to reoffend. In terms of severity, Wong and Burt (2007) demonstrated that psychopathic offenders do have more criminogenic needs than non-psychopathic offenders.

Responsivity General responsivity outlines the importance of employing cognitive-behavioral treatment interventions with the goal of reducing procriminal behaviors. Certainly, among general offender populations, such interventions have demonstrated significant reductions in recidivism (Gendreau & Andrews, 1990; McGuire et al., 2008). Unfortunately, the evidence for psychopathic offenders seems to suggest that these offenders do not experience the same level of treatment change as their non-psychopathic counterparts. In an early summary of the literature on psychopathy and cognitive-behavioral (CBT) programs, Thornton and Blud (2007) outlined several key findings: (1) psychopathic offenders demonstrated less treatment change overall, especially in the short-term; (2) retention in the program was related to better post-treatment outcomes; and (3) participation in some cognitive-behavioral programs resulted in worse post-treatment outcomes for some psychopathic offenders. More recently, Olver (2016) outlined the treatment responsivity of a sample of men who underwent an intensive violence-reduction program; all four facets of psychopathy were related to less treatment change. Therefore, the effectiveness of cognitive-behavioral programs for psychopathic offenders is a complex issue and likely depends on the specific combination of psychopathic traits and the ability of treatment staff to retain psychopathic offenders within the treatment program.

Andrews and Bonta (2010) explicitly state that psychopathy should be considered within the specific responsivity principle. Certainly, it is not difficult to envision that psychopathic offenders would be considered "difficult" clients. Indeed, evidence for the relationship between psychopathic traits and poor treatment compliance abound (see Hemphill & Hart, 2002). In a meta-analysis examining predictors of treatment attrition, Olver et al. (2011) identified psychopathy scores as being significantly related to treatment dropout. Psychopathic offenders are also more likely to be disruptive in treatment settings (Barbaree, 2005; Hughes et al., 1997) and lacking in overall motivation (Ogloff et al., 1990). There is also evidence that psychopathic offenders are less able to form appropriate, high-quality relationships with service providers, which is identified as a core practice within the RNR framework (Andrews & Bonta, 2010). In a study on the relationship between psychopathy and working alliance, DeSorcy et al. (2020) demonstrated that psychopathy, especially the affective features, was related to a diminished capacity to bond emotionally with treatment providers.

Part of the suggested solution to dealing with "difficult" or "weakly motivated" clients within the specific responsivity principle is to "reduce personal and situational barriers to full participation in treatment...[and to]...establish high-quality relationships" (Andrews & Bonta, 2010, p. 46). Given the consistent finding that psychopathic offenders are unable or unwilling to fully participate in treatment or to form the necessary social bonds with treatment providers, it seems that a more specific proscriptive approach to incorporating psychopathy within the specific responsivity principle is needed.

13.5 Re-thinking the RNR Model: Two-Component Model

Although Andrews and Bonta (2010) included a delineation between Factor 1 and Factor 2 traits in their description of the criminogenic need of APP, and that psychopathy is mentioned within the specific responsivity principle, Wong (2015) and colleagues (Wong & Hare, 2005, Wong et al., 2012) have formalized the incorporation of psychopathic traits within RNR principles in their Two-Component Model of offender rehabilitation. At the core of the argument for the adoption of the Two-Component Model, is the idea that in order to see positive effects of treatment, psychopathic offenders must be retained within that treatment (Wong, 2015; Wong et al., 2012). Furthermore, the goal of the treatment is not the modulation of psychopathic traits (especially those encompassed within Factor 1), but rather the ultimate reduction of criminal behavior (Wong & Burt, 2007; Wong & Hare, 2005; Wong et al., 2012).

Component 1 Based on evidence that Factor 1 traits are more weakly related to reoffending compared to Factor 2 traits (e.g., Yang et al., 2010), and that Factor 1 traits are associated with a variety of difficult treatment behaviors (DeSorcy et al., 2020; Olver et al., 2011; Wong & Hare, 2005), it is most appropriate to treat Factor 1 as a specific responsivity issue. The goal of Component 1, or the Interpersonal Component, is to treat Factor 1 traits and behaviors as responsivity issues that must be addressed to ensure that the psychopathic offender does not engage in behaviors that will disrupt the treatment program or result in treatment dropout (Wong et al., 2012). Particular attention should be paid to attempts to manipulate treatment providers or antagonize providers and other clients.

In addressing these traits and behaviors, Wong and Hare (2005) outline several key strategies that treatment providers can adopt. In overcoming treatment resistance, program staff are instructed to emphasize psychopathic offenders' own interests in remaining crime-free, a strategy that plays well towards psychopathic offenders' increased narcissism and self-centeredness. In forming appropriate working alliances, the goal should not be on forming warm, caring, emotional bonds, but rather on emphasizing task-related bonds that require less emotional investment. Other techniques include closely monitoring attempts at manipulation and staff splitting and to deal with these issues openly and proactively (Wong, 2015; Wong & Hare, 2005; Wong et al., 2012).

Component 2 Component 2, or the Criminogenic Component, outlines that Factor 2 traits and behaviors should be treated as criminogenic needs, based on the assumption that they represent a persistent and entrenched antisocial behavior pattern (Wong, 2015; Wong et al., 2012). For example, it is assumed that while some aspects of Factor 2 are static and unchangeable (i.e., early behavioral problems), others are approximate representations of established criminogenic needs (e.g., poor behavioral controls; parasitic lifestyle). The application of Component 2 is not expected to differ based on the presence of psychopathic traits. The goal is the delivery of an evidence-based rehabilitation program that reliably assesses and targets dynamic, criminogenic needs (Wong, 2015).

Therefore, the application of Component 2 requires that the dynamic, criminogenic needs of clients, including those with psychopathic traits, be assessed and monitored throughout the treatment program for indications of positive change. Wong (2015) recommends the use of the Violence Risk Scale (VRS; Wong & Gordon, 2006) as it can identify appropriate treatment targets and incorporates a stages-of-change (Prochaska et al., 1992) component to measure a client's progression on these treatment targets (e.g., going from contemplation to action). The VRS incorporates these changes as reductions in the overall risk of reoffending. The take-away message is that psychopathic clients have the same criminogenic needs as non-psychopathic clients, even if they may have more of them.

13.5.1 Evidence for the Two-Component Model

Several studies now provide evidence for the effectiveness of the Two-Component Model of offender rehabilitation. These studies focused on assessing the level of change in criminogenic needs that occurred during the program and whether these changes were related to changes in recidivism. Olver and Wong (2009) assessed changes in criminogenic needs using the Violence Risk Scale-Sex Offender version (VRS-SO; Wong et al., 2003) in a sample of 156 federal sex offenders; a cut-score of 25 on the PCL-R was used to identify the high psychopathy group. Consistent with the responsivity principle of the RNR model, offenders underwent a high intensity CBT program. Results indicated that psychopathy was a significant predictor of treatment dropout; however, consistent with Component 1, focusing on treatment motivation reduced treatment attrition in that the majority of psychopathic offenders completed the treatment program. Controlling for sexual offending risk, after a 10-year follow-up period psychopathic offenders who did not complete treatment were more likely to violently reoffend (but not sexually reoffend) compared with psychopathic offenders who completed treatment ($d = .98$). Consistent with Component 2, more treatment change among psychopathic offenders was associated with less violent recidivism.

More recently, Olver et al. (2013) examined the effect of a high-intensity CBT program aimed at reducing violent recidivism. This sample was particularly high risk with over 25% scoring at or above 30 on the PCL-R. The Violence Risk Scale (VRS; Wong & Gordan, 2006) was used to assess treatment change from pre- to post-treatment. Factor 1 traits (especially the Affective facet) were significantly related to *less* therapeutic change. After controlling for Factor 1, however, there was a significant relationship between treatment change and reductions in violent recidivism. This study specifically demonstrated that Factor 1 traits and behaviors act as treatment barriers; once addressed, even offenders scoring high on psychopathy can benefit from a structured CBT program.

13.6 The Good Lives Model

The Good Lives Model (GLM) is a strength-based theoretical framework that incorporates effective strategies of other frameworks with an emphasis on the engagement of participants in the rehabilitation process (Willis & Ward, 2013). Developed by Ward and colleagues (Laws & Ward, 2011; Ward, 2002; Ward & Maruna, 2007), the overarching goal of the GLM is to provide clients with resources to live a 'good or better life' that is both socially acceptable and personally meaningful (Ward & Brown, 2004; Willis & Ward, 2013).

According to the GLM, all human beings, including those involved in the criminal justice system, are goal-directed and are predisposed to attain a number of primary human goods. 'Primary goods' refer to certain states of mind, personal characteristics, and experiences that represent an individual's core values and life priorities (Willis & Ward, 2013). Currently, 11 classes of primary goods have been proposed by Ward and colleagues (e.g., knowledge, community, happiness; see Ward & Gannon, 2006). From this perspective, criminal behavior results from maladaptive strategies, called secondary or instrumental goods, used to attain these life goals (Willis & Ward, 2013). Thus, the problem does not lie with the life goals of an individual, but rather with how they attempt to achieve them. The GLM further proposes that criminal behavior results from an individual lacking the means, capacity, or capability to attain a primary good, paying little attention to some needs while paying too much attention to others, or having conflicting goals that lead to problems in attaining primary goods (Ward & Stewart, 2003).

Treatment under the GLM framework is similar to risk management frameworks in many ways, including the use of CBT interventions (Ward & Gannon, 2006). However, the GLM focuses both on promoting goods and managing or reducing risk. This twin focus is achieved mainly through equipping clients with the skills, values, attitudes, and resources (i.e., internal and external conditions) they need to lead a more prosocial life that still meets their prioritized needs (Whitehead et al., 2007). The emphasis is on approach rather than avoidance goals. That is, instead of focusing on the behaviors that a client cannot engage in (avoidance), treatment assists individuals in finding more appropriate ways to attain their primary goods (approach; Willis & Ward, 2013). For example, interventions would focus on how an individual can achieve autonomy without violence towards others or how they can achieve inner peace without the use of substances (Yates, 2013).

The GLM frames criminogenic needs as internal or external obstacles to living a good life that block the acquisition of primary goods (Ward & Brown, 2004). In other words, risk factors distort or omit competencies or opportunities that are required to live a "good" life. Through the GLM framework, an individual can relate their risk factors, either directly or indirectly, to their ability to attain valued goals (Whitehead et al., 2007). By doing so, the individual can become motivated to address his or her criminogenic needs in order to obtain primary goods. An assessment of criminogenic needs therefore allows clinicians to identify the primary good that is not being satisfied appropriately, and to develop an understanding of what competencies or opportunities are required for the client to meet their needs without harming others (Ward & Brown, 2004).

According to Willis and Ward (2013), the core RNR principles are incorporated within the GLM, however, the GLM also attempts to address some perceived flaws of RNR-based programs, particularly their focus on individual deficits, risk management, and avoidance goals. These latter characteristics are thought to interfere with the treatment engagement of clients (Mann et al., 2004; Ward & Gannon, 2006; Willis & Ward, 2013). Thus, the GLM aims to ground the goals of risk management strategies within a model that is more motivating and meaningful for individuals engaged in treatment (Whitehead et al., 2007).

Research on the effectiveness of the GLM is still in its infancy, however, preliminary results generally suggest that the model may enhance the efficacy of treatment programs that adhere to RNR principles. Specifically, current research suggests that the GLM may improve treatment engagement and enhance motivation (Barnett et al., 2014; Gannon et al., 2011; Harkins et al., 2012; Lindsay et al., 2007; Mann et al., 2004; Ware & Bright, 2008; Willis et al., 2014; Whitehead et al., 2007). It is important to note, however, that the current evidence is based mainly on case studies, non-randomized samples, and small sample sizes (Netto et al., 2014). As such, results should be interpreted with caution until more rigorous studies can be conducted. Further, although it is a general theory of rehabilitation, the GLM has mainly been applied to sex offending treatment programs (Willis & Ward, 2013).

In one of the only experimental studies examining the GLM, Mann et al. (2004) compared an approach goal oriented (GLM) relapse prevention (RP) program to an avoidance goal oriented (risk-reduction) RP program among 47 individuals convicted of a sexual offense. Results suggested that clients in the approach-oriented intervention were more engaged in treatment as measured by homework compliance, more willing to disclose lapses, and seen as more motivated by therapists compared to participants in the avoidance-oriented programs. However, the study did not examine any form of recidivism, meaning that while the approach-oriented intervention appeared to have benefits, the extent to which the program addressed criminal offending is unknown.

Two additional studies have compared individuals with histories of sexual offending who either attended a GLM-consistent intervention or a risk-focused RP intervention (Barnett et al., 2014; Harkins et al., 2012) on pre- to post-treatment changes to attrition rates, views of offenders and facilitators, and a variety of psychometric measures that the authors believed to be relevant to treatment (e.g., interpersonal reactivity, loneliness, under-assertiveness, sexual interest in children, relapse prevention, victim empathy). In both studies, no significant differences in treatment attrition or treatment change were found in either program types. However, Harkins et al. (2012) reported that facilitators and participants of the GLM-consistent program saw the intervention as more positive and future-focused. Barnett et al. (2014) found that participants of the GLM-based program attained post-treatment scores similar to those of non-offending individuals on several of the measures of pro-offending attitudes and socio-affective functioning.

13.6.1 Psychopathy and the GLM

Currently, there is only one case study examining the GLM with an individual with psychopathic traits. Whitehead et al. (2007) described the implementation of the GLM with an individual deemed at high risk to reoffend. The case study included detailed guidelines for assessment, treatment planning, and monitoring. The individual had a history of violent offending, demonstrated many psychopathic traits, and, despite attending and completing several high-intensity treatment programs, reoffended on release. Having exhausted all treatment options with little progress, the GLM was implemented in order to complement and enhance the risk management interventions already in place. The GLM was meant to facilitate treatment readiness and promote long-term reintegration goals by getting the client to focus on defining and then achieving a meaningful and fulfilling life. This, in turn, would help keep the client engaged in the treatment process and actively address his criminogenic needs. Examples of goals for this particular client included attending university, improving relationships with the opposite sex, and making his family proud.

The authors' emphasized that the success of using the GLM with this high-risk individual was partly due to focusing the therapy sessions on goals associated with the individual's well-being instead of on moral ideas of right and wrong. This way, clients can be equipped with capabilities to achieve *their* goals, but in socially acceptable ways (Whitehead et al., 2007). This would seem to indicate that psychopathic offenders may have different primary goals than non-psychopathic offenders. The point of treatment should therefore be on identifying personally endorsed goals for this particular population and encouraging prosocial ways to attain those goals. Lalumière et al. (2005) supported this notion when they argued that individuals with considerable psychopathic traits would continue to recidivate unless they were able to manipulate others in a non-criminal way. Additionally, this approach is in line with the concept of helping clients with psychopathy move away from self-interest and towards 'qualified self-interest', where they learn to consider their impact on others so that they can achieve their goals, whatever those goals may be (Hemphill & Hart, 2002).

The case study described by Whitehead et al. (2007) is also very analogous to Wong's (2015) Two-Component Model. For example, the solution for the appropriate rehabilitation of psychopathic offenders based on the GLM was to focus simultaneously on treatment readiness and retention (Component 1) while also continuing to address criminogenic needs (Component 2). Ogloff and Davies (2004) also reconceptualised the GLM to fit within the RNR model. The authors postulated that the GLM may address treatment responsiveness, thus being a part of the responsivity principle, by being an important mediating factor for change. Applying the GLM in this manner is also simply another description of the Two-Component model. The GLM would be used to address Factor 1 traits as they relate to treatment readiness and motivation while also addressing important criminogenic needs.

A few features of the GLM may, however, be detrimental to the treatment of psychopathic offenders. The collaborative nature of interventions that follow the

GLM may give psychopathic offenders the opportunity to manipulate and control others. Certainly, this aspect of therapeutic communities has shown to be particularly problematic for people with psychopathic traits (e.g., Rice et al., 1992). Additionally, although addressing treatment motivation is a positive aspect of GLM, the success of such attempts would greatly depend on the actual strategies employed. Any attempt to build a positive therapeutic relationship has the potential to result in worse outcomes for clients with psychopathic traits.

13.7 Desistance Frameworks

There are various definitions of desistance in the literature, although crime desistance generally refers to an individual's cessation of criminal behavior and is viewed as a dynamic process and not an event *per se*, as lapses, relapses, and recoveries are normal (Burnett, 2004; Porporino, 2010; Ward & Laws, 2010). While an individual may stop offending for any given period, this does not necessarily mean that they have permanently stopped offending behaviors (Piquero, 2004). In contrast, an individual who has reoffended may also cease offending at any point. Desistance research attempts to understand the natural change processes associated with an individual turning away from crime and successfully reintegrating into the community (McNeill et al., 2005).

Many theories of desistance exist, although they generally focus on one or all of the following factors: (1) age and maturation, (2) life transitions and social bonds, and (3) changes in identity (Maruna, 2001). Briefly, theories that focus on the relationship between age and desistance emphasize the age-crime curve. The age-crime curve, derived from plotting age by crime rates, shows that crime rates rise during adolescence, peak in early adulthood before dropping in later adulthood (Moffitt, 1993; Stolzenberg & D'Alessio, 2008). Gottfredson and Hirschi (1990) proposed that the decline in offending rates in adulthood is likely due to the biological effects of ageing. This notion of "burn out" with age has also been proposed by Collins (2004).

Theories emphasizing social bonds include the age-graded theory of informal social control by Sampson and Laub (1993), which suggests that salient life events and social ties in adulthood could, to some extent, interrupt a criminal career. Thus, despite criminal propensity, the presence of key 'turning points' and strong social bonds could lead to desistance from crime for any individual (Sampson & Laub, 1993; Laub & Sampson, 2001). Examples of turning points include strong relationships, stable work, and transformation of identity (Laub & Sampson, 2001). While the theory initially focused little on personal factors, it was later revised to emphasize the role of personal agency in desistance trajectories (Laub & Sampson, 2003).

Conversely, theorists such as Maruna (2001) emphasize the contribution of cognitive transformations to desistance. Through interviews, Maruna (2001) discovered that both persisters (i.e., those that admitted to continued criminal behavior) and desisters (i.e., those that claimed to have stopped all criminal behavior) developed what he called 'scripts'. Persisters saw themselves as helpless and dependent on circumstances whereas desisters had a more optimistic outlook on both their ability to control their own lives and be productive, contributing members of society. Although events such as marriage and stable employment have important roles in the process of desistance, Maruna (2001) posits that human agency is the key factor. Other investigations have also supported the unique influence of internal factors of desistance (Giordano et al., 2002; Lebel et al., 2008; Maruna & Roy, 2007; Paternoster & Bushway, 2009). In other words, while turning point events are important, they may have a different impact depending on an individual's level of motivation, perceptions of self, openness to change, and maturation (Giordano et al., 2007; Lebel et al., 2008).

Therefore, individuals are more likely to desist from crime when they have reached a point of maturation, when they have strong bonds with family and their community, fulfilling employment, when they abstain from drugs and alcohol, have feelings of hope and self-efficacy, a sense of meaning and purpose, and recognition of their worth from others (see Farrall & Calverley, 2005; Maruna & Mann, 2019; Rocque, 2017). Notably, desistence research has focused mainly on the natural course of crime desistence and not on how interventions may help with the process (Maruna, 2010). There is also no singular desistance intervention or treatment program. A desistance-focused intervention typically means that the design and delivery of the intervention are drawn from the findings of desistance research and/or the expertise of individuals whom themselves have desisted from crime (Maruna & Mann, 2019).

Many recommendations for how interventions, as well as community supervision, can incorporate the findings from desistance research are available (see Farrall, 2004; Maguire & Raynor, 2006; Maruna et al., 2004; Maruna & Mann, 2019; McNeill, 2003; Porporino, 2010; Rex. 1999; Ward & Laws, 2010). For instance, desistance research has demonstrated that employment and meaningful relationships can lead to the cessation of crime (Lebel et al., 2008; Sampson & Laub, 1993), thus any social initiatives that make these events more possible should be encouraged (Ward & Laws, 2010). Further, the existence of various social, vocational, academic, parenting, and relationship skill-building courses already available to individuals to help increase their social capital aligns with the desistance framework (Maguire & Raynor, 2006; Martín et al., 2010). Evidence-based programs that teach offenders problem-solving, coping and planning skills are also consistent with desistance theory. By emphasizing practical reasoning over more abstract, theoretical reasoning skills, Porporino (2010) suggests that programs could become more desistance supportive.

Additionally, Ward and Laws (2010) have suggested that the GLM, which provides clear guidelines for interventions, can integrate desistance ideas into treatment programs because of the overlapping theoretical background of the two frameworks. Similarly, emphasizing the importance of protective factors, which are defined as personal or situational factors that can reduce the risk of reoffending (de Vogel et al., 2009), in addition to risk factors may be another way to incorporate more desistance-supportive strategies. Protective factors have demonstrated incremental predictive validity over risk factors alone (de Vries Robbé et al., 2013), with some noted protective factors mirroring those related to desistance, such as social support (Ullrich & Coid, 2011), employment (de Vogel et al., 2011), and motivation (de Vogel et al., 2011).

Proponents of desistance frameworks have also suggested that rehabilitation efforts should be more strength-focused (Maruna & LeBel, 2003), emphasize relationships (e.g., therapeutic relationships, relationships with significant others; Burnett & McNeill, 2005; McNeill, 2006), develop and maintain motivation and hope (Farrall & Calverly, 2006), and acknowledge and accommodate issues of identity and diversity (Weaver & McNeill, 2010). Empirical validation of these recommendations is still needed to determine how effective assisted desistance is in reducing recidivism.

13.7.1 Psychopathy and Desistance

The construct of psychopathy has mainly been described as a barrier to desistance (McCuish, 2016). This characterization is not surprising given that the core features of psychopathy, especially Factor 1 traits and behaviors, would hinder the effects of informal social controls (Cernkovich & Giordano, 2001; McCarthy et al., 2012; McCuish, 2016, 2019). Features of psychopathy such as sensation seeking (Cooke et al., 2012), impulsivity (Morgan et al., 2011), and being unattached and uncommitted (Cooke et al., 2004) may increase the likelihood of engaging in high risk and dangerous offending as well as decrease the likelihood of considering the consequences of offending or being affected by factors considered as deterrents from crime (e.g., risk of injury, lengthy prison sentences, deaths of criminal associates; Caldwell et al., 2006; McCuish, 2016; Vaughn et al., 2008). Individuals high in psychopathic traits may also experience sources of informal social controls (e.g., marriage, employment), but in a way that may increase their opportunities for criminal behavior rather than leading to desistance (e.g., domestic abuse, theft from work; McCuish, 2019; Steels et al., 1998). Psychopathy is also significantly associated with chronic offending (Piquero et al., 2012), even when controlling for several risk and protective factors (e.g., substance abuse, family dynamics; Corrado et al., 2015).

Although high levels of psychopathic traits present a barrier to desistance, there are still individuals who never come into contact with the law and some who stop criminal behavior altogether, despite possessing numerous psychopathic traits. Focusing on the three main desistance factors (i.e., age, life transitions and social bonds, and the transformation of identity; Maruna, 2001), there appears to be some support that theories based on these factors may apply to individuals with high levels of psychopathy. For example, there is evidence to suggest that age is a natural source of desistance for those with psychopathy, albeit, appearing to have a delayed effect. Hare et al. (1988) found that individuals with high PCL scores committed more crimes than people with low scores between the ages of 16 and 40, but that after the age of 40, conviction rates decreased considerably. Similarly, Shaw and

Porter (2012) found that the number of nonviolent offenses committed by those with high PCL-R scores declined after the age of 30 relative to violent offenses; violence offenses similarly declined, then rebounded in the late 30s before declining considerably. Research has also demonstrated that Factor 2 traits can change more readily over time, while Factor 1 traits remain relatively stable (Harpur & Hare, 1994). It is therefore plausible that age is a natural form of desistance for criminal behaviors associated with Factor 2 traits, rather than Factor 1 traits.

Examinations of protective factors can be used to assess the role of informal social controls (i.e., life transitions, social bonds) for those with psychopathic traits. In a study examining the association between protective factors and measures of psychopathy and antisocial behavior among community members with and without criminal histories, DeMatteo et al. (2005) found no significant relationships between protective factors and psychopathy. In contrast, Burt et al. (2016) examined 123 individuals with PCL-R scores of 25 or higher who had completed a minimum of 4 months in a violent offender treatment program and found that those that had not received a new conviction for a violent offense after 5 years were older at release and had better community support than those that violently recidivated. Those who desisted also had significantly lower PCL-R Factor 2 scores, but higher Factor 1 scores (Burt et al., 2016).

Noted as key factors to desistance, the transformation of identity (i.e., motivation, perceptions of self, openness to change) may be difficult to foster in individuals high in psychopathy because interpersonal traits are generally stable across the lifespan (Blonigen et al., 2006; Harpur & Hare, 1994). Therefore, it makes sense that psychopathy is a barrier for desistance if human agency influences the effect of other forms of desistance. Motivation is a major obstacle in individuals demonstrating many psychopathic traits (Hemphill & Hart, 2002; Ogloff et al., 1990), however, there are also high-risk individuals that want to stop offending, and those that can find motivation and show changes in treatment are more likely to desist (Looman et al., 2005; Olver & Wong, 2009; Polaschek & Yesberg; 2015). Consistent with the Two-Component Model, motivation and other interpersonal traits may need to be addressed as specific responsivity factors before antisocial tendencies can be addressed.

Overall, there is little research that has explicitly examined the process of desistance for individuals high on psychopathy and the research that does exist appears to be quite pessimistic (i.e., psychopathy as an obstacle). Yet interestingly, when examined as a whole, it appears that, despite representing a barrier to desistance, there is some evidence that individuals with psychopathic traits can desist from crime, even if they do so more slowly. Moreover, research based on desistance theories appears to provide further support for the Two-Component Model. More specifically, the studies described above appear to support the focus on Factor 2 traits in interventions, as they seem to be more directly linked to persistence or desistance of crime (i.e., criminal trajectories, the influence of protective factors, and informal social controls). However, Factor 1 traits may still need to be addressed in treatment, although to a lesser extent, as they may act as obstacles (i.e., responsivity issues) to the influence of natural desistance factors.

13.8 Gender Considerations

Psychopathy is a relevant construct to examine and treat in women (Klein Tuente et al., 2014), however, there are gender-specific considerations and limitations that must be acknowledged. First and foremost, research has suggested that psychopathy occurs less frequently in women (Wynn et al., 2012). Yet, the extent to which the observed differences in the prevalence of psychopathy in men and women are due to physical differences in frequency (i.e., women are less likely to demonstrate high levels of psychopathy), or due to limitations in the diagnostic tools and terminology used (i.e., the assessment of psychopathy is male-orientated), is still debated (Forouzan & Cooke, 2005; Nicholls & Petrila, 2005; Rogstad & Rogers, 2008; Wynn et al., 2012).

The validity of using measures such as the PCL-R in assessing women has been questioned, as both the predictive validity (Dolan & Vøllm, 2009; Neumann & Hare, 2008; Salekin et al., 1998; Singh et al., 2011; Weizmann-Henelius et al., 2015) and factor structure (Dolan & Vøllm, 2009; Jackson et al., 2002; Warren et al., 2003) have shown to be inconsistent in populations of women. Thus, caution in using psychopathy measures originally validated on men is warranted, with some researchers suggesting that we should also focus on total scores instead of factor scores and that we should view psychopathy as dimensional rather than using any cut-off scores to ensure that women with significant psychopathic traits are not missed (Jackson et al., 2002; Kreis & Cooke, 2012).

There is also evidence that psychopathy might be expressed differently in women compared to men. Certain interpersonal features such as grandiose self-image and superficial charm are rarely seen in women (Rogstad & Rogers, 2008), yet other features such as impulsivity, poor behavioral controls, and emotional instability appear more frequently (Kreis & Cooke, 2012; Strand & Belfrage, 2005; Weizmann-Henelius et al., 2015; Wennberg, 2012). Typical markers for psychopathy may also have different underlying motivational factors depending on gender. For example, while a man high in psychopathy may use force and violence, a woman may resort to manipulation, flirtation, or coercion (Nicholls & Petrila, 2005).

Additional gender differences have been found while comparing offense and offender characteristics. Current studies have suggested that women commit fewer sexual offenses (de Vogel et al., 2016; Strand & Belfrage, 2005), engage in more self-destructive behaviors (e.g., self-harm, neglect; de Vogel et al., 2016; Wennberg, 2012), have different drug-use trajectories (Schulz et al., 2016), express more relational or verbal aggression (Carroll et al., 2010; Crick, 1995; Kistner et al., 2010), have high rates of history of victimization (de Vogel et al., 2016), engage in more antisocial behavior in the home (Robbins et al., 2003), and target known victims (e.g., family, friends, acquaintances) rather than strangers (Robbins et al., 2003).

Currently, there are very few programmes available for women with psychopathic traits, and even fewer with published accounts of their effectiveness (Nicholls & Petrila, 2005; Richards et al., 2003). While programs and interventions need to be sensitive to gender-specific needs, they should still focus on enhancing treatment motivation, fostering collaborative working relationships, and using cognitive-behavioral principles, even if the majority of support for these recommendations come from studies on men (Logan, 2009). In applying the Two-Component model, women seem to express higher Factor 2 traits (e.g., poor behavioral controls, impulsivity) and lower Factor 1 traits (e.g., grandiose sense of self) which may mean that they present with fewer treatment barriers for motivation and retention. As research focusing on women high in psychopathy continues to grow, our understanding of how the construct manifests itself in women as well as the best treatment approach in this population will strengthen.

13.9 Conclusion

Taken together, the evidence for the treatment of psychopathic traits indicates that it is important to assess and address the underlying factors instead of focusing on psychopathy total scores. It is also clear that intervention programs should focus on addressing behavioral outcomes and not on changing actual psychopathic traits. Although evidence for changing Factor 1 traits are almost non-existent (see Baskin-Sommers et al., 2015 for a novel cognitive intervention approach), there is now a growing body of research for the ability of evidence-based offender rehabilitation programs to address the behavioral aspects of psychopathy that lead to criminal offending (i.e., Two-Component Model; Wong, 2015). Another key component to treating people with psychopathic traits is addressing treatment motivation. Both the Two-Component Model and the GLM emphasize the importance of retaining these individuals in the treatment program in order to see any benefit. Both models also identify Factor 1 traits as being particularly relevant to treatment motivation, often acting as treatment barriers. Factor 2 traits, on the other hand, make appropriate treatment targets that, when addressed, will produce reductions in risk for reoffending.

Placing psychopathy within established correctional paradigms results in several findings that should be cause for treatment optimism as opposed to the pessimism that is often cited. Studies examining the Two-Component model have shown that psychopathic offenders, even those that are high risk, can benefit from treatment interventions resulting in lowered risk and less serious offending (e.g., Olver & Wong, 2009). Although evidence for the application of the GLM to psychopathic offenders is premature, given the GLM's focus on treatment motivation and achieving offender-specific goals, positive outcomes similar to those found with the Two-Component Model could be posited. In terms of desistance, despite the overall pessimism, the examination of individual studies of desistance components has identified that maturation (e.g., Shaw & Porter, 2012) and the presence of protective factors (Burt et al., 2016) can have positive effects on psychopathic offenders. Overall, there is a growing body of research that indicates that, while psychopathic individuals are difficult to treat, positive behavioral outcomes can be achieved.

References

Acheson, S. K. (2005). Review of the Hare Psychopathy Checklist-Revised. In R. A. Spies & B. S. Plake (Eds.), *The sixteenth mental measurements yearbook* (pp. 429–431). Buros Institute of Mental Measurements.

Andrews, D. A., & Bonta, J. (1994). *The psychology of criminal conduct*. Anderson.

Andrews, D. A., & Bonta, J. (2010). *The psychology of criminal conduct* (5th ed.). Anderson.

Andrews, D. A., & Dowden, C. (2007). The Risk-Need-Responsivity model of assessment and human service in prevention and corrections: Crime-prevention jurisprudence. *Canadian Journal of Criminology and Criminal Justice, 49*, 439–464. https://doi.org/10.3138/cjccj.49.4.439

Andrews, D. A., Bonta, J., & Hoge, R. D. (1990). Classification for effective rehabilitation: Rediscovering psychology. *Criminal Justice and Behavior, 17*, 19–52. https://doi.org/10.1177/0093854890017001004

Andrews, D. A., Bonta, J., & Wormith, S. J. (2006). The recent past and near future of risk and/or need assessment. *Crime and Delinquency, 52*, 7–27. https://doi.org/10.1177/0011128705281756

Barbaree, H. E. (2005). Psychopathy, treatment behavior, and recidivism: An extended follow-up of Seto and Barbaree. *Journal of Interpersonal Violence, 20*, 1115–1131. https://doi.org/10.1177/0886260505278262

Barnett, G. D., Manderville-Norden, R., & Rakestrow, J. (2014). The Good Lives Model or relapse prevention: What works better in facilitating change? *Sexual Abuse: A Journal of Research and Treatment, 26*, 3–33. https://doi.org/10.1177/1079063212474473

Baskin-Sommers, A. R., Curtin, J. J., & Newman, J. P. (2013). Emotion-modulated startle in psychopathy: Clarifying familiar effects. *Journal of Abnormal Psychology, 122*, 458–468. https://doi.org/10.1037/a0030958

Baskin-Sommers, A. R., Curtin, J. J., & Newman, J. P. (2015). Altering the cognitive-affective dysfunctions of psychopathic and externalizing offender subtypes with cognitive remediation. *Clinical Psychological Science, 3*, 45–57. https://doi.org/10.1177/2167702614560744

Blais, J., & Forth, A. E. (2014). Prosecution-retained versus court-appointed experts: Comparing and contrasting risk assessment reports in preventative detention hearings. *Law and Human Behavior, 38*, 531–543. https://doi.org/10.1037/lhb0000082

Blais, J., Solodukhin, E., & Forth, A. E. (2014). A meta-analysis exploring the relationship between psychopathy and instrumental versus reactive violence. *Criminal Justice and Behavior, 41*, 797–821. https://doi.org/10.1177/0093854813519629

Blonigen, D. M., Hicks, B. M., Krueger, R. F., Patrick, C. J., & Iacono, W. G. (2006). Continuity and change in psychopathic traits as measured via normal-range personality: A longitudinal–biometric study. *Journal of Abnormal Psychology, 115*, 85–95. https://doi.org/10.1037/0021-843X.115.1.85

Bonta, J., & Andrews, D. A. (2017). *The psychology of criminal conduct* (6th ed.). Taylor & Francis.

Burnett, R. (2004). To re-offend or not to re-offend? The ambivalence of convicted property offenders. In S. Maruna & R. Immarigeon (Eds.), *After crime and punishment: Pathways to offender reintegration* (pp. 152–180). Willan.

Burnett, R., & McNeill, F. (2005). The place of the officer–offender relationship in assisting offenders to desist from crime. *Probation Journal, 52*, 247–268. https://doi.org/10.1177/0264550505055112

Burt, G. N., Olver, M. E., & Wong, S. C. P. (2016). Investigating characteristics of the nonrecidivating psychopathic offender. *Criminal Justice and Behavior, 43*, 1741–1760. https://doi.org/10.1177/0093854816661215

Caldwell, M., Skeem, J., Salekin, R., & van Rybroek, G. (2006). Treatment response of adolescent offenders with psychopathy features: A 2-year follow-up. *Criminal Justice and Behavior, 33*, 571–596. https://doi.org/10.1177/0093854806288176

Carroll, J. S., Nelson, D. A., Yorgason, J. B., Harper, J. M., Ashton, R. H., & Jensen, A. C. (2010). Relational aggression in marriage. *Aggressive Behavior, 6*, 315–329. https://doi.org/10.1002/ab.20349

Caspi, A. (1998). Personality development across the life course. In W. Damon (Series Ed.) & N. Eisenberg (Vol. Ed.), *Handbook of child psychology: Vol. 3 Social, emotional, and personality development* (5th ed., pp. 311–388). Wiley.

Caspi, A., & Silva, P. A. (1995). Temperamental qualities at age three predict personality traits in young adulthood: Longitudinal evidence from a birth cohort. *Child Development, 66*, 486–498. https://doi.org/10.2307/1131592

Caspi, A., Roberts, B. W., & Shiner, R. L. (2005). Personality development: Stability and change. *Annual Review of Psychology, 56*, 453–484. https://doi.org/10.1146/annurev.psych.55.090902.141913

Cernkovich, S. A., & Giordano, P. C. (2001). Stability and change in antisocial behavior: The transition from adolescence to early adulthood. *Criminology, 39*, 371–410. https://doi.org/10.1111/j.1745-9125.2001.tb00927.x

Clarkin, J. F., Livesley, W. J., & Dimaggio, G. (2016). A case study of integrated treatment. In J. Livesley, G. Dimaggio, & J. Clarkin (Eds.), *Integrated treatment of personality disorders: A modular approach* (pp. 439–449). Guildford.

Cleckley, H. (1976). *The mask of sanity: An attempt to clarify some issues about the so-called psychopathic personality* (5th ed.). Mosby, Inc. (Original work published 1941).

Coid, J., & Yang, M. (2011). The impact of psychopathy on violence among the household population of Great Britain. *Social Psychiatry and Psychiatric Epidemiology, 46*, 473–480. https://doi.org/10.1007/s00127-010-0212-4

Coid, J., Ullrich, S., Roberts, A., & Hare, R. D. (2009). Prevalence and correlates of psychopathic traits in the household population of Great Britain. *International Journal of Law and Psychiatry, 32*, 65–73. https://doi.org/10.1016/j.ijlp.2009.01.002

Collins, R. E. (2004). Onset and desistance in criminal careers: Neurobiology and the age-crime relationship. *Journal of Offender Rehabilitation, 39*, 1–19. https://doi.org/10.1300/J076v39n03_01

Cooke, D. J., & Michie, C. (2001). Refining the construct of psychopathy: Towards a hierarchical model. *Psychological Assessment, 13*, 171–188. https://doi.org/10.1037111040-3590.13.2.171

Cooke, D. J., Michie, C., Hart, S. D., & Clark, D. A. (2004). Reconstructing psychopathy: Clarifying the significance of antisocial and socially deviant behavior in the diagnosis of psychopathic personality disorder. *Journal of Personality Disorders, 18*, 337–357. https://doi.org/10.1521/pedi.2004.18.4.337

Cooke, D. J., Hart, S. D., Logan, C., & Michie, C. (2012). Explicating the construct of psychopathy: Development and validation of a conceptual model, the Comprehensive Assessment of Psychopathic Personality (CAPP). *International Journal of Forensic Mental Health, 11*, 242–252. https://doi.org/10.1080/14999013.2012.746759

Corrado, R. R., DeLisi, M., Hart, S. D., & McCuish, E. C. (2015). Can the causal mechanisms underlying chronic, serious, and violent offending trajectories be elucidated using the psychopathy construct? *Journal of Criminal Justice, 43*, 251–261. https://doi.org/10.1016/j.jcrimjus.2015.04.006

Crick, N. (1995). Relational aggression: The role of intent attributions, feelings of distress, and provocation type. *Development and Psychopathology, 7*, 313–322. https://doi.org/10.1017/S0954579400006520

de Oliveira-Souza, R., Hare, R. D., Bramati, I. E., Garrido, G. J., Azevedo Ignácio, F., Tovar-Moll, F., & Moll, J. (2008). Psychopathy as a disorder of the moral brain: Fronto-temporo-limbic grey matter reductions demonstrated by voxel-based morphometry. *NeuroImage, 40*, 1202–1213. https://doi.org/10.1016/j.neuroimage.2007.12.054

de Vogel, V., de Ruiter, C., Bouman, Y., & de Vries Robbé, M. (2009). *SAPROF. Guidelines for the assessment of protective factors for violence risk*. Forum Educatief.

de Vogel, V., de Vries Robbé, M., de Ruiter, C., & Bouman, Y. H. A. (2011). Assessing protective factors in forensic psychiatric practice: Introducing the SAPROF. *International Journal of Forensic Mental Health, 10*, 171–177. https://doi.org/10.1080/14999013.2011.600230

de Vogel, V., Stam, J., Bouman, Y. H., Horst, P. T., & Lancel, M. (2016). Violent women: A multicentre study into gender differences in forensic psychiatric patients. *The Journal of Forensic Psychiatry & Psychology, 27*, 145–168. https://doi.org/10.1080/14789949.2015.1102312

de Vries Robbé, M., de Vogel, V., & Douglas, K. S. (2013). Risk factors and protective factors: A two-sided dynamic approach to violence risk assessment. *Journal of Forensic Psychiatry & Psychology, 24*, 440–457. https://doi.org/10.1080/14789949.2013.818162

DeMatteo, D., Heilbrun, K., & Marczyk, G. (2005). Psychopathy, risk of violence, and protective factors in a noninstitutionalized and noncriminal sample. *International Journal of Forensic Mental Health, 4*, 147–157. https://doi.org/10.1080/14999013.2005.10471220

DeSorcy, D. R., Olver, M. E., & Wormith, J. S. (2020). Working alliance and psychopathy: Linkages to treatment outcome in a sample of treated sexual offenders. *Journal of Interpersonal Violence, 35*, 1739–1760. https://doi.org/10.1177/0886260517698822

Dolan, M., & Vøllm, B. (2009). Antisocial personality disorder and psychopathy in women: A literature review on the reliability and validity of assessment instruments. *International Journal of Law and Psychiatry, 32*, 2–9. https://doi.org/10.1016/j.ijlp.2008.11.002

Dowden, C., & Andrews, D. (1999). What works for female offenders: A meta-analytic review. *Crime & Delinquency, 45*, 438–452. https://doi.org/10.1177/0011128799045004002

Dowden, C., & Andrews, D. A. (2000). Effective correctional treatment and violent reoffending: A meta-analysis. *Canadian Journal of Criminology, 42*, 449–468. https://doi.org/10.3138/cjcrim.42.4.449

Farrall, S. (2004). Supervision, motivation and social context: What matters most when probationers desist. In G. Mair (Ed.), *What matters in probation* (pp. 187–209). Willan.

Farrall, S., & Calverley, A. (2005). *Understanding desistance from crime*. McGraw-Hill Education (UK).

Farrall, S., & Calverley, A. (2006). *Understanding desistance from crime: Theoretical directions in resettlement and rehabilitation*. Open University Press.

Forouzan, E., & Cooke, D. J. (2005). Figuring out la femme fatale: Conceptual and assessment issues concerning psychopathy in females. *Behavioral Sciences & the Law, 23*, 765–778. https://doi.org/10.1002/bsl.669

Gannon, T. A., King, T., Miles, H., Lockerbie, L., & Willis, G. (2011). Good lives sexual offender treatment for mentally disordered offenders. *The British Journal of Forensic Practice, 13*, 153–168. https://doi.org/10.1108/14636641111157805

Gendreau, P., & Andrews, D. A. (1990). Tertiary prevention: What the meta-analyses of the offender treatment literature tell us about "what works". *Canadian Journal of Criminology, 32*, 173–184. https://heinonline-org.proxy.library.carleton.ca/HOL/Page?lname=&handle=hein.journals/cjccj32&collection=&page=173&collection=journals

Giordano, P. C., Cernkovich, S. A., & Rudolph, J. L. (2002). Gender, crime, and desistance: Toward a theory of cognitive transformation. *American Journal of Sociology, 107*, 990–1064. https://doi.org/10.1086/343191

Giordano, P. C., Schroeder, R. D., & Cernkovich, S. A. (2007). Emotions and crime over the life-course: A neo-median perspective on criminal continuity and change. *American Journal of Sociology, 112*, 1603–1661. https://doi.org/10.1086/512710

Glenn, A. L., Raine, A., Yaralian, P. S., & Yang, Y. (2010). Increased volume of the striatum in psychopathic individuals. *Biological Psychiatry, 67*, 52–58. https://doi.org/10.1016/j.biopsych.2009.06.018

Gottfredson, M. R., & Hirschi, T. (1990). *A general theory of crime*. Stanford University Press.

Gray, J. A., & McNaughton, N. (2000). *The neuropsychology of anxiety: An enquiry into the functions of the septo-hippocampal system* (2nd ed.). Oxford University Press.

Gretton, H. M., McBride, M., Hare, R. D., O'Shaughnessy, R., & Kumka, G. (2001). Psychopathy and recidivism in adolescent sex offenders. *Criminal Justice and Behavior, 28*, 427–449. https://doi.org/10.1177/009385480102800403

Guay, J. P., Ruscio, J., Knight, R. A., & Hare, R. D. (2007). A taxometric analysis of the latent structure of psychopathy: Evidence for dimensionality. *Journal of Abnormal Psychology, 116*, 701–716. https://doi.org/10.1037/0021-843X.116.4.701

Guy, L. S., Edens, J. F., Anthony, C., & Douglas, K. S. (2005). Does psychopathy predict institutional misconduct among adults? A meta-analytic investigation. *Journal of Consulting and Clinical Psychology, 73*, 1056–1064. https://doi.org/10.1037/0022-006X.73.6.1056

Hanson, R. K., & Morton-Bourgon, K. E. (2009). The accuracy of recidivism risk assessments for sexual offenders: A meta-analysis of 118 prediction studies. *Psychological Assessment, 21*, 1–21. https://doi.org/10.1037/a0014421

Hanson, R. K., Bourgon, G., Helmus, L., & Hodgins, S. (2009). The principles of effective correctional treatment also apply to sexual offenders: A meta-analysis. *Criminal Justice and Behavior, 36*, 865–891. https://doi.org/10.1177/0093854809338545

Hare, R. D. (1991). *The Hare Psychopathy Checklist—Revised*. Multi-Health Systems.

Hare, R. D. (2003). *Manual for the Revised Psychopathy Checklist* (2nd ed.). Multi-Health Systems.

Hare, R. D., & Neumann, C. S. (2008). Psychopathy as a clinical and empirical construct. *Annual Review of Clinical Psychology, 4*, 217–246. https://doi.org/10.1146/annurev.clinpsy.3.022806.091452

Hare, R. D., McPherson, L. M., & Forth, A. E. (1988). Male psychopaths and their criminal careers. *Journal of Consulting and Clinical Psychology, 56*, 710–714. https://doi.org/10.1037/0022-006X.56.5.710

Hare, R. D., Neumann, C. S., & Mokros, A. (2017). The PCL-R assessment of psychopathy: Development, properties, debates and new directions. In C. J. Patrick (Ed.), *Handbook of psychopathy* (2nd ed., pp. 39–79). Guilford Press.

Harkins, L., Flak, V. E., Beech, A. R., & Woodhams, J. (2012). Evaluation of a community-based sex offender treatment program using a Good Lives Model approach. *Sexual Abuse: A Journal of Research and Treatment, 24*, 519–543. https://doi.org/10.1177/1079063211429469

Harpur, T. J., & Hare, R. D. (1994). Assessment of psychopathy as a function of age. *Journal of Abnormal Psychology, 103*, 604–609.

Hart, S. D., Kropp, P. R., & Hare, R. D. (1988). Performance of male psychopaths following conditional release from prison. *Journal of Consulting and Clinical Psychology, 56*, 227–232. https://doi.org/10.1037/0022-006x.56.2.227

Hawes, S. W., Boccaccini, M. T., & Murrie, D. C. (2013). Psychopathy and the combination of psychopathy and sexual deviance as predictors of sexual recidivism: Meta-analytic findings using the Psychopathy Checklist-Revised. *Psychological Assessment, 25*, 233–243. https://doi.org/10.1037/a0030391

Hemphill, J. F., & Hart, S. D. (2002). Motivating the unmotivated: Psychopathy, treatment, and change. In M. McMurran (Ed.), *Motivating offenders to change: A guide to enhancing engagement in therapy* (pp. 193–219). Wiley.

Hughes, G., Hogue, T., Hollin, C., & Champion, H. (1997). First-stage evaluation of a treatment programme for personality disordered offenders. *Journal of Forensic Psychiatry, 8*(3), 515–527. https://doi.org/10.1080/09585189708412273

Hurducas, C. C., Singh, J. P., de Ruiter, C., & Petrila, J. (2014). Violence risk assessment tools: A systematic review of surveys. *International Journal of Forensic Mental Health, 13*, 181–192. https://doi.org/10.1080/14999013.2014.942923

Jackson, R. L., Rogers, R., Neumann, C. S., & Lambert, P. L. (2002). Psychopathy in female offenders. *Criminal Justice and Behavior, 29*, 692–704. https://doi.org/10.1177/009385402237922

Kennealy, P. J., Skeem, J. L., Walters, G. D., & Camp, J. (2010). Do core interpersonal and affective traits of PCL-R psychopathy interact with antisocial behavior and disinhibition to predict violence? *Psychological Assessment, 22*, 569–580. https://doi.org/10.1037/a0019618

Kiehl, K. A., & Hoffman, M. B. (2011). The criminal psychopath: History, neuroscience, and economics. *Jurimetrics Journal, 51*, 355–397. https://www.ncbi.nlm.nih.gov/pmc/articles/PMC4059069/

Kistner, J., Counts-Allan, C., Dunkel, S., Drew, C. H., David-Ferdon, C., & Lopez, C. (2010). Sex differences in relational and overt aggression in the late elementary school years. *Aggressive Behavior, 36*, 282–291. https://doi.org/10.1002/ab.20350

Klein Tuente, S., de Vogel, V., & Stam, J. (2014). Exploring the criminal behavior of women with psychopathy: Results from a multicenter study into psychopathy and violent offending in female forensic psychiatric patients. *International Journal of Forensic Mental Health, 13*, 311–322. https://doi.org/10.1080/14999013.2014.951105

Koehler, J. A., Humphreys, D. K., Akoensi, T. D., Sánchez de Ribera, O., & Lösel, F. (2014). A systematic review and meta-analysis on the effects of European drug treatment programmes on reoffending. *Psychology, Crime & Law, 20*(6), 584–602. https://doi.org/10.1080/1068316X.2013.804921

Kreis, M. K. F., & Cooke, D. J. (2012). The manifestation of psychopathic traits in women: An exploration using case examples. *International Journal of Forensic Mental Health, 11*, 267–279. https://doi.org/10.1080/14999013.2012.746755

Lalumière, M. L., Harris, G. T., Quinsey, V. L., & Rice, M. E. (2005). *The causes of rape: Understanding individual differences in male propensity for sexual aggression*. American Psychological Association.

Langton, C. M., Hogue, T. E., Daffern, M., Mannion, A., & Howells, K. (2011). Personality traits as predictors of inpatient aggression in a high-security forensic psychiatric setting: Prospective evaluation of the PCL-R and IPDE dimension ratings. *International Journal of Offender Therapy and Comparative Criminology, 55*, 392–415. https://doi.org/10.1177/0306624X10370828

Laub, J., & Sampson, R. J. (2001). Understanding desistance from crime. *Crime and Justice: A Review of Research, 28*, 1–70. https://doi.org/10.1086/652208

Laub, J. H., & Sampson, R. J. (2003). *Shared beginnings, divergent lives: Delinquent boys to age 70*. Harvard University Press.

Laws, D. R., & Ward, T. (2011). *Desistance and sexual offending: Alternatives to throwing away the keys*. Guilford.

LeBel, T., Burnett, R., Maruna, S., & Bushway, S. (2008). The 'Chicken and Egg' of subjective and social factors in desistance from crime. *European Journal of Criminology, 5*, 131–159. https://doi.org/10.1177/1477370807087640

Leistico, A. R., Salekin, R. T., DeCoster, J., & Rogers, R. (2008). A large-scale meta-analysis relating the Hare measures of psychopathy to antisocial conduct. *Law and Human Behavior, 32*, 28–45. https://doi.org/10.1007/s10979-007-9096-6

Lindsay, W. R., Ward, T., Morgan, T., & Wilson, I. (2007). Self-regulation of sex offending, future pathways and the Good Lives Model: Applications and problems. *Journal of Sexual Aggression, 13*, 37–50. https://doi.org/10.1080/13552600701365613

Lipsey, M. W. (1992). Juvenile delinquency treatment: A meta-analytic inquiry into the variability of effects. In T. D. Cook, H. Cooper, D. S. Cordray, H. Hartmann, L. V. Hedges, R. J. Light, T. A. Louis, & F. Mosteller (Eds.), *Meta-analysis for explanation: A casebook* (pp. 83–127). Russell Sage Foundation.

Lipsey, M. W. (1995). What do we learn from 400 studies on the effectiveness of treatment with juvenile delinquents? In J. McGuire (Ed.), *What works: Reducing reoffending* (pp. 63–78). Wiley.

Logan, C. (2009). Psychopathy in women: Conceptual issues, clinical presentation and management. *Neuropsychiatrie, 23*(S1), 1–9.

Looman, J., Abracen, J., Serin, R., & Marquis, P. (2005). Psychopathy, treatment change, and recidivism in high-risk, high-need sexual offenders. *Journal of Interpersonal Violence, 20*, 549–568. https://doi.org/10.1177/0886260504271583

Lykken, D. T. (1995). *The antisocial personalities*. Lawrence Erlbaum Associates, Inc.

Lynam, D. R. (1997). Pursuing the psychopath: Capturing the fledgling psychopath in the nomological net. *Journal of Abnormal Psychology, 106*, 425–438. https://doi.org/10.1037/0021-843X.106.3.425

Maguire, M., & Raynor, P. (2006). How the resettlement of prisoners promotes desistance from crime: Or does it? *Criminology and Criminal Justice, 6*, 19–38. https://doi.org/10.1177/1748895806060665

Mailloux, D. L., Abracen, J., Serin, R., Cousineau, C., Malcolm, B., & Looman, J. (2003). Dosage of treatment to sexual offenders: Are we overprescribing? *International Journal of Offender Therapy and Comparative Criminology, 47*, 171–184. https://doi.org/10.1177/0306624X03251096

Mann, R. E., Webster, S. D., Schofield, C., & Marshall, W. L. (2004). Approach versus avoidance goals with sexual offenders. *Sexual Abuse: A Journal of Research and Treatment, 16*, 65–75. https://doi.org/10.1177/107906320401600105

Martín, A. M., Hernández, B., Hernández-Fernaud, E., Arregui, J. L., & Hernández, J. A. (2010). The enhancement effect of social and employment integration on the delay of recidivism of released offenders trained with the R & R programme. *Psychology, Crime & Law, 16*, 401–413. https://doi.org/10.1080/10683160902776835

Martinson, R. (1974). What works? Questions and answers about prison reform. *The Public Interest, 35*, 22–54. https://search-proquest-com.proxy.library.carleton.ca/docview/1298113963?accountid=9894

Maruna, S. (2001). *Making good: How ex-Convicts reform and rebuild their lives*. American Psychological Association.

Maruna, S. (2010). *Understanding desistance from crime*. A report for the Ministry of Justice and National Offender Management Services. http://www.safeground.org.uk/wp-content/uploads/Desistance-Fact-Sheet.pdf

Maruna, S., & LeBel, T. (2003). Welcome home? Examining the 're-entry court' concept from a strengths-based perspective. *Western Criminology Review, 4*, 91–107. https://heinonline.org/HOL/LandingPage?handle=hein.journals/wescrim4&div=12&id=&page=

Maruna, S., & Mann, R. (2019). *Reconciling "desistance" and "what works."* HM Inspectorate of Probation. Academic Insights 19/1.

Maruna, S., & Roy, K. (2007). Amputation or reconstruction? Notes on the concept of "knifing off" and desistance from crime. *Journal of Contemporary Criminal Justice, 23*, 104–124. https://doi.org/10.1177/1043986206298951

Maruna, S., LeBel, T. P., Mitchell, N., & Naples, M. (2004). Pygmalion in the reintegration process: Desistance from crime through the looking glass. *Psychology, Crime & Law, 10*, 271–281. https://doi.org/10.1080/10683160410001662762

McCarthy, L., Huband, N., Patel, S., Banerjee, P., & Duggan, C. (2012). Personality disorder and psychopathy as predictors of psychosocial and criminological outcome in mentally disordered offenders. *International Journal of Forensic Mental Health, 11*, 227–237. https://doi.org/10.1080/14999013.2012.739262

McCuish, E. C. (2016). *Bringing psychopathy into research on offending trajectories: Understanding the construct's role as a barrier to desistance*. Unpublished doctoral dissertation. https://summit.sfu.ca/item/16705

McCuish, E. C. (2019). Psychopathy and offending trajectories. In M. DeLisi (Ed.), *Handbook of psychopathy and crime* (pp. 447–461). Routledge International.

McGuire, J., Bilby, C. A. L., Hatcher, R. M., Hollin, C. R., Hounsome, J., & Palmer, E. J. (2008). Evaluation of structured cognitive-behavioural treatment programmes in reducing criminal recidivism. *Journal of Experimental Criminology, 4*, 21–40. https://doi.org/10.1007/s11292-007-9047-8

McMain, S. F., Links, P. S., Gnam, W. H., Guimond, T., Cardish, R. J., Korman, L., & Streiner, D. L. (2009). A randomized trial of dialectical behavior therapy versus general psychiatric management for borderline personality disorder. *American Journal of Psychiatry, 166*, 1365–1374. https://doi.org/10.1176/appi.ajp.2009.09010039

McNeill, F. (2003). Desistance based practice. In W. H. Chui & M. Nellis (Eds.), *Moving probation forward: Evidence, arguments and practice* (pp. 146–162). Pearson Education.

McNeill, F. (2006). A desistance paradigm for offender management. *Criminology and Criminal Justice, 6*, 39–62. https://doi.org/10.1177/1748895806060666

McNeill, F., Batchelor, S., Burnett, R., & Knox, J. (2005). *21st century social work. Reducing re-offending: Key practice skills*. The Scottish Executive.

Moffitt, T. E. (1993). Adolescence-limited and life-course-persistent antisocial behavior: A developmental taxonomy. *Psychological Review, 100*, 674–701. https://doi.org/10.1037/0033-295X.100.4.674

Morgan, J. E., Gray, N. S., & Snowden, R. J. (2011). The relationship between psychopathy and impulsivity: A multi-impulsivity measurement approach. *Personality and Individual Differences, 51*, 429–434. https://doi.org/10.1016/j.paid.2011.03.043

Müller, J. L., Sommer, M., Wagner, V., Lange, K., Taschler, H., Röder, C. H., Schuierer, G., Klein, H. E., & Hajak, G. (2003). Abnormalities in emotion processing within cortical and subcortical regions in criminal psychopaths: Evidence from a functional magnetic imaging study using pictures with emotional content. *Biological Psychiatry, 15*, 152–162. https://doi.org/10.1016/S0006-3223(02)01749-3

Neal, T. M. S., & Grisso, T. (2014). Assessment practices and expert judgment methods in forensic psychology and psychiatry: An international snapshot. *Criminal Justice and Behavior, 41*, 1406–1421. https://doi.org/10.1177/0093854814548449

Netto, N. R., Carter, J. M., & Bonell, C. (2014). Systematic review of interventions that adopt the 'good lives' approach to offender rehabilitation. *Journal of Offender Rehabilitation, 53*, 403–432. https://doi.org/10.1080/10509674.2014.931746

Neumann, C. S., & Hare, R. D. (2008). Psychopathic traits in a large community sample: Links to violence, alcohol use, and intelligence. *Journal of Consulting and Clinical Psychology, 76*, 893–899. https://doi.org/10.1037/0022-006X.76.5.893

Neumann, C. S., Hare, R. D., & Newman, J. P. (2007). The super-ordinate nature of the Psychopathy Checklist-Revised. *Journal of Personality Disorders, 21*, 102–117. https://doi.org/10.1521/pedi.2007.21.2.102

Newman, J. P., MacCoon, D. G., Vaughn, L. J., & Sadeh, N. (2005). Validating a distinction between primary and secondary psychopathy with measures of Gray's BIS and BAS constructs. *Journal of Abnormal Psychology, 114*, 319–323. https://doi.org/10.1037/0021-843X.114.2.319

Nicholls, T. L., & Petrila, J. (2005). Gender and psychopathy: An overview of important issues and introduction to the special issue. *Behavioral Sciences & the Law, 23*, 729–741. https://doi.org/10.1002/bsl.677

Ogloff, J. R. P., & Davis, M. R. (2004). Advances in offender assessment and rehabilitation: Contributions of the risk-needs-responsivity approach. *Psychology, Crime & Law, 10*, 229–242. https://doi.org/10.1080/10683160410001662735

Ogloff, J. R. P., Wong, S., & Greenwood, A. (1990). Treating criminal psychopaths in a therapeutic community program. *Behavioral Sciences & the Law, 8*, 181–190. https://doi.org/10.1002/bsl.2370080210

Olver, M. E. (2016). Treatment of psychopathic offenders: Evidence, issues, and controversies. *Journal of Community Safety & Well-Being, 1*, 75–82. https://doi.org/10.35502/jcswb.25

Olver, M. E., & Wong, S. C. P. (2009). Therapeutic responses of psychopathic sexual offenders: Treatment attrition, therapeutic change, and long-term recidivism. *Journal of Counseling and Clinical Psychology, 77*, 326–336. https://doi.org/10.1037/a0015001

Olver, M. E., & Wong, S. (2011). Predictors of sex offender treatment dropout: Psychopathy, sex offender risk, and responsivity implications. *Psychology, Crime & Law, 17*, 457–471. https://doi.org/10.1080/10683160903318876

Olver, M. E., Lewis, K., & Wong, S. C. P. (2013). Risk reduction treatment of high-risk psychopathic offenders: The relationship of psychopathy and treatment change to violent recidivism. *Personality Disorders: Theory, Research, and Treatment, 4*(2), 160–167. https://doi.org/10.1037/a0029769

Olver, M. E., Stockdale, K. C., & Wormith, J. S. (2011). A meta-analysis of predictors of offender treatment attrition and its relationship to recidivism. *Journal of Consulting and Clinical Psychology, 79*, 6–21. https://doi.org/10.1037/a0022200

Paternoster, R., & Bushway, S. (2009). Desistance and the feared self: Toward an identity theory of criminal desistance. *The Journal of Criminal Law & Criminology, 99*, 1103–1156. https://pdfs.semanticscholar.org/12a3/bea05f8eb3c15584ca8d5de9b40e20501169.pdf

Piquero, A. (2004). Somewhere between persistence and desistance: The intermittency of criminal careers. In S. Maruna & R. Immarigeon (Eds.), *After crime and punishment: Pathways to offender reintegration* (pp. 102–125). Willan.

Piquero, A. R., Jennings, W. G., & Barnes, J. C. (2012). Violence in criminal careers: A review of the literature from a developmental life-course perspective. *Aggression and Violent Behavior, 17*, 171–179. https://doi.org/10.1016/j.avb.2012.02.008

Polaschek, D. L. L., & Yesberg, J. A. (2015). Desistance in high-risk prisoners: Pre-release self-reported desistance commitment and perceptions of change predict 12-month survival. *Practice: The New Zealand Corrections Journal, 3*, 24–29. https://scholar.google.ca/scholar?cluster=17467535750009824603&hl=en&as_sdt=0,5

Porporino, F. J. (2010). Bringing sense and sensitivity to corrections: From programmes to 'fix' offenders to services to support desistance. In J. Brayford, F. Cowe, & J. Deering (Eds.), *What else works? Creative work with offenders and other social excluded people* (pp. 61–85). Willan.

Porter, S., Birt, A., & Boer, D. P. (2001). Investigation of the criminal and conditional release profiles of Canadian federal offenders as a function of psychopathy age. *Law and Human Behavior, 25*, 647–661. https://doi.org/10.1023/A:1012710424821

Prochaska, J. O., DiClemente, C. C., & Norcross, J. C. (1992). In search of how people change: Applications to addictive behaviors. *Journal of Addictions Nursing, 5*, 2–16. https://doi.org/10.1037//0003-066x.47.9.1102

Reidy, D. E., Kearns, M. C., DeGue, S., Lilienfeld, S. O., Massetti, G., & Kiehl, K. A. (2015). Why psychopathy matters: Implications for public health and violence prevention. *Aggression and Violent Behavior, 24*, 214–225. https://doi.org/10.1016/j.avb.2015.05.018

Rex, S. (1999). Desistance from offending: Experiences of probation. *The Howard Journal of Criminal Justice, 36*, 366–383. https://doi.org/10.1111/1468-2311.00141

Rice, M. E., Harris, G. T., & Cormier, C. A. (1992). An evaluation of a maximum security therapeutic community for psychopaths and other mentally disordered offenders. *Law and Human Behavior, 16*, 399–412. https://doi.org/10.1007/BF02352266

Richards, H. J., Casey, J. O., & Lucente, S. W. (2003). Psychopathy and treatment response in incarcerated female substance abusers. *Criminal Justice and Behavior, 30*, 251–276. https://doi.org/10.1177/0093854802251010

Robbins, P., Monahan, J., & Silver, E. (2003). Mental disorder, violence, and gender. *Law and Human Behavior, 27*, 561–571. https://doi.org/10.1023/B:LAHU.0000004886.13268.f2

Roberts, B. W., Luo, J., Briley, D. A., Chow, P. I., Su, R., & Hill, P. L. (2017). A systematic review of personality trait change through intervention. *Psychological Bulletin, 143*, 117–141. https://doi.org/10.1037/bul0000088

Rocque, M. (2017). *Desistance from crime: New advances in theory and research*. Springer.

Rogstad, J. E., & Rogers, R. (2008). Gender differences in contributions of emotions to psychopathy and antisocial personality disorder. *Clinical Psychology Review, 28*, 1472–1484. https://doi.org/10.1016/j.cpr.2008.09.004

Salekin, R., Rogers, R., & Sewell, K. (1996). A review and meta-analysis of the Psychopathy Checklist and Psychopathy Checklist-Revised: Predictive validity of dangerousness. *Clinical Psychology: Science and Practice, 3*, 203–215. https://doi.org/10.1111/j.1468-2850.1996.tb00071.x

Salekin, R. T., Rogers, R., Ustad, K. L., & Sewell, K. W. (1998). Psychopathy and recidivism among female inmates. *Law and Human Behavior, 22*, 109–128. https://doi.org/10.1023/A:1025780806538

Sampson, R. J., & Laub, J. H. (1993). *Crime in the making: Pathways and turning points through life*. Harvard University Press.

Schulz, N., Murphy, B., & Verona, E. (2016). Gender differences in psychopathy links to drug use. *Law and Human Behavior, 40*, 159–168. https://doi.org/10.1037/lhb0000165

Shaw, J., & Porter, S. (2012). Forever a psychopath? Psychopathy and the criminal career trajectory. In H. Häkkänen-Nyholm & J. Nyholm (Eds.), *Psychopathy and law: A practitioner's guide* (pp. 201–221). Wiley.

Singh, J. P., Grann, M., & Fazel, S. (2011). A comparative study of violence risk assessment tools: A systematic review and metaregression analysis of 68 studies involving 25,980 participants. *Clinical Psychology Review, 31*, 499–513. https://doi.org/10.1016/j.cpr.2010.11.009

Steels, M., Roney, G., Larkin, E., Jones, P., Croudace, T., & Duggan, C. (1998). Discharged from special hospital under restrictions: A comparison of the fates of psychopaths and the mentally ill. *Criminal Behavior and Mental Health, 8*, 39–55. https://doi.org/10.1002/cbm.210

Stolzenberg, L., & D'Alessio, S. J. (2008). Co-offending and the age-crime curve. *Journal of Research in Crime and Delinquency, 45*, 65–86. https://doi.org/10.1177/0022427807309441

Strand, S., & Belfrage, H. (2005). Gender differences in psychopathy in a Swedish offender sample. *Behavioral Sciences & the Law, 23*, 837–850. https://doi.org/10.1002/bsl.674

Swogger, M. T., Walsh, Z., & Kosson, D. S. (2007). Domestic violence and psychopathic traits: Distinguishing the antisocial batterer from other antisocial offenders. *Aggressive Behavior, 33*, 253–260. https://doi.org/10.1002/ab.20185

Thornton, D., & Blud, L. (2007). The influence of psychopathic traits on response to treatment. In H. Hervé & J. C. Yuille (Eds.), *The psychopath: Theory, research and practice* (pp. 141–170). Lawrence Erlbaum Associates, Inc.

Ullrich, S., & Coid, J. (2011). Protective factors for violence among released prisoners: Effects over time and interactions with static risk. *Journal of Consulting and Clinical Psychology, 79*, 381–390. https://doi.org/10.1037/a0023613

Vaughn, M. G., Howard, M. O., & DeLisi, M. (2008). Psychopathic personality traits and delinquent careers: An empirical examination. *International Journal of Law and Psychiatry, 31*, 407–416. https://doi.org/10.1016/j.ijlp.2008.08.001

Wallace, J. F., Malterer, M. B., & Newman, J. P. (2009). Mapping Gray's BIS and BAS constructs onto Factor 1 and Factor 2 of Hare's Psychopathy Checklist–Revised. *Personality and Individual Differences, 47*, 812–816. https://doi.org/10.1016/j.paid.2009.06.019

Walters, G. D. (2003a). Predicting criminal justice outcomes with the Psychopathy Checklist and Lifestyle Criminality Screening Form: A meta-analytic comparison. *Behavioral Sciences & the Law, 21*, 89–102. https://doi.org/10.1002/bsl.519

Walters, G. D. (2003b). Predicting institutional adjustment and recidivism with the psychopathy checklist factor scores: A meta-analysis. *Law and Human Behavior, 27*, 541–558. https://doi.org/10.1023/A:1025490207678

Ward, T. (2002). Good lives and the rehabilitation of offenders: Promises and problems. *Aggression and Violent Behavior, 7*, 513–528. https://doi.org/10.1016/S1359-1789(01)00076-3

Ward, T., & Brown, M. (2004). The good lives model and conceptual issues in offender rehabilitation. *Psychology, Crime & Law, 10*, 243–257. https://doi.org/10.1080/10683160410001662744

Ward, T., & Gannon, T. A. (2006). Rehabilitation, etiology, and self-regulation: The comprehensive good lives model of treatment for sexual offenders. *Aggression and Violent Behavior, 11*, 77–94. https://doi.org/10.1016/j.avb.2005.06.001

Ward, T., & Laws, D. R. (2010). Desistance from sex offending: Motivating change, enriching practice. *International Journal of Forensic Mental Health, 9*, 11–23. https://doi.org/10.1080/14999011003791598

Ward, T., & Maruna, S. (2007). *Rehabilitation: Beyond the risk paradigm*. Routledge.

Ward, T., & Stewart, C. (2003). The treatment of sex offenders: Risk management and good lives. *Professional Psychology: Research and Practice, 34*, 353–360. https://doi.org/10.1037/0735-7028.34.4.353

Ware, J., & Bright, D. A. (2008). Evolution of a treatment programme for sex offenders: Changes to the NSW Custody-Based Intensive Treatment (CUBIT). *Psychiatry, Psychology and Law, 15*, 340–349. https://doi.org/10.1080/13218710802014543

Warren, J. I., Burnette, M. L., South, S. C., Chauhan, P., Bale, R., Friend, R., & Van Patten, I. (2003). Psychopathy in women: Structural modeling and comorbidity. *International Journal of Law and Psychiatry, 26*, 223–242. https://doi.org/10.1016/S0160-2527(03)00034-7

Weaver, B., & McNeill, F. (2010). Travelling hopefully: Desistance research and probation practice. In J. Brayford, F. Cowe, & J. Deering (Eds.), *What else works? Creative work with offenders and other social excluded people* (pp. 36–60). Willan.

Weizmann-Henelius, G., Virkkunen, M., Gammelgård, M., Eronen, M., & Putkonen, H. (2015). The PCL-R and violent recidivism in a prospective follow-up of a nationwide sample of female offenders. *The Journal of Forensic Psychiatry & Psychology, 26*, 667–685. https://doi.org/10.1080/14789949.2015.1049192

Wennberg, T. (2012). *There are differences between men and women with psychopathic personality traits regarding sub-types of psychopathy, criminality, aggression and victimization*. Örebro University. http://www.diva-portal.org/smash/record.jsf?pid=diva2%3A607742&dswid=747

Whitehead, P. R., Ward, T., & Collie, R. M. (2007). Time for a change: Applying the good lives model of rehabilitation to a high-risk violent offender. *International Journal of Offender Therapy and Comparative Criminology, 51*, 578–598. https://doi.org/10.1177/0306624X06296236

Willis, G. M., & Ward, T. (2013). The good lives model: Does it work? Preliminary evidence. In L. Craig, L. Dixon, & T. A. Gannon (Eds.), *What works in offender rehabilitation* (pp. 305–317). Wiley.

Willis, G. M., Ward, T., & Levenson, J. S. (2014). The Good Lives Model (GLM): An evaluation of the GLM operationalization in North American treatment programs. *Sexual Abuse: A Journal of Research and Treatment, 26*, 58–81. https://doi.org/10.1177/1079063213478202

Wong, S. (2015). Treatment of violence prone individuals with psychopathic personality traits. In J. Livesley, G. Dimaggio, & J. Clarkin (Eds.), *Integrated treatment of personality disorders: A modular approach* (pp. 345–376). Guildford.

Wong, S. C. P., & Burt, G. (2007). The heterogeneity of incarcerated psychopaths: Differences in risk, need, recidivism and management approaches. In H. Hervé & J. C. Yuille (Eds.), *The psychopath: Theory, research and practice* (pp. 461–484). Lawrence Erlbaum Associates, Inc.

Wong, S. C. P., & Gordon, A. (2006). The validity and reliability of the Violence Risk Scale: A treatment friendly violence risk assessment scale. *Psychology, Public Policy, and Law, 12*, 279–309. https://doi.org/10.1037/1076-8971.12.3.279

Wong, S., & Hare, R. D. (2005). *Guidelines for a psychopathy treatment program*. Multi-Health System.

Wong, S., Olver, M. E., Nicholaichuk, T. P., & Gordon, A. (2003). *The Violence Risk Scale: Sexual Offender version (VRS-SO)*. Saskatoon, SK: Regional Psychiatric Centre and University of Saskatchewan.

Wong, S. C. P., Gordon, A., Gu, D., Lewis, K., & Olver, M. E. (2012). The effectiveness of violence reduction treatment for psychopathic offenders: Empirical evidence and a treatment model. *International Journal of Forensic Mental Health, 11*, 336–349. https://doi.org/10.1080/14999013.2012.746760

Wynn, R., Høiseth, M. H., & Pettersen, G. (2012). Psychopathy in women: Theoretical and clinical perspectives. *International Journal of Women's Health, 4*, 257–263. https://doi.org/10.2147/IJWH.S25518

Yang, Y., & Raine, A. (2017). The neuroanatomical bases of psychopathy: A review of brain imaging studies. In C. J. Patrick (Ed.), *Handbook of psychopathy* (2nd ed., pp. 380–400). Guilford Press.

Yang, Y., Raine, A., Lencz, T., Bihrle, S., LaCasse, L., & Colletti, P. (2005). Volume reduction in prefrontal gray matter in unsuccessful criminal psychopaths. *Biological Psychiatry, 57*, 1103–1108. https://doi.org/10.1016/j.biopsych.2005.01.021

Yang, Y., Raine, A., Colletti, P., Toga, A. W., & Narr, K. L. (2009). Abnormal temporal and pre-frontal cortical gray matter thinning in psychopaths. *Molecular Psychiatry, 14*, 561–562. https://doi.org/10.1038/mp.2009.12

Yang, M., Wong, S. P., & Coid, J. (2010). The efficacy of violence prediction: A meta-analytic comparison of nine risk assessment tools. *Psychological Bulletin, 136*, 740–767. https://doi.org/10.1037/a0020473

Yates, P. M. (2013). Treatment of sexual offenders: Research, best practices, and emerging models. *International Journal of Behavioral Consultation and Therapy, 8*, 89–95. https://doi.org/10.1037/h0100989

Chapter 14
Therapeutic Considerations and Interventions for Psychopathy

Corine de Ruiter and Martin Hildebrand

Abstract Psychopathic offenders present a challenge to treatment providers. By definition, they experience limited distress that might motivate them for treatment. Because of their attitudes and behaviors, psychopathic offenders have been predominantly seen as unresponsive to treatment. In this chapter, we provide a review of existing empirical research on the treatment of psychopathy. We take a historical approach, starting with early treatment approaches and empirical studies into their effects, up until more recently developed interventions. Our review suggests that there is no empirical evidence to support the thesis that psychopathic offenders are generally unresponsive to treatment. In fact, several common "myths" that psychopathic patients are unable to form a working alliance with a therapist or that they cannot develop empathy, are refuted by recent evidence. We end our chapter with a set of "lessons learned" and "pointers to the future" concerning the treatment of psychopathy.

Keywords Psychopathy · Psychopathic personality disorder · Treatment · Cognitive-behavioral therapy · Therapeutic alliance · Dialectical behavior therapy · Schema therapy · Therapeutic community

14.1 Psychopathy and Therapeutic Pessimism

The diagnosis of psychopathy does not promise much good in the eyes of lay people and professionals alike. The therapeutic nihilism that used to be characteristic of the offender rehabilitation literature more generally, the so-called "Nothing Works" doctrine (Farabee, 2005; Martinson, 1974), has in recent decades been replaced by the

C. de Ruiter (✉)
Maastricht University, Maastricht, the Netherlands
e-mail: corine.deruiter@maastrichtuniversity.nl

M. Hildebrand
Private Practice, De Bilt, the Netherlands

J. E. Vitale (ed.), *The Complexity of Psychopathy*, Dangerous Behavior in Clinical and Forensic Psychology, https://doi.org/10.1007/978-3-030-83156-1_14

"What Works" approach to offender treatment. The latter development should be credited to the groundbreaking scholarly work of Andrews and Bonta, who developed the Risk-Need-Responsivity (RNR) model of offender rehabilitation (Andrews & Bonta, 1994, 2010; Andrews et al., 1990). The RNR model purports that high-risk offenders should receive the most intensive treatment and risk management interventions, to maximize (violent) crime reduction (Polaschek et al., 2016). Psychopathic offenders are, by definition, high-risk offenders, consequently in need of the most intensive treatment (Skeem & Polaschek, 2020). In reality, high-risk psychopathic offenders are often the least likely to receive the most intensive treatment because they are usually assumed to be the most hardened and unlikely to respond to treatment (Skeem & Polaschek, 2020). Because of their dangerousness as a subgroup of the offender population, they are more likely to receive the death penalty in the US (DeMatteo et al., 2020), partly due to the pejorative connotations this diagnostic label holds (Edens et al., 2018).

Treatment approaches to psychopathic offenders can be distinguished into rehabilitating, risk-reducing treatment and treatment of psychopathy in its essence (Polaschek & Skeem, 2018). In the former type of treatment, the focus lies on reduction of risk factors for reoffending, such as substance use problems, criminal thinking styles, and poor anger management. A recently developed treatment that belongs to this type is Wong and Hare's psychopathy treatment program (Wong, 2013; Wong & Hare, 2005). The second type of treatment is directed at changing the core features of psychopathic personality disorder (PD), such as limited affect and affect dysregulation (Chakhssi et al., 2014b; Galietta & Rosenfeld, 2012; de Ruiter et al., 2016).

In this chapter, we will provide a review of the existing research base on the treatment of psychopathy. We will take a historical approach, starting with early treatments and empirical studies into their effects, up until more recently developed interventions. The knowledge base on treatment effects on psychopathy in adults is limited and the research methodology applied is often less than optimal. The scarcity of empirical research into psychopathy treatment stands in great contrast to the database on the treatment of other PDs, for instance, borderline PD. A recent Cochrane meta-analysis and review on psychological treatments for BPD (Storebø et al., 2020) included 75 randomized controlled trials with a total of 4507 participants, which tested 16 different kinds of psychotherapy, dialectical behavior therapy (DBT) and mentalisation-based treatment (MBT) being the most frequently used. Our review is necessarily much more limited in scope. Our goal is to separate some wheat from the chaff, so this bit of wheat might be useful in generating future crops which hopefully result in more effective treatment for individuals with psychopathic PD in the future.

14.2 Early Treatment Approaches (1990–2006): Therapeutic Communities

The therapeutic community (TC) has been one of the experimental treatments for psychopathy (Harris & Rice, 2006). The TC is based on the premise that a milieu or environment that is therapeutic can be created which is useful to effect positive behavior change. However, how this is implemented varies dramatically and not all TCs are created equal. Some early reports, prior to the 1980s (e.g., Copas et al., 1984; Copas & Whitely, 1976; Kiger, 1967; see also Dolan, 1998), reported positive results regarding the effectiveness of the TC at reducing violence and other disruptive behavior in psychopathic patients. However, methodological limitations, including poor definitions of psychopathy and lack of control groups (e.g., no comparative data for untreated psychopaths), made findings very difficult to interpret (Lösel, 1998).

Ogloff et al. (1990) were the first to explore the impact of contemporarily defined psychopathy (i.e., defined by the Psychopathy Checklist [PCL]; Hare, 1985) on treatment behavior in a TC treatment program in a Canadian forensic hospital ($N = 80$). In this often-cited study, the primary treatment modality was a large therapeutic group that met on weekdays for approximately two hours. The group was described as unstructured and relied strongly on the input of patients. PCL scores were used to divide patients into high (total score of 27 or more), moderate (18–26), and low (score of 17 and below) psychopathy groups. The outcome variables included: length of time spent in the TC program; ratings (on a 4-point scale) of degree of motivation/effort put into the program; and ratings (also on a 4-point scale) of degree of clinical improvement shown during treatment. Note that degree of motivation and degree of clinical improvement were coded from clinical and institutional files. Patients diagnosed as psychopathic (PCL $\geq$ 27) performed significantly poorer on all three outcome criteria than patients with moderate or low PCL scores. On average, psychopathic patients remained in the program for a shorter period, showed less motivation and clinical improvement than each of the other groups (Ogloff et al. 1990).

The now classic study conducted by Rice et al. (1992) of a TC operated through the Penetanguishine Mental Health Centre in Ontario, Canada, undeniably has had the greatest impact on the idea that TCs for psychopaths are set up for failure. The authors retrospectively evaluated the 1960s Oak Ridge Social Therapy Unit, a hospitalization program for mentally disordered offenders thought to be especially suitable for psychopaths. It operated for over a decade and drew worldwide attention for its novelty.[1] Treatment was intensive and highly unconventional, to say the least. It was largely peer operated and involved intensive group therapy for up to 80 hours per week, in which the men would be locked in groups in small rooms, left to discuss their issues and to confront each other on their behavior. There was little input from staff, with the patients left essentially to run their own treatment. Hallucinogens

[1] Extensive descriptions of the program can be found elsewhere (e.g., Barker & Mason, 1968; Barker, 1980; Barker & McLaughlin, 1977; Harris et al., 1994; Nielsen, 2000; Quinsey, 1981; Weisman, 1995). In fact, in the 1970s, the Oak Ridge regimen was described extremely positively by both a panel of experts and a Canadian government report, claiming "here psychopaths are treated with success" (Quinsey et al., 1998). In 2000, however, a class lawsuit was raised against the institution and its practitioners because the treatment program was so degrading and inhumane. In May 2017, a Canadian judge ruled in favor of the plaintiffs, stating that Oak Ridge ran therapeutic programs for years that amounted to torture for the patients involved (Fine, 2017).

and sedatives were administered to lessen defenses or to augment disclosure, often at the direction of other patients. The men were subjected to group pressures, nude encounter groups, and deprivation in various forms. Thus, the key components of the treatment were highly experimental, based on principles of brainwashing in a Chinese prison camp (Harris et al., 1994) and judged by the authors themselves as violating patients' rights by 1992 standards (Rice et al., 1992).

In the Rice et al. (1992) study, 146 treated offenders who had spent at least two years in the program were matched with an equal number of untreated offenders (controls). The offenders were matched for age, criminal history, and index offense. All offenders were scored on the Psychopathy Checklist-Revised (PCL-R; Hare, 2003) based on file information (gathered in the 1970s) and a cutoff score of 25 or higher was set for classifying offenders as psychopathic. The results of a follow-up roughly 10.5 years posttreatment showed that there was very little overall difference between the two groups (i.e., treated and untreated offenders), despite the rather lengthy and intensive treatment program that the treated offenders had received. However, when the groups were divided into psychopathic (PCL-R ≥ 25) and non-psychopathic (PCL-R < 25), it was found that more treated psychopathic offenders recidivated with a violent offense compared to untreated psychopaths (77% versus 55%). The opposite was true for nonpsychopathic participants—that is, more untreated than treated nonpsychopathic offender failed (39% versus 22%). Thus, treatment was associated with a *reduction* in violent recidivism among nonpsychopathic offenders but with an *increase* in violent recidivism among psychopathic offenders. In addition, with regard to possible differences in treatment responsiveness between treated psychopathic and nonpsychopathic offenders, it was found that those classified as psychopathic showed poorer adjustment in terms of problem behavior while in the institution than the nonpsychopathic individuals, although they were just as likely as nonpsychopathic offenders to receive positive staff recommendations and achieve positions of trust. The authors speculated that the treatment provided a learning opportunity (e.g., learning about the feelings of others, behaving in socially skilled ways) for both psychopathic and nonpsychopathic participants alike. Whereas the nonpsychopathic individuals used the information to behave prosocially, the psychopathic individuals used it to manipulate and exploit others (Harris & Rice, 2006; Rice et al., 1992). According to Rice et al. (1992), "The results strongly suggest that the kind of therapeutic community described in this article is the wrong program for serious psychopathic offenders" (p. 408). "Community treatment programs that generally seek to cultivate pro-social empathic and caring qualities might inadvertently make psychopaths better equipped to 'facilitate the manipulation and exploitation of others,' and such treatment efforts could, therefore, be 'associated with novel ways to commit violent crime'" (p. 409). Notably, during their stay in the TC, psychopathic offenders were significantly more likely than nonpsychopathic offenders to be referred to a 'disciplinary subprogram', to remedy noncompliance and to be written up and placed in seclusion for disruptive or violent behavior (Rice et al., 1992). These indices of misbehavior and punishment were, in turn, significantly predictive of recidivism. However, the effect of the TC on recidivism, after statistically controlling for these disciplinary sanctions (which may have resulted in a lower treatment intensity), apparently has not been examined.

Results of other studies conducted in TCs also suggested that TC approaches are not likely to benefit psychopathic offenders. Hobson et al. (2000) evaluated a TC in Grendon prison, England, and found a significant relationship between PCL-R Factor 1 scores and negative behaviors in therapy groups and on the ward. The authors found a particularly strong relationship between negative treatment behaviors and the PCL-R items 'glibness/superficial charm', 'grandiosity', and 'failure to take responsibility'. Thus, Hobson et al. (2000) concluded that PCL-R Factor 1 scores should be considered when assessing an offenders' suitability for participation in a therapeutic community. Finally, in a study of a TC for female substance abusers, Richards et al. (2003) found that, although 'true' psychopaths (PCL-R score > 30) were excluded from the treatment program, psychopathy scores were still significantly associated with poor treatment response (in terms of avoidance of urine tests, violent and disruptive rule violations, sporadic attention, failing to stay in the program), and upon release, fewer days in the community prior to receiving a new criminal charge. Factor 1 scores in particular were associated with increased risk for general recidivism.

Overall, the preponderance of evidence indicates that TC treatment approaches are not likely to benefit psychopathic offenders in terms of recidivism reduction. Other than by means of official recidivism data, the TC programs were not evaluated. For example, there was no measure of change in clinical outcomes, most importantly, there was no measure of change in psychopathic traits or other dynamic risk factors for violent recidivism. The early optimism regarding the effectiveness of the TC in treating psychopathy obviously diminished. However, the TC studies reviewed above, which suggested support for the thesis that psychopathy is not amenable to treatment, had significant methodological and conceptual flaws that bring into question the validity of their results.

14.3 Cognitive-Behavioral Treatment Approaches

Besides TCs, treatment programs based on cognitive–behavioral theory have been recommended for psychopathic offenders (e.g., Andrews & Bonta, 1994; Brown & Gutsch, 1985; Serin & Kuriychuk, 1994). Below, we will review studies that examined the effectiveness of cognitive–behavioral treatment approaches in the treatment of psychopathy.

A number of studies have examined the effectiveness of cognitive-behavioral treatment of sex offenders with high vs. low scores on psychopathy. Seto and Barbaree (1999) were the first to examine the association of PCL-R psychopathy, behavior during treatment, and recidivism among a sample of 216 sex offenders in a cognitive–behavioral and relapse prevention program at the Warkworth Sexual Behavior Clinic (WSBC), located in a medium secure federal penitentiary in Ontario, Canada. The treatment involved daily 3-hour group sessions over a period of 5 months. The treatment focused on the identification and understanding of individual offense chains by sequencing the thoughts, feelings, and behaviors preceding the commission of a sexual offense. In addition, a relapse prevention plan was developed for each individual offender (for a detailed description of the treatment program, see Barbaree et al., 1998). Notably, the treatment was not designed to target psychopathy. Offenders were assigned to one of four groups based on their scores on the PCL-R and a measure of treatment behavior (including attendance, participation in group sessions, disruptive behavior, global clinician ratings of motivation and change achieved in treatment) based on a median-split for each measure (median PCL-R score = 15). Results revealed that offenders scoring 15 or higher on the PCL-R who behaved well in treatment were much more likely to commit a new offense during an average follow-up period of 32 months than offenders in the other three groups. Among the more psychopathic offenders, those rated as participating well in treatment were five times more likely to commit a new serious (violent or sexual) offense as those who were rated as participating poorly. No such 'paradoxical' pattern was found for offenders scoring low (i.e., < 15) on the PCL-R. Based on their results, Seto and Barbaree (1999) suggested that "good treatment behavior should not be considered when making management decisions, especially for men who score higher on the PCL-R" (p. 1245). At the time this study was published, it caused considerable concern (Barbaree et al., 2006) because the findings echoed with Rice et al.'s (1992) evaluation of the Penetanguishine TC program. Even a treatment program that followed the principles of best-evidence correctional treatment (Andrews & Bonta, 1994; Andrews et al., 1990)—e.g., highly structured and cognitive-behavioral, matching the learning style of most offenders—could possibly make some psychopathic offenders worse.

However, subsequent follow-up research of the same sample provided a different and more complex picture. Barbaree (2005) examined the same sample using a longer follow-up period (mean of 62 months instead of 32) and more comprehensive (and less biased) recidivism data. In addition, he used a PCL-R score of 25 to split the sample, which is obviously more appropriate to identify a high psychopathy group. With the extended follow-up period and new outcome data, Barbaree (2005) found that there was no significant difference in serious recidivism rates between psychopathic offenders who showed good in-treatment behavior and psychopathic offenders who showed poor in-treatment behavior (34% versus 30%). Neither treatment behavior nor the psychopathy—treatment behavior interaction was a significant predictor of recidivism at any of the fixed follow-up times (follow-up periods of 3, 5, and 6 years). Barbaree (2005) concluded there was no evidence that justified Seto and Barbaree's (1999) earlier conclusion that treatment made psychopathic sex offenders worse. He also stressed the importance of awaiting an accumulation of evidence over a number of studies before making major changes in policy and practice regarding treatment of psychopathy (Barbaree, 2005).

Langton et al. (2006) expanded the WSBC sample to 418 treated sex offenders and followed the sample up for 5 years post-release. The authors used a cut-off of 25 (instead of 15) to characterize PCL-R psychopathy in this sample. In contrast to the previous findings of Seto and Barbaree (1999) and Barbaree (2005), Langton et al. (2006) found a significant psychopathy x in-treatment behavior interaction effect, such that psychopathic offenders who displayed *poor* treatment behavior had a significantly higher and faster rate of sexual recidivism over the follow-up period than psychopathic offenders who behaved well during treatment. Finally, Looman et al. (2005) used a similar design as Seto and Barbaree (1999) to examine recidivism outcomes for a sample of 102 sex offenders who had participated in an institutional treatment program for sex offenders at the Regional Treatment Centre Sex Offender Treatment Program in Kingston, Ontario, Canada. The program was a 7-month high-intensity treatment program providing both group therapy and individual therapy to sexual offenders who are assessed as being high risk for reoffending and having high treatment needs. Looman et al. (2005) examined two indicators of treatment change: (1) had the offenders made good vs. poor treatment progress, and (2) were the offenders evaluated as having lowered their risk level at the end of treatment or not? The authors found that psychopathic offenders (PCL-R score > 25) with ratings of good progress in treatment reoffended seriously (i.e., violently or sexually) at a significantly faster rate than did either of the groups with lower PCL-R scores. High psychopathy participants with ratings of poor treatment behavior did not differ from either group of low PCL-R participants with regard to sexual and violent recidivism. The recidivism rate for the two high PCL-R groups did not differ, indicating a main effect for the PCL-R rather than an interaction effect. In addition, among high PCL-R offenders, those rated as lower risk at posttreatment in fact reoffended at a lower rate (30%) than those whose risk was rated as unchanged (50%), although this difference failed to reach significance, probably due to the small cell sizes and concomitant low statistical power. Thus, both Langton et al. (2006) and Looman et al. (2005) found that one of their two groups of psychopathic offenders—split into good and poor treatment behavior—reoffended at a statistically equivalent rate to the two low psychopathy groups — also split by quality of treatment behavior. According to Polaschek and Daly (2013), this result could be interpreted as indicating that some psychopathic offenders might have benefitted from the treatment program, since in each study one group of psychopathic offenders had a comparable outcome to non-psychopathic offenders, although this improved result was found for the better treatment progress group in the Langton et al. (2006) study, and for the poorer treatment progress group in the study conducted by Looman et al. (2005). This difference may be explained by the use of different operationalizations of treatment process/treatment progress in both studies. Nevertheless, according to Polaschek and Daly (2013), the contradictory results in these studies provide some support for the idea that the heterogeneity of PCL-psychopaths extends to their response to treatment.

Further doubts regarding the efficacy of cognitive-behavioral treatment programs for psychopathic offenders emerged from outcome studies conducted outside Canada. For example, Hughes et al. (1997) described preliminary results for a very small sample of offenders who had participated in a program for mentally disordered offenders in an English high-secure forensic psychiatric hospital. The authors found that PCL-R scores (specifically, Factor 1 scores) were significantly inversely correlated with overall clinical change, even though patients with PCL-R scores over 30 were excluded from the study as it was assumed that they would not benefit from treatment. The authors concluded that, "the degree of therapeutic change was strongly mediated by level of psychopathy" (Hughes et al., 1997, p. 524). However, since 'true' psychopaths were excluded from treatment, this study does not provide an adequate test of the effect of treatment for psychopathic offenders. In another study, Hare et al. (2000) evaluated cognitive-behavioral prison programs for psychopathic and nonpsychopathic offenders in several English prisons. Offenders participated in a short-term anger management program involving social skills training. Two-year general reconviction rates for 278 offenders released into the community were determined for those who took part in at least one of the programs and for those who did not. A strong treatment effect was found for offenders in the high PCL-R Factor 1 group, but in the wrong direction. Treated offenders who scored high on Factor 1 had significantly higher rates of recidivism compared to high PCL-R F1 offenders who did not receive treatment (i.e., 85.7% vs. 58.8%). According to the authors, Factor 1 psychopaths may have increased their manipulative skills while in treatment. Hare et al. (2000) also called into question the appropriateness of the interventions because these programs showed very little benefit, even for nonpsychopathic offenders. In fact, no clear description of the treatment in this study is given, and it is possible that it varied across settings (Salekin et al., 2010).

14.4 Salekin's Meta-Analytic Reviews of Research on the Treatment of Psychopathy

Taken together, the early treatment research that used the PCL(-R) to define offenders low versus high in psychopathy not only supported the long held notion that psychopathic individuals were untreatable, but further suggested that treatment might actually make them worse. As noted by Polaschek and Daly (2013), the study by Rice et al. (1992) effectively "slammed the lid shut for many on the advisability of even attempting treatment" (p. 195). In fact, a number of treatment programs began denying treatment to people with high PCL scores based on the evidence that treatment would fail to help them or make them worse (e.g., D'Silva et al., 2004; Hughes et al., 1997; McCarthy & Duggan, 2010; Richards et al., 2003).

In 2002, Salekin published a meta-analysis[2] that challenged the general pessimism about the treatment of psychopathy. He reviewed 42 studies that he identified

[2] There were some attempts at reviewing the treatment literature on psychopathy before the Salekin (2002) meta-analysis. For instance, a study by Garrido et al. (1995) reported on two separate meta-analyses, though without providing the needed detail on references and methods. Also, Wong (2000) found that very few studies satisfied the criteria of a well-designed study. That is, few studies used validated assessments of psychopathy, adequately described the treatment approaches used, or employed control groups and appropriate outcome measures. A few years later, a subsequent systematic review of the treatment literature, conducted by D'Silva et al. (2004), came to a similar conclusion.

as evaluating the effectiveness of some form of therapy for psychopathic patients. The designs of the studies varied from large-scale evaluations of programs featuring several hundred patients to single case studies. Salekin (2002) found that, on average, approximately 62% of patients benefited from treatment, and 60% when case studies were removed. The most effective treatment modality was cognitive-behavioral (average success rate = 62%), followed closely by psychoanalytic psychotherapy (success rate = 59%). Additionally, treatment was found to be especially effective when delivered for a longer period (success rate = 91% for treatments > 12 months; 61% for treatments < 6 months), and for youths (96% success rate for juveniles vs. 63% for adults). The results also showed that many studies included in the meta-analysis contained serious methodological flaws. For example, many had very small sample sizes (i.e., 10 were case studies with 1 to 2 participants; 11 had sample sizes of 10 or less), only four of the 42 studies used the PCL-R as the objective measure of psychopathy, many treatment programs used approaches that were not supported by evidence, few studies had control groups, few studies followed up their clients post-treatment or used recidivism or violent behavior as an outcome variable, and most relied on clinical impressions to determine treatment effectiveness (Harris & Rice, 2006). Indeed, Salekin (2002) noted the poor quality of much of the research, "Though the studies in the current review may be less than optimal in scientific rigor, their inclusion is considered to be both necessary and important given our current state of knowledge on psychopathy" (p. 106). There were also serious methodological issues with the meta-analysis itself, such as questionable estimates used to determine treatment outcomes of the control groups (Harris & Rice, 2006). All these limitations notwithstanding, Salekin concluded that "therapeutic pessimism with regard to the psychopathy–treatment relation is not warranted" (p. 105).

It is legitimate to question the optimistic conclusion of Salekin's (2002) review. For lack of well-designed and adequately powered effectiveness studies (D'Silva et al., 2004; Harris & Rice, 2006), a more appropriate and accurate conclusion could have been that the jury is still out on whether psychopathy can be effectively treated. A more recent review by Salekin et al. (2010) provided at least partial support for the treatability of psychopathy. Using 13 studies (eight treatment studies on adult samples and five on child and youth samples) that all used a contemporary and coherent operationalization of psychopathy (e.g., PCL-R) and that employed a contemporary model of intervention, such as cognitive-behavioral therapy, Salekin et al. (2010) investigated treatment outcome in terms of forensically relevant criteria. The authors found that treatment for adults showed low to moderate success with three out of eight studies demonstrating treatment benefits. Treatment of youth appeared to be more promising with six of eight studies showing treatment gains. However, as noted by Olver (2016), not all treatment programs were equally evidence-informed, and some published studies of well-known treatment programs were not included in the review (e.g., Looman et al., 2005), or only the earlier versions (e.g., Seto & Barbaree, 1999) of subsequently updated studies (Barbaree, 2005; Langton et al., 2006) were reviewed. Although there were less than optimal success rates with adults, the authors concluded that "bright line distinctions" regarding the treatability of psychopathic individuals from non-psychopathic individuals cannot be determined at this time (Salekin et al., 2010, p. 235).

14.5 More Recent Treatment Studies

Several quasi-experimental studies conducted in Dutch maximum secure forensic psychiatric hospitals concur with Salekin et al.'s (2010) conclusion that there is no clear-cut evidence for the nontreatability of psychopathic individuals relative to nonpsychopaths. The Netherlands has a long history of treating severely personality disordered offenders deemed diminished responsible for the crimes they committed. Dutch criminal law has permitted mandated treatment and secure confinement of mentally disordered offenders under the so-called TBS order since 1928 (van Marle, 2002). More than two-thirds of the patients committed under TBS legal statute have a PD without a concomitant major mental disorder, in contrast to forensic hospitals in North America (de Ruiter & Trestman, 2007).

Dutch forensic psychiatric hospitals mostly offer cognitive-behavioral treatment with a focus on behavioral chain analysis of the moment-to-moment experience of the individual during the offense, and relapse prevention (e.g., Laws et al., 2000). Chakhssi et al. (2010) investigated change during CBT treatment delivered in forensic psychiatric center De Rooyse Wissel to personality disordered offenders high vs. low on PCL-R diagnosed psychopathy. Seventy-four personality disordered offenders were divided into high-psychopathic and low-psychopathic cases (high-psychopathic traits was defined as PCL-R total score ≥ 26; 26 is the common European cutoff criterion; Cooke et al., 2005). Over a period of 20 months of forensic treatment, all offenders were assessed repeatedly by psychiatric nurses on risk-related behaviors. Group- and individual level analyses showed few significant differences between patients scoring high vs. low on psychopathy, in terms of treatment effect. Both high and low PCL-R scorers showed significant improvements in adaptive social behavior, communication skills, insight and taking responsibility. A subgroup of high PCL-R scorers (22%) got worse on nurse ratings of physical aggression during treatment, whereas none of the low PCL-R patients did. Post hoc analyses did not reveal differences on the four PCL-R facet scores between the psychopathic offenders who deteriorated and those who improved (Chakhssi et al., 2010, p. 675).

A somewhat comparable study was reported by Hildebrand and de Ruiter (2012) who examined change during forensic CBT treatment in 87 forensic patients, all mandated under the TBS-order, with different degrees of psychopathy [a median split (PCL-R = 22) was used to create the two groups][3] in another Dutch forensic hospital, the Van der Hoeven Kliniek. The outcome measures used were different from the nurse-rated tool in the Chakhssi et al. (2010) study. Nurse ratings of

[3] Twenty-seven (63%) patients in the high-psychopathic traits group ($N = 43$) were diagnosed with PCL-R ≥ 26.

interpersonal behavior, as well as self-report inventories and the Rorschach Inkblot Method were used upon admission and after 20 months of treatment. Findings showed no significant differences between patients high on psychopathic traits compared to those low on psychopathic traits in degree of change between the two time points on any of the indicators of dynamic risk (e.g., impulsivity, egocentrism, distrustful attitudes and hostility) as measured with self-report, performance- and observation based assessment tools (Hildebrand & de Ruiter, 2012).

Two earlier North-American studies had also shown that psychological treatment may be helpful to psychopathic offenders. For example, in an evaluation of treatment in 871 civil psychiatric patients (Skeem et al., 2002), psychopathy, defined as a score of 18 and higher on the PCL:SV,[4] did not moderate the effect of treatment involvement and subsequent violence during a post-discharge follow-up of one year. Similar findings were reported for a sample of 156 PCL-R assessed sex offenders. After a 10-year post-treatment follow-up, sex offenders who demonstrated positive therapeutic responses during a cognitive-behavioral program with a relapse prevention component were less likely to recidivate in violent and sexual crimes (Olver & Wong, 2009), regardless of their psychopathy scores.

To date, no randomized controlled trials of treatment effectiveness studies for psychopathy have been published in the literature. Most existing treatment approaches are cognitive-behavioral and focus on reducing psychopaths' recidivism risk by addressing their antisocial cognitions, teaching them more effective coping skills and enhancing their motivation towards pro-social goals and behaviors (Polaschek & Skeem, 2018).

14.6 Treatments Designed for Psychopathic Offenders

As already mentioned previously, two types of psychopathy treatment can be distinguished: risk-reduction and PD focused. In this section, we will briefly review more recently developed treatment models that reflect these two types of treatment.

14.6.1 Risk-Reduction Approaches: Wong & Hare (2005) Psychopathy Treatment Program (PTP)

Wong et al. (Wong & Hare, 2005; Wong et al., 2012) proposed a two-component model for psychopathy treatment. Component 1 is termed the Interpersonal Component and entails managing the Factor 1 traits as a responsivity factor, while Component 2 is termed the Criminogenic Component and involves treating the criminogenic needs associated with Factor 2, per the risk and need principles of the RNR model. The rationale behind this treatment rests on the assumption that the

[4] In the PCL: SV manual, Hart et al. (1995) state that a score of 18 or above on the Screening Version strongly suggests psychopathy.

primary objective in the treatment of psychopathic offenders is to reduce their risk for violence or other serious antisocial behavior.

The PTP is more a strategy for behavioral self-management rather than a cure for psychopathy. Participants of the PTP should be assisted in developing deeper insights into their lifelong psychopathology and to accept the fact that they will require long-term and continuing self-management for most aspects of their lives to keep them from recidivating. Community support upon re-entry into the community is crucial to help them refrain from a return to a criminal lifestyle (Wong & Burt, 2007).

To the best of our knowledge, there are no studies that provide a direct test of the effectiveness of the PTP program. Wong et al. (2012) presented three studies on the effectiveness of two RNR-based risk reduction programs (one for violent offenders and one for sexual offenders) that they deem consistent with the two-component model. The results showed that, for both violent and sexual offenders with significant psychopathic traits, risk reductions assessed during treatment by means of the Violence Risk Scale (Wong & Gordon, 2006), a file-based risk measure, were linked to significant reductions in sexual and violent recidivism after release into society. For one of the studies, the effect of the treatment was only revealed in the severity of reoffending, not in its frequency (Wong et al., 2012).

Sewall and Olver (2019) tested the two-component model in a long-term follow-up study (17.6 years post release) among a sample of 302 sex offenders, who had participated in an 8-month high-intensity sexual violence reduction treatment program, based on CBT and relapse prevention. They conducted many different analyses to examine interaction effects between psychopathy level, treatment completion, and therapeutic change (measured by scores on the Violence Risk Scale-Sexual offense version). High-psychopathy men (PCL-R $\geq$ 25) had significantly higher rates of treatment noncompletion (30%) compared to low psychopathy men (6%), but they did not show less therapeutic change. The authors also found support for the interpersonal/affective facet as a responsivity factor, in that the Affective facet correlated with decreased treatment progress, although they also found a significant correlation between the Lifestyle facet and treatment noncompletion, which was not predicted by the PTP model. Interestingly, there were no significant differences in sexual recidivism rates as a function of psychopathy and treatment completion status, even after controlling for pretreatment sexual reoffending risk score. Perhaps the most interesting finding from this study was that men who were high in psychopathy, high risk, and showed large therapeutic change, had a modest rate of sexual, but also violent, recidivism (Sewall & Olver, 2019).

Olver (2016) and Wong et al. (2012) do not see a role for personality change in psychopathy treatment: "Attempting to do so would be akin to an attempt to transform these individuals into warm, empathic, considerate beings who experience the normal range and intensities of human emotion. Not only are such attempts likely to fail, but there is little evidence that targeting the psychopath's personality in treatment is linked to reductions in violence and other forms of recidivism" (Olver, 2016, p. 79).

14.6.2 Personality Disorder Approaches: Galietta & Rosenfeld (2012) Dialectical Behavior Therapy (DBT) for Psychopathy

Galietta and Rosenfeld's (2012) motivation to develop an adapted version of DBT (Linehan, 1993) for psychopathic patients arose from their observation that effects (in terms of recidivism reduction) of most risk-reduction programs were rather modest (Tyrer et al., 2009). In their opinion, the focus on changing cognitions and behaviors in risk-reduction programs leaves the crucial problem of emotion dysregulation (both over- and underregulation) among psychopathic individuals untreated. Their choice of DBT, as opposed to other treatment models, was based on DBT's proven effectiveness with borderline PD (Linehan et al., 1999, 2002, see also the recent Cochrane review by Storebø et al., 2020) and the conceptual overlap between borderline PD and psychopathic PD.

In Linehan's (1993) treatment model, aversive childhood environments are viewed as important in explaining the etiology of borderline PD. Caregivers are seen as "invalidating" their child when they ignore the child's emotional distress and punish emotional expression and emotionally driven behaviors. Empirical research provides support for the role of childhood trauma in the development of psychopathy: in offender samples, self-reported childhood trauma is associated with higher PCL-R scores (Graham et al., 2012; Kolla et al., 2013; Marshall & Cooke, 1999; Poythress et al., 2006; Weizmann-Henelius et al., 2010). The evidence appears strongest for Factor 2 psychopathic traits, but some studies also find associations between childhood trauma and Factor 1 traits, such as blunted affect and lack of empathy (e.g., Graham et al., 2012; Marshall & Cooke, 1999).

Galietta and Rosenfeld (2012) share a number of relevant experiences in adapting DBT for psychopathic patients. First, creating commitment to treatment appears to be a crucial component. Second, a focus on the complete range of emotions, not just anger and hostility, is needed, because they observed that reactive anger was often a secondary response "to a brief flash of fear or vulnerability, particularly in individuals who have a history of childhood trauma" (p. 328). Similar to DBT for borderline PD, the treatment consists of weekly individual and group sessions, and telephone coaching in between sessions. Tailored, individualized treatment targets are based on a behavioral chain analysis (BCA) of the index offense and if necessary, prior violent offenses. Compared to Linehan's original model for borderline PD, the skills group is modified to include simpler language, more emphasis on problem recognition and problem solving, and mindfulness techniques to recognize and develop emotions as well as compassion for others. Telephone coaching is much more structured and scheduled in advance, instead of the on-demand set-up for borderline PD. The case study reported by Galietta and Rosenfeld (2012) points at the importance of the therapeutic alliance in fostering treatment motivation and commitment to DBT for psychopathy. The challenging nature of the population requires active emotional and practical support for DBT therapists (Galietta & Rosenfeld (2012).

14.6.3 *Schema Therapy for Forensic PD Patients, Including Those with Psychopathy*

Schema Therapy (ST) was developed for patients with severe PDs who are considered difficult to treat with traditional cognitive-behavioral therapy (Young et al., 2003). ST builds on the cognitive-behavioral approach developed by Beck et al. (1990), but places more emphasis on the processing of childhood origins of mental health problems, on experiential techniques, on the therapeutic alliance, and on maladaptive coping styles (Young et al., 2003). ST has already shown effectiveness for borderline PD (for a recent review, see Storebø et al., 2020), and Bernstein et al. (2007) designed an ST adaptation for use with forensic patients with severe PD. They stated explicitly that a high PCL-R score is not an exclusion criterion for treatment with ST (Bernstein et al., 2007). The forensic ST model hypothesizes that criminal and violent behavior can be explained by an unfolding sequence of maladaptive schema modes, or moment-to-moment states, that comprise emotions, cognitions, and behavior.

Schema Mode Work is the preferred form of ST with more severe PDs (Young et al., 2003). Young defined 11 maladaptive schema modes, to which Bernstein et al. (2007) added 4 "forensic" modes: Angry Protector Mode, Predator Mode, Conning and Manipulative Mode, and Over-Controller Mode (Obsessive and Paranoid subtypes). Ideally, an individual also has a strong Healthy Adult Mode that is aware of the various maladaptive modes and can moderate and integrate them (Young et al., 2003). Schema Mode Work consists of a set of techniques to help the patient mitigate or eliminate his individual maladaptive Schema Modes, and to develop a stronger Healthy Adult Mode that can assist in meeting basic emotional needs in a more prosocial manner. Similar to DBT, ST has a strong focus on emotion recognition and regulation, but in addition, ST tries to link maladaptive modes (including the emotions that go with them) to failures of early caregivers to meet the child's basic needs for warmth, guidance and limit setting. With the "limited re-parenting" technique, the ST therapist attempts to meet these thwarted developmental needs within the confines of the therapeutic relationship. Regular supervision and support for the therapists are needed to ensure the quality of ST delivery to forensic patients (Bernstein et al., 2007).

Research suggests that early maladaptive schemas, assessed with self-report, are common in patients with psychopathic traits (Chakhssi et al., 2014a). Keulen-de Vos et al. (2016) tested the underlying theory of forensic ST, which states that offending behavior can be understood as a sequence of maladaptive schema modes. The authors coded schema modes on the basis of descriptions of forensic patients' ($N = 95$) offenses in their charts, which typically included statements by the patient as well as victims' and witnesses' statements. For the sample as a whole, vulnerable child modes, accompanied by feelings of abandonment or shame, were evident in the events leading up to the offenses, while over-compensatory modes, such as bully and attack and predator modes, had a stronger presence during the offenses. This finding concurs with forensic ST's view that states involving aggression compensate for contrary emotional states, such as those involving feelings of weakness, fear, humiliation, or helplessness. The associations between schema modes and PCL-R psychopathy revealed a number of interesting findings. The bully and attack mode and the conning and manipulative mode were positively correlated with the interpersonal facet. The affective facet showed negative correlations with vulnerable child modes, during events leading up to the offense. The detached self-soother mode, i.e., alcohol or drug use, was positively related to the lifestyle facet, both before and during the offense (Keulen-de Vos et al., 2016).

Preliminary findings of a multicenter randomized clinical trial (RCT) using ST with forensic patients with PD suggests treatment reduces future violence risk and improves the ability to be open and vulnerable during treatment (Bernstein et al., 2012). This paper did not report interaction effects of psychopathy and treatment, however, because of limited sample size. A single case study documented the process of individual Schema Therapy (ST) in a Dutch forensic patient with psychopathic traits (Chakhssi et al., 2014b). The patient had been a victim of extreme physical and emotional abuse as a child and the therapist used different ST techniques in an attempt to alter the resultant maladaptive schema modes of the patient. After the ST treatment, the antisocial modes, such as the predator, bully and attack, and self-aggrandizer modes, were clearly less prevalent than at the beginning. There was also more room for healthy adult modes of being and for vulnerable emotions, although mistrust schemas could still be easily triggered. The case study also showed the patient's PCL-R total score changed from 27 at baseline to 14 after four years of intensive ST; pre- and post PCL-R ratings were performed by two independent assessors who were not involved in the patient's treatment. Remarkably, the Affective facet showed the largest change: from 7 to 1; the Interpersonal facet decreased from 4 to 1. This finding, although just an $N = 1$ result, challenges the notion that the affective and interpersonal 'core' of psychopathy is immutable (Olver, 2016).

14.7 The Future of Psychopathy Treatment

We started to work as scientist-practitioners in a forensic psychiatric hospital in 1995. The first author had just spent the first nine years of her career in general outpatient psychiatry, assessing and treating patients with anxiety and mood disorders. We were struck by the lack of evidence-based treatments for forensic psychiatric patients, including those with psychopathic PD, compared to the empirical knowledge base that informed psychiatric treatments for anxiety and depressive symptoms at the time. Considering the social cost of psychopathy to society, both in terms of human emotional and physical suffering, it would appear wise to invest in the development of effective treatments for this disorder. Now, twenty-five years later, science still cannot provide a clear answer to the question of what works for psychopathy. Obviously, conducting effectiveness research within criminal justice environments is a huge challenge; controlled research in these settings is difficult and requires cooperation at many levels (e.g., institutional leadership, treatment staff engagement and supervision, and patient/offender cooperativeness). RCTs are virtually impossible to conduct, because the legal system and ethical considerations make random allocation to treatment vs. no-treatment undesirable.

14.8 Lessons Learned

With these thoughts in mind, we would like to end our contribution with a set of "lessons learned" and "pointers to the future" concerning the treatment of psychopathy:

Lesson #1. Psychopathy is not untreatable. For treatment to be effective, it will have to be more tailored than most current "one-size-fits-all" offender (group) treatments and require a longer duration, which includes working through past traumatic experiences and a period of aftercare.

Lesson #2. Negatively toned misconceptions about psychopathy and psychopathic behaviors among professionals lead to diminished hope for change. As an example, it is rather widely assumed that high psychopathy offenders seek treatment to manipulate others and reach desired outcomes, such as early release from detention. However, a recent study tested this idea in a sample of 217 jail inmates and failed to find an association between PCL:SV total, Factor 1 and Factor 2 scores and treatment seeking (including psycho-educational and support groups and substance use treatment while detained (Schrader et al., 2018). As a second example, many authors contend that psychopathy, and Factor 1 in particular, has a negative effect on the therapeutic alliance. However, several studies that examined relationships between psychopathy scores and working alliance scores, as reported by both therapists and clients, do not find significant associations (Polaschek & Ross, 2010; Walton et al., 2018).

Lesson #3. Psychopathic patients are able to engage in a therapeutic alliance. To achieve this, therapists need to be nonjudgmental and validate the clients' thoughts, feelings and behaviors (Chakhssi et al., 2014b; Galietta & Rosenfeld, 2012). Obviously, violent and harmful behavior are never to be validated, but the underlying feelings and thoughts, such as "I felt belittled by that remark" may have validity. In the words of Gullhaugen and Nøttestad (2012): "Empathy may be taught through the process of considering the psychopathic offender's needs, which herein lays the irony in treatment of psychopathy" (p. 648).

Lesson #4. Psychopathic patients are a heterogeneous group. Any type of treatment should start with a thorough assessment of the patient's offending behavior through methods such as behavioral chain analysis or schema mode sequences. An interesting case study of a male violent offender with a PCL-R score of 38, demonstrated the utility of the Adult Attachment Interview and the Rorschach Performance Assessment System in identifying underlying unresolved loss and trauma, as well as strong denial of fear and vulnerability, counteracted by extreme outbursts of anger (Nørbech et al., 2013).

14.9 Pointers to the Future

Pointer #1. Positive, strengths-focused interventions, such as mindfulness meditation, yoga, and aerobic exercise could serve as a positive adjunctive treatment to present-day risk-reduction approaches (for a discussion and underlying rationale, see de Ruiter, 2018). Some of these are already part of therapeutic interventions, such as DBT.

Pointer #2. Because RCTs will remain an exception for effectiveness studies in offender treatment, we believe alternative, quasi-experimental designs, including case series analysis, can be helpful in moving the field of psychopathy treatment forward. Of note, not only treatment "successes", but also treatment "failures" can be informative.

Pointer #3. A non-repressive, therapeutic climate is an essential component of any offender rehabilitation program. In forensic ST, it is made explicit that its effectiveness depends on an institutional environment that is sufficiently safe and supportive of the patient's recovery (Bernstein et al., 2007). In the ST model, a harsh institutional environment would reinforce precisely the kinds of aggressive, maladaptive Schema Modes in forensic patients that ST is attempting to change. A recent, qualitative study of opiate maintenance treatment (OMT) in a Norwegian prison demonstrated that repressive and collective control measures clearly undermined the rehabilitative aims of the OMT (Mjåland, 2015). This will apply *a fortiori* to offenders high in psychopathy, who are particularly sensitive to feeling controlled, and will likely respond with higher than average levels of resistance and aggression.

14.10 Conclusion

Present-day psychopathy research can be traced back to Hervey Cleckley's (1941/1988) *The Mask of Sanity*, and Robert Hare's operationalization of the disorder in the Psychopathy Checklist and allied instruments. Cleckley's view that psychopaths were unable to develop an emotional attachment needed for effective psychotherapy and therefore failed to benefit from treatment, lingers on until today. We believe it is time to leave this view behind, given present-day evidence to the contrary. We do not claim treating patients with psychopathic PD is easy, on the contrary, a high level of experience and theoretical sophistication on the part of treatment developers and implementers is needed. The efforts made by the scientist-practitioners in this field, as summarized in the present chapter, will hopefully inspire professionals involved in the treatment of this fascinating disorder.

References

Andrews, D. A., & Bonta, J. (1994). *The psychology of criminal conduct*. Anderson.

Andrews, D. A., & Bonta, J. (2010). *The psychology of criminal conduct* (5th ed.). Routledge.

Andrews, D. A., Zinger, I., Hoge, R. D., Bonta, J., Gendreau, P., & Cullen, F. T. (1990). Does correctional treatment work? A clinically relevant and psychologically informed meta-analysis. *Criminology, 28*, 369–404. https://doi.org/10.1111/j.1745-9125.1990.tb01330.x

Barbaree, H. E. (2005). Psychopathy, treatment behavior, and recidivism: An extended follow-up of Seto and Barbaree. *Journal of Interpersonal Violence, 20*, 1115–1131. https://doi.org/10.1177/0886260505278262

Barbaree, H. E., Peacock, E. J., Cortini, F., Marshall, W. L., & Seto, M. (1998). Ontario penitentiaries' program. In W. L. Marshall, Y. M. Fernandez, S. M. Hudson, & T. Ward (Eds.), *Sourcebook of treatment programs for sexual offenders* (pp. 59–77). Plenum.

Barbaree, H. E., Langton, C. M., & Peacock, E. J. (2006). Sexual offender treatment for psychopaths: Is it harmful? In W. L. Marshall, Y. M. Fernandez, & L. E. Marshall (Eds.), *Sexual offender treatment: Controversial issues* (pp. 159–171). Wiley.

Barker, E. (1980). The Penetanguishene Program: A personal review. In H. Toch (Ed.), *Therapeutic communities in corrections* (pp. 73–81). Praeger.

Barker, E. T., & Mason, M. H. (1968). Buber behind bars. *Canadian Psychiatric Association Journal, 13*, 61–72. https://doi.org/10.1177/070674376801300111

Barker, E., & McLaughlin, A. J. (1977). The total encounter capsule. *Canadian Psychiatric Association Journal, 22*, 355–360. https://doi.org/10.1177/070674377702200705

Beck, A. T., Freeman, A., & Associates. (1990). *Cognitive therapy of personality disorders*. Guilford.

Bernstein, D. P., Arntz, A., & de Vos, M. (2007). Schema Focused Therapy in forensic settings: Theoretical model and recommendations for best clinical practice. *International Journal of Forensic Mental Health, 6*, 169–183. https://doi.org/10.1080/14999013.2007.10471261

Bernstein, D. P., Nijman, H., Karos, K., Keulen-de Vos, M. E., de Vogel, V., & Lucker, T. (2012). Treatment of personality disordered offenders in the Netherlands: Initial findings of a multicenter randomized clinical trial on the effectiveness of Schema Therapy. *International Journal of Forensic Mental Health, 11*, S312–S324. https://doi.org/10.1080/14999013.2012.746757

Brown, H. J., & Gutsch, K. U. (1985). Cognitions associated with a delay of gratification task: A study with psychopaths and normal prisoners. *Criminal Justice and Behavior, 12*, 453–462. https://doi.org/10.1177/0093854885012004004

Chakhssi, F., de Ruiter, C., & Bernstein, D. (2010). Change during forensic treatment in psychopathic versus nonpsychopathic offenders. *Journal of Forensic Psychiatry & Psychology, 21*, 660–682. https://doi.org/10.1080/14789949.2010.483283

Chakhssi, F., Bernstein, D., & de Ruiter, C. (2014a). Early maladaptive schemas in relation to facets of psychopathy and institutional violence in offenders with personality disorders. *Legal and Criminological Psychology, 19*, 356–372. https://doi.org/10.1111/lcrp.12002

Chakhssi, F., Kersten, T., de Ruiter, C., & Bernstein, D. P. (2014b). Treating the untreatable: A single case study of a psychopathic inpatient treated with schema therapy. *Psychotherapy, 51*, 447–461. https://doi.org/10.1037/a0035773

Cleckley, H. M. (1941). *The mask of sanity: An attempt to reinterpret the so-called psychopathic personality*. Mosby.

Cleckley, H. M. (1988). *The mask of sanity: An attempt to clarify some issues about the so-called psychopathic personality* (5th ed.). Emily S. Cleckley.

Cooke, D. J., Michie, C., Hart, S. D., & Clark, D. (2005). Searching for the pan-cultural core of psychopathic personality disorder: Continental Europe and North America compared. *Personality and Individual Differences, 39*, 283–295. https://doi.org/10.1016/j.paid.2005.01.004

Copas, J. B., & Whiteley, J. S. (1976). Predicting success in the treatment of psychopaths. *British Journal of Psychiatry, 129*, 388–392. https://doi.org/10.1192/bjp.129.4.388

Copas, J. B., O'Brien, M., Roberts, J., & Whiteley, J. S. (1984). Treatment outcome in personality disorder: The effect of social psychological and behavioural variables. *Personality and Individual Differences, 5*, 565–573. https://doi.org/10.1016/0191-8869(84)90031-X

de Ruiter, C. (2018). Modifying risk factors—Building strengths. In A. R. Beech, A. J. Carter, R. E. Mann, & P. Rothstein (Eds.), *The Wiley-Blackwell handbook of forensic neuroscience, Volume 2* (pp. 553–573). Wiley.

de Ruiter, C., & Trestman, R. L. (2007). Prevalence and treatment of personality disorders in Dutch forensic mental health services. *Journal of the American Academy of Psychiatry and the Law, 35*, 92–97.

de Ruiter, C., Chakhssi, F., & Bernstein, D. P. (2016). Treating the untreatable psychopath. In C. G. Gacono (Ed.), *The clinical and forensic assessment of psychopathy: A practitioner's guide* (2nd ed., pp. 388–402). Taylor & Francis.

D'Silva, K., Duggan, C., & McCarthy, L. (2004). Does treatment really make psychopaths worse? A review of the evidence. *Journal of Personality Disorders, 18*, 163–177. https://doi.org/10.1521/pedi.18.2.163.32775

DeMatteo, D., Hart, S. D., Heilbrun, K., Boccaccini, M. T., Cunningham, M. D., Douglas, K. S., Dvoskin, J. A., Edens, J. F., Guy, L. S., Murrie, D. C., Otto, R. K., Packer, I. K., & Reidy, T. J. (2020). Statement of concerned experts on the use of the Hare Psychopathy Checklist—Revised in capital sentencing to assess risk for institutional violence. *Psychology, Public Policy, and Law, 26*, 133–144. https://doi.org/10.1037/law0000223

Dolan, D. (1998). Therapeutic community treatment for severe personality disorders. In T. Millon, E. Simonsen, M. Birket-Smith, & R. D. Davis (Eds.), *Psychopathy: Antisocial, criminal and violent behavior* (pp. 407–430). Guilford.

Edens, J. F., Petrila, J., & Kelley, S. E. (2018). Legal and ethical issues in the assessment and treatment of psychopathy. In C. J. Patrick (Ed.), *Handbook of psychopathy* (2nd ed., pp. 732–751). Guilford.

Farabee, D. (2005). *Rethinking rehabilitation: Why can't we reform our criminals?* AEI Press.

Fine, S. (2017, June 7). Doctors tortured patients at Ontario Mental-Health Centre, judge rules. *The Globe and Mail.* Retrieved from https://www.theglobeandmail.com/news/national/doctors-at-ontario-mental-health-facility-torturedpatients-court-finds/article35246519/

Galietta, M., & Rosenfeld, B. (2012). Adapting Dialectical Behavior Therapy (DBT) for the treatment of psychopathy. *International Journal of Forensic Mental Health, 11*, 325–335. https://doi.org/10.1080/14999013.2012.746762

Garrido, V., Esteban, C., & Molero, C. (1995). The effectiveness in the treatment of psychopathy: A meta-analysis. *Issues in Criminological and Legal Psychology, 24*, 57–59.

Graham, N., Kimonis, E. R., Wasserman, A. L., & Kline, S. M. (2012). Associations among childhood abuse and psychopathy facets in male sexual offenders. *Personality Disorders: Theory, Research, and Treatment, 3*, 66–75. https://doi.org/10.1037/a0025605

Gullhaugen, A. S., & Nottestad, J. A. (2012). Testing theoretical models for future clinical practice in the treatment of psychopathy. *The Journal of Forensic Psychiatry & Psychology, 23*, 635–653. https://doi.org/10.1080/14789949.2012.729390

Hare, R. D. (1985). *The psychopathy checklist.* Unpublished manuscript, University of British Columbia.

Hare, R. D. (2003). *Manual for the Hare psychopathy checklist–revised* (2nd ed.). Multi-Health Systems.

Hare, R. D., Clark, D., Grann, M., & Thornton, D. (2000). Psychopathy, and the predictive validity of the PCL-R: An international perspective. *Behavioral Sciences & the Law, 18*, 623–645. https://doi.org/10.1002/1099-0798(200010)18:5<623::AID-BSL409>3.0.CO;2-W

Harris, G. T., & Rice, M. E. (2006). Treatment of psychopathy: A review of empirical findings. In C. J. Patrick (Ed.), *Handbook of psychopathy* (pp. 555–572). Guilford.

Harris, G. T., Rice, M. E., & Cormier, C. A. (1994). Psychopaths: Is a therapeutic community therapeutic? *Therapeutic Communities, 15*, 283–300.

Hart, S. D., Cox, D. N., & Hare, R. D. (1995). *Manual for the Hare Psychopathy Checklist: Screening Version (PCL:SV)*. Multi-Health Systems.

Hildebrand, M., & de Ruiter, C. (2012). Psychopathic traits and change on indicators of dynamic risk factors during inpatient forensic psychiatric treatment. *International Journal of Law and Psychiatry, 35*, 276–288. https://doi.org/10.1016/j.ijlp.2012.04.001

Hobson, J., Shine, J., & Roberts, R. (2000). How do psychopaths behave in a prison therapeutic community? *Psychology, Crime, and Law, 6*, 139–154. https://doi.org/10.1080/10683160008410838

Hughes, G., Hogue, T., Hollin, C., & Champion, H. (1997). First-stage evaluation of a treatment programme for personality disordered offenders. *The Journal of Forensic Psychiatry, 8*, 515–527. https://doi.org/10.1080/09585189708412273

Keulen-de Vos, M. E., Bernstein, D. P., Vanstipelen, S., de Vogel, V., Lucker, T. P. C., Slaats, M., Hartkoorn, M., & Arntz, A. (2016). Schema modes in criminal and violent behaviour of forensic cluster B PD patients: A retrospective and prospective study. *Legal and Criminological Psychology, 21*, 56–76. https://doi.org/10.1111/lcrp.12047

Kiger, R. S. (1967). Treating the psychopathic patient in a therapeutic community. *Hospital and Community Psychiatry, 18*, 191–196.

Kolla, N. J., Malcolm, C., Attard, S., Arenovich, T., Blackwood, N., & Hodgins, S. (2013). Childhood maltreatment and aggressive behaviour in violent offenders with psychopathy. *Canadian Journal of Psychiatry, 58*, 487–494.

Langton, C. M., Barbaree, H. E., Harkins, L., & Peacock, E. J. (2006). Sex offenders' response to treatment and its association with recidivism as a function of psychopathy. *Sexual Abuse: A Journal of Research and Treatment, 18*, 99–120. https://doi.org/10.1177/107906320601800107

Laws, D. R., Hudson, S. M., & Ward, T. (2000). *Remaking relapse prevention with sex offenders: A sourcebook*. Sage.

Linehan, M. M. (1993). *Cognitive behavioral treatment of borderline personality disorder*. Guilford.

Linehan, M. M., Schmidt, H., Dimeff, L. A., Craft, J. C., Kanter, J., & Comtois, K. A. (1999). Dialectical behavior therapy for patients with borderline personality disorder and drug-dependence. *The American Journal on Addictions, 8*, 279–292. https://doi.org/10.1080/105504999305686

Linehan, M., Dimeff, L., Reynolds, S., Comtois, K., Welch, S., Heagerty, P., & Kivlahan, D. R. (2002). Dialectical behavior therapy versus comprehensive validation therapy plus 12-step for the treatment of opioid dependent women meeting criteria for borderline personality disorder. *Drug and Alcohol Dependence, 67*, 13–26. https://doi.org/10.1016/s0376-8716(02)00011-x

Looman, J., Abracen, J., Serin, R., & Marquis, P. (2005). Psychopathy, treatment change and recidivism in high risk high need sexual offenders. *Journal of Interpersonal Violence, 20*, 549–568. https://doi.org/10.1177/0886260504271583

Lösel, F. (1998). Treatment and management of psychopaths. In D. J. Cooke, R. D. Hare, & A. E. Forth (Eds.), *Psychopathy: Theory, research, and implications for society* (pp. 303–354). Kluwer.

Marshall, L. A., & Cooke, D. J. (1999). The childhood experiences of psychopaths: A retrospective study of familial and societal factors. *Journal of Personality Disorders, 13*, 211–225. https://doi.org/10.1521/pedi.1999.13.3.211

Martinson, R. (1974). What works? Questions and answers about prison reform. *The Public Interest, 35*, 22–54.

McCarthy, L., & Duggan, C. (2010). Engagement in medium secure personality disorder service: A comparative study of psychological functioning and offending outcomes. *Criminal Behavior and Mental Health, 20*, 112–128. https://doi.org/10.1002/cbm.758

Mjåland, K. (2015). The paradox of control: An ethnographic analysis of opiate maintenance treatment in a Norwegian prison. *International Journal of Drug Policy, 26*, 781–789. https://doi.org/10.1016/j.drugpo.2015.04.020

Nielsen, R. F. (2000). *Total encounters: The life and times of the Mental Health Centre Penetanguishene*. McMaster University Press.

Nørbech, P. C. B., Crittenden, P. M., & Hartmann, E. (2013). Self-protective strategies, violence and psychopathy: Theory and a case study. *Journal of Personality Assessment, 95*, 571–584. https://doi.org/10.1080/00223891.2013.823441

Ogloff, J. R. P., Wong, S., & Greenwood, A. (1990). Treating criminal psychopaths in a therapeutic community program. *Behavioral Sciences & the Law, 8*, 181–190. https://doi.org/10.1002/bsl.2370080210

Olver, M. E. (2016). Treatment of psychopathic offenders: Evidence, issues, and controversies. *Journal of Community Safety and Well-Being, 1*, 75–83. https://doi.org/10.35502/jcswb.25

Olver, M. E., & Wong, S. C. (2009). Therapeutic responses of psychopathic sexual offenders: Treatment attrition, therapeutic change, and long term recidivism. *Journal of Consulting and Clinical Psychology, 77*, 328–336. https://doi.org/10.1037/a0015001

Polaschek, D. L., & Daly, T. E. (2013). Treatment and psychopathy in forensic settings. *Aggression and Violent Behavior, 18*, 592–603. https://doi.org/10.1016/j.avb.2013.06.003

Polaschek, D. L., & Ross, E. C. (2010). Do early therapeutic alliance, motivation, and change readiness predict therapy outcomes for high risk violent prisoners? *Criminal Behaviour and Mental Health, 20*, 100–111. https://doi.org/10.1002/cbm.759

Polaschek, D. L., & Skeem, J. L. (2018). Treatment of adults and juveniles with psychopathy. In C. J. Patrick (Ed.), *Handbook of psychopathy* (2nd ed., pp. 710–731). Guilford.

Polaschek, D. L. L., Yesberg, J. A., Bell, R. K., Casey, A. R., & Dickson, S. R. (2016). Intensive psychological treatment of high-risk violent offenders: Outcomes and pre-release mechanisms. *Psychology, Crime & Law, 22*, 344–365. https://doi.org/10.1080/1068316X.2015.1109088

Poythress, N. G., Skeem, J. L., & Lilienfeld, S. O. (2006). Associations among early abuse, dissociation, and psychopathy in an offender sample. *Journal of Abnormal Psychology, 115*, 88–297. https://doi.org/10.1037/0021-843X.115.2.288

Quinsey, V. L. (1981). The long term management of the mentally disordered offender. In S. J. Hucker, C. D. Webster, & M. H. Ben-Aron (Eds.), *Mental disorder and criminal responsibility* (pp. 137–155). Butterworths.

Quinsey, V. L., Harris, G. T., Rice, M. E., & Cormier, C. A. (1998). *Violent offenders: Appraising and managing risk*. American Psychological Association.

Rice, M. L., Harris, G. T., & Cormier, C. A. (1992). An evaluation of a maximum security therapeutic community for psychopaths and other mentally disordered offenders. *Law and Human Behavior, 16*, 399–412. https://doi.org/10.1007/BF02352266

Richards, H. J., Casey, J. O., & Lucente, S. W. (2003). Psychopathy and treatment response in incarcerated female substance abusers. *Criminal Justice and Behavior, 30*, 251–276. https://doi.org/10.1177/0093854802251010

Salekin, R. T. (2002). Psychopathy and therapeutic pessimism: Clinical lore or clinical reality? *Clinical Psychology Review, 22*, 79–112. https://doi.org/10.1016/s0272-7358(01)00083-6

Salekin, R. T., Worley, C., & Grimes, R. D. (2010). Treatment of psychopathy: A review and brief introduction to the mental model approach for psychopathy. *Behavioral Sciences & the Law, 28*, 235–266. https://doi.org/10.1002/bsl.928

Schrader, S. W., Tangney, J. P., & Stuewig, J. B. (2018). Does psychopathy differentially predict treatment-seeking during incarceration versus postrelease? *Journal of Offender Rehabilitation, 57*, 207–221. https://doi.org/10.1080/10509674.2017.1400487

Serin, R. C., & Kuriychuk, M. (1994). Social and cognitive processing deficits in violent offenders: Implications for treatment. *International Journal of Law and Psychiatry, 17*, 431–441. https://doi.org/10.1016/0160-2527(94)90018-3

Seto, M. C., & Barbaree, H. E. (1999). Psychopathy, treatment behavior, and sex offenders recidivism. *Journal of Interpersonal Violence, 14*, 1235–1248. https://doi.org/10.1177/088626099014012001

Sewall, L. A., & Olver, M. E. (2019). Psychopathy and treatment outcome: Results from a sexual violence reduction program. *Personality Disorders: Theory, Research, and Treatment, 10*, 59–69. https://doi.org/10.1037/per0000297

Skeem, J. L., & Polaschek, D. L. (2020). High risk, not hopeless: Correctional intervention for people at risk for violence. *Marquette Law Review, 103*, 1129–1148.

Skeem, J. L., Monahan, J., & Mulvey, E. (2002). Psychopathy, treatment involvement, and subsequent violence among civil psychiatric patients. *Law and Human Behavior, 26*, 577–603. https://doi.org/10.1023/A:1020993916404

Storebø, O. J., Stoffers-Winterling, J. M., Völlm, B. A., Kongerslev, M. T., Mattivi, J. T., Jørgensen, M. S., Faltinsen, E., Todorovac, A., Sales, C. P., Callesen, H. E., Lieb, K., & Simonsen, E. (2020). Psychological therapies for people with borderline personality disorder. *Cochrane Database of Systematic Review, 5,* Art. No.: CD012955. https://doi.org/10.1002/14651858.CD012955.pub2

Tyrer, P., Cooper, S., Rutter, D., Seivewright, H., Duggan, C., Maden, T., Barrett, B., Joyce, E., Rao, B., Nur, U., Cicchetti, D., Crawford, M., & Byford, S. (2009). The assessment of dangerous and severe personality disorder: Lessons learned from a randomized controlled trial linked to qualitative analysis. *Journal of Forensic Psychiatry & Psychology, 20*, 132–146. https://doi.org/10.1080/14789940802236872

van Marle, H. J. C. (2002). The Dutch entrustment act (TBS): Its principles and innovations. *International Journal of Forensic Mental Health, 1*, 83–92. https://doi.org/10.1080/14999013.2002.10471163

Walton, A., Jeglic, E. L., & Blasko, B. L. (2018). The role of psychopathic traits in the development of the therapeutic alliance among sexual offenders. *Sexual Abuse, 30*, 211–229. https://doi.org/10.1177/1079063216637859

Weisman, R. (1995). Reflections on the Oakridge experiment with mentally disordered offenders, 1965–1968. *International Journal of Law and Psychiatry, 18*, 265–290. https://doi.org/10.1016/0160-2527(95)00011-6

Weizmann-Henelius, G., Grönroos, M., Putkonen, H., Eronen, M., Lindberg, N., & Häkkänen-Nyholm, H. (2010). Psychopathy and gender differences in childhood psychosocial characteristics in homicide offenders—A nationwide register-based study. *Journal of Forensic Psychiatry & Psychology, 6*, 801–814. https://doi.org/10.1080/14789949.2010.506616

Wong, S. (2000). Treatment of criminal psychopaths. In S. Hodgins & R. Muller-Isberner (Eds.), *Violence, crime and mentally disordered offenders: Concepts and methods for effective treatment and prevention* (pp. 81–106). Wiley.

Wong, S. C. P. (2013). Treatment of psychopathy in correctional settings. In O. Thienhaus & M. Piasecki (Eds.), *Textbook on correctional psychiatry* (pp. 1–26). Civic Research Press.

Wong, S. C. P., & Burt, G. (2007). The heterogeneity of incarcerated psychopaths: Differences in risk, need, recidivism and management approaches. In J. Yuille & H. Hervé (Eds.), *The psychopath: Theory, research and practice* (pp. 461–484). Erlbaum.

Wong, S. C. P., & Gordon, A. (2006). The validity and reliability of the violence risk scale: A treatment friendly violence risk assessment scale. *Psychology, Public Policy and Law, 12*, 279–309. https://doi.org/10.1037/1076-8971.12.3.279

Wong, S. C. P., & Hare, R. D. (2005). *Guidelines for a psychopathy treatment program*. Multi-Health Systems.

Wong, S. C. P., Gordon, A., Gu, D., Lewis, K., & Olver, M. E. (2012). The effectiveness of violence reduction treatment for psychopathic offenders: Empirical evidence and a treatment model. *International Journal of Forensic Mental Health, 11*, 336–349. https://doi.org/10.1080/14999013.2012.746760

Young, J. E., Klosko, J. S., & Weishaar, M. E. (2003). *Schema therapy: A practitioner's guide*. Guilford.

Chapter 15
Psychoanalytic Perspectives on Psychopathy

Jessica Yakeley

Abstract The neuroscientific understanding of the brain of the psychopath is gathering apace. But to guide empirical research, a theory of the psychopath's mind is also important. One such theory of mind is the psychoanalytic. Contemporary psychoanalytic theorists offer an explanatory model of the psychopath's personality, which encompasses the dynamic nature of his mind and its developmental origins. Such a model needs to take into account attitudes and behaviours that may appear to be antithetical to human nature – the lack of empathy and emotional attachment, the inversion of moral values, the addiction to violence, cruelty and extreme states of excitement, the triumphant manipulation and deception of others, and the stance of arrogance, grandiosity and omnipotence. It also specifies the motivation and meaning of the psychopath's behaviour, understand his subjective experience of the world, and informs our realistic perception of the risks he poses to himself and others (Meloy & Yakeley, 2021)

Keywords Affect · Aggression · Anxiety · Attachment · Countertransference · Defense mechanisms · Gene-environment interactions · Group therapy · Mentalization · Object-relations theory · Personality organization · Psychoanalytic · Psychopathy · Psychodynamic psychotherapy · Risk-assessment · Therapeutic community · Trauma

J. Yakeley (✉)
Portman Clinic Tavistock and Portman NHS Foundation Trust, London, UK
e-mail: JYakeley@tavi-port.nhs.uk

J. E. Vitale (ed.), *The Complexity of Psychopathy*, Dangerous Behavior in Clinical and Forensic Psychology, https://doi.org/10.1007/978-3-030-83156-1_15

15.1 Introduction

The neuroscientific understanding of the brain of the psychopath is gathering apace. But to guide empirical research, a theory of the psychopath's mind is also important. One such theory of mind is the psychoanalytic. Contemporary psychoanalytic theorists offer an explanatory model of the psychopath's personality, which encompasses the dynamic nature of his[1] mind and its developmental origins. Such a model needs to take into account attitudes and behaviours that may appear to be antithetical to human nature – the lack of empathy and emotional attachment, the inversion of moral values, the addiction to violence, cruelty and extreme states of excitement, the triumphant manipulation and deception of others, and the stance of arrogance, grandiosity and omnipotence. It also specifies the motivation and meaning of the psychopath's behaviour, understand his subjective experience of the world, and informs our realistic perception of the risks he poses to himself and others (Meloy & Yakeley, 2021).

This chapter is divided into two main sections reviewing the psychoanalytic theories of psychopathy and the psychoanalytically-informed management and treatment of the psychopath, respectively. The first part reviews the historical psychoanalytic theories of psychopathy that laid the conceptual foundations for the contributions of more recent psychoanalytic thinking. It then examines the empirical evidence for genetic, neurobiological, and environmental factors in the development of psychopathy, and describes how attachment theory provides an integrated aetiological model that links these biological and environmental influences to inform a contemporary psychoanalytic understanding of the workings of the psychopathic mind. The second section of the chapter describes in detail a psychoanalytic approach to the assessment, management and treatment of individuals with psychopathy. Although most psychopaths will not be suitable for conventional psychoanalytic psychotherapy, a psychoanalytically informed framework may be helpful in guiding the effective management of patients and offenders with psychopathy. Any treatment planning should include assessment of the psychopath's risk, consideration of how his personality characteristics influence his response to treatment, general principles of treatment, and specific therapeutic approaches.

15.2 Historical Psychoanalytic Perspectives of Psychopathy

Since the French psychiatrist Pinel described in 1801 a group of patients who behaved in impulsive and aggressive ways with no apparent loss of reasoning – 'manie sans delire', the history of the concept of psychopathy has been mired in controversies and dichotomies: moral condemnation versus clinical objectivity; the role of biology in its aetiology versus that of the environment; a degenerative condition versus one that has adapted to a hostile environment; and sociological

[1] As psychopathy is more common in men, the male pronoun will be used throughout, which is not to minimise the occurrence and significance of female psychopathy.

influences versus familial disturbance in its developmental origins. During the late nineteenth century and early twentieth century a series of influential psychiatrists construed psychopathy as biologically-rooted entity that was degenerative in moral stature, reflected in a trend of pejorative diagnostic terminology: Koch's (1891) concept of 'psychopathic inferiority', Meyer's (1904) 'constitutional inferiority', Kraepelin's (1915) notions of 'degeneration', and Prichard's (Prichard, 1835) 'moral insanity'. An exception was Birnbaum (1930) who emphasised the psychogenic nature of the disorder, stressing the influence of social learning and environmental failures, and introduced the term 'sociopathic'.

Thus the advent of psychoanalytic interest in the criminal mind was in the context of two major currents of scientific philosophy at the time: the corruption of neutral observation by moral judgement, and the divergence of the biogenic and the psychogenic approaches to psychopathy that are in fact both legitimate and complementary (Meloy, 1992). Psychoanalytic theorists entering this arena endeavoured to maintain a clinical and objective attitude divorced from moral judgement, and to explore the role of both constitutional and environmental factors in psychopathy's developmental trajectory.

15.2.1 Criminals from a Sense of Guilt

In his 1916 paper *'Some character-types met with in psycho-analytic work',* Freud described a group of people whom he referred to as 'criminals from a sense of guilt'. These were individuals who were drawn to committing forbidden antisocial deeds to relieve a pre-existing unconscious sense of guilt which he believed stemmed from the Oedipus Complex and the criminal wishes of killing the father and having sexual relations with the mother. However, although he believed that the majority of criminals unconsciously wished to be punished for parricide and maternal incest, he recognised a sub-group of individuals we would characterise as psychopaths: "Among adult criminals we must no doubt except those who commit crimes without any sense of guilt, who have either developed no moral inhibitions or who, in their conflict with society, consider themselves justified in their action" (Freud, 1916, p. 333). He wrote further in 1928, "two traits are essential in a criminal: boundless egoism and a strong destructive urge. Common to both of these, and a necessary condition for their expression, is absence of love, lack of an emotional appreciation of (human) objects" (Freud, 1928,. p. 178).

15.2.2 Developmental Deficits

Freud highlighted several fundamental characteristics of the psychopath – his lack of moral conscience, narcissism, aggression and inability to form loving attachments. These ideas were taken up by subsequent psychoanalytic writers in the first half of the twentieth century who, influenced by the human-inflicted atrocities of the first and second world wars, identified individuals engaged in antisocial and delinquent behaviour which they attributed to failures of the superego, deficits in early identifications, and early disturbed parent-child relations. These analysts include Alexander (1923, 1930, 1935), who explored in a series of papers both the biogenic and psychological roots of psychopathy; Aichhorn (Aichorn, 1925), who wrote a seminal book *'Wayward Youth'* which conceptualised psychopathy as a disturbance of Oedipal conflicts, failures of identification and narcissism; Horney (1945), who proposed that the psychopath's exploitation of others gives him an omnipotent sense of triumph that obscures a sense of barrenness; Fenichel (1945), who highlighted early deficits in identification with others, resulting in a superego that was free of inhibiting influences and thus the person was able to fulfil instinctual urges without constraints; and Reich (1945), who described the psychopath as a 'phallic narcissistic character' who was arrogant, openly aggressive and sadistic, derogatory towards women and revenge towards an internalised mother figure.

15.2.3 Psychopathy as a Defence Against Trauma

These analytic writers emphasised developmental deficits evident in the mind of the psychopath, but others proposed that psychopathy was a defensive structure that had developed due to the impact of early trauma. Thus, Winnicott (1956) distinguished between 'privation', where the child had never had any good experiences, which can only lead to hopelessness; and 'deprivation' where there have been some early good experiences, but which are subsequently lost, producing 'antisocial tendencies' of anger, resentment and violence in the child, which are seen as a more hopeful, albeit unconscious, communication to regain the early care which he had received. Similarly, Bowlby (1944) coined the term 'affectionless psychopaths' for children whose apparent indifference to others concealed their fear of 'the risk of their hearts being broken again' (p.124). Karpman (1946), an American psychiatrist and proponent of psychoanalysis, distinguished between primary and secondary psychopaths. He proposed that primary psychopaths display an absence of conscience, guilt, attachment and emotionality, the disorder being primarily constitutional in aetiology, whereas the antisocial behaviour of secondary psychopaths arises as a response to underlying neurotic conflicts and parental rejection.

15.2.4 The Mask of Sanity

Meanwhile, although sceptical of psychoanalysis, in 1941 American psychiatrist Cleckley published his classic work *The Mask of Sanity,* in which he proposed that psychopathy concealed an underlying psychotic condition. This idea was later elaborated by the American psychoanalyst Kernberg (1984) in his conceptualisations of personality organisations. The clarity of Cleckley's description of the psychopath's primary traits (e.g., guiltlessness, lack of remorse and shame, incapacity for object love, emotional shallowness, impulsivity, egocentricity, inability to learn from experience, and lack of insight) refined the clinical depiction of psychopathy. Although the term is not included in either the DSM or ICD categorical diagnostic classifications of mental disorders, its validity as a dimensional personality construct received support from Hare's empirical investigation of Cleckley's diagnostic criteria, and development of his widely-used assessment tool, the Psychopathy Checklist- Revised (Hare, 1991).

15.2.5 Object Relations Theory

Cleckley's insight into the mind and behaviour of the psychopath lent itself to further psychodynamic explorations within the psychoanalytic school of object relations. Object relations theory was developed by psychoanalytic theorists such as Klein, Winnicott and Fairbairn, and later by others, most notably Kernberg, and proposes that the child's experience, perceptions and fantasies about their relationships with significant caregivers become internalised and incorporated in the mind at an early stage of development to become 'internal objects', or prototypical mental constructs, which influence the individual's ways of relating to others in adulthood (Yakeley, 2010). The mother is usually the first object in the infant's life and the relationship established with her is incorporated into the infant's mind, and is then modified by subsequent relationships with significant others as the child develops. Object relations theory differs from Freud's belief that the focus of the infant was on mastering sexual and aggressive instincts, in proposing that the primary focus of the child is on developing relationships with caregivers; in other words, instead of being primarily pleasure-seeking, the infant is object-seeking. In normal development, the infant is gradually able to integrate different experiences of the mother – e.g. good experiences from being fed and bad experiences of being hungry and not fed immediately – from a 'part-object' representation of her to a 'whole object' representation, and similarly becomes able to differentiate representations of himself as a 'self-object' from representations of others. However, when the baby persistently experiences the mother as persecutory, absent, or neglectful, the gradual integration of different parts of the self is impaired, resulting in splitting of the ego and fragmented sense of self (Klein, 1946). Winnicott stressed the importance of the 'good-enough' mother in being able to provide what he called a 'facilitating maternal environment' necessary for normal infant development, including a sense of basic trust which enabled the child to understand people as separate beings, and failures of good enough parenting led to failures in the internalisation of objects and distrust of the environment (Winnicott, 1965).

15.2.6 Personality Organisations

Klein (1957, 1964), Mahler (1968, 1979) and Jacobson (1964, 1971) made significant contributions to understanding psychopathy from an object relational perspective, but Kernberg (1975, 1976, 1984) has been most influential in the fields of psychiatry and personality disorder in advancing the notion that psychopathy is a severe variant of narcissistic personality disorder. Kernberg's concept of personality organisation is helpful in understanding the development of personality traits that predispose an individual to develop psychopathy. Kernberg takes a dimensional approach and proposes that there are three levels of severity of any individual's personality organisation, ranging from reasonably healthy to seriously ill: the neurotic level, the borderline level and the psychotic level. These levels are differentiated on the basis of identity integration, the nature of the individual's defence mechanisms, and reality testing.

The neurotic level is the most mature and healthiest type of personality organization (Kernberg, 1984). The person has intact reality testing and capacity for insight, an integrated and consistent sense of themselves and of other people, and generally relies on mature defence mechanisms, such as repression, when stressed. At the opposite end of the personality organization dimension is the psychotic level, which describes people with severely disorganized personalities who find it difficult to distinguish the boundary between themselves and other people, and between experiences and perceptions that originate within their own mind from those that originate in the real world. They also primarily use immature defences such as denial, projection, and splitting, which are normal in young children but when they predominate in adult life are pathological.

Between the neurotic and psychotic dimension are personalities organized at the borderline level (Kernberg, 1984). Unlike the more severe psychotic level, in these people, reality testing is generally intact, but they have a fragmented sense of self and others and a diffuse and incoherent identity resulting in relationships that tend to be superficial, narcissistically-driven, and characterised by lack of empathy and awareness of people as separate individuals with differing needs and opinions. They also predominantly use primitive defence mechanisms such as splitting, projective identification, idealisation, denigration, and omnipotent control. Kernberg (1984) proposes that the psychopath's character is organised at the more severe end of the borderline level. The psychopath may appear to function at a more sophisticated level – the mask of sanity – but this conceals serious and pervasive deficits in psychological structure and functioning. Meloy (2001) has described this as "when one gazes upon the psychopath, there is less there than meets the eye" (p.13).

We can see how the psychoanalytic theories of psychopathy have shifted from Freud and his early followers' view that psychopathy was the result of fundamental deficits in the psychopath's mind and development, to the idea that psychopathy was a defence against early trauma, to more recent object relations psychoanalytic theorists who examined the psychogenic and intrapsychic origins of psychopathy with an increasing emphasis on the importance of narcissistic psychopathology and disturbances in early object relations. Meanwhile, researchers from other disciplines in the field of psychopathy became more interested in genetic and neuroscientific empirical research that validated constitutional and organic theories of psychopathic character development and identified neurobiological vulnerabilities that predispose the individual to developing psychopathy. It is worth reviewing the evidence here, as these findings are not antithetical to the hypotheses regarding the origins of psychopathy proposed by these various psychoanalysts.

15.3 Aetiology: Genetics, Neurobiology, and Environment

There is convincing evidence that psychopathic traits have a moderate to high heritability and that there is a biological basis to psychopathy (Glenn & Raine, 2014). Numerous twin studies in childhood and adolescence document that psychopathic tendencies or callous unemotional traits—which are thought to be the precursors of psychopathy in adulthood—have a genetic origin (Larsson et al., 2006; Taylor et al., 2003; Viding et al., 2005, 2009; Viding & Larsson, 2010). This has called into question the belief that a neglectful and abusive environment is central to the development of the psychopath. Marshall and Cooke (1999) found a negative curvilinear relationship between early adverse experiences and psychopathy. They found that for adult psychopaths, as their psychopathic traits as measured by the PCL-R increased into the mild to moderate range, there was a historical increase in neglect and abuse in their childhood experiences; however, as psychopathy increases into the severe range, there was a decrease in neglect and abuse while growing up. This suggests that the more severe the psychopathy, the more psychobiologically rooted is the cause. Similarly, studies have shown that aggressive and antisocial behaviour in children with callous and unemotional traits show a strong heritability compared to children with antisocial behaviour but an absence of callous and unemotional traits (Viding et al., 2005).

There is now a wealth of empirical evidence demonstrating the neurobiological underpinnings of psychopathy, focussing on core features including underarousal and lack of fear. Early studies of the psychopath's underarousal, particularly in response to punishment, demonstrated peripheral autonomic hyporeactivity to aversive events, as measured by skin conductance, or galvanic skin response (Hare, 1970). This work has been replicated by other researchers throughout the world (Raine, 2013) in many studies that have found that habitual criminals are chronically cortically underaroused and show abnormal physiological responses to threat (e.g. Lilienfeld et al., 2018; López et al., 2013; Patrick, 2018; Raine, 1993, 2013). Low levels of cortical arousal have also been implicated in research with children and adolescents who display callous-unemotional traits (Frick et al., 2003). These children exhibit thrill-seeking behaviour and fearlessness, show deficits in responding to negative stimuli, habituate more easily to distress in others (Kimonis et al., 2006), and show lower autonomic reactivity to negative emotional stimuli (Blair, 1999). These physiological responses have been linked to structural and functional brain abnormalities, predominantly in the limbic system, in particular the amygdala (e.g. Blair, 2018; Glenn & Raine, 2014; Yang & Raine, 2018).

However, it is important to note that these neurobiological abnormalities in the brains of psychopaths may not solely be the result of genetic or constitutional factors but may also be due to the effects of early environmental experiences that have affected the structure and function of the developing brain. Numerous studies have shown a positive link between high levels of psychopathy and adverse childhood experiences and family disruption, including physical, sexual and emotional abuse, neglect, harsh parenting, parental mental illness or alcoholism, parental criminality, institutional deprivation, malnutrition, and smoking in pregnancy (e.g. Borja & Ostrosky, 2013; Dargis et al., 2016; Farrington et al., 2006; Graham et al., 2012;

Grönroos et al., 2010; Kolla et al., 2013; Ometto et al., 2016; Schraft et al., 2013; Sevecke et al., 2016; Sonuga-Barke et al., 2010). These research findings corroborate the clinical experience of working with psychopaths, the majority of whom report traumatic events and disturbed relationships with significant others in childhood.

15.3.1 Primary Versus Secondary Psychopathy, the Role of Anxiety and Diagnostic Confusion

Psychopathy is not classified as a diagnostic category in the current psychiatric classification systems of mental disorders – *International Classification of Mental and Behavioural Disorders, Tenth Edition* (ICD-10; World Health Organisation, 1992) and *Diagnostic and Statistical Manual of Mental Disorders* (DSM-5; American Psychiatric Association, 2013). The diagnoses that most closely approximate psychopathy associated with antisocial behaviour are dissocial personality disorder in the ICD-10 and antisocial personality disorder (ASPD) within the DSM-5. However, these diagnostic categories describe a heterogeneous population and do not distinguish between those individuals with mild, moderate, or severe psychopathy, as measured on the PCL-R (Hare, 2003). A substantial body of research has shown that, at most, only one out of three patients with ASPD has severe psychopathy, and this latter group has a significantly poorer treatment prognosis than do patients with mild to moderately psychopathic ASPD (Hare, 1991, 2003). There is evidence to show that these different sub-groups have different aetiological and developmental pathways and show different responses to treatment (e.g., Caspi et al., 2002).

De Brito and Hodgins (2009) emphasize the importance of co-occuring anxiety in subtyping ASPD. Based on studies of children and adults, they propose that around half of the ASPD population are characterized by anxiety as well as persistent antisocial behaviour and have low levels of callous unemotional traits as children and low levels of psychopathic traits as adults. This group is more likely to have experienced physical abuse as children and resort to violence as a compensatory response to underlying emotional conflict and distress. The other half have normal to low levels of anxiety, and varying levels of psychopathy, but include a sub-group with high levels of psychopathy. This group shows high levels of callous and unemotional traits as children, low levels of anxiety, more predatory violence and are less amenable to treatment.

Moreover, even those diagnosed with high psychopathy scores as measured on the PCL-R may show variable levels of anxiety (Blackburn, 2009). Although psychopathy represents a continuous dimension (Hare & Neumann, 2005), the PCL-R is multi-factorial and measures both traits and criminal behaviour. The two subfactors F1 (reflecting selfish and callous use of others) and F2 (reflecting socially deviant traits and lifestyle) are associated with different patterns of personality traits and deviant behaviour (Hare, 2003). Recent evidence (e.g. Mealey, 1995; Porter, 1996) substantiates Karpman's (1946) original distinction between primary and secondary psychopaths, the former group displaying no anxiety and the latter group exhibiting some anxiety potentially originating in childhood as a defence against trauma and abuse. Differences have been shown between primary and secondary groups of psychopaths who are equated on an overall measure of psychopathy but differ in levels of anxiety (e.g, Brinkley et al., 2004; Newman et al., 2005). Where anxiety is included as a clustering variable in cluster analyses of high-scoring PCL-R offenders, more and less anxious subtypes emerge, supporting the primary-secondary distinction (Blackburn, 2009). These differences are important to identify when considering the psychopath's amenability to treatment.

15.3.2 Gene-Environmental Interactions

These studies delineating different subgroups of psychopathic individuals reflect the earlier psychoanalytic debates regarding whether psychopathic characteristics were due to deficits in the person's ego that were constitutional in origin as proposed by Freud and early post-Freudians, or whether they were the manifestation of unconscious defence mechanisms formed in early childhood in order to cope with the anxiety generated by experiencing adversity, as advocated by Klein, Winnicott and other psychoanalysts working within an object relations framework. However, it is unlikely that genetic and environmental factors act independently in the development of psychopathy. Behavioural-genetic research has attempted to estimate the extent to which genetic factors, shared environmental factors, and nonshared environmental factors explain variance in psychopathic personality traits (Waldman & Rhee, 2006), and an increasing number of behavioural-genetic studies have demonstrated significant gene-environment interactions, where a person's genotype influences the degree of exposure to environmental risk factors (Beaver et al., 2011; Hicks et al., 2012; Hyde et al., 2016; Waldman & Rhee, 2006).

Contemporary psychoanalytic writers such as Meloy (Meloy, 1992; Meloy & Yakeley, 2021) have sought to integrate these two divergent paths into a biopsychogenic model that proposes that although neuroanatomical, neurophysiological, and twin and adoption studies suggest biological and genetic factors are operant in the development of psychopathy, early disturbed object relations and other environmental influences are also involved. Attachment theory provides an explanatory aetiological framework that links these biological and environmental influences in the development of the disorder and provides empirical evidence to validate a psychoanalytic object relational approach to understanding the dynamics of the mind of the psychopath (Meloy & Yakeley, 2021).

15.4 Attachment

Attachment is a species-specific behavioural system serving the survival of the infant, in which the infant is biologically programmed to ensure close proximity to his primary attachment figure (usually the mother) and feel secure in her presence, via a range of attachment behaviours. Based on the work of Bowlby (1969) and expanded by researchers such as Main and Goldwyn (1994) and Ainsworth (George et al., 1996), attachment theory proposes that the human need for significant relationships is universal and established at a psychobiological level. Normal secure attachments are necessary for the development of affect regulation, impulse control, empathy and the capacity to reflect or mentalize. Early disruptions in attachment caused by child abuse, neglect, emotional deprivation, parental separation or loss can have serious adverse effects on the developing attachment relationship between the infant and his caregivers and produce long-term pathological effects giving rise to personality difficulties, disturbed relationships and mental disorders in adult life. Bowlby was influenced by Klein and Winnicott, and findings from attachment research provide empirical evidence for the ideas of these and subsequent psychoanalytic object relations theorists, such as Kernberg, which propose that that if the child suffers early adverse experiences of his primary caregivers, his further development will become impaired.

There is increasing evidence that disturbed attachment experiences are implicated in the development of psychopathy. Four distinct pathological or insecure attachment styles have been identified and measured in adults: fearful, preoccupied, disorganized and dismissive (George et al., 1996). A recent meta-analysis of 12 studies with a total of 1876 participants looking at the relationship between attachment styles and psychopathic traits showed a positive association between psychopathy and insecure and disorganised attachment. The strongest associations were found in forensic and prison samples (van der Zouwen et al., 2018), which is consistent with evidence that offenders in prisons or secure forensic institutions are more likely to report having experienced disruptions in attachment due to separations, abuse and neglect from their early caregivers than in the general population (Coid, 1992; Heads et al., 1997; Weeks & Widom, 1998).

In a study of adolescents, Taubner et al. (2012) found that the ability to mentalize moderated the relationship between psychopathic traits and psychopathy. Mentalization is the capacity to reflect and to think about mental states, including thoughts, beliefs, desires and affects, to be able to distinguish one's own mental states from others, and to be able to interpret the actions and behaviour of oneself and others as meaningful and based on intentional mental states (Allen et al., 2008). Mentalizing is an essential human capacity underpinning interpersonal relations that develops in the first few years of life in the context of safe and secure child-caregiver attachment relationships (Bateman & Fonagy, 2004). In this study, individuals with psychopathic traits who had a higher ability to mentalize showed less proactive aggression than those with a lower capacity for mentalization.

15.5 A Contemporary Psychoanalytic Understanding of the Mind of the Psychopath

How do the primary traits of the psychopath – his lack of attachment, anxiety and empathy, his egocentricity and grandiosity, and his lack of moral conscience – emerge? Meloy & Yakeley (2021) integrate findings from attachment research and object relations theory to propose a psychoanalytic theory of the mind of a psychopath. This proposes that very early disturbances in separation and identification processes set the scene for the development of his pathological behaviours and attitudes.

15.5.1 *Failures of Internalisation*

Meloy (1992) suggests that early disruptions in attachment due to abuse and adversity from primary caregivers expose the infant psychopath to overly harsh sensory-perceptual experiences which predispose to the construction of a narcissistic outer shell that protects the inner more vulnerable self. This is similar to Winnicott's (1960) notion of a 'false self' that develops prematurely at the expense of the hidden 'true self', and Cleckley's (1941) mask of sanity concealing a hidden core of psychosis. In the absence of consistent and reliable nurturing experiences, the infant develops an early organismic distrust in the environment that impedes the processes of internalisation of and identification with good objects or experiences that are necessary for normal development. The predominance of harsh and malign objects and paucity of soothing internalisation experiences lead the child to unconsciously deny the need for the latter, and instead identifies with the hard, aggressive objects experienced externally, a defence mechanism which was first described by Anna Freud as identification with the aggressor (Freud, 1936). Meloy (1992) stresses that these hostile objects may be the result of real abuse from caretakers, or they may be re-internalised projections of the psychopath's own aggressive impulses in the absence of abuse.

15.5.2 *Primitive Internalised Object Relations and the Grandiose Self*

The psychopath's mind is organised at the borderline level as described by Kernberg (1975, 1976, 1984). His failures to internalise and identify with whole object relationships means that his internal world is two-dimensional and populated by primitive internal objects, or 'part-objects', in which good and bad are not integrated, and self and object are not fully differentiated into whole, separate and meaningful individuals. The psychopath's relationships with others are narcissistically-driven and determined by a paradigm of dominance and control in which external objects are experienced as existing only for gratification. His object relationships have a dyadic structure – predator /prey, dominance/submission – and are maintained through the use of primitive defences, such as splitting, denial, omnipotence and projection, so that self-representations are always enhanced, and object representations are always devalued. More mature defence mechanisms such as repression and sublimation are lacking. Similarly, his affective life is shallow and with a range and depth of feeling akin to that of a toddler who has not yet learned to socialise with others. Consciously felt emotions are those more concerned with the self and do not require an appreciation of others as whole objects, but are related to part-objects – envy, shame, dysphoria boredom, frustration, rage and excitement. His modulation of affects is unstable with emotions that are felt intensely and quickly dissipate. More mature emotions such as anger, guilt, fear, sadness, gratitude, sympathy, and remorse, which are deeper and more complex and which involve an appreciation of others as whole objects and a capacity for secure attachment are missing. His emotional life is centred on the internal management of envy and shame, two primitive affects which are felt to be unbearable and therefore have to be projected into others, often triggering violence and intentional destruction of the object in real life.

At the core of the psychopath is the grandiose self (Meloy, 1988). This is an unconscious pathological defensive structure which is a variant of the grandiose self-structure described by Kernberg (1976) in his theory of narcissistic personality disorders. The grandiose self-structure is present in all narcissistic personality disorders but is the primary identification in the psychopath, an idealisation of himself as a predator dominating and denigrating others as prey and constitutes the cognitive and affective core of the self. The grandiose self is formed from the coalescence of the abnormal internalisations of the psychopath as described above but is a tenuous structure that must be sustained at all cost to preserve the psychopath's narcissistic equilibrium. This is achieved by continually experiencing his own self-representations as positive and projecting all bad objects, negative affects and representations into others.

However, unlike individuals with more benign types of narcissistic personality disorder, maintaining the grandiose self as the primary identification by elevating himself and denigrating others in fantasy is not sufficient. The grandiose self can only be conserved by actually belittling, defaming and abusing others in reality, including the use of violence. Meloy (1988, 1992) suggests that this failure of his omnipotent fantasy in containing violence is because the psychopath becomes immune to his own fantasies, which are exacerbated by chronic autonomic low arousal, so that intolerable emotions of emptiness, shame and envy start to reach consciousness and can only be evacuated by damaging the object. The denigrated object diminishes the psychopath's envy since there are no longer any qualities worth possessing and diminishes shame since it no longer serves as a source of humiliation.

15.5.3 The Psychopathic Superego

One of the hallmarks of psychopathy is the lack of guilt, remorse and moral values, which psychoanalysts have attributed to abnormalities in the psychopath's superego, or moral conscience. The superego is the third component of Freud's (1923) tripartite structural model of the mind, the other two being the ego and the id. He saw the superego as an intrapsychic structure that develops from the ego after the resolution of the Oedipus complex by identification with the father to avert castration anxiety, and identification with the mother to avoid loss of her love. The concept has been developed in many different ways since Freud, but a broad generalisation would understand the superego to be the internalisation of parental values, goals, and restrictions to form the conscience of the individual, and can be experienced as supportive, punitive or absent. Failure to achieve these moral standards gives rise to feelings of guilt. Freud (1923) believed that the superego was absent in psychopaths, whereas the psychoanalyst Fenichel (1931) believed there was some evidence of primitive superego functioning in such individuals, and Klein (1927), by contrast, viewed the superego as being present but overly harsh and punitive.

Subsequent object relation theorists such as and Kernberg (1984) propose that in the psychopath the superego is not fully developed but is formed of sadistic precursors that are fragments of the early harsh and persecutory objects that he internalised and identified with in infancy. These aggressive identifications, which have replaced those based on normal parental ideals, become organised into a pathological superego that rewards malevolent intents and destructive behaviours and denigrates positive goals and behaviours, thus accounting for the reversal of values or inverse conscience of the psychopath (Richards, 1998; Svrakic et al., 1991). The psychopath attributes negative value to notions such as attachment, morality, love and empathy, and positive value to aggression, sadism, deception and greed. Moreover, his identification with badness or evil means that he lacks the internal constraints that normally inhibit gratification of impulses. As the pre-psychopathic child grows older, he increasingly identifies with older peers and mentors outside of the family who are aggressive and destructive, and such identifications consolidate the sadistic superego.

15.5.4 Imitation and Simulation

The psychopath's inability to form deep and meaningful identifications with others means that he resorts to simulation or imitation of other's attitudes and behaviour in order to appear to fit in to society. The psychoanalyst Greenacre (1958) referred to the psychopath as an imposter, possessing an 'as-if' quality and lack of authenticity. Early unconscious simulatory processes develop in later childhood and adolescence into a more conscious imitation of acceptable behaviour to gain social advantage, whilst at the same time honing his manipulative skills. This explains the psychopath's ability to exploit, dupe, deceive, and defraud others whilst appearing beguiling, charming, and sincere.

Certain people may be particularly vulnerable to becoming victims of the psychopath's deceptions, exploitations and betrayals (Howell, 2018). Successful fraudsters or conmen may carefully select their victims by recognising subtle narcissistic vulnerabilities – a longing for love and acceptance or a wish for wealth or success that he promises. The psychopath may create a false feeling of resonance in the victim, which Meloy (1988) has termed 'malignant pseudoidentification', where the psychopath feigns admiration and simulates certain behaviours of the victim to create the illusion of a special bond between them by appealing to the victim's narcissism. The British psychoanalyst Symington (1980) goes further in proposing that we are all susceptible to disbelieve the psychopath's greed and destructiveness, as recognising his sadism requires us to recognise our own propensity for sadism and destructiveness.

15.5.5 Psychopathic Aggression

Not all psychopaths are actually violent, but when they are, violence is not normally felt to be conflictual with the psychopath's sense of self, as the impulse for aggression is either acted out immediately or remains a source of aggressive fuelling of the grandiose self-structure. His lack of attachment and capacity to empathise with the victim, as well as his inverse conscience means that he does not possess the normal internal inhibitory mechanisms that prevent most people from being violent to others. The psychoanalyst Glasser (Glasser, 1998) proposed a useful distinction between what he called 'self-preservative violence' and sadomasochistic violence, both of which arise from an early pathological relationship with the mother where aggression is unconsciously used in order to create space and separate from an overwhelming maternal object.

Self-preservative violence is a primitive response triggered by any perceived threat to the physical or psychological self. These threats include attacks on a person's self-esteem, frustration, humiliation or an insult to an ideal to which the person is attached; but also include internal threats such as feeling attacked by a sadistic superego or fearing a loss of identity by feelings of disintegration and internal confusion as may arise in psychotic illness. The violent response in self-preservative violence is fundamental, immediate, and aimed at destroying the source of danger.

Sadomasochistic violence, by contrast, is not an immediate response, but is planned and calculated to achieve violent purposes, including the torture and control of victims. A crucial distinction between the two modes is how they differ in their relationship to the object or victim. In self-preservative violence, the object at the time of violence is perceived as an immediate danger but holds no other personal significance and its emotional responses as a whole person are of no interest – it just needs to be eliminated. By contrast, in sadomasochistic violence, the responses of the object or victim are crucial: the object must be seen to suffer, but to do so it must be kept alive, rather than eliminated as in the case of self-preservative violence. Sadomasochistic violence also involves pleasure, which is not a component of self-preservative violence, where anxiety is always present. Glasser (Glasser, 1998) gives a simple example of the difference between the two types of violence: the soldier who kills the enemy in a battle, believing that such an action is necessary to prevent himself from being killed, is exhibiting self-preservative violence, whereas the soldier who captures the enemy and tortures him to make him suffer is acting out sadomasochistic violence.

During the same period that Glasser was formulating his ideas concerning self-preservative and sadistic aggression with colleagues at the Portman Clinic, Meloy

(1988, 1992, 2006) applied object relations theory and attachment theory to a bimodal model of violence that originated in the animal physiology literature a half century earlier. Meloy and others, including Eichelman (1988), McEllistrem (2004), and Siegel and Victoroff (2009), elaborated upon the physiological, pharmacological and forensic distinction between two psychobiologically different modes of violence 'affective' and 'predatory'. Affective, sometimes called emotional or reactive aggression, corresponds to Glasser's self-preservative aggression, and is a mode of violence that is accompanied by high levels of sympathetic arousal and emotion (usually anger or fear) and is a reaction to an imminent threat. Predatory, sometimes called instrumental violence, corresponds to Glasser's sadomasochistic violence, and is characterized by a lack of emotion, careful planning and preparation. It is also frequent among psychopaths and facilitated by their lack of autonomic arousal, such that anxiety and fear are not consciously felt and do not interfere with predation (Meloy, 2006). Predatory violence may be enhanced by the use of psychostimulant drugs, which heighten and expand the grandiose self-structure, increasing its propensity for violent action to sustain it. The execution of homicides, sexual homicides, and serial killings, which a minority of psychopaths commit, often involve predatory violence and are preceded by rehearsal fantasies of grandiosity and omnipotence, and private rituals in which the planned culmination of violence may be acted out in lesser forms. Psychopathic criminals are more likely than other criminals to engage in both affective and predatory violence (Cornell et al., 1996; Serin, 1991; Walsh, 1999; Williamson et al., 1987; Woodworth & Porter, 2002).

To summarise, a contemporary psychoanalytic understanding of the psychopath proposes that his character structure is organised at a borderline level, with the use of predominantly primitive defence mechanisms such as projection and splitting, failures of internalisation and identificatory processes to produce superego abnormalities, and the defensive construction of a grandiose self that must be maintained by continual idealisation of himself and behavioural denigration and manipulation of others, including violence. His attraction to sadistic or predatory violence is facilitated by his lack of empathy, his low level of emotional arousal, his identification with sadistic objects, and the use of stimulant drugs that bolster his psychopathic ego (Yakeley, 2010).

15.6 Psychoanalytically-Informed Management and Treatment of Psychopathy

A psychoanalytic approach to risk assessment enhances rather than replaces more conventional methods of the evaluation of risk of patients or offenders with psychopathic traits seen in mental health or criminal justice settings. Several factors, amongst others, are important to assess in estimating the person's risk of antisocial behaviour or violence towards others, and towards the person himself. The degree of psychopathy should be evaluated with an instrument such as the Psychopathy Checklist- Revised (PCL-R; Hare, 1991, 2003), as patients with severe psychopathy have a significantly poorer treatment prognosis than do patients with mild to moderately psychopathic traits as measured on the PCL-R.

Current thinking on risk assessment and management is that it should be less concerned with prediction (which is notoriously unreliable) and more concerned with making a formulation about risk (Blumenthal et al., 2010). This would be asking, in what circumstances would the risk of what be increased for this particular individual, and why. Understanding the meaning of the antisocial act can help anticipate when the offender might be dangerous again. The formulation would also aim to assist clinical thinking about whether and under what clinical conditions a psychological intervention can take place safely.

It is important in thinking about risk to look at different types of violence that the person uses. Blair et al. (2005) has noted that "no biologically based disorder other than psychopathy is associated with an increased risk of instrumental aggression" (p. 155). However, psychopaths also engage in affective aggression more than non-psychopathic offenders. Going back to Glasser's (1998) distinction between self-preservative and sadomasochistic violence, self-preservative (affective) violence is a response to an immediate threat where the patient is anxious and operates in fight/flight mode, and as such more primitive and more dangerous – but if the perceived threat to the self is understood, future triggers may be anticipated. On the other hand, sadomasochistic (predatory) violence may pose less immediate risk because it is planned, where the person might groom his victim, but it is much more difficult for the perpetrator to relinquish because it is a source of pleasure.

Countertransference There are many risk assessment instruments used in forensic settings that utilise a combination actuarial factors and structured clinical judgement, such as the PCL-R (Hare, 2003), the Violence Risk Appraisal Guide (VRAG; Quinsey et al., 2006) and the Historical Clinical Risk Management-20 (HCR-20; Webster et al., 1997) to evaluate a patient's or offender's risk of violence to others. However, it has been shown that the emotional responses of experienced professionals who are well trained in structured and actuarial risk assessment may affect their predication of risk, in that they often unconsciously ignore actuarial risk factors and overestimate or underestimate the patient's risk according to their subjective judgement (Blumenthal et al., 2010). How do we understand this subjective response?

Countertransference refers to the thoughts and feelings that the therapist, clinician or other professional has towards the patient. Whilst these may reflect the individual professional's own conflicts and personal history, they may also be a reflection of what the patient feels, or is doing to, the therapist consciously or unconsciously. Awareness of the therapist's countertransference has become an essential part of the process and technique of modern psychoanalytic therapy and can be used to inform the therapist's therapeutic interventions and interpretations. Careful examination of one's countertransference is not only important in psychotherapy, but may be very helpful in understanding the psychopathology of the offender and the risk that he poses. Common countertransference reactions towards offender patients include moral outrage and beliefs that the person is untreatable; feelings of hopelessness and guilt when change does not occur; disgust; excessive fear, and its counterpart, the denial of real dangerousness; devaluation and loss of professional identity; excessively punitive and sadistic responses, such as overestimating a patient's risk; and sexual excitement which is rarely admitted or spoken about, but can lead to boundary violations (Meloy & Yakeley, 2013).

It is frequently thought that having feelings towards patients and clients, let alone admitting them, is unprofessional and unacceptable, particularly if these feelings are negative, for example feelings of hatred towards the patient. However, it is inevitable that such disturbed individuals will evoke emotional responses in those trying to manage or treat them, and if these feelings are not acknowledged, or they are denied completely, the professional is more likely to act in inappropriate ways.

Inadequate analysis of the clinician's emotional responses or countertransference to the patient can contribute to faulty risk assessment that may, in itself, increase risk. For example, patients' actions can provoke anger, fear or disgust, which may elicit punitive or sadistic responses in professionals, so that risk is overestimated and inappropriate and possibly unnecessary interventions such as prolonged incarceration or physical restraint are instituted. The patient's subsequent anger and resentment at feeling punished and mistreated may lead to an increased risk of his behaving dangerously. Other offenders may elicit sympathy and present themselves as innocent victims who are not responsible for their actions, which may resonate with a clinician's 'rescue fantasies' in their desire to treat patients whom they perceive have been misunderstood and mistreated by other professionals, so that the risk here is underestimated.

Setting Where therapy takes place is crucial. Unless this is secure, treatment cannot occur. In forensic institutions, the staff may feel physically safe due to the locked wards and high walls, but emotionally insecure, because of the dangerous and disturbed patients with whom they work, and they may need help to acknowledge and contain the anxieties provoked in them. Although a culture of bravado and camaraderie is common, the reality that many staff have difficulty in coping is reflected in the high rates of sickness, burnout and staff turnover in such secure institutions. As described above, patients and their offences will inevitably have an emotional impact, sometimes unconsciously, on the staff around them and this will influence how the staff react towards them. The treatment setting must be secure enough to ensure the safety of both patients and staff before treatment planning can begin – the anxieties of both need to be contained.

A safe environment can be achieved by not only creating consistent, clearly defined and controlled external structures – the physical environment – but also by creating a healthy emotional environment through understanding the unconscious communications between patients and staff, and between different members of the multi-disciplinary team or institution. Such a focus on the relationships between patients/offenders and staff has been referred to as 'relational security' (Department of Health XE "Health" , 2010). Adequate staff training, supervision and support is essential to prevent the high levels of staff turnover, sick leave and 'burn-out' that are rife in forensic institutions. The institution itself may become sick and fragmented as a result of the staff group unconsciously employing pathological group defences to protect themselves against the intense anxieties generated by working with highly disturbed patients.

How may these problems be addressed? Here, a psychoanalytic approach is in treating the group as a whole, rather than targeting individual staff members. What is needed are integrative interventions aimed at restoring the healthy cohesion of the group – whether this group comprises the members of the ward, the multidisciplinary team, or the whole institution. The aim is to facilitate and promote reflective forums in which staff can come together in a non-threatening and creative way to think about their emotional reactions to patients and how these are enacted within the organization. Such groups may be in the form of case discussions where individual patients are discussed, including talking about their emotional impact on the staff, or reflective practice groups where the dynamics between staff- both healthy and unhealthy – are talked about. These groups can help staff consider and reflect upon their interactions with patients and each other, allowing them to admit to uncomfortable feelings about their work, and to introduce them to psychoanalytic concepts such as the unconscious, countertransference, and projection. This fosters the development of a psychological atmosphere that will benefit both staff and patients, in which the capacity to think rather than act is promoted. In the UK, reflective practice has been adopted by many forensic services and prisons.

Meaning of Violence Between the Offender and Others In order to assess risk, it is also important to understand the meaning of the person's antisocial behaviour in relation to his history and current relationships. Violence is not a senseless act 'out of the blue' but represents a communication with unconscious meaning. For example, a seemingly inexplicable and unprovoked attack on a female stranger may represent, at least in part, the patient's unconscious rage at his mother turning a blind eye to the abuse inflicted upon him by his stepfather in childhood. Consciously, the patient reports having a good relationship with his mother and sees her as a victim of domestic abuse. This patient, however, may be particularly sensitive to having a female therapist, whom he may initially idealise, but then respond to aggressively when he feels rejected or ignored, for example when sessions are cancelled.

It is therefore important to understand the dynamic relationship between the offender and others, and how this is related to early significant object relationships. This can be examined more closely in the dynamic or transference relationship between the offender and the professionals involved in his care, because the offender will repeat his habitual patterns of relating with the people who are treating him, as with all his relationships. Understanding these relationships as well as the feelings and anxieties in both offender and those around him in the context of the patient's early history and offending behaviour can facilitate a more accurate evaluation of the risk a person might pose.

Changes in the Therapeutic Frame Relational security is present when the professional team around the offender can form a supportive containing framework, which is essential in providing a safe environment in which therapeutic work can take place. Any change or violation in this containment or therapeutic frame, on the part of offender or therapist, however seemingly insignificant, may indicate increased risk, for example breaks in treatments, or a change of mental health worker. Professionals are often unaware how breaks in the treatment, for example due to holidays or the clinician leaving the job, may trigger intense feelings of loss and rejection in the patient who has unconsciously become dependent on the therapist, key worker, or even institution, and such feelings are not acceptable in consciousness and so will be acted out in violence. When considering risk assessment and psychotherapeutic treatment, it is therefore important to understand such anxieties in the patient and be alert to their appearance in the transference, which reflects how the patient unconsciously experiences the therapist, or other professionals, influenced by his early relationships with others (Yakeley & Williams, 2014).

To summarise, a comprehensive, psychoanalytically-informed risk assessment of the psychopath includes measuring the degree of psychopathy; consideration of the setting where any treatment is proposed to take place; awareness of the clinician's countertransference and how this can help understand the psychopathology of the offender and the risk that he poses; understanding of the meaning, including unconscious meaning, of the antisocial act to anticipate when the offender might be dangerous again; and awareness of how any changes in the therapeutic frame might affect his risk.

15.7 Personality Characteristics and Treatment Prognosis

In any mental health assessment, it is important to identify the presence of any mental disorder(s) to determine which treatments are most appropriate and effective. However, psychopathy in itself does not constitute a formal diagnostic category, and the diagnosis most associated with psychopathic traits is ASPD. Nevertheless, particular personality attributes of the psychopathic individual may specifically affect how he responds to treatment and his prognosis and are therefore important to identify.

Anxiety ASPD, including those with psychopathy, is associated with considerable and complex co-morbidity with other mental disorders (Swanson et al., 1994), particularly substance misuse (Compton et al., 2005; Robins et al., 1991). At least half of those with ASPD have co-occurring anxiety disorders (Goodwin & Hamilton, 2003) and a quarter have a depressive disorder (Lenzenweger et al., 2007). The presence of anxiety or depression is associated with a better response to treatment and prognosis as the patient's distress from the symptoms of these conditions means they are more likely to engage in treatment (Gabbard & Coyne, 1987). Moreover, anxiety is indicative of some capacity for healthier internalized object relations and ability to form an attachment to others, and is a necessary correlate of any successful mental health treatment that depends on interpersonal methods, such as psychodynamic psychotherapy.

Attachment and Object Relations Psychoanalytic and psychodynamic treatments use the therapeutic relationship that develops between the patient and therapist, with the unconscious transference-countertransference dynamics within forming the fulcrum of therapeutic change. However, psychopathic patients, who lack the capacity for attachment, are likely to fail to benefit from any treatment that depends on the development of a meaningful relationship with the therapist. Moreover, they may pose an explicit danger to the professional because their lack of empathy for the therapist will not inhibit aggression. The severely psychopathic patient is unable to represent others as whole, real, and meaningful individuals deserving of respect and empathy, instead viewing them as objects to dominate and exploit. The more severe the psychopathy, the more the patient will relate to others on the basis of power rather than affection (Meloy, 1988). This may include attempts to control staff and other patients in the treatment setting, which bolster his grandiose self and defend against anxieties by being controlled himself by professionals.

Psychological Affects and Defences Similarly, the psychopath's lack of ability to feel meaningful, more mature emotions that involve appreciation of another person, such as affection, guilt, remorse, sympathy and loss, presents difficulties for modalities that depend on emotional access to the patient such as psychoanalytic and psychodynamic approaches that require a capacity to feel emotion in relation to the psychotherapist and talk about it. However, psychopaths' capacity for simulation may make them adept at imitating certain emotional states for secondary gain or to manipulate the psychotherapist, which may be difficult to detect. As described earlier, the psychopath most predictably uses primitive defence mechanisms such as projection, devaluation, denial, projective identification, omnipotence, and splitting (Gacono & Meloy, 1994; Hare, 2003) which become operant in relation to the treating clinician. For example, the psychopathic patient may use projective identification by unconsciously projecting or attributing negative characteristics of his personality, such as envy, aggression or fear, to the clinician, which are then viewed as a threat that must be diminished, attempting to control the clinician through overt or covert intimidation.

Superego Characteristics The presence of any superego development, such as evidence of a socially desirable need to rationalize antisocial acts, is a positive prognostic sign. Some mild to moderately psychopathic patients may show evidence of harsh and punitive attitudes toward the self which signify some internalized values. Patients with severe psychopathy are likely to behave sadistically toward others and feel no need to justify their behaviours. These individuals should not be considered for treatment as they pose a risk to both staff and genuinely mentally ill patients. Therapy of any kind is likely to be of no benefit and should not be offered to psychopathic patients who manifest any of the following features: sadistic aggressive behaviour resulting in serious injury, complete absence of remorse or justification for such behaviour, very superior intelligence or mildly intellectual disability, a historical absence of emotional attachments, and unexpected fear felt by the experienced clinician in the patient's presence (Meloy & Yakeley, 2010).

15.8 General Treatment Considerations

Regardless of the specific therapeutic intervention offered, the psychopath's deficient capability in developing meaningful attachment relationships with others, which will include professionals involved in his treatment, poses particular problems in his engagement and responses to therapy. Special consideration should be given to factors relevant to motivation for therapy. In addition, boundary setting and breaks from treatment present additional challenges.

Motivation for and Engagement in Therapy When assessing a patient with psychopathy, there may be discrepancies between the motives for referral of the psychopathic individual, and those of professionals involved with the individual. For example, whereas the primary motivation of the latter is to reduce the psychopath's risk to others, the psychopath himself, if indeed he wants help at all, may only want to engage with treatment to be seen to comply with conditions imposed by professionals in order to achieve personal goals such as being released from prison or being contact with children. Some may be troubled by symptoms of anxiety, depression, or other mental disorders, but many psychopathic individuals may not accept a traditional sick role or consider themselves as psychotherapy patients. It is therefore important to assess the individual's motivation for treatment and whether this is at odds with that of the referrer.

The minority of antisocial or psychopathic patients who may eventually benefit from psychodynamic psychotherapy may need an extended period of engagement or motivational work. Therapists treating such individuals should anticipate numerous challenges, including lateness or missed sessions, verbal aggression and social disruption, frequent crises, and substance abuse (Dowsett & Craissati, 2008). Therapists should consider preparing patients carefully for treatment, which may include giving practical advice, psychoeducation about their personality traits, some explanation about the treatment model, and in general fostering as collaborative a relationship as possible. To reduce drop-out and noncompliance with treatment, therapists should also be proactive in their follow up of patients, such as calling the patient to remind him of appointments and addressing factors known to reduce compliance such substance misuse, self-harm, and a chaotic life-style.

Boundaries Psychopathic individuals experience relationships within a paradigm of power and control, and issues of dominance and hierarchy will inevitably pervade any treatment offered. Due to their distrust or contempt for authority, often based on their own negative experiences of parental figures, they will inevitably rebel against the rules and boundaries that are necessary to any therapeutic intervention. Boundary violations are therefore to be anticipated and therapists must be prepared to tolerate some expression of anti-authoritarian attitudes. At the same time, such individuals may be involved in gangs, organised crime or other criminal subcultures with their own codes of conduct, and how these might differ from and offer greater gain from more socially acceptable boundaries are important to explore in therapy. The psychopath's capacity to charm, seduce and manipulate others for their own gain may also draw professionals into boundary violations, which include inappropriate and risky social or sexual relationships.

Breaks in Therapy Psychopathic patients who have some capacity for attachment may find breaks in treatment difficult as this may trigger negative feelings, such as anxiety, anger, shame and humiliation, associated with rejections and losses experienced earlier in their lives. Such feelings may be difficult to acknowledge, tolerate, and process and are instead acted out in violence. Thus, periods when therapists are absent are associated with increased risk. The erratic attendance of the patients and their conscious denial of attachment needs and rejection of treatment may impede clinicians' awareness of the impact of interruptions in therapy. Ambivalent feelings in relation to the ending of therapy should also be expected and explored, if possible, to avert premature drop-out.

To summarise, some of the common features that arise in the treatment of patients of psychopathy that are important to consider whatever the specific treatment modality include the motivation of the patient in his wish for therapeutic change, how to engage the person in therapy, how boundaries are negotiated and the effects of breaks in treatment.

15.9 Specific Treatment Approaches

Treatment of the patient needs to consider both the modality and model of therapy. The modality is the vehicle through which therapy is delivered, and may be individual therapy, group, or democratic therapeutic community. Different therapeutic interventions or models may be delivered within each mode and will include psychoanalytic or psychodynamic psychotherapy with certain modifications of technique. Although methodologically robust studies of the efficacy of psychodynamic treatments for antisocial and psychopathic patients to date are lacking, there is a growing evidence base for the effectiveness of psychodynamic psychological therapies developed specifically for individuals with personality disorder such as mentalization-based treatment and democratic therapeutic communities (e.g., Bateman & Fonagy, 2008b; Capone et al., 2016; Newbury, 2010).

15.9.1 Individual Psychodynamic Psychotherapy

Despite the many therapeutic risks inevitably encountered, experienced psychodynamic and psychoanalytic clinicians, and those under their supervision, continue to embark on individual psychodynamic psychotherapy with forensic patients and offenders, including those with ASPD and psychopathy. Psychotherapy should ideally commence while the patient is in an institutional setting so that he is contained within a structured environment. If such a setting is not available, sufficient community support should be organized so that the appropriate professionals are accessible to respond to crises. This may prove difficult to organize in practice, given the reluctance that many general psychiatrists and community mental health teams continue to exhibit towards providing care for individuals diagnosed with ASPD in the absence of concurrent mental illness.

The therapist must be prepared to adopt a technique that is flexible and sensitively attuned to the patient's manifest and unconscious anxieties, which will inevitably involve some modification of more conventional psychoanalytic techniques that may be appropriate for less disturbed patients but proves ineffective or even counter-productive in forensic patients. The more anxious or paranoid patient is likely to experience silences as persecutory and may also not tolerate the full length of a session. Therapeutic interventions should be carefully timed and worded, and centred around the affective focus of the patient's communications. Many therapists (e.g. Bateman, 1999; Fonagy, 1999; Gabbard, 2005; Yakeley, 2010) working with violent and antisocial patients advocate the avoidance of free association and early interpretations of unconscious conflicts and fantasies, as these are not understood by patients with poor representational capacity and deficits in symbolic thinking. Instead, the therapist may need to put words to the patient's concrete thoughts and feelings and use basic metaphors to introduce him to symbolic thinking. Similarly, premature interpretations of transference, especially the negative transference, should be avoided, as these may be perceived by patient as critical and retaliatory as they find it difficult or impossible to experience the 'as if' quality of the transference, instead identifying with the concrete content of interpretations, not their symbolic meaning. Instead, it is more useful to provide brief and simple descriptive comments about the patient's state of mind (Bateman, 1999; Fonagy & Target, 1995). The aims of the therapist are to help the patient connect his internal state of mind to his behavioural actions and to gradually understand how acts of violence or misuse of substances may defend against the awareness of more painful thoughts and feelings. The therapist, therefore, should adopt a flexible stance in which she is consistent, boundaried, and able to confront the patient's denials and minimization of his antisocial behaviour, yet remain empathic and nonjudgmental. This is challenging and long-term work that should not be carried out in isolation. The therapist will inevitably be subject to the full onslaught of the patient's projections, and rigorous and continual monitoring of her countertransference is necessary to avoid being drawn into enactments in the therapeutic encounter. Appropriate and on-going supervision is essential to provide a thinking space for the therapist and to allow a third perspective into the workings of therapeutic dyad.

15.9.2 Group-Analytic Therapy

Many different group treatments for people with mental health and psychological problems now exist in an array of settings, including the forensic field. In the UK, regular group therapy was started in high secure hospitals in the 1970s (Cox, 1976), and since then there have been group therapy programmes based on different therapeutic approaches, including psychoanalytic approaches, delivered to offenders and forensic patients in criminal justice and health settings in the UK. Group-analytic psychotherapy specifically utilises psychoanalytic concepts and techniques as applied to the group treatment of such individuals.

For many psychopathic and antisocial patients, group therapy may be the treatment of choice. There may be several reasons for this. For patients who are terrified of losing control of their emotions and being violent, group therapy can be less arousing than individual therapy where the intensity of the relationship with the therapist may feel overwhelming. In a group, the multiple transferences amongst the different group members offer each patient more than one target for their aggression, which may decrease their levels of anxiety and arousal. Group therapy also offers more opportunities for mentalization in there being several minds in the room, as well as providing the modelling of more appropriate behaviour and interpersonal interactions that may be internalized by the patient. The triggers to potential interpersonal violent behaviour may be more easily recognised and confronted in a group, which can act as a socio-familial microcosm in which the offender's interactions with other group members can be understood as reflecting the pathological dynamics of their original familial experiences (Welldon, 1996). Patients whose activities involve secretiveness and deception, such as perpetration of sexual abuse, can be more effectively challenged in a group, and similarly, more psychopathic patients will find it more difficult to con others in a group of similar patients who can recognize, challenge and penetrate their pervasive patterns of deception.

15.9.3 Therapeutic Communities

The term therapeutic community refers to a structured psychologically-informed treatment programme where a range of activities, including specific psychotherapies and social interaction, form the treatment programme. The group relations of peers within the community and the community itself, rather than any single element, form the primary key agents of therapy to help individuals acquire social skills and learn social norms. Therapeutic communities were originally developed in health settings, and stem from the pioneering work in the UK of the psychoanalysts Bion, Rickman, Main, and Maxwell-Jones and the group analyst Foulkes who worked with shell-shocked soldiers in the second world war (Yakeley et al., 2016).

Therapeutic communities are based on a number of psychoanalytic concepts and theories, including Bowlby's (1969) work on attachment in feeling connected and belonging to the therapeutic group; Bion's (1962) concept of containment, in feeling safe; Main's (1983) 'culture of enquiry' in feeling heard in a culture of openness; Foulkes' (1964) notion of inclusion in feeling involved as part of the whole; and Sullivan's (1953) theory of agency in feeling empowered with an effective sense of self. Therapeutic communities may be residential or delivered in the community as day programmes, and have been increasingly established in forensic health settings including prisons and probation. Grendon Underwood prison was the first therapeutic community to be developed in a custodial setting in the UK in 1962.

There are a number of outcome studies of therapeutic communities in both health and forensic settings, although many lack methodological rigour and are based on small samples sizes with mixed findings in relation to reducing risk. However, as a whole the evidence points to an improvement in interpersonal outcomes and a reduction in offending, particularly for people with personality disorder (Capone et al., 2016; Lees et al., 1999, 2004; Newbury, 2010).

15.9.4 Mentalization-Based Treatment

In recent years, specific therapies have been developed and empirically supported for the treatment of severe personality disorders, mostly in the treatment of patients with borderline personality disorder. One of the most prominent of such therapies to emerge in the UK from the psychoanalytic school is mentalization-based treatment (MBT; Bateman & Fonagy, 2004). MBT is a structured, time-limited, evidence-based psychological therapy that was originally developed in the 1990s to treat patients with borderline personality disorder in a partial (day) hospital setting. It is a psychodynamic therapy that incorporates relational and cognitive elements and its theoretical frame of reference includes developmental psychology, attachment theory and a theory about the mechanism of therapeutic action (Bateman & Fonagy, 2012). MBT is specifically focused on increasing the capacity to mentalize. As described above, individuals with ASPD and psychopathy show marked deficits in mentalizing which negatively impact on their relationships with others and increases their capacity for violence.

MBT was initially shown to be effective in a randomized controlled trial in patients with borderline personality disorder (Bateman & Fonagy, 1999) where it diminished suicidal and self-injurious behaviours, significantly improved interpersonal functioning and reduced the number of hospitalisations and use of medication compared to the control group. Follow-up studies report that these gains were maintained post treatment (Bateman & Fonagy, 2001, 2008a). MBT has subsequently been adapted for other disorders, including ASPD (Bateman et al., 2013; Bateman & Fonagy, 2008b, 2009), with increasing interest in applying MBT to patients in forensic in-patient settings. Evidence that MBT might be effective in treating patients with ASPD emerged from a trial in which MBT was found to be more effective than structured clinical management for BPD patients comorbid with ASPD. Outcome measures included improvements in symptoms related to aggression (e.g., the reduction of anger, hostility, paranoia), frequency of self-harm and suicide attempts, improvement of negative mood, general psychiatric symptoms, interpersonal problems, and social adjustment (Bateman et al., 2016). MBT is currently being evaluated in a large-scale community multi-site randomised control trial in the UK criminal justice system comparing MBT with other services currently offered by probation to adult male offenders with a diagnosis of ASPD, including those with psychopathy.

15.10 Conclusion

Psychoanalytic thinking is neither obsolete nor solipsistic but offers a particular theory of mind that is complementary, not contradictory, to that of other disciplines, and which is continuously evolving in line with empirical research into the structure and functioning of the human brain and its pathologies. It offers a perspective on the inner life of the individual – his subjective experience of the world and how he relates to himself and others – and puts flesh on the bones of the neuroscientific discoveries of the nature of the brain. Inherent in a psychoanalytic approach to psychopathy is a theory of development that traces how environmental circumstances modify and interact with genetic factors to shape the psychopath's character and the underlying psychological structures and processes of his mind. Building a picture of his internal world – his object relations, unconscious fantasies, superego characteristics and defence mechanisms – and illuminating how the psychopath thinks and feels, and how his perceptions of and actions towards himself and others are driven by unconscious, as well as conscious factors, gives us insight into his motivations and creates a dynamic map of the ways in which he will respond to interventions aimed at reducing risk or alleviating distress.

In a psychoanalytic approach to the management of psychopathic patients or offenders, interventions are not solely aimed at the psychopath himself, but are also for the staff group or institution as a whole in creating reflective spaces in which they can identify and reflect on their countertransference – the emotional responses and collective defence mechanisms that are unconsciously mobilised to defend against the anxieties of work with such disturbed individuals. Understanding how these reactions in professionals reflect the projection of unwanted thoughts and feelings of the psychopath not only gives insight into the inner workings of his mind, but anticipates and averts non-professional behaviours which may parallel the destructive behaviours of the psychopath.

Working with psychopathic individuals in any capacity or setting is arduous and beset with risks, and such work should not be carried out in isolation but should take place with others in a team where the anxieties of staff can be contained. A psychoanalytic framework offers such containment in facilitating an exploration of the dark reaches of the human psyche and interpreting its discoveries into coherent theory and practice within the security of others.

References

Aichorn, A. (1925). *Wayward youth*. Viking.

Alexander, F. (1923). *Psychoanalysis of the total personality* English translation. Nervous and Mental Disease Publications, 1930.

Alexander, F. (1930). The neurotic character. *International Journal of Psycho-Analysis, 11*, 292–313.

Alexander, F. (1935). *Roots of crime*. Knopf.

Allen, J. G., Fonagy, P., & Bateman, A. (2008). *Mentalizing in clinical practice*. American Psychiatric Press.
American Psychiatric Association (Ed.). (2013). *Diagnostic and statistical manual of mental disorders* (5th ed.). American Psychiatric Association.
Bateman, A. W. (1999). Narcissism and it relation to violence and suicide. In R. Perelberg (Ed.), *Psychoanalytic understanding of violence and suicide*. Routledge.
Bateman, A. W., & Fonagy, P. (1999). Effectiveness of partial hospitalization in the treatment of borderline personality disorder: A randomized controlled trial. *American Journal of Psychiatry, 156*, 1563–1569.
Bateman, A. W., & Fonagy, P. (2001). Treatment of borderline personality disorder with psychoanalytically oriented partial hospitalization: An 18 -month follow-up. *American Journal of Psychiatry, 158*, 36–42.
Bateman, A. W., & Fonagy, P. (2004). *Psychotherapy for borderline personality disorder: Mentalization-based treatment*. Oxford University Press.
Bateman, A. W., & Fonagy, P. (2008a). 8-year follow-up of patients treated for borderline personality disorder: Mentalization-based treatment versus treatment as usual. *American Journal of Psychiatry, 165*, 631–638.
Bateman, A. W., & Fonagy, P. (2008b). Comorbid antisocial and borderline personality disorders: Mentalization-based treatment. *Journal of Clinical Psychology, 64*, 181–194.
Bateman, A. W., & Fonagy, P. (2009). Randomized controlled trial of outpatient mentalization-based treatment versus structured clinical management for borderline personality disorder. *American Journal of Psychiatry, 166*, 1355–1364.
Bateman, A. W., & Fonagy, P. (Eds.). (2012). *Handbook of mentalizing in mental health practice*. American Psychiatric Publishing, Inc.
Bateman, A. W., Bolton, R., & Fonagy, P. (2013). Antisocial personality disorder: A mentalizing framework. *FOCUS: Journal of Lifelong Learning in Psychiatry, 11*, 178–186.
Bateman, A. W., O'Connell, J., Lorenzini, N., Gardner, T., & Fonagy, P. (2016). A randomised controlled trial of mentalization-based treatment versus structured clinical management for patients with comorbid borderline personality disorder and antisocial personality disorder. *BMC Psychiatry, 16*, 304.
Beaver, K., Barnes, J. C., May, J., & Schwartz, J. (2011). Psychopathic personality traits, genetic risk, and gene-environment correlations. *Criminal Justice and Behavior, 38*, 896–912.
Bion, W. R. (1962). *Learning from experience*. Heinemann. [Reprinted London: Karnac Books, 1984.].
Birnbaum, K. (1930). The social significance of the psychopath. *The Annals of the American Academy of Political and Social Science, 149*, 70–79.
Blackburn, R. (2009). Subtypes of psychopath. In M. McMurran & R. Howard (Eds.), *Wiley series in forensic clinical psychology. Personality, personality disorder and violence: An evidence based approach* (pp. 113–132). Wiley-Blackwell.
Blair, R. J. R. (1999). Responsiveness to distress cues in the child with psychopathic tendencies. *Personality and Individual Differences, 27*, 135–145.
Blair, J., Mitchell, D., & Blair, K (2005). *The Psychopath: Emotion and the Brain*. Oxford, UK, Blackwell.
Blair, R. J. R. (2018). Traits of empathy and anger: Implications for psychopathy and other disorders associated with aggression. *Philosophical Transactions of the Royal Society London B Biological Sciences, 373*. https://doi.org/10.1098/rstb.2017.0155:20170155
Blumenthal, S., Huckle, C., Czornyj, R., Craissati, J., & Richardson, P. (2010). The role of affect in the estimation of risk. *Journal of Mental Health, 19*, 444–451.
Borja, K., & Ostrosky, F. (2013). Early traumatic events in psychopaths. *Journal of Forensic Sciences, 58*, 927–931.
Bowlby, J. (1944). Forty-four juvenile thieves: Their characters and home life. *International Journal of Psycho-Analysis, 25*, 19–53.
Bowlby, J. (1969). *Attachment and loss, vol. 1, attachment*. Basic Books.

Brinkley, C. A., Newman, J. P., Widiger, T. A., & Lynam, D. R. (2004). Two approaches to parsing the heterogeneity of psychopathy. *Clinical Psychology: Science and Practice, 11*, 69–94.
Capone, G., Schroder, T., Clarke, S., & Braham, L. (2016). Outcomes of therapeutic community treatment for personality disorder. *Therapeutic Communities: The International Journal of Therapeutic Communities, 37*, 84–100.
Caspi, A., McClay, J., Moffitt, T. E., Mills, S., Martin, J., Craig, I. W., Taylor, A., & Poulton, R. (2002). Role of genotype in the cycle of violence in maltreated children. *Science, 297*, 851–854.
Cleckley, H. (1941). *The mask of sanity*. C.V. Mosby.
Coid, J. (1992). DSM-III diagnosis in criminal psychopaths: A way forward. *Criminal Behaviour and Mental Health, 2*, 78–94.
Compton, W. M., Conway, K. P., Stinson, F. S., Colliver, J. D., & Grant, B. F. (2005). Prevalence, correlates, and comorbidity of DSM-IV antisocial personality syndromes and alcohol and specific drug use disorders in the United States: Results from the national epidemiologic survey on alcohol and related conditions. *Journal of Clinical Psychiatry, 66*, 677–685.
Cornell, D., Warren, J., Hawk, G., Stafford, E., Oram, G., & Pine, D. (1996). Psychopathy in instrumental and reactive violent offenders. *Journal of Consulting and Clinical Psychology, 64*, 783–790.
Cox, M. (1976). Group psychotherapy in a secure setting. *Proceedings of the Royal Society of Medicine, 69*, 215–220.
Dargis, M., Newman, J., & Koenigs, M. (2016). Clarifying the link between childhood abuse history and psychopathic traits in adult criminal offenders. *Personality Disorders, 7*, 221–228.
De Brito, S. A., & Hodgins, S. (2009). Antisocial personality disorder. In M. McMurran & R. Howard (Eds.), *Personality, personality disorder and violence* (pp. 133–153). Wiley.
Department of Health. (2010). *Your guide to relational security: See, think, act*. Department of Health.
Dowsett, J., & Craissati, J. (2008). *Managing personality disordered offenders in the community: A psychological approach*. Routledge.
Eichelman, B. (1988). Toward a rational pharmacotherapy for aggressive and violent behavior. *Hospital and Community Psychiatry, 1*, 31–39.
Farrington, D., Coid, J., Harnett, L., Jolliffe, D., Soteriou, N., Turner, R., & West, D. (2006). *Criminal careers up to age 50 and life success up to age 48: New findings from the Cambridge study in delinquent development*. Home Office Report, 299.
Fenichel, O. (1931). The pre-genital antecedents of the Oedipus complex. *International Journal of Psycho-Analysis, 12*, 412–430.
Fenichel, O. (1945). *The psychoanalytic theory of neurosis*. Norton.
Fonagy, P. (1999). Final remarks. In R. Perelberg (Ed.), *Psychoanalytic understanding of violence and suicide*. Routledge.
Fonagy, P., & Target, M. (1995). Understanding the violent patient: The use of the body and the role of the father. *International Journal of Psycho-Analysis, 76*, 487–501.
Foulkes, S. H. (1964). *Therapeutic group analysis*. Karnac Books. [Reprinted 2002, London.].
Freud, S. (1916). Some character-types met with in psycho-analytic work: III criminals from a sense of guilt. In J. Strachey (Ed.), *The standard edition of the complete psychological works of Sigmund Freud* (Vol. 14). Hogarth Press and the Institute of Psychoanalysis.
Freud, S. (1923). The ego and the id. In J. Strachey (Ed.), *The standard edition of the complete psychological works of Sigmund Freud* (Vol. 19). Hogarth Press and the Institute of Psychoanalysis.
Freud, S. (1928). *Dostoevsky and parricide* (Vol. XXI, Standard ed.). Hogarth Press.
Freud, A. (1936). *The ego and the mechanisms of defence*. Hogarth Press.
Frick, P., Cornell, D., Barry, C., Bodin, S. D., & Dane, H. E. (2003). Callous-unemotional traits and conduct problems in the prediction of conduct problem severity, aggression, and self-report of delinquency. *Journal of Abnormal Child Psychology, 31*, 457–470.

Gabbard, G. (2005). *Psychodynamic psychiatry in clinical practice* (4th ed.). American Psychiatric Press.
Gabbard, G., & Coyne, L. (1987). Predictors of response of antisocial patients to hospital treatment. *Hospital and Community Psychiatry, 38*, 1181–1185.
Gacono, C. B., & Meloy, J. R. (1994). *The Rorschach assessment of aggressive and psychopathic personalities*. Erlbaum.
George, C., Kaplan, N., & Main, M. (1996). *Adult attachment interview*. Unpublished manuscript, University of California at Berkeley.
Glasser, M. (1998). On violence: A preliminary communication. *International Journal of Psycho-Analysis, 79*, 887–902.
Glenn, A. L., & Raine, A. (2014). *Psychology and crime. Psychopathy: An introduction to biological findings and their implications*. New York University Press.
Goodwin, R. D., & Hamilton, S. P. (2003). Lifetime comorbidity of antisocial personality disorder and anxiety disorders among adults in the community. *Psychiatry Research, 117*, 159–166.
Graham, N., Kimonis, E. R., Wasserman, A. L., & Kline, S. M. (2012). Associations among childhood abuse and psychopathy facets in male sexual offenders. *Personality Disorders: Theory, Research, and Treatment, 3*, 66–75.
Greenacre, P. (1958). The imposter. *Psychoanalytic Quarterly, 27*, 359–383.
Hare, R. D. (1970). *Psychopathy: Theory and research*. John Wiley & Sons.
Hare, R. D. (1991). *Manual of the revised psychopathy checklist*. Multi Health Systems.
Hare, R. D. (2003). *Hare psychopathy checklist—Revised (PCL-R): 2nd edition technical manual*. Multi Health Systems.
Hare, R. D., & Neumann, C. S. (2005). Structural models of psychopathy. *Current Psychiatry Reports, 7*, 57–64.
Heads, T., Taylor, P., & Leese, M. (1997). Childhood experiences of patients with schizophrenia and a history of violence: A special hospital sample. *Criminal Behaviour and Mental Health, 7*, 117–130.
Hicks, B. M., Carlson, M. D., Blonigen, D. M., Patrick, C. J., Iacono, W. G., & MGue, M. (2012). Psychopathic personality traits and environmental contexts: Differential correlates, gender differences, and genetic mediation. *Personality Disorders: Theory, Research, and Treatment, 3*, 209–227.
Horney, K. (1945). *Our inner conflicts*. Norton.
Howell, E. F. (2018). Outsiders to love: The psychopathic character and dilemma. *Contemporary Psychoanalysis, 54*, 17–39.
Hyde, L. W., Waller, R., Trentacosta, C. J., Shaw, D. S., Neiderhiser, J. M., Ganiban, J. M., Reiss, D., & Leve, L. D. (2016). Heritable and nonheritable pathways to early callous-unemotional behaviors. *The American Journal of Psychiatry, 173*, 903–910.
Jacobson, E. (1964). *The self and the object world*. International University Press.
Jacobson, E. (1971). *Depression*. International University Press.
Karpman, B. (1946). Psychopathy in the scheme of human typology. *Journal of Nervous and Mental Disease, 103*, 276–288.
Kernberg, O. F. (1975). *Borderline conditions and pathological narcissism*. Jason Aronson.
Kernberg, O. F. (1976). *Object relations theory and clinical psychoanalysis*. Jason Aronson.
Kernberg, O. F. (1984). *Severe personality disorders*. Yale University Press.
Kimonis, E. R., Frick, P. J., Fazekas, H., & Loney, B. R. (2006). Psychopathy, aggression, and the processing of emotional stimuli in non-referred girls and boys. *Behavioral Sciences & the Law, 24*, 21–37. [Published correction appears in *Behavioral Sciences and the Law, 24*, 407].
Klein, M. (1927). Criminal tendencies in normal children. *British Journal of Medical Psychology, 7*, 177–192.
Klein, M. (1946). Notes on some schizoid mechanisms. In M. Klein (Ed.), *Envy and gratitude and other works*. Hogarth.
Klein, M. (1957). Envy and gratitude. In M. Klein (Ed.), *Envy and gratitude and other works*. Hogarth.

Klein, M. (1964). *Contributions to psychoanalysis: 1920–1945*. McGraw Hill.

Koch, J. L. (1891). *Die Psychopathischen Minderwertigkeiten*. Maier.

Kolla, N. J., Malcolm, C., Attard, S., Arenovich, T., Blackwood, N., & Hodgins, S. (2013). Childhood maltreatment and aggressive behaviour in violent offenders with psychopathy. *The Canadian Journal of Psychiatry/La Revue canadienne de psychiatrie, 58*, 487–494.

Kraepelin, E. (1915). *Psychiatrie: Ein Lehrbuch* (8th ed.). Barth.

Larsson, H., Andershed, H., & Lichtenstein, P. (2006). A genetic factor explains most of the variation in the psychopathic personality. *Journal of Abnormal Psychology, 115*, 221–230.

Lees, J., Manning, N., & Rawlings, B. (1999). *Therapeutic community effectiveness: A systematic international review of therapeutic community treatment for people with personality disorders and mentally disordered offenders* (CRD Report no. 17). NHS Centre for Reviews and Dissemination, University of York.

Lees, J., Manning, N., & Rawlings, B. (2004). A culture of enquiry: Research evidence and the therapeutic community. *Psychiatric Quarterly, 75*, 279–294.

Lenzenweger, M. F., Lane, M. C., Loranger, A. W., & Kessler, R. C. (2007). DSM-IV personality disorders in the National Comorbidity Survey Replication. *Biological Psychiatry, 62*, 553–564.

Lilienfeld, S. O., Watts, A. L., Smith, S. F., & Latzman, R. D. (2018). Boldness: Conceptual and methodological issues. In C. J. Patrick (Ed.), *Handbook of psychopathy* (pp. 165–186). The Guilford Press.

López, R., Poy, R., Patrick, C. J., & Moltó, J. (2013). Deficient fear conditioning and self-reported psychopathy: The role of fearless dominance. *Psychophysiology, 50*, 210–218.

Mahler, M. S. (1968). *On human symbiosis and the vicissitudes of individuation. Vol. I. Infantile psychosis*. International Universities Press.

Mahler, M. S. (1979). *Selected papers of Margaret S. Mahler*. Jason Aronson.

Main, T. F. (1983). The concept of a therapeutic community – Variations and vicissitudes. In M. Pines (Ed.), *The evolution of group analysis*. Routledge/Kegan.

Main, M., & Goldwyn, R. (1994). *Adult attachment scoring and classification system version 6*. Unpublished work, Department of Psychology, University of California at Berkeley Berkeley CA.

Marshall, L., & Cooke, D. (1999). The childhood experiences of psychopaths: A retrospective study of familial and societal factors. *Journal of Personality Disorders, 13*, 211–225.

McEllistrem, J. (2004). Affective and predatory violence: A bimodal classification system of human aggression and violence. *Aggression and Violent Behavior, 10*, 1–30.

Mealey, L. (1995). The sociobiology of sociopathy: An integrated evolutionary model. *Behavioural and Brain Sciences, 18*, 523–599.

Meloy, J. R. (1988). *The psychopathic mind: Origins, dynamics and treatment*. Jason Aronson.

Meloy, J. R. (1992). *Violent attachments*. Jason Aronson.

Meloy, J. R. (2001). *The mark of Cain*. The Analytic Press.

Meloy, J. R. (2006). The empirical basis and forensic application of affective and predatory violence. *Australian and New Zealand Journal of Psychiatry, 40*, 539–547.

Meloy, J. R., & Yakeley, J. (2010). Treatment of cluster B disorders: Antisocial personality disorder. In J. Clarkin, P. Fonagy, & G. Gabbard (Eds.), *Psychodynamic psychotherapy for personality disorders: A clinical handbook* (pp. 349–378). American Psychiatric Press.

Meloy, J. R., & Yakeley, J. (2013). Antisocial personality disorder. In G. O. Gabbard & J. Gunderson (Eds.), *Gabbard's treatments of psychiatric disorders*. American Psychiatric Publishing.

Meloy, J. R., & Yakeley, A. (2021). A psychoanalytic view of the psychopath. In A. R. Felthous & H. Saβ (Eds.), *International handbook on psychopathic disorders and the law* (2nd ed.). Wiley.

Meyer, A. (1904). A review of recent problems of psychiatry. In A. Church & F. Peterson (Eds.), *Nervous and mental diseases* (4th ed.). Williams and Wilkins.

Newbury, M. (2010). A synthesis of outcome research at Grendon therapeutic community prison. *Therapeutic Communities, 31*, 356–371.

Newman, J. P., MacCoon, D. G., Vaughn, L. J., & Sadeh, N. (2005). Validating a distinction between primary and secondary psychopathy with measures of Gray's BIS and BAS constructs. *Journal of Abnormal Psychology, 114*, 319–323.

Ometto, M., de Oliveira, P. A., Milioni, A. L., Dos Santos, B., Scivoletto, S., Busatto, G. F., Nunes, P. V., & Cunha, P. J. (2016). Social skills and psychopathic traits in maltreated adolescents. *European Child & Adolescent Psychiatry, 25*, 397–405.
Patrick, C. J. (2018). Cognitive and emotional processing in psychopathy. In C. J. Patrick (Ed.), *Handbook of psychopathy* (pp. 422–455). The Guilford Press.
Porter, S. (1996). Without conscience or without active conscience? The etiology of psychopathy revisited. *Aggression and Violent Behavior, 1*, 179–189.
Prichard, J. C. (1835). *A treatise on insanity and other disorders affecting the mind*. Sherwood, Gilbert and Piper.
Quinsey, V. L., Harris, G. T., Rice, M. E., & Cormier, C. A. (2006). *The law and public policy. Violent offenders: Appraising and managing risk* (2nd ed.). American Psychological Association.
Raine, A. (1993). *The psychopathology of crime*. Academic.
Raine, A. (2013). *The anatomy of violence*. Pantheon.
Reich, W. (1945). *Character analysis* (2nd ed.). Farrar, Strauss and Giroux.
Richards, H. (1998). Evil intent: Violence and disorders of the will. In T. Millon, E. Simonson, M. Birket-Smith, & R. D. Davis (Eds.), *Psychopathy: Antisocial, criminal and violent behavior*. The Guildford Press.
Robins, L. N., Tipp, J., & Przybeck, T. (1991). Antisocial personality. In L. N. Robins & D. A. Regier (Eds.), *Psychiatric disorders in America: The epidemiological catchment area study* (pp. 258–290). The Free Press.
Schraft, C. V., Kosson, D. S., & Mcbride, C. K. (2013). Exposure to violence within home and community environments and psychopathic tendencies in detained adolescents. *Criminal Justice and Behavior, 40*, 1027–1043.
Serin, R. (1991). Psychopathy and violence in criminals. *Journal of Interpersonal Violence, 6*, 423–431.
Sevecke, K., Franke, S., Kosson, D., & Krischer, M. (2016). Emotional dysregulation and trauma predicting psychopathy dimensions in female and male juvenile offenders. *Child and Adolescent Psychiatry and Mental Health, 10*, 43.
Siegel, A., & Victoroff, J. (2009). Understanding human aggression: New insights from neuroscience. *International Journal of Law and Psychiatry, 32*, 209–215.
Sonuga-Barke, E. J., Schlotz, W., & Kreppner, J. (2010). Differentiating developmental trajectories for conduct, emotion and peer problems following early deprivation. *Monographs of the Society for Research in Child Development, 75*, 102–124.
Sullivan, H. S. (1953). *The interpersonal theory of psychiatry*. Norton.
Svrakic, D., McCallum, K., & Milan, P. (1991). Developmental, structural and clinical approach to narcissistic and antisocial personalities. *American Journal of Psychoanalysis, 51*, 413–432.
Swanson, M. C., Bland, R. C., & Newman, S. C. (1994). Epidemiology of psychiatric disorders in Edmonton. Antisocial personality disorders. *Acta Psychiatrica Scandinavica. Supplementum, 376*, 63–70.
Symington, N. (1980). The response aroused by the psychopath. *International Review of Psycho-Analysis, 7*, 291–298.
Taubner, S., White, L. O., Zimmermann, J., Fonagy, P., & Nolte, T. (2012). Mentalization moderates and mediates the link between psychopathy and aggressive behavior in male adolescents. *Journal of the American Psychoanalytic Association, 60*, 605–612.
Taylor, J., Loney, B. R., Bobadilla, L., Iacono, W. G., & McGue, M. (2003). Genetic and environmental influences on psychopathy trait dimensions in a community sample of male twins. *Journal of Abnormal Child Psychology, 31*, 633–645.
van der Zouwen, M., Hoeve, M., Hendriks, A. M., Asscher, J. J., & Stams, G. J. (2018). The association between attachment and psychopathic traits. *Aggression and Violent Behavior, 43*, 45–55.
Viding, E., & Larsson, H. (2010). Genetics of child and adolescent psychopathy. In R. T. Salekin & D. R. Lynam (Eds.), *Handbook of child and adolescent psychopathy* (pp. 113–134). Guilford.
Viding, E., Blair, R. J., Moffitt, T. E., & Plomin, R. (2005). Evidence for substantial genetic risk for psychopathy in 7-year-olds. *Journal of Child Psychology & Psychiatry and Allied Disciplines, 46*, 592–597.

Viding, E., Fontaine, N. M., Oliver, B. R., & Plomin, R. (2009). Negative parental discipline, conduct problems and callous-unemotional traits: A monozygotic twin differences study. *British Journal of Psychiatry, 195*, 414–419.

Waldman, I. D., & Rhee, S. H. (2006). Genetic and environmental influences on psychopathy and antisocial behavior. In C. J. Patrick (Ed.), *Handbook of psychopathy* (pp. 205–228). Guilford.

Walsh, T. C. (1999). Psychopathic and nonpsychopathic violence among alcoholic offenders. *International Journal of Offender Therapy and Comparative Criminology, 43*, 34–48.

Webster, C. D., Douglas, K. S., Eaves, D., & Hart, S. T. (1997). *HCR-20: Assessing risk for violence, version 2*. Mental Health, Law and Policy Institute, Simon Fraser University.

Weeks, R., & Widom, C. S. (1998). Self-report of early childhood victimization among incarcerated adult male felons. *Journal of Interpersonal Violence, 13*, 346–361.

Weizmann-Henelius, G., Grönroos, M., Putkonen, H., Eronen, M., Lindberg, N., & Häkkänen-Nyholm, H. (2010). Psychopathy and gender differences in childhood psychosocial characteristics in homicide offenders – A nationwide register-based study. *The Journal of Forensic Psychiatry & Psychology, 21*, 801–814.

Welldon, E. (1996). Group-analytic psychotherapy in an out-patient setting. In C. Cordess & M. Cox (Eds.), *Forensic psychotherapy: Crime, psychodynamics and the offender patient*. Jessica Kingsley.

Williamson, S., Hare, R. D., & Wong, S. (1987). Violence: Criminal psychopaths and their victims. *Canadian Journal of Behavioral Science, 19*, 454–462.

Winnicott, D. W. (1956). The anti-social tendency. In *Through paediatrics to psychoanalysis*. Hogarth Press. [Reprinted 1984].

Winnicott, D. W. (1960). Ego distortion in terms of true and false self. In *The maturational processes and the facilitating environment*. Hogarth Press. [Reprinted London: Karnac Books, 1990].

Winnicott, D. W. (1965). *The maturational processes and the facilitating environment*. Hogarth Press. [Reprinted London: Karnac Books, 1990].

Woodworth, M., & Porter, S. (2002). In cold blood: Characteristics of criminal homicides as a function of psychopathy. *Journal of Abnormal Psychology, 111*, 436–445.

World Health Organisation (WHO). (1992). *International classification of mental and Behavioural disorders, tenth edition (ICD-10)*. WHO.

Yakeley, J. (2010). *Working with violence – A contemporary psychoanalytic approach*. Palgrave Macmillan.

Yakeley, J., & Williams, A. (2014). Antisocial personality disorder: New directions. *Advances in Psychiatric Treatment, 20*, 132–143.

Yakeley, J., Johnston, J., Adshead, G., & Allison, L. (Eds.). (2016). *The Oxford specialist handbook of medical psychotherapy*. Oxford University Press.

Yang, Y., & Raine, A. (2018). The neuroanatomical bases of psychopathy: A review of brain imaging findings. In C. J. Patrick (Ed.), *Handbook of psychopathy* (2nd ed., pp. 380–400). The Guilford Press.

Chapter 16
Existential Perspectives of Psychopathy

Stephen Arthur Diamond

Abstract *Psychopathy*, also known diagnostically as *sociopathy* and *antisocial* or *dyssocial personality disorder,* can be described as a chronic constellation of callous, immoral, manipulative, aggressive, or violent personality traits and behaviors. While antisocial tendencies have historically been extensively studied through various lenses, exceedingly little has been written regarding psychopathy from the perspective of existential psychology and psychotherapy (see Diamond SA, Anger, madness, and the daimonic: the psychological genesis of violence, evil, and creativity. Foreword by Rollo May. State University of New York Press, 1996; Diamond SA, J Appl Psychoanal Stud 5:21–45, 2003; Diamond SA, Violence as secular evil: forensic evaluation and treatment of violent offenders from the viewpoint of existential depth psychology. In: Mason T (ed) Forensic psychiatry: influences of evil, Humana Press, pp 179–206, 2006). Thus, this chapter explores the phenomenon of psychopathy from the frame of reference of contemporary existential therapy and seeks to shed light on how the existentially inclined forensic clinician evaluates, conceptualizes, and conducts treatment with psychopathic or antisocial patients. It provides brief definitions and descriptions of both psychopathy and existential therapy, examines the existential roots of the frustration, anger, rage, resentment, hostility, and hatred that can lead to psychopathic cruelty, malevolence, depravity, and destructiveness, and considers how the existential approach to psychopathy differs fundamentally from most mainstream therapies today. Further, this exploration delves deeply into psychopathy not only from the standpoint of existential psychotherapies in general (see, for example, Cooper M, Existential therapies, 2nd edn. SAGE. (Original work published 2003), 2016), but from that of a specific form of existential therapy the author refers to as "existential depth psychology" (Diamond SA, Anger, madness, and the daimonic: the psychological genesis of violence, evil, and creativity. Foreword by Rollo May. State University of New York Press, 1996). Drawing and building upon the existential psychoanalysis of Rollo May and the author's own more than four decades of professional experience as a clinical and forensic psychologist and practicing psychotherapist (see Diamond SA, Anger,

S. A. Diamond (✉)
Clinical and Forensic Psychologist, Marina del Rey, CA, USA

J. E. Vitale (ed.), *The Complexity of Psychopathy*, Dangerous Behavior in Clinical and Forensic Psychology, https://doi.org/10.1007/978-3-030-83156-1_16

madness, and the daimonic: the psychological genesis of violence, evil, and creativity. Foreword by Rollo May. State University of New York Press, 1996; Diamond SA, Existential Analysis, 10, 27–41, 1999; Diamond SA, J Appl Psychoanal Stud 5:21–45, 2003; Diamond SA, Violence as secular evil: forensic evaluation and treatment of violent offenders from the viewpoint of existential depth psychology. In: Mason T (ed) Forensic psychiatry: influences of evil, Humana Press, pp 179–206, 2006; Existential therapy: confronting life's ultimate concerns. In Tinsley H, Lease S, Giffin Wiersma N (eds) Contemporary theory and practice in counseling and psychotherapy. SAGE, pp 323–352, 2016; Diamond SA, J Humanist Psychol, 2018), existential depth psychology synthesizes, integrates and reconciles the "depth psychology" of Freud, Adler, Rank, and particularly, Carl Jung's analytical psychology, with existential analysis or existential therapy (Diamond SA, J Humanist Psychol, 2018, online).

Keywords Existential therapy · Psychopathy · Antisocial personality disorder · Sociopathy · Dyssocial personality disorder · Psychopathic narcissism · Nihilism · Guilt · Anxiety · Rollo May · Irvin Yalom · Viktor Frankl · J.-P. Sartre · C.G. Jung · Sigmund Freud · Existentialism · Existential analysis · Existential psychotherapy · Existential depth psychology · Phenomenology · Anger · Rage · Violence · Evil · The daimonic · Serial killers · Mass shootings

16.1 Introduction

Psychopathy, also known diagnostically as sociopathy and antisocial or dyssocial personality disorder, can be described as a chronic constellation of callous, immoral, manipulative, aggressive, or violent personality traits and behaviors. While antisocial tendencies have historically been extensively studied through various lenses, exceedingly little has been written regarding psychopathy from the perspective of existential psychology and psychotherapy (see Diamond, 1996, 2003, 2006). Thus, this chapter explores the phenomenon of psychopathy from the frame of reference of contemporary existential therapy and seeks to shed light on how the existentially inclined forensic clinician evaluates, conceptualizes, and conducts treatment with psychopathic or antisocial patients. It provides brief definitions and descriptions of both psychopathy and existential therapy, examines the existential roots of the frustration, anger, rage, resentment, hostility, and hatred that can lead to psychopathic cruelty, malevolence, depravity, and destructiveness, and considers how the existential approach to psychopathy differs fundamentally from most mainstream therapies today. Further, this exploration delves deeply into psychopathy not only from the standpoint of existential psychotherapies in general (see, for example, Cooper, 2016), but from that of a specific form of existential therapy the author refers to as "existential depth psychology" (Diamond, 1996). Drawing and building upon the existential psychoanalysis of Rollo May and the author's own more than four decades of professional experience as a clinical and forensic psychologist and practicing psychotherapist (see Diamond, 1996, 1999, 2003, 2006, 2016, 2018), existential depth psychology synthesizes, integrates and reconciles the "depth psychology" of Freud, Adler, Rank, and particularly, Carl Jung's analytical psychology, with existential analysis or existential therapy (Diamond, 2018, online).

16.2 What Is Psychopathy?

The diagnostic term *psychopath* has been kicking around since the nineteenth century, but was popularized by psychiatrist Hervey Cleckley (1941) in *The Mask of Sanity: An Attempt to Clarify Some Issues About the So-Called Psychopathic Personality*. For Cleckley, the psychopathic personality was initially defined by the presence of a relatively high-functioning, aggressively narcissistic, extraverted *persona* (see Jung, 1961), disguising an antisocial and latent psychotic core—although, as Cleckley later recognized, whether, despite a remarkable lack of insight regarding the reality and severity of their problems, most psychopaths are truly psychotic in the classic sense (e.g., experience hallucinations and/or delusions with impaired reality testing) is debatable. While it can be said that we all normally put on and need some sort of facade designed to hide our socially unacceptable tendencies or *personal shadow* (see Jung, 1961; see also Diamond, 1991, 1996, 2009b, c, 2018), the so-called psychopath is especially skilled at doing so, outwardly camouflaging a considerably more morbid, malevolent, disturbed, and destructive dark-side or shadow within than most of the general population. The DSM-5 diagnosis of Antisocial Personality Disorder focuses primarily on observable or well-documented long-standing patterns of behavior such as blatant disregard for social norms, pathological lying, impulsivity, irresponsibility, recklessness, cruelty, violence, lawbreaking, and lack of guilt or remorse for such behaviors. Psychopathy and dyssocial personality disorder, however, emphasize somewhat more subjective and inferred personality traits like lack of interpersonal warmth, caring, or empathy, easily formed but short-lived superficial attachments, low tolerance for frustration, chronically irritable mood, absence of conscience, failure to learn from negative consequences, and defensive projection and deflection of blame onto others. For example, Hare's Psychopathy Checklist- Revised (1991) emphasizes specific characteristics such as glibness or charismatic charm, narcissistic grandiosity, need for constant stimulation, shallow affect, parasitic lifestyle, sexual promiscuity, serial marriages, and habitual lying, manipulativeness, conning, or deceitfulness.

Although it is not formally included in DSM-5, psychopathy is, by definition, a "personality disorder." Personality disorders are, "an enduring pattern of inner experience and behavior… [that is] inflexible and pervasive across a broad range of personal and social situations" (DSM-5, p.321). For this reason, all personality disorders are relatively difficult to treat, due in part to the deeply rooted defense mechanisms, embedded behavioral patterns, and entrenched traits. From an existential perspective, psychopathy is a specific way of being-in-the-world, and this socially inappropriate way of existing provides the psychopath with his or her sense of identity, significance, self-esteem, purpose, security, control, and power. For these damaged individuals, psychopathic behavior serves as a means of overcoming chronic feelings of helplessness, insecurity, shame, and inferiority. It is the only lifestyle and way of being in the world the psychopath has ever known, and, despite extremely negative consequences such as recurring arrests and incarceration, psychopathy has helped the person *survive* so far. So, existentially speaking, we can think of psychopathy as a complex primitive *survival mechanism* without which the person does not know how to otherwise exist and participate in society.

16.2.1 Psychopathy as an Anger Disorder

I have elsewhere proposed (Diamond, 1996, 2003, 2006) that psychopathy, like many other mental disorders, is, fundamentally, an anger *disorder*. The central role of chronically repressed anger or rage in a multitude of different pathological mental phenomena such as mania, major depression, psychosis, and, psychopathy, is vastly underappreciated by most contemporary clinicians (See Diamond, 1996). Antisocial personality disorder generally includes a chronic and pathological anger, rage, resentment, and hostility toward others. On this matter, I find myself in agreement with psychoanalyst Otto Kernberg's (1992) assertion that "hatred derives from rage, the primary affect around which the drive of aggression clusters," and that this intense and chronic hatred is "the core affect of severe psychopathological conditions, particularly severe personality disorders, perversions, and functional psychoses" (p. 21).

Psychopathy, like APD, consists of an unconscious core of chronically repressed anger, rage, resentment, enmity, hostility, and the unremitting urge for revenge, retaliation, and retribution. The psychopath is possessed and driven by this compulsion to avenge the perceived unfair or hurtful fate he or she has been subjected to. As we will later see, this neurotic (and sometimes psychotic) unrelenting obsessive need for retaliation is at the very heart of the psychopath's problem, and, therefore, must, along with the underlying narcissistic rage that drives it, be explicitly acknowledged and addressed in his or her treatment, something most current mainstream therapies fail to adequately do. Indeed, during this century we have been virtually bombarded daily with reports of horrific mass shootings and other grotesque eruptions of so-called senseless violence (See Diamond, 1996). Most of these murderous acts are committed by males, which likely corresponds to the statistical fact that, among diagnosed cases of APD, men outnumber women by a ratio of more than 3:1 (American Psychiatric Association, 2013). While such appalling, cruel, and vicious acts of aggression are clearly antisocial in nature, the perpetrators do not necessarily always meet the full diagnostic criteria for antisocial personality disorder, dyssocial personality disorder, sociopathy, or psychopathy per se. Nor does every person exhibiting such antisocial syndromes engage in outwardly violent or homicidal behavior. But given the terrifying reality and ubiquity of our raging epidemic of violence in America and with greater frequency elsewhere around the world, forensic psychologists, psychiatrists, and other mental health professionals must try to better understand and treat these escalating psychopathic trends in society, and the deeply disturbed and dangerous individuals who increasingly come to the attention of the forensic clinician for both evaluation and treatment (See Diamond, 1996, 2006).

16.2.2 Psychopathic Narcissism: A New Diagnosis?

In order to more deeply comprehend the phenomenon of psychopathy—and the anger, rage, hate, and hostility at its heart— it is necessary to explore not only the existential roots of antisocial personality but additionally, the dynamic psychology underlying the pervasive problem of *pathological narcissism.* What precisely do we mean by "narcissism"? Psychologist Stephen Johnson (1987) notes that, "The narcissist has buried his (or her) true self-expression in response to early injuries and replaced it with a highly developed, compensatory, 'false self'" (p. 39). It is exactly this "false self" (Winnicott, 1960) in *extremis* that we witness in the psychopath. Kohut (1978) proposes that pathological narcissism stems from the mishandling by parents or caretakers of the child's normal or natural narcissism. Neurotic narcissism can stem from receiving either too little or too much "narcissistic supply" during childhood or adolescence. Children naturally need love, support, and attention. But they also need firm limit-setting, boundaries, appropriate and consistent consequences for bad behavior, and what developmental psychologists call "optimal frustration." *Optimal frustration* is how children learn to delay gratification, persevere at tasks, develop inner strength and independence, and adapt to what Freud (1966, pp. 402–403) famously referred to as the "reality principle."

Children are innately narcissistic and self-centered, and must be taught by and learn from their parents or caretakers that the world does not revolve around them, that we must be considerate of and cooperative with others, and that there are some selfish behaviors that are wrong, unacceptable, and will not be tolerated. When a child does not receive such moral education at home, he or she is ill-prepared to deal with the world at large. In such cases, we see an unchecked infantile egoism or narcissism never sufficiently socialized, and therefore, never moderated. Indeed, overindulgence, lack of discipline, and overprotectiveness can be as deeply wounding and destructive as its polar opposite. Such "spoiling" of the child, as it is called colloquially, is in itself a traumatizing type of deprivation and abandonment in which one's basic needs for structure, guidance, limit-setting, reality testing, and parental authority are neglected and frustrated. In a sense, the child feels instinctively that the parent does not care enough to provide the essential limit-setting and structure. He or she is at first deeply hurt by, and then resentful and infuriated at this tragic parental failure. This festering anger, having no real positive outlet, tends to be chronically repressed, turning over time into toxic resentment, embitterment, and narcissistic rage (Diamond, 1996).

Otto Kernberg (1992) described *malignant narcissism* as a syndrome characterized by a combination of narcissistic personality disorder (NPD), antisocial features, paranoid traits, and sadistic or egosyntonic aggression. Other symptoms may include an absence of conscience, a psychological need for power, and a grandiose sense of importance. The difference between what I call psychopathic narcissism and Kernberg's notion of *malignant narcissism* may be the degree to which the person's pathological narcissism has become psychopathic, insofar as her or his symptoms meet the diagnostic criteria for both antisocial and narcissistic personality disorders. For Kernberg, malignant narcissism lies somewhere on the spectrum between psychopathy and narcissistic personality disorder, and is, therefore, comprised of a somewhat less destructive form of pathological narcissism than that typically found in what I am calling psychopathic narcissism. Patients exhibiting psychopathic narcissism would likely embody all four personality traits referred to by some psychologists as the "dark tetrad" (Book et al., 2015; Međedović & Petrović, 2015): extreme pathological narcissism, psychopathy, sadistic cruelty, and Machiavellianism. Thus, psychopathic narcissism, like malignant narcissism, lies somewhere between antisocial personality disorder and narcissistic personality disorder, though nearer to APD than NPD. The diagnostic boundary between these two problematic personality disorders is blurry at best, and sometimes non-existent, which presents to the clinician as a highly amorphous mixture of both narcissistic and psychopathic traits.

To sum up, there can be a very fine, sometimes imperceptible line dividing pathological narcissism and psychopathy, a line which can be crossed at any time. The psychopath lives on the far side of this line, having bitterly turned against society, repeatedly and often impulsively engaging in illegal activity leading to multiple arrests, as well as in lying, manipulating, conning, and aggressive behavior aimed at repaying a slight and resisting being "pushed around" or told what to do by others, particularly legitimate authority figures. The pathological narcissist, on the other hand, is typically better adapted to the culture. These individuals frequently function at a higher level, are often financially and socially more successful, skirt the law more skillfully, choose to work within the system, ostensibly accept rather than reject society, yet still play by their own self-serving, nihilistic, and rebellious rules. Somewhere in between these two distinct but closely related personalities lies what I have described here as the "psychopathic narcissist." In some ways, psychopathic narcissism may prove to be the most difficult disorder to diagnose, since it is neither clearly one nor the other, fish nor fowl, but rather a deeply complex and deceptively "normal" looking blend of both.

16.3 What Is Existential Therapy?

Existential therapy is an attitude or approach to treatment not easily summarized and defined, and likely not as familiar to most readers as certain other theoretical orientations (See, for instance, Yalom, 1980; May, 1983; Cooper, 2016; van Deurzen et al., 2019). Thus, meaningfully discussing this matter requires some brief, basic, concise description of existential philosophy, psychology, and psychotherapy for the uninitiated reader. As I have elsewhere written, "Existential therapy is rooted in a set of distinctive philosophical, theoretical, and methodological orientations to treatment. [However,] [f]rom this basic conceptual framework, an increasingly heterogeneous collection of existentially based approaches has emerged, rendering … existential therapy rather difficult to define" (Diamond, 2016, p. 324; See also, Cooper, 2016; van Deurzen et al., 2019). For the specific purposes of this chapter, we will be exploring the complex problem of psychopathy primarily from three different but related perspectives: what pioneering European practitioners such as Binswanger, Boss, and Frankl first called "existential analysis": what in America subsequently evolved into today's "existential therapy" as articulated mainly by May, Bugental, and Yalom; and, thirdly, an integrative variation of existential therapy I practice and refer to as existential depth psychology.

Though divergent in both theory and practice, each of these three therapeutic approaches share the same fundamental focus on and concern with the subjective experience of human existence, which is what truly makes them *existential:* "The term *existential* refers to those naturally occurring, universal, and inescapable elemental realities characterizing the human condition" (Diamond, 2016, p. 324). There is no denying that in psychology and psychiatry, our theoretical paradigms strongly shape how we conceptualize such complex phenomena as aberrant human behavior, psychopathology in general, and psychopathy specifically. For example, the existential practitioner's perspective on the etiology and significance of psychopathic patterns of behavior will differ significantly from that of the cognitive-behaviorist, Rogerian, neurobiologist, psychoanalyst, or psychopharmacologist. In turn, these perceptions explicitly and implicitly influence the diagnosis, prognosis, and particular treatment approach recommended or taken.

16.3.1 Existential Therapy and Psychiatric Diagnosis

It must preliminarily be noted here that most (though not all) existentially inclined psychotherapists today vehemently oppose psychiatric diagnosis, primarily on philosophical and ethical grounds. For these clinicians, diagnosing, and thereby medicalizing and pathologizing psychological distress and difficulties dealing with human existence and postmodern life seems fundamentally antithetical to the phenomenological, humanistic, and philosophical approach upon which existential analysis or therapy is founded. They argue, often eloquently, that diagnosing human beings based on our present psychiatric nosological systems is unreliable, reductionistic, dehumanizing, stigmatizing, not valid, and unnecessary. More broadly, there is among existential therapists a strong philosophical objection to the simplistic application of psychiatry's reductionistic, mechanistic, and materialistic "medical model" to the theory and practice of psychotherapy. Indeed, this growing resistance to psychodiagnosisis is not limited to existential therapists per se, but is shared by a diversity of mental health practitioners, including many Jungians, Rogerians, and positive psychologists, among others (see, for example, Kamens et al., 2017, 2019).

In my judgment, this radical antipsychiatric movement (spearheaded by the existentially informed late-twentieth century writings of Thomas Szasz, R.D. Laing,

David Cooper, and others) represents both a major weakness and corrective strength of contemporary existential therapy. The strength of this rebellious stance is that in disavowing and rejecting the reductionistic, materialistic, technological, and deterministic application of the medical model to psychology and psychotherapy, existential therapy also rejects the dehumanizing tendency to pathologize and pigeon-hole human beings, behavior, and subjective experiences into preconceived, artificial, and constrictive categories and constructs. Whenever clinicians diagnose someone, we run the risk of perceiving that person merely as some "disorder" or collection of symptoms, rather than as a unique, complex, autonomous, free, and responsible person existing and inextricably embedded in an intrinsically contextual world. In contrast, existential therapy lends itself to taking a more phenomenological, unpresupposing, holistic, systemic, caring, humane, dignified, and, therefore, hopefully more efficacious approach toward helping troubled individuals live more productive, fulfilling, and meaningful lives.

On the other hand, the major weakness of this radical rejection of psychiatric or psychological diagnosis is ignoring or discounting the cumulative and hard-won clinical wisdom contained and encoded in diagnostic terminology. Such ignorance does not serve the best interests of either therapist or patient, and can be potentially disastrous for both. For example, accurately diagnosing psychopathy or APD brings to bear the wealth of prior research and clinical experience of professional colleagues, which can help the counselor, psychotherapist, or forensic practitioner avoid, or at least be better prepared for, some of the predictable pitfalls that working with these extremely challenging individuals inevitably presents. Clearly, for the forensic clinician in particular, such negativity, hostility, or resistance toward diagnosing and lack of proficient diagnostic skills, would be unethical, impractical, and professionally unacceptable. This begs a crucial question in the context of this chapter and volume, one which we will attempt to address here: *How can an existential orientation or approach be relevant to forensic practice?*

16.3.2 Existential Analysis

Existential analysis emerged during the late 1930s in Europe, and in America some two decades later, thanks primarily to psychologist and psychoanalyst Rollo May and the groundbreaking publication in 1958 of *Existence: A New Dimension in Psychiatry and Psychology*. Its iconoclastic founders, physicians and psychoanalysts Ludwig Binswanger and Medard Boss, were profoundly dissatisfied with the perceived dogmatism and literalism of both Freudian and Jungian analysis, which they felt prevented the analyst from accurately comprehending and knowing the patient or analysand *as that person actually experiences existing in his or her own subjective world.*

Strongly influenced by and drawing heavily upon European existential philosophy—especially that of Husserl's celebrated student, Martin Heidegger—the "existential analysts" asserted that it was the psychoanalyst's unintended tendency to see the patient through the distorted lens of his or her own preexisting theoretical orientation, thus unwittingly forcing the person to fit onto a Procrustean bed made solely of preformed Freudian or Jungian notions and constructs. In other words, both Binswanger and Boss felt that psychoanalysts were not truly encountering, attending to, and accurately revealing the actual living person in his or her unique contextual reality—that is, what Heidegger (1927/2010) called *being-in-the-world* (*Dasein*). For example, in dogmatically keeping with the theoretical doctrines underlying and informing these therapies, the Freudian seeks and finds unconscious sexual or aggressive material to comprehend, interpret, or explain the patient's symptoms; and the Jungian analyst looks predominantly for spiritual, mythological, and archetypal interpretations (See May's (1983) discussion in *The Discovery of Being;* also Sartre's (1953/1962) existential critique of Freudian analysis titled *Existential* Psychoanalysis; for further discussion of some of the similarities and differences between Jungian analysis and existential therapy, see Diamond, 2018).

In order to preclude this clinical pitfall, the existential analyst or therapist deliberately chooses to refrain from applying such preconceived reductionistic notions in an effort to be more receptive, open to, and informed by the patient's own reported subjective experience of reality in the present moment. The existential therapist seeks to see the person not merely as some mechanistic collection of disparate symptoms but as a sentient *human* being, existing and embedded in an interpersonal and contextual world. Indeed, existential therapy is primarily concerned with discovering, disclosing, and more deeply understanding the *individual behind the symptom*, the subjectivity of this "existing person," i.e., in his or her unique *being*, which can be understood as the existential source and ground of the person's sense of self, agency, identity, awareness, power, will, personal freedom, and responsibility. Thus, the core existential concept of *being* goes far beyond the Freudian *ego* or Jungian *persona*, and its essential experience has been described by May (1983) as the "'I am' experience" (p. 100). This basic subjective experience of one's own existence or *being*, writes May (1983), "is not in itself the solution to a person's problems; it is rather the *precondition* [and *prerequisite*] for their [therapeutic] solution" (p. 100), and is, therefore precisely what existential therapy aspires to promote. But, how exactly is this done? The fundamental technique or method of existential analysis or psychotherapy is phenomenology (see, for example, Spinelli, 2005; Diamond, 2016, 2018; Langle & Klaassen, 2019). Phenomenology is the therapeutic practice of purposely setting aside or bracketing off as many preconceptions or presuppositions as possible immediately prior to and during each session, so as to be more receptive, true, and fully present to the here-and-now encounter with the suffering or perplexed person sitting before us. Philosopher Edmund Husserl is generally credited with introducing phenomenology around the same time Freud first published his seminal work *The Interpretation of Dreams* in 1900; Husserl's method was subsequently modified by Heidegger, and enthusiastically adopted by the early European existential analysts. For most contemporary existential therapists, "phenomenology" refers to the disciplined philosophical method by which certain elemental "ultimate concerns" (Tillich, 1952) or existential "givens" (Yalom, 1980) such as death, anxiety, responsibility, aloneness, suffering, freedom, and meaninglessness are illuminated, and through which the person's basic experience of being-in-the-world can best be clearly revealed, and thus, more adeptly apprehended and addressed.

16.3.3 Existential Therapy

Like the continental existential analysis from which it was derived, today's existential therapy is a philosophically-informed phenomenological approach primarily focused upon the universal human experience of finding oneself "thrown" or suddenly inserted into existence, being-in-the-world of physicality, finitude, facticity, and of others (Heidegger, 1927/2010). It is especially concerned with the individual's potentiality and personal responsibility for authentically willing and exercising the inherent freedom to choose, to find or create meaning and purpose, and to courageously, constructively, and unequivocally be in the world despite life's intrinsic suffering, frustration, negativity, and absurdity. While existential therapy has historically been closely linked with American humanistic psychology and shares some of its basic values and methodology, there are significant philosophical and pragmatic differences between the two, particularly as regards acknowledging and dealing clinically with the problem of human evil (See, for example, the philosophical debate between May, 1982; Rogers, 1982).

While existential analysis was never initially intended to be a total rejection of the rich psychoanalytic theory and practice from which it arose as much as an effort to make the profound and penetrating "depth psychology" of Freud and Jung more therapeutic, perceptive, and humane, existential therapy today has, for some, evolved into a distinct and self-contained clinical approach based almost exclusively on existential and phenomenological philosophy rather than psychology. However, others, including myself, consider contemporary existential therapy to be as much derived from depth psychology and the contributions of iconoclastic clinicians like Freud, Jung, Rank, Adler, Frankl, Laing, Perls, May, and Yalom as from academic continental philosophy, and remains more of an attitude and orientation to psychotherapy rather than yet another dogmatic, insular, rigid, and doctrinaire approach to treatment. Because of this, existential *therapy* is, in my view, essentially different from existential *philosophy*: the former is and has, since its inception, always been a psychodynamically informed practical approach to conducting clinical work with suffering patients or clients, whereas the latter consists mainly of a more esoteric, intellectual, technical, academic, and arcane philosophical discourse (Diamond, 2016).

A key concept in the theory and practice of existential therapy is the *existential crisis*: "Central to existential therapy is the concept of an *existential crisis* as both a perilous passage and a precious opportunity for transformation and growth… In general, [a]n existential crisis is some subjective or objective stressor that threatens our basic sense of security, self-esteem, identity, or survival" (Diamond, 2016, p. 325). Commonly, it is some sort of existential crisis that motivates someone to seek psychotherapy. An existential crisis can be precipitated by or underlie normal developmental stages (e.g., adolescence, mid-life, aging), or transitions having to do with career, marriage, parenthood, or retirement. Moreover, adverse life events like divorce, loss, sickness, financial stress, unemployment, or moral, ethical, or spiritual confusion can trigger an existential crisis; as can profoundly traumatizing events such as tragic accidents, being the victim of violent crime, terrorism, or war, and destructive natural disasters such as tornadoes, earthquakes, floods, famine, hurricanes, or global pandemics. Confrontations with death and one's own mortality can evoke an existential crisis. However, the person seeking treatment is often unaware that an existential crisis has been constellated. Instead, the suffering patient tends to experience and complain of sundry symptoms such as anxiety, depression, addiction, or relationship problems. But, from the perspective of existential therapy, such distressing phenomena are frequently symptomatic of a latent existential crisis or conflict crying out to be confronted if these symptoms are to be more or less resolved without depending solely and interminably on psychiatric drugs and/or endless psychotherapy.

Existential therapy is essentially a humanistic and *relational* approach to treatment. Thus, it is not some strict adherence to a particular theoretical orientation or technical methodology that matters most in existential therapy, but rather *the real relationship between patient and therapist itself.* The existential therapist tries to be fully present to the momentous face-to-face encounter between two living human beings in which both actively participate and dynamically interact. As Yalom (2009) succinctly states it, "*Therapy should not be theory-driven but relationship-driven*" (p. xviii). Nor should it be technique-driven, as is the state of affairs in most psychotherapy today. Existential therapy, according to Yalom and Josselson (2013, p. 286) is, at least to some significant extent, "always an alternating sequence of interaction and reflection on that interaction." It consists of a collaborative dialogue and intimate discussion, not only of the patient's concerns and problems, but of the nature and quality of the therapeutic relationship itself. This supportive, empathic, caring commitment to focusing on and constantly reinforcing the quality of the working alliance, faithfully apprehending, acknowledging, and validating the person's subjective *being* in the here-and-now, and accompanying him or her as faithful companion, midwife, fellow traveler, and guide through their personal existential crises is fundamental to the efficacy of the therapy process.

Creating and maintaining such a therapeutic relationship is perhaps the primary challenge in the treatment of psychopathy. These individuals, by definition, tend to form only superficial or casual relationships that are based mainly on Machiavellianism, objectification, distrust, callousness, and narcissistic self-interest. Thus, paradoxically, it is precisely the existential clinician's humanistic, caring, and receptive attitude that can at times render treatment ineffectual due to the psychopath's uncanny capacity to "con," charm, persuade, intimidate, and manipulate the naïve, well-intentioned, or even seasoned psychotherapist. Further, how can the forensic clinician in particular willingly enter into and cultivate a close relationship with the predatory murderer, rapist, pedophile, necrophile, misogynist, career criminal, i.e. the psychopath? To do so requires not only taking a phenomenological approach, temporarily placing our reflexive moral judgments, revulsions, countertransference, and preconceptions aside, but, at the same time, acknowledging the harsh reality of the evil deeds he or she may have allegedly or actually committed with an attitude of empathy, compassion, caring, and acceptance. From an existential stance, "while extreme psychopathic behavior seems monstrous to us, at bottom, sociopathy is a human affliction, manifested in a suffering fellow human being, not some inhuman monster" (Diamond, 2003, p. 32). Yet, the cruel, depraved, and destructive acts of the sociopath or psychopath may seem monstrous to us, and this leads us to defensively dehumanize and demonize these violent offenders—which makes us a little monstrous too. In taking this existential approach to forensic evaluation over the years, my own sometimes initially negative countertransferential fantasies, expectations of, or reactions to certain defendants prior to meeting with them—something I see as a deeply human and natural response to being confronted with the stark and disturbing reality of evil, which can itself at times be diagnostic— dissipated upon actually encountering them face-to-face. What came across invariably was rather their raw humanity, their desperate existential battle to be in the world, to exist, to survive, to assert and empower themselves, to seek some sense of significance and recognition, more or less masked by their maladaptive defense mechanisms, malevolent behavior, aggressive attitude, prior criminal record, and typically extensive psychiatric history.

Indeed, this existential relationship between patient and therapist is different than the considerably more detached "classic psychoanalytical notion of providing a passive 'blank screen' onto which patients can project or transfer their unconscious conflicts" (Diamond, 2016, p. 335). Though existential depth psychology, for example, acknowledges and addresses this meaningful phenomenon when necessary, we could describe the existential relationship, like all human interactions, as containing both a *transferential* and *real interpersonal* component, each being of equal importance in the treatment process. In existential therapy, the real human relationship between patient and therapist always takes precedence over manualized interventions or technical tricks. In clinical practice, existential treatment may look very similar to various other contemporary "talking cures," insofar as it consists essentially of an ongoing interactive verbal exchange between a client or patient and psychotherapist. However,

> Contemporary existential therapy differs radically from more technically based approaches in that the individual practitioner's decision of what (if any) intervention to use must be a continual and conscious choice in response to whatever is phenomenologically emerging in the moment. Sometimes simple *presence*, being as intently and fully focused on the here-and-now encounter as possible, precludes the need for applying any specific technique, leading to existential therapy's enigmatic yet effective *technique of no technique* (Diamond, 2016, p. 331).

As Rollo May (1983) helpfully explains, "existential technique should have flexibility and versatility, varying from patient to patient and from one phase to another in treatment with the same patient" (p. 153).

Finally, of ultimate concern for virtually every existential clinician, despite their divergence, is how best to discover, deepen, and comprehend the subjective experience of the person sitting before them, to illuminate and reveal his or her unique being-in-the-world. Thus, existential therapy is essentially an *experiential* approach: it encourages, values, and stresses subjective *experience* over analytical interpretation, explanation, or insight (which, of course, includes an immediate awareness of *physical* embodiment as well as *emotional* subjectivity), and what is really happening here-and-now in the patient's world rather than what took place in the remote or recent past. Unlike psychoanalysts, existential therapists generally do not routinely offer Freudian or Jungian interpretations or seek to focus intensively on early childhood during each and every weekly or biweekly session, but rather attend mindfully with empathy, *presence*, curiosity, caring, and genuine *encounter* to what is happening in the moment without attempting to explain or interpret it for the patient, thus leaving it largely to the person him or herself to make sense of, or come to terms with.

16.3.4 Existential Depth Psychology

Existential depth psychology, the unique existential approach developed and practiced by the author (see Diamond, 1996, 1999, 2016, 2018) is a controversial and, for some, seemingly theoretically incompatible (see e.g., Cohn, 1999) synthesis of existential therapy with the "depth psychology" of Freud, Adler, Rank, and specifically C.G. Jung's Analytical Psychology and Rollo May's (1970) existential psychoanalysis, with their focus on the "unconscious," "shadow," the "daimonic," and the perennial problem of human evil (See the section below for more on the fundamental existential paradigm of the *daimonic*.). In particular, the pervasive, and vexing phenomenon of pathological anger and rage in the human experience is an ultimate concern and primary focus of treatment. This core concern in existential depth psychology with rooting out and revealing the source of anger, rage, destructiveness, and evil is especially pertinent to the problem of psychopathy.

To begin with, in contradistinction to most existential therapies today, existential depth psychology considers psychodiagnosis a potentially helpful and even essential part of the treatment process, providing a powerful way of "acknowledging and naming a person's *existential suffering*...," one that serves to "proffer some meaning and significance for the person's suffering" (Diamond, 2016, p. 340). Indeed, from the perspective of existential depth psychology, psychopathology in general and so-called mental disorders specifically represent, distinct, capsulized, and distilled descriptions of universal or archetypal (Jung, 1961) human patterns of subjective experience and objective behaviors such as those typically seen in depressive or anxiety disorders, psychosis, and psychopathy or antisocial personality disorder. Expertly diagnosing such archetypal experiences and behaviors—while not taking the diagnostic label itself too literally, definitively, deterministically, or concretely—provides the clinician an indispensable means of acknowledging and describing patients' symptoms as something that they share in common with countless others across cultures throughout millennia, as well as a concise and convenient means of communicating about the presence and severity of these pathological patterns to other professionals.

In existential depth psychology, "in addition to a definite emphasis on facing forthrightly the existential facts of life—anxiety, freedom, destiny, responsibility, will, aloneness, meaninglessness, and mortality—techniques would be employed for the express purpose of cultivating the daimonic rather than suppressing, defusing, or eradicating it" (Diamond, 1996, pp. 221–222). In distinction to existential analysis or therapy per se, existential depth psychology, while employing much of the same methodology, can be best distinguished by the "degree to which it directly addresses the daimonic" (Diamond, 1996, p. 219). More generally, "In existential depth psychology, we seek to understand and interact with our patients in ways that transcend—or underlie—the dogmas and doctrines of different school of psychotherapy, while at the same time making use of these various potentially helpful concepts and techniques when appropriate" (Diamond, 1996, p. 223). The ultimate aim is to "provide a process by which patients could not only engage the daimonic, but, by discerning their deepest intentionality, govern … [it] with greater integrity" (Diamond, 1996, p. 233).

Of special concern for existential depth psychology is the central role of repressed anger or rage in psychopathology, and the importance of consciously acknowledging, confronting, and learning to express such daimonic emotions constructively or creatively rather than denying or suppressing them. This is particularly relevant to the treatment of psychopathy, in which chronically repressed anger or rage plays such a prominent part. For existential depth psychology, the key to working effectively with anger-based disorders such as psychopathy, sociopathy, dyssocial or antisocial personality is facilitating and encouraging the patient's ability and willingness to consciously confront and redirect the daimonic—especially the anger or rage— into more constructive activity. The daimonic—especially anger, sex, and the desire for power and control in the case of psychopathic personalities—will inevitably be expressed: if not constructively, creatively, or productively, then negatively, cruelly, and destructively. This difficult and risky work comprises the primary thrust of existential depth psychology (See Diamond, 1996).

The secret, as May (in Diamond, 1996) states, is to try "to shift or redirect the anger and the rage into those positive pursuits that the person has been omitting from his or her life" (p. xxii). And how is this pragmatically accomplished? By helping the patient to incrementally become more aware of how he or she truly feels and what he or she truly wants in life. Typically, these long-standing desires, dreams, or goals from childhood or adolescence are repressed, and replaced with that of simply surviving day-to-day or achieving success, notoriety, or recognition by committing shocking crimes. By consistently directing the psychopath's attention to her or his subjectivity in the here-and-now over time, a rediscovery of this long-lost inner *self*, as Jung (1961) called it, becomes possible. It is precisely this original and authentic self that *preexisted and preceded their pathology*, that psychopaths must become reacquainted with if therapy is to succeed in any real sense. The psychopath may ultimately decide to return to school, seek a meaningful vocation or career, volunteer for some valued cause, commit to finding a spouse and starting a family, devote him or herself to some spiritual or religious lifestyle, or take up painting, sculpture, writing, filmmaking, or another means of expressing the daimonic more creatively in the world. But ultimately, whatever path is chosen by the psychopath, it must be his or her own decision, as opposed to something imposed from without. In the absence of the freely chosen creation and willing integration, of, and total commitment to, this "new life," the psychopathic patient will almost always eventually regress to his or her former mode of existence.

The elemental yet exceedingly difficult to define notion of "will" is key to existential depth psychology and its core emphasis on personal freedom and choice.

Referring to psychoanalyst Otto Rank, one of the, until recently, under-recognized forerunners of existential therapy and creator of "Will Therapy," May (1939) writes: "Rank holds that… the individual creates his own personality by creative willing, and that neurosis is due precisely to the fact that the patient cannot will constructively" (p. 52). According to Rank (1936), chronically thwarted, repressed, or frustrated *will* frequently expresses itself as "counter-will," such as in rebellious, obstinate, oppositional, irresponsible, hostile, defiant, illegal, and sometimes violent—i.e., antisocial or psychopathic—behavior. In existential depth psychology, *will* is understood as the essential power that makes us both free and responsible beings. But free will always exists in dialectical relationship with fate or determinism (i.e., those things in life over which we have little or no control). Psychopathy, therefore, can be perceived as a furious, petulant protest against fate or existential reality, a self-defeating and destructive assertion of will, power, and personal freedom. However, this same willfulness, when more constructively expressed and directed, is what potentially empowers the psychopath (or any patient) to change his or her destiny. (For further discussion on this subject, see Rank's *Will Therapy* (1936) and *May's Love and Will* (1969)).

We could say that more so than other existential therapies, existential depth psychology equally utilizes both *experiential* and *cognitive* interventions. Existential depth psychology is, like all existential therapies, fundamentally experiential in practice; but it equally values and incorporates cognitive restructuring, insight, understanding, integration, and meaning-making. For instance, in existential depth psychology, judicious use of interpretation to foster awareness of those forgotten or repressed childhood experiences, unconscious conflicts, and painful emotional demons that continue to constrain and torment the patient today is indispensable. In conjunction with experiential interventions, cognitive integration of the patient's traumatic, frustrating, and confusing subjective experiences, past, present, and future, is considered essential to coming to terms with them. Thus, in practice, on occasion we might see some discussion of psychological concepts and philosophical or mythological motifs, the existential questions of "free will," personal responsibility, authenticity, and nihilism, or classic Jungian notions such as *introversion* and *extraversion*, *anima* and *animus*, *persona*, ego, self, and *shadow*. However, though such cognitive conversations can unquestionably be useful at certain points in the process with specific patients, as a general rule, therapy sessions are not overly laden with intellectual discussions of existential, Freudian, or Jungian themes, but focus more experientially on the patient's emotions and subjectivity in the here-and-now.

Lastly, in existential depth psychology in particular, we would likely see some spontaneous and in-depth discussion of dreams (see, for instance, Jung, 1964/1968; May et al., 1958; Perls, 1971; Moustakas, 1994). The dream, may, as Freud (1900) posited, contain disguised symbolic references to unfulfilled wishes, repressed desires, sexual and aggressive impulses, unconscious conflicts, and unresolved past trauma, but can also simultaneously and literally depict and speak to the patient's present (and future) existential anxieties, concerns, frustrations, and aspirations. Or, it could, as Jung (1964/1968) suggested, serve as a compensatory counterbalance to consciousness, provide valuable guidance, or indicate what attitudinal or behavioral changes would, if chosen, make us more whole, individuated, and balanced beings. The patient may spontaneously choose to share his or her dreams with the therapist, or at times might be invited by the therapist to do so, though this is not done routinely as in psychoanalysis. In any case, the patient or client is initially encouraged to present the dream exactly as it was, without interpretation or conscious censoring, and to elaborate on its contents. Working with dream material might involve inquiring about the patient's own associations and interpretations, and, in some cases, the therapist sharing his or her own subjective responses or speculations regarding the possible significance or relevance of the dream. In existential depth psychology, the therapist does not prejudge or place his or her own theoretical preconceptions on the dream. The patient is permitted the "last word" as to the possible meaning of the dream, if any, and bears the sole responsibility for deciding how he or she will respond to it (Diamond, 1996).

Consider, for example, the following dream of a former psychotherapy patient, which illustrates the psychopathic potentialities lurking below the surface in him at that particular time, and in each of us:

> I had this wild dream last night.... I wasn't going to tell you.... It was so ugly.... I was afraid to tell you. In my dream, I wanted to see what it was like to *kill*; so I took my shotgun and wiped out twelve little kids ... It was such a random act of violence that nobody had a clue where to start looking, why it was done, or who did it. There were no traces. I kept vacillating back and forth whether to keep my mouth shut and go on living with the demons: it was obviously haunting, because I was ashamed and disgraced with what I did.... What I got out of ... [the dream] is that there's this dark side to me—to *everyone*—and acting on it and then taking responsibility for it was the question: whether I would do that or not. I chose not to. I chose to flee from it.... The dark side was very powerful. I let it go and then I wished I hadn't. (Diamond, 1996, pp. 245–246)

16.4 Some Existential Perspectives on Psychopathy: Confronting Life's Ultimate Concerns

According to the World Confederation for Existential Therapy (2016), existential therapy is founded, at least partly, upon certain "philosophies of existence" that stress specific "ultimate concerns." Existential philosopher and theologian Paul Tillich (1952) informs us that, for him, an "ultimate concern" is something—e.g., a belief, value, interest, pursuit, role, responsibility, caring, commitment, conviction, quality, or way of life—that is taken or approached with utmost "unconditional seriousness"; "What, for instance, would you be ready to suffer or even die for?" (p. 8). Adopting a somewhat different usage, Yalom (1980) contends that for existential therapy, an "ultimate concern" has to do with those intrinsically ineluctable or existentially "given" aspects of the human predicament we all share in common and find most mysterious, significant, frightening, confounding, challenging, and inspiring. Choice, freedom, personal and social responsibility, courage, commitment, integrity, dignity, and authentically facing rather than evading existential anxiety, anger, despair, guilt, alienation, and the perennial problem of evil are ultimate concerns for existential therapy; as are the enormous challenges of finding meaning, purpose, and personal fulfillment in a seemingly absurd and meaningless world wherein death, suffering, loss, anxiety, frustration, and aloneness are inevitable. How, then, can the psychopath be understood from this distinctly existential perspective? How can these so-called ultimate concerns shed light on the psychopathic personality's complex psychology? And, in what ways might such profound philosophical perspectives pragmatically inform and facilitate the psychological comprehension required for the efficacious forensic treatment of this notoriously refractory and pernicious population?

16.4.1 Freedom and Responsibility

Let us start our existential exploration of psychopathy by examining one of the central tenets of existentialism as famously stated by French philosopher Jean-Paul Sartre (1946/2007, p. 349): "Existence precedes essence." Sartre, who was heavily influenced by Heidegger, radically asserted that despite deterministic forces, such as biology and environment, the human being exists, has freedom, and is thus ultimately solely responsible for what he or she becomes: "I *am* my choices" (Sartre, 1953/1962, p. 5). According to Sartre (1953/1962) we are "condemned to be free" (p. 353) and must bravely bear this fateful burden of freedom and responsibility. There is no inherent "human nature," no divinely imbued purpose or *raison d'etre*, no "higher power" or "ultimate rescuer" (Yalom, 1980) to save us. Human beings are existentially alone and "abandoned" (or, as Nietzsche (1883/2019) proclaimed, "God is dead."), and we have nothing and nobody to depend upon, thank, or blame for our behaviors and decisions or their consequences but ourselves.

For existential therapy, this congenital and inescapable personal freedom is present even in presumably "autonomous" complexes and unconscious defense mechanisms such as denial, dissociation, or repression. That is to say, at some existential level of awareness, we always *choose* what to preclude from consciousness, and what not to. What to know about ourselves and what we wish not to know. And it is we who are responsible for these choices. Try as we may, we can never escape from our existential freedom and responsibility for it. This is why Sartre (1946/2007) insists that freedom, and freedom only, is the very quintessence of being human: "Man is freedom" (p. 353).

This philosophical but also clinically relevant question of radical freedom and responsibility plays a pivotal role in the problem of psychopathy. As Viennese existential analyst Viktor Frankl (1946/1985) concludes, "Freedom, however, is not the last word.... Freedom is in danger of degenerating into mere arbitrariness [and evil] unless it is lived in terms of responsibleness" (pp. 155–156). Freedom and responsibility are inextricably linked. In psychopathy—for reasons we will soon be discussing—the person's innate existential freedom is consistently negatively exercised, without regard or respect for the well-being, integrity, and safety of society and other sentient beings, and personal responsibility is repeatedly evaded, denied, and rejected outright.

Indeed, the key philosophical question of *personal responsibility* seems quite pertinent to the problem of psychopathy or antisocial personality disorder, in which two of the DSM-5 (2013) diagnostic criteria specifically refer to "consistent irresponsibility, as indicated by repeated failure to sustain consistent work behavior or honor financial obligation…. [and] lack of remorse, as indicated by being indifferent to or rationalizing having hurt, mistreated, or stolen from another" (p. 325). Psychopaths tend to be socially and interpersonally irresponsible, and, when caught or confronted, often flatly deny responsibility for their illegal or irresponsible behavior, compulsively and creatively lying and prevaricating to avoid being forced to accept responsibility and consequences for their actions, even in the face of irrefutable evidence to the contrary.

Today, psychopathy or antisocial personality, like most other mental disorders, is perceived by mainstream psychiatry and psychology as primarily a neurobiologically-based condition predetermined (or at least strongly predisposed to) by genetics (see, for instance, Blair, 2003; Dolan, 2018; Tiihonen et al., 2020). But, in fact, both adopted *and* biological offspring of antisocial or psychopathic parents run an increased risk of developing this disorder (American Psychiatric Association, 1994, p. 648). Further, while monozygotic twins are approximately twice as likely as dizygotic twins to develop psychopathy, concordance rates across studies tend not to exceed 50% for identical twins, indicating nurture to be at least as significant a factor as nature in the etiology of this disorder (e.g., see Raine, 1993; Millon & Simonsen, 1998). So, there is little doubt that despite certain neurological or genetically inherited traits characteristic of psychopathy, family, cultural, contextual, and collective environment play a prominent role in its etiology and development.

To this point, psychopaths have never learned to take responsibility for their behavior, a lesson that normally begins being inculcated in early childhood and adolescence. All children require some moral education and to be trained to obey the rules and laws, first of the family, then the educational system, and later, of society. In that sense, we human beings, as Freud (1929/2002) held, are all born with certain primitive antisocial or psychopathic potentialities, which must be discouraged and suppressed in the interest of civilization and socialization. Children, not in reality the seemingly innocent and angelic creatures we wish to see them as, must be instructed not to lie, cheat, steal, manipulate, tease, push, punch, bully, or otherwise harm or even kill other children or animals, to resist any tendencies to engage in such asocial behaviors, and to be polite, cooperative, and productive members of society. But, due often to inadequate (too little *or* too much) parental limit-setting, punishment, moral or religious education, and discipline, psychopaths seem to have never assimilated this crucial life lesson.

From an existential standpoint, "Freedom is like a muscle that must be developed and regularly exercised, a blessing but also a burden" (Diamond, 2016, p. 328). Ultimately, our freedom is never free or without cost. One price we human beings pay for possessing freedom is the experience of existential anxiety and guilt. However, since psychopaths apparently tend to feel less anxiety, guilt, and responsibility regarding their actions, in some significant ways psychopathic patients actually experience *less* freedom than others due, perhaps, to the deeply compulsive quality of their antisocial behavior patterns. The psychopath demonstrates a perverse kind of existential freedom, choosing to act without restraint on certain fantasies or impulsions all human beings inherently possess the capacity to experience, but normally resist. The difference is that for psychopaths these dark and dangerous fantasies tend to be stronger, more intrusive, obsessive, compelling, and eventually are malevolently enacted in the world. Nevertheless, as Frankl (1946/1985) a trained psychiatrist and neurologist, reminds us,

> …every human being has the freedom to change at any instant… the individual personality…remains essentially unpredictable… There is nothing conceivable which would so condition a man as to leave him without the slightest freedom. Therefore, a residue of freedom, however limited it may be, is left to man in neurotic and even psychotic cases (p. 156).

Indeed, "One of the most confounding issues that patients bring to psychotherapy, whether explicitly or not, is that of personal responsibility. Commonly, patients make the mistake of taking either too little or too much responsibility for life events" (Diamond, 2016, p. 328). In the case of antisocial or psychopathic patients, outwardly this inclination tends heavily toward the former, i.e., taking insufficient or no responsibility for what happens to them and their victims. But inwardly, they often feel victimized by and overly responsible for their unfortunate childhood circumstances, and this sense of hyper-responsibility becomes the source of toxic shame and low self-esteem. As for most psychotherapy patients, existential treatment of psychopaths requires them to become mature, insightful, and courageous enough to accept total responsibility for their bad behavior and its consequences; but, at the same time, not to take on too much responsibility for those things in life over which they had—or still have—little or no control (e.g., childhood neglect, abuse, deprivation, parental psychopathology, racial, religious, or gender discrimination, etc.) In short, to take full responsibility for their *destiny*, but not for their *fate*.

16.4.2 Fate and Destiny

The powerful influence of being raised in an environment where the child's basic needs for love, attention, affection, understanding, dignity, and discipline are either severely neglected or routinely overindulged, or in which the child is repeatedly abused, rejected, or abandoned, cannot be minimized. "Studies in youth and adults have demonstrated a strong association between early traumatic incidents and later dissocial behavior" (Sevecke et al., 2016). Such impoverished, hostile, or sometimes toxically narcissistic settings are found frequently in the psychopath's painful family history. In this regard, we can conceive of psychopathy, like most other mental disorders, as resulting from some intricate interplay between nature and nurture, or from the dialectical interaction of *fate* and *destiny:*

> Traditionally, the term *fate* refers to the existential givens of life, those aspects of existence over which we can exert little or no control (See Yalom, 1980, who somewhat simplistically categorizes these core existential facts of life as freedom, meaninglessness, isolation, and death). *Destiny*, in contrast, 'is related to the word *destination*' (Lowen, 1980, p. 49). It refers to what we may become. We are responsible for our destiny but not our fate (Diamond, 2016, p. 328).

Fate can be compared to the playing cards one is randomly dealt by existence; and *destiny* to the way one chooses to play them. Our genetics and the predispositions to which they render us susceptible are certainly part of our fate; our destiny is how we deal with our inherited biological and genetic makeup (i.e., what we do or do not do to manage our vulnerabilities and to cultivate our strengths; Diamond, 2016). Of course, the philosophical concept of *fatalism* or *predestination* can be misused to evade responsibility for one's actions and decisions, to diminish one's existential freedom, and to see oneself as fate's hapless victim. But, conversely, to blame ourselves for all misfortune or take credit for good luck and deny the influence of fate makes us guilty of what the ancient Greeks called *hubris*: excessive human pride, egoism, or what we today would diagnose as *narcissism*.

Hence, it is never exclusively *essence*, some innate defining quality or nature, as Sartre would presumably say, that genetically determines psychopathy, but rather the specific choices and decisions made by the person in dealing with these idiosyncratic contextual factors and existential "givens" (Yalom, 1980). This existential perspective can at least partially explain why some individuals with similar or identical genetic influences—and even with the same or very similar parental, family, and contextual factors– become psychopaths and some do not. Therefore, existentially speaking, it is not genetics nor environment that determine whether psychopathy occurs, but ultimately the ways in which individuals decide to exercise their existential *freedom* in coping with their *fate,* and the degree to which they are willing to accept *responsibility* for choosing, willing, and creating their own *destiny*.

16.4.3 Anxiety and Guilt

The phenomenon of anxiety is a universal human experience. Existential therapy places special emphasis on the experience of *anxiety* as central to the problem of psychopathology, both the psychotherapy and creative process, and the human condition generally. Unlike mainstream Western medicine, psychiatry, and clinical psychology today, which reflexively strive to swiftly suppress anxiety with sundry psychotropic drugs and anxiety-quelling cognitive and behavioral interventions, existential therapy does not perceive anxiety solely as some entirely negative experience to avoid or eliminate in any way possible. Rather, anxiety is seen as an ultimately inescapable, existential, enlivening, meaningful (see May, 1977), and potentially positive and growth-promoting phenomenon: "Although painful and at times debilitating, anxiety signifies the existential struggle for [significance], meaning, integrity, [selfhood], and authenticity" (Diamond, 2016, p. 325). As existential philosopher Soren Kierkegaard (1884/1980) put it, anxiety can become our greatest teacher—if we are willing to listen carefully to what it has to say rather than reflexively running away from it.

Kierkegaard (1884/1980) saw *Angst* (anxiety or dread) as nothing less than "the dizziness of freedom" (p. 61). When we become cognizant of our existential freedom to choose what to do with our lives and of our responsibility for making these decisions and for their possible consequences, *Angst* arises in us. *Angst* is best translated from the Danish and German as a profound sense of anguish, apprehension, insecurity, and anxiety regarding this heavy existential burden of freedom and responsibility, and the inherent tenuousness, groundlessness, meaninglessness, and absurdity of human existence. Existential therapy holds that this type of *Angst* or anxiety can motivate, excite, and make us more keenly aware of our own being.

Anxiety actually has numerous sources and manifestations. Mortality and the acute anxiety that accompanies it, i.e., *death anxiety*, are ultimate concerns in existential therapy. May (1950/1977) defined *existential anxiety* as "the experience of Being affirming itself against Nonbeing. The latter is that which would reduce or destroy Being, such as aggression, fatigue, boredom, [illness,] and, ultimately death" (p. xv). Anxiety can also stem from intrapsychic and interpersonal conflict, confusion, irrational thinking, cognitive distortions, guilt feelings, and the dread of abandonment, rejection, punishment, humiliation, exposure, annihilation, loss, suffering, alienation, or aloneness. On the one hand, anxiety is an intrinsic part of our intrapsychic defense system, serving to preserve integrity of the ego and personality structure. On the other, it signifies the human being's instinctive existential struggle to survive, thrive, and assert ourselves in a world in which we are beset by forces that threaten to prevent us from finding and fulfilling our destiny.

Anxiety, from the standpoint of existential therapy, is often trying to tell us something vitally important about ourselves and our way of being in the world: it can be a sign or warning that we are somehow out of balance, in "bad faith" with, or at odds with our authentic self, and that there is something we need to *do* about that or somehow change within ourselves or world. Like a fever, anxiety lets us know that there is some inner war raging, a mortal struggle not merely for survival, but for a more meaningful, fulfilling, purposeful, and creative existence. As we see daily in the practice of psychotherapy, such existential anxiety commonly and inescapably accompanies what Jung (1961) termed the *individuation* process.

May (1950/1977) drew a distinction between "normal" (ontological or existential) and pathological (neurotic or psychotic) anxiety. While *existential anxiety* (*Angst*) is typically experienced as vague discomfort or tension, *pathological anxiety* (e.g., panic attacks, phobias, obsessive-compulsive disorder, social or generalized anxiety disorders) can be an extraordinarily painful, chronic, and debilitating experience, often requiring clinical intervention such as psychotherapy, medication, or both. What is the source of such severe pathological anxiety according to existential theory? *A core concept in existential therapy is that pathological neurotic (or sometimes psychotic) anxiety is the direct result of chronically repressing, avoiding, or denying ontological or existential anxiety*. Thus, for existential therapy, to experience some existential anxiety is to experience being human. That is to say, anxiety is not inherently pathological, but intrinsic to the human condition. All of which begs the question: *Do psychopath's feel anxiety?*

Karpman (1948) proposed two different types of psychopathy: primary and secondary. *Primary* psychopathy corresponds closely with Cleckley's (1941) early descriptions of the callous psychopathic personality (Murphy & Vess, 2003), and is still considered to be genetically determined. This primary psychopath was believed by Cleckley (1941) and others (e.g., Lykken, 1995) to be totally devoid of and incapable of feeling anxiety, and some research suggests that primary psychopaths do show reduced autonomic responses in response to threatening or fearful stimuli, as well as deficits in recognizing fear-related cues (Karasavva, 2019; Lykken,

1995). *Secondary* psychopathy is seen as more psychologically and circumstantially influenced, impulsive, emotionally unstable, and anxiety prone (Frick et al., 1999; Sandvik et al., 2015; Skeem et al., 2011). Psychodynamically, the secondary psychopath's subjective experience of anxiety can be seen as indicative of a less successful defense mechanism against feeling than is present in the primary psychopath, and, therefore, from an existential standpoint, of a better prognosis in treatment than those with seemingly no or minimal anxiety. But the majority of psychopaths (primary and secondary) can, in my estimation, generally successfully repress or suppress anxiety, along with various other painful or uncomfortable emotions such as sadness, guilt, remorse, empathy, tenderness, compassion, caring, or love.

Normally, some anxiety is necessary, and can serve as a warning signal (see Freud's (1926) seminal notion of *signal anxiety*) and deterrent regarding dangerous, inappropriate, immoral, or evil impulses, fantasies, and behaviors. Without this inner psychobiological alarm system, the psychopath is free to act on such impulsions with little to no natural inhibition. As with the effects of alcohol or other disinhibiting substances, the psychopath's relative lack of anxiety allows him or her to do what most of us dread and resist doing. It gives psychopaths a curious kind of *pathological courage*, seemingly unrestrained by normal feelings of fear, reticence, remorse, shame, guilt, or anxiety, an uninhibited impulsivity, which can lead to extremely negative consequences, for both themselves and their victims. This same psychopathic fearlessness applies also to risk-taking and the willingness (or inner need) to court injury or even death, as seen in a reckless, death-defying disregard for their own safety and that of others (DSM-5). This apparent absence of death anxiety in particular permits the psychopath to act in ways which are extremely hazardous, socially unacceptable, illegal, or unethical, but, at the same time, potentially advantageous. When these high-risk behaviors are externally rewarded in some way—be it with financial gain, fame, excitement, pleasure, pride, sex, or notoriety— they are, in the lingo of behaviorism, at least intermittently, and therefore, powerfully reinforced, rendering them exceedingly resistant to extinction.

Guilt, closely correlated to anxiety, is another ultimate concern in existential therapy, one associated with the concept of *conscience* and phenomenon of *shame*. As with anxiety, from an existential perspective, there are both existential and pathological forms of guilt: *existential* guilt is experienced when we fail to acknowledge our personal potentialities, to honor our authentic values and true selves, or to courageously find and fulfill our destiny; *pathological* guilt results from the chronic refusal to acknowledge, accept, and constructively address one's ontological or existential guilt. Existentially speaking, guilt is perceived as the direct consequence of choosing to be in an inauthentic state of self-deception that Sartre (1953/1962) referred to as "bad faith" (*mauvaise foi*). Like existential anxiety, existential guilt has something important to tell us, and it is our responsibility to ourselves and those around us to carefully listen and respond to it. Guilt is traditionally associated with what organized religion— something most psychopaths reject (Jack et al. 2015)—deems sinful, immoral, or evil, Such religiously-based guilt tends to be neurotic, as Freud found, but still serves an important, archetypal purpose in human morality and ethics (e.g., the Old Testament's Ten Commandments). For some, guilt feelings may be morbid, masochistic, or misguided, often requiring therapeutic resolution—as, for instance, in the case of inordinate sexual guilt—existential guilt or shame is nonetheless an essential part of one's innermost "moral compass," without which we are apt to dangerously lose our way in the world. But if guilt, be it existential, religious, or pathological, is in fact such an inescapable, archetypal, and universal component of the human condition, how can it be possible for the psychopath never to know it?

It is true that the psychopath's deceptive, exploitative, and manipulative behavior can and frequently is described as "shameless." Psychopaths are true masters of deception in their dealings with others. But they are equally guilty of habitually deceiving themselves. Being in *bad faith* with oneself is the antithesis of being genuine, real, or *authentic*. *Authenticity* requires courage, insight, integrity, and a willingness to be brutally honest with oneself, which is the polar opposite of—and ultimately, the antidote to—self-deception. Psychopaths, who, at some level of their being *know* they are guilty of committing certain crimes or evil deeds, must constantly lie to themselves in order to preserve their tenuous sense of self, worth, integrity, and dignity. Certainly, we all participate in some degree of self-deception. But distortion of reality by the psychopath, while not typically as severe as that of the psychotic, is almost always part of the clinical picture. In order to avoid feeling or appearing guilty, reality is distorted to comport with the psychopath's compensatory narcissistic, grandiose, false, and inflated self-image or *persona* (Jung, 1961), and those around him or her are pressured directly and indirectly to perceive reality in precisely the same way. Hence, the psychopath's notoriously self-serving tendency to exaggerate, manipulate, confabulate, or invent his or her own truth, and to strive to convince others of its reality, veracity, and legitimacy.

Guilt feelings are related to emotions of regret or remorse, which psychopaths are presumed to be unable to experience. They seem simply not to care, to lack empathy or conscience. However, decades of clinical experience and recent research (e.g., Baskin-Sommers et al., 2016) suggest otherwise. As I have elsewhere written (Diamond, 2003), "it has long been presumed that the antisocial personality—the psychopath—subsequent to having committed a crime, has no real sense of conscience or guilt, owing perhaps to some genetic anomalie or insufficient superego" (p. 31). Still, I would argue that these deeply damaged individuals do indeed suffer from feelings of existential guilt, in the form of a latent anger, rage, or resentment toward themselves regarding their own bad behavior and abject failure to actualize their better selves. They are very adept at repressing, projecting, or redirecting that rage externally, and, thereby, avoiding any feelings of guilt, shame, or responsibility for their actions.

Nonetheless, the psychopathic conscience is—like the deeper feelings belonging to their long-denied and dissociated "true self"—still present, I would argue, but figuratively frozen and buried beneath the thick, cold ice of the defensive "false self" (Winnicott, 1960). So, it is not true, in my opinion, that the psychopath has no congenital *capacity* for guilt; but rather that he or she has become highly proficient at burying and suppressing any sense of shame or guilt, along with most other vulnerable feelings (e.g., love, empathy, regret, etc.). Despite the skill with which the psychopath suppresses any feelings of guilt, shame, or remorse, from the standpoint of existential depth psychology it remains present because there is a recognition that, despite the congenital capacity for evil, all people possess an innate, instinctive, and teleological inclination toward good, balance, or wholeness which, when thwarted, generates existential guilt feelings (Diamond, 2003). Therefore, in the existential treatment of psychopathy, this chronically dissociated guilt—and the intrinsic tendency toward goodness from which it stems— must be exhumed, resurrected, experienced, tolerated, assimilated, and integrated into the personality so as to further humanize the uncaring, cold, and callous psychopathic persona.

16.4.4 Suffering and Death

Suffering—be it physical, emotional, or spiritual—and *death* are both ultimate concerns for existential therapy. Suffering is an inextricable, intrinsic, and tragic part of human existence; an inevitable, existential fact of life (see Diamond, 2018). The sources of human suffering are legion. Some human misery and suffering has its source in man's inhumanity to man (see, for example, Frankl's (1946/1985) recounting of his own suffering and that of fellow death camp prisoners in *Man's Search for Meaning*); in everyday interpersonal hostility, hatred, and cruelty; and some stems from the malicious and deliberate "disregard for and violation of the rights of others" (American Psychiatric Association, 2013, p. 291), destructiveness, and violence of severe personality disorders such as psychopathy or APD.

The universal experience of suffering, and, ultimately, death, stimulate some of life's farthest-reaching existential, spiritual, scientific, and religious queries: Why must we suffer and eventually die? What is death? Is there a God? If so, what kind of deity would condone suffering? Does suffering have any purpose, significance, value, or meaning? Can suffering be avoided? Is life really worth living despite suffering? These are some ultimate concerns which existential therapy attempts to assist patients or clients to courageously confront and seek to answer for themselves.

As with the experience of anxiety or guilt, we can distinguish between *pathological suffering* and *existential suffering*. Indeed, as Jung (1938) so succinctly and perceptively put it, the pathological suffering of "neurosis is always a substitute for legitimate suffering" (p. 75). That is to say, we pay a painful price for habitually avoiding, denying, or repressing rather than accepting existential suffering. This applies to psychopathology in general, and to psychopathy in particular. Indeed, the nineteenth century term *psychopath*—like the contemporary term *psychopathology*—stems from the Greek root meaning "mental disease," "sick spirit," or "suffering soul." There is every reason to believe that psychopaths suffer, as do all sentient beings. As Martens (2014), a psychiatrist who stresses the therapeutic importance of recognizing the psychopath's suffering, states, "The current picture of the psychopath is incomplete because emotional suffering and loneliness are ignored. When these aspects are considered, our conception of the psychopath goes beyond the heartless and becomes more human." However, while there is some truth to this statement—which serves to remind us that psychopathy is fundamentally a *human* affliction—the paradox is that *psychopaths suffer—and often inflict unspeakable suffering on others—mainly from their refusal to allow themselves to become more aware of and fully experience their own existential suffering.*

Like every human being, psychopaths suffer on both the *personal* and *existential* levels; in the latter case, they suffer from existential alienation, purposelessness, meaninglessness, anomie, etc. Indeed, typically, the psychopath has suffered his or her whole life from feelings of inferiority, insecurity, anxiety, resentment, rage, inadequacy, failure, and rejection. However, as is widely known, psychopaths rarely seek psychotherapy on their own, preferring to keep private their illegal, immoral, and antisocial activities, and to cope in their own dysfunctional way with their severe emotional suffering. Many manage to avoid detection, arrest, incarceration, and other sources of suffering potentiated by their antisocial lifestyle. But, in most (though not all) cases, even these clever criminals eventually experience negative consequences. That is when the psychopath's defensive persona begins to break down, and her or his subjective suffering starts to surface. It is not until then, following repeated and increasingly noxious negative consequences, that psychopaths finally start to suffer sufficiently to either seek help or come to the attention of mental health professionals. Tragically, for most—and particularly for those unfortunate victims upon whom they sadistically prey and have already inflicted immense suffering—that is a little late in the game.

Indeed, psychopaths seem obsessed with inflicting suffering on their unsuspecting victims, and frequently report feeling compelled to do so (Diamond, 2003). Such *sadism*—taking pleasure in causing or observing physical or psychological suffering in others— is a prominent feature of psychopathy in general. *Sexual sadism*—which links sadism with intense sexual arousal—can be frequently seen in psychopathic serial killers like Ted Bundy, Edmund Kemper, John Wayne Gacy, Dennis Rader, and Jeffrey Dahmer, each of whom were reportedly sexually aroused by the feelings of power that intentionally inflicting injury, suffering, and death upon their victims engendered. Kemper, for instance, the so-called Co-ed Killer, engaged in degrading sexual activity with his own despised dead mother's decapitated head after brutally dispatching her. Ted Bundy—like Dahmer, who dismembered his male lovers, storing their genitalia, skulls, and other preserved body parts in his apartment as sentimental keepsakes—is said to have spent time with his tortured and deceased female victims, biting and sexually violating them.

Such extreme sadism or sexual sadism is an outward expression of the psychopathic serial killer's inner suffering and rage, resentment, hostility, and hatred toward his or her victims, who sometimes serve as symbolic representations or surrogates for parents, siblings, former love interests, authority figures, and society at large. Most psychopaths, though outwardly grandiose, glib, charming, and narcissistic, suffer inwardly from low self-esteem, shame, and self-loathing. Contrary to what Cleckley (1941) claimed, from an existential standpoint, some classic psychopaths *do* retain the capacity to suffer from painful feelings such as regret, remorse, shame, guilt, and anxiety, but defensively and reflexively *choose—and are responsible for choosing—* to suppress or dissociate such emotions from consciousness, thereby excluding them from the decision-making process that informs their behavior. Their suffering is well-disguised by their callous or, in some cases, charismatic psychopathic persona, but it is nonetheless covertly present and pervasive. This neurotic suffering is rooted not only in their repeated narcissistic wounding during childhood and adolescence, but derives also from their subsequent evil deeds as adults, and the existential guilt they unconsciously harbor regarding having committed such atrocities. In this sense, we can presume that psychopaths suffer from an *unconscious conscience:* they suffer silently from profound feelings of shame, anger, guilt, and anxiety about their past, present, and future. As in the psychotherapeutic treatment of most mental disorders, but the personality disorders in particular, the clinician's task is to try to encourage the psychopath to admit to and consciously experience, accept, and tolerate his or her legitimate existential and personal suffering, rather than symbolically or literally acting it out so as to avoid facing and feeling it.

Two prime sources of suffering, and areas of special concern and clinical focus for existential therapy are *death* and *death anxiety.* Throughout human history, people have been obsessed with the inexorable phenomenon of death and its significance. Death tends to be a taboo subject in Western culture, as Ernest Becker (1973) brilliantly explains in his book *The Denial of Death*. There, he argues that almost everything we do (or do not do) in life is designed to avoid consciously confronting the terrifying and terrible reality of mortality. As Freud himself (1915) mused, "Our own death is indeed unimaginable… ," concluding that "*in the unconscious every one of us is convinced of his own immortality* [my emphasis] (pp. 304–305).

Most of the time, we manage to keep the awareness of our own mortality at bay. But when this bare existential reality threatens to become conscious, we experience painful *death anxiety*. Death anxiety is not limited solely to the threat of literally losing one's psychological, spiritual, and physical existence, but refers symbolically to the dread of total annihilation, negation, non-being, and the loss of any and all future possibilities. Death anxiety, *whether conscious or not,* is a universal source of significant human suffering, frequently underlying various psychiatric symptoms such as panic attacks, phobias, and generalized anxiety, yet is often not recognized, acknowledged, or adequately addressed by mainstream psychotherapies.

For existential therapists, the reality of death, though profoundly anxiety provoking, must ultimately be consciously confronted, accepted, and even embraced, for he or she who cannot face and accept the existential facts of finitude and death cannot fully appreciate and commit to existence in its totality. Some death anxiety is instinctual and necessary (e.g., the "fight or flight" response in the face of imminent existential threat), and intrinsic to the human condition. However, excessive fear of death leads to neurotic (or sometimes psychotic) fear and debilitating avoidance of life.

Do psychopaths ever experience death anxiety? Based on their extreme risk-taking behaviors and "reckless disregard for safety of self or others" (American Psychiatric Association, 2013, p.325), it would appear they do not. Further, in the psychopath, this dearth of death anxiety is sometimes coupled with a morbid attraction to sadism, destructiveness, and death. Thus, psychopaths seem to harbor an ambivalent attitude toward death. On the one hand, they, like all living creatures, instinctively fear death, and try desperately to avoid their own annihilation; but, on the other, they are driven by a powerful and perverse morbid fascination with death, reflected, for instance, in their cruel and sadistic torture and killing of insects and animals as children. Moreover, some violent psychopaths are not only homicidal, but suicidal as well. These psychopathic killers seek not only to cause the suffering and death of as many innocent victims as possible, but also desire their own demise by suicide or "suicide by cop." For many, suicidality is sought solely in an effort to avoid suffering the negative consequences of their evil deeds, which would be consistent with the psychopath's life-long pattern of evading personal responsibility. But other psychopaths seem to truly harbor a hidden death wish, which is, like their murderous urges, usually a destructive expression of their chronic existential frustration, rage, depression, suffering, and despair.

16.4.5 Depression and Despair

Despair is a universal human experience and yet another core concern in existential therapy. When no significance or purpose can be found regarding life's inevitable existential suffering, or when chronic meaninglessness and existential frustration itself are the source of such suffering, *existential despair* sets in. We see widespread symptoms of both existential and pathological despair surging today, individually and collectively, not only in dramatically escalating suicide rates in recent decades (Hedegaard et al., 2018), but in the alarming proliferation of frustration, anger, resentment, nihilism, materialism, hedonism, addiction, and depression in postmodern Western society.

We all experience existential despair at times as part of the human condition, but for most it tends to dissipate relatively quickly. *Existential* depression (Berra, 2021), a deeper and more prolonged type of existential despair, commonly occurs as the consequence of some existential crisis, for instance a sudden confrontation with life's absurdity, meaninglessness, or with mortality. When, over time, existential despair and depression remain unresolved, they can turn into pathological depression or *clinical despair*, which "consists of a deep discouragement and loss of faith in one's ability to find meaning and fulfillment and to create a satisfactory future" (Diamond, 2016, pp. 328–329).

Psychopaths suffer frequently from a profound feeling of existential despair and an underlying clinical depression. Research demonstrates heightened rates of mood disorder, substance use disorder, suicidal ideation, and suicide attempts among individuals diagnosed with APD (Werner et al., 2015; see also Gómez-Leal et al., 2019, on the positive correlation between psychopathy and depression.). This *psychopathic* depression is avoided and self-medicated through the compulsive seeking of intense stimulation, including lawbreaking, risk-taking, intoxication, enragement, sadistic cruelty, and violence (Diamond, 2003). The psychopath's veiled depression or clinical despair stems, in part, from inadequate parenting, neglect, abandonment, and abuse during childhood, and is one of the underlying conditions that must be directly confronted during the existential treatment of antisocial patients.

Another possible way of comprehending the psychopath's excessive need for constant stimulation may be related to the existential reality, and, to some extent, inevitability of a certain degree of tedium, routine, and boredom in life. (See Camus; 1955; Diamond, 2016 on the Greek myth of Sisyphus, for example). For the psychopath, the "conventional," "ordinary," "normal," or "straight" life—being a law-abiding, responsible citizen who rises early every morning to go to work, pays his or her bills and taxes on time, has committed, long-term relationships or remains faithfully married to the same spouse for life, etc., is only for "suckers." Psychopaths believe that they–often by dint of their self-perceived superiority—do not need to conform to such a mundane and pedestrian existence. Psychopaths choose instead to disobey the rules set by societal authority and to seek excitement and stimulation in their rebellious and furious refusal to conform to cultural standards and norms. While there is certainly nothing inherently wrong with desiring a more exciting, stimulating, unconventional, creative, free, and fulfilling lifestyle, something existential therapy encourages, the problem is that the psychopath seeks such stimulation in dyssocial or antisocial activities of various kinds, willfully disrespecting the rights of others and rules of civilized society with a reckless disregard for limits, boundaries, decency, or responsibility.

16.4.6 Nihilism and Meaninglessness

Central to existential therapy is the monumental matter of *meaning* and *meaninglessness*. Much like Jung's analytical psychology, with its emphasis on archetypes, symbols, mythology, and meaning (Jung, 1968), existential therapy similarly concerns itself with the crucial task of finding or making meaning in life. Frankl (1946/1985), an existential analyst, held that human beings possess an innate, existential, or instinctual "will to meaning" (pp. 121–122). When that basic need for meaning goes unmet despite one's best efforts or due to some detrimental circumstance we experience "existential frustration" (p. 123) and a loss of meaning and purpose Frankl calls an "existential vacuum" (p. 128). Since, as we know from physics, nature abhors a vacuum, this void, emptiness, nothingness, or so-called *existential vacuum* is prone to being invaded by sundry psychiatric symptoms, irrational notions, obsessional fantasies, intrusive thoughts, and can lead to compulsive activities such as sexual promiscuity, workaholism, substance abuse, and, sometimes psychotic symptomatology (Frankl, 1946/1985). The therapeutic solution proffered by Frankl, is rather to consciously find and fill this inner emptiness with some existential, personal or spiritual sense of meaning and purpose in life.

Indeed, existential analysis or therapy can be partly described as a meaning-making process, in which, with the therapist's assistance, the patient struggles to make sense of the seeming senselessness of existence. There are myriad ways in which to find meaning in life, but perhaps the most important and relevant for our purposes here is described by Frankl (1946/1985) as "the attitude we take toward unavoidable suffering" (p. 133). Such existential suffering includes loss, illness, aging, and, inevitably, death. Meaning can be found or made by exercising one's existential freedom to consciously choose the attitude taken toward unavoidable suffering and fate. This existential path to meaning could explain why some victims of dysfunctional families and desperate circumstances become psychopaths and some do not. Despite their unfortunate fate, the latter have managed to find or create meaning or some sense of significance via some more positive or constructive avenue; they have discovered and adopted a helpful psychological, philosophical, or spiritual attitude toward life; they have courageously and creatively come to terms with their fate and taken control of their destiny.

The traditional psychoanalytic, or especially, Jungian approach to assisting patients to find meaning is through the methods of *interpretation* and discussion of archetypes or *myths,* "narrative patterns that give significance to our existence" (May, 1991, p. 15). Similarly, in existential depth psychology, myths are seen as archetypal or universal patterns or repositories of existential truth, and can provide a constructive way to attribute meaning to our existence (Diamond, 1996). However, what happens when we have no myths or other means to help us make sense of life's suffering, senselessness, and absurdity? One negative or destructive way of dealing with the problem of *mythlessness* or meaninglessness is to consciously or unconsciously adopt a nihilistic attitude or philosophy of life, something we frequently find in the psychopath. Indeed, the underlying presence of nihilism is quite common in psychopathy, clinical depression, pathological narcissism, and many other mental disorders, but is seldom recognized as such by psychotherapists.

For the nihilist, nothing matters or has any real meaning or value in life, in part due to his or her acute awareness of, anxiety about, and fixation on, the daunting existential facts of finitude, death, nothingness, and life's intrinsic unfairness, senselessness, and absurdity. Nihilists seize upon the existential perception of existence as finite, transitory, groundless, and meaningless to justify their amoral and anarchic worldview and destructive behavior. Thus, ironically, some sociopaths take pleasure and find meaning or satisfaction in creating anarchy, confusion, and chaos. For the nihilist, the inexorable existential reality of mortality utterly nullifies life, and with it, any possible meaning, purpose, or significance it could conceivably contain. As a result of this philosophical nullification, the nihilist, like the psychopath, angrily chooses to play by his or her own rules—or by none at all. Such existential nihilism can initially evoke an exhilarating sense of freedom and liberation, but leads inevitably to a morass of meaninglessness, "an angry, bitter and resentful refusal and failure to accept … [existential] reality" (Diamond, 1996, p. 309).

Nihilism is never the goal nor intended result of existential therapy, as some of its critics mistakenly suppose. Rather, for many patients, it serves as the starting point from which the arduous quest for meaning, purpose, and significance proceeds. Before this search for meaning can begin, it is essential for the existential therapist to explicitly recognize and acknowledge the patient's underlying, latent, and often unconscious, unarticulated nihilistic attitude toward life, and the legitimate reasons for having adopted and maintained it until now. This holds particularly true in the treatment of psychopathy. "Courage," writes Tillich (1952), "is the power of life to affirm itself in spite of … ambiguity, while the negation of life because of its negativity is an expression of cowardice" (p. 27). It can be said that, despite all their fearless risk-taking and dare-devil activities, the psychopath lacks the requisite courage to unequivocally accept and affirm existential reality, instead bitterly rejecting life, and any possibility of finding meaning or purpose. They angrily lash out at society, the world, others, God, and at existence itself in violent protest: "Frustrated, wounded, and … furious, they have sullenly withdrawn from the proverbial field of battle we call life, becoming further alienated and isolated from the world. Their existence seems meaningless and without purpose" (Diamond, 2016, p. 331).

Nonetheless, from an existential stance, psychopaths, like all human beings, remain motivated by the same basic need for meaning and purpose in life. Paradoxically and perversely, it is even conceivable that some psychopaths, having failed to find any constructive, culturally acceptable, or creative purpose in life, may seek some sense of significance, specialness, personal identity, and purpose by *choosing* to become mass or serial killers. This freely chosen role becomes their own personal *myth*, an identity or narrative in which they discover some sense of meaning and purpose. We all have some conscious or unconscious myth of ourselves, a way of conceptualizing who we are and our context in the cosmos (May, 1991). And it is precisely psychopaths' self-perpetuating and extraordinarily problematic myth of themselves that must be addressed during existential treatment. To relinquish this myth without finding one to replace it would leave the psychopath devoid of all meaning or purpose. Hence, the emphasis on helping psychopaths discover or create and commit to some positive alternative source of significance and meaning, some new myth, as part of their rehabilitation process and potential reintegration into society.

16.4.7 Alienation and Aloneness

For existential therapy, another of life's ultimate concerns is the sometimes excruciating experience of aloneness, isolation, and alienation (Yalom, 1980; Moustakas, 1990). Many psychopaths appear to share a pervasive sense of loneliness and alienation. But this sense of isolation and aloneness, of feeling like a stranger in a strange world, is, to some extent, an existential reality for us all. Existentially speaking, as Heidegger (1927/2010) holds, we are each involuntarily thrust or "thrown" into this already existing world alone, often must walk through it alone, and, in the end, die alone. We exist in a contextual collective world of other beings surrounding and relating to us, but try as we may, can never be completely free of or permanently transcend our own isolated consciousness, subjectivity, interiority, and individuality. Yalom (1980) refers to this fundamental aloneness or individuality as *existential isolation*— the inherent and ultimately unbridgeable schism of separateness between human beings—distinguishing it from *interpersonal* and *intrapersonal isolation.*

Despite our inescapable existential aloneness, we are at the same time instinctively social animals, interdependent, existing within an intricate social web of relatedness with other creatures like ourselves. Everyone, even *introverted* types (Jung, 1971), need some sustained degree of social contact and interpersonal interaction. When we are chronically frustrated in fulfilling this basic need for human warmth, compassion, camaraderie, love, and intimacy, a sullen rage accrues over time, manifesting itself in psychopathology, and, in the most extreme cases, culminates in cruelty, destructiveness, and violence. Violence, avers May (1969),

> is the ultimate destructive substitute which surges in to fill the vacuum where there is no related-ness. …When inward life dries up, when feeling decreases and apathy increases, when one cannot affect or even genuinely *touch* another person, violence flares up as a daimonic necessity for contact, a mad drive forcing touch in the most direct way possible (pp. 30–31).

For some of the most severe psychopaths, like mass shooters and serial killers, such social violence can be seen as "a desperate, last-ditch attempt to break out of their self-imposed state of social isolation.… Once one has publicly committed a high-profile violent crime, he or she is no longer alone, anonymous, and ignored; violence, in such instances, serves as an absurd, evil vehicle to infamy" (Diamond, 1996, p. 28).

Psychopaths can experience existential, interpersonal, and intrapersonal isolation even more acutely than most. The majority tend to be loners, partly due to their inability to form close and lasting connections. For some psychopaths, sadism, cruelty, and violence serve, to some extent, as a way of indirectly expressing their profound sense of existential alienation and aloneness, and the immense rage they feel regarding their inability to overcome this moribund state of isolation. Serial killer Jeffrey Dahmer's bizarre homicidal, necrophilic, and cannibalistic behavior, for instance, appears to have been directly related to his profound feelings of loneliness, social isolation, dread of abandonment, and desperate search for lasting companionship, love, and acceptance. Even more fundamentally, psychopaths are almost always totally alienated from themselves. They exhibit a schizoid-like detachment from their emotions. This *intrapersonal isolation* may be part of the reason that psychopaths—especially so-called *primary psychopaths*—seek extraordinary degrees of stimulation, seem not to learn from experience, and have no apparent sense of anxiety, shame, or remorse. They are pathologically out of touch with their inner being as well as with that of their fellow beings. This exaggerated sense of estrangement or alienation from people and society makes it much easier for psychopaths to dehumanize others, objectify them, and treat them so cruelly. Of course, we all have the capacity for such dehumanizing distortion of others, but the psychopath takes this intrinsic capacity to dehumanize others to another level. As Yalom (1980) contends, one way of mitigating and making more bearable our existential aloneness is to create and maintain intimate relationships with others. However, this poses a significant problem for the psychopathic personality, who engages solely in superficial relationships, often has a history of sexual promiscuity, brief serial marriages, and who tends to selfishly exploit others for financial, sexual, or other personal gain. The psychopath's pathological lying, conning, infidelity, and Machiavellian need for power and control make intimate relationships all but impossible (Hare, 1998). This incapacity to form and sustain supportive, healthy, respectful human relationships forces the psychopath to cope with his or her aloneness, anonymity, and existential isolation differently than most of us. In this regard, the psychopath may actually suffer even more from such interpersonal isolation than those who are better able to assuage their existential aloneness through mutually intimate connections with others.

16.4.8 Power and Impotence

It is near impossible to speak meaningfully about psychopathy without acknowledging its close connection with the conscious or unconscious striving for *power* or what existential philosopher Friedrich Nietzsche (1883/2019) referred to as the "will to power." For Nietzsche, the individual's instinctive "will to power" was a primarily positive force associated with self-actualization, affirmation, perpetuation, and assertion, but became dangerous when denied. Alfred Adler, in his own Individual Psychology, adopted this Nietzschean "will to power" as the primal motivation in human beings, "a drive toward fighting for satisfaction which I call 'aggression drive'" (Adler, in Ansbacher & Ansbacher, p. 34). While we all seek some sense of power, mastery, and control in life, the psychopath is consumed, possessed, and driven by this craving. Psychopaths consistently seek to assert power and control over others, and this power drive can be compulsive and unrelenting, fueled by an unquenchable desire to compensate for profound feelings of powerlessness, insignificance, inferiority, and helplessness.

This psychopathic pursuit of power can be expressed in a broad spectrum of symptoms, ranging from oppositional and defiant behaviors, property destruction, stealing, teasing or bullying, to inflicting intense physical suffering on insects or animals, to the violent abduction, torture, rape, and sadistic killing of human victims. When psychopathic individuals seek and successfully attain to positions of power in industry, academia, or politics, the results can be catastrophic, since it is especially in the psychopathic person that "absolute power corrupts absolutely." But this same ruthlessness and unbridled longing for power is also played out in the daily lives of petty criminals, wreaking havoc and causing suffering to all those within their smaller sphere of influence.

The psychopath's wielding of power and control derives frequently from feelings of having been powerless during childhood or adolescence, as well as into adulthood. Children are relatively impotent compared to their parents and other adults, and when neglected or abused, feel totally out of control of their immediate world. Such helpless feelings, coupled with an unremitting rage toward the perceived perpetrators of their suffering, sow the poisonous seeds of psychopathy, which can take root and grow when these toxic circumstances persist without relief, and which is why early intervention is so essential in preventing or mitigating psychopathy and other serious mental disorders. We see this striving for power and control, for example, in the negative acting out behaviors of children and adolescents in both Oppositional Defiant Disorder and Conduct Disorder, both of which can and often do foreshadow the development of adult APD.

The traumatic experience of having been in some way unfairly victimized remains at the very heart of the psychopathic or antisocial personality disorder. Indeed, psychopaths were, in my own professional experience as a forensic evaluator, almost invariably the powerless victims of an extraordinarily difficult and painful fate during their most formative and vulnerable years. This tragic victimhood plays a central part in how psychopaths eventually come to see themselves, their place in the world, and how they choose to act in it. In psychopathy, the victim becomes the victimizer; the powerless become the predator. Victimizing others within one's immediate environment is an attempt by the psychopath to overcome these feelings of helplessness from childhood and adolescence, and to vent his or her hatred, resentment, and rage. For the psychopath, such destructive predatory behavior is the only way he or she has found to experience and express some measure of power and control in the world—or, at least, in his or her "little world"—and it is tragically a malignant, negative, destructive, and, ultimately, self-defeating and disempowering way of doing so.

16.4.9 Existential Frustration, Anger, and Rage

Anger and rage may be the most difficult of all human emotions to constructively manage (Diamond, 1996). *Anger*—and rage, the epitome of anger—can be both destructive and constructive. It is a primal emotion essential to the integrity, power, vitality, and dignity of the personality. While the roots of anger range widely, and can generally include the psychobiological response to some actual or perceived insult or threat to one's integrity or dignity (Diamond, 1996), the existential phenomenon of *frustration* is perhaps its primary source: "Frustration is an existential concomitant of the human condition to which few—if any—are immune" (Diamond, 1996, p. 25). What are the existential or universal sources of the psychopath's frustration, anger, or rage? By *existential frustration*, I refer to a universal underlying feeling of deep dissatisfaction, annoyance, irritation, anger, rage, or resentment with the reality of one's existence, resulting from a perceived lack of freedom, power, or control, love and acceptance, unfulfilled desires, unresolved difficulties, or a failure to find some sense of meaning and purpose in life. Indeed, existential frustration can occur regarding any or all of these "ultimate concerns." The chronic repression or denial of existential frustration and the feelings it incurs, including anger or rage, amplify and make it even more dangerous and destructive. When existential frustration and the anger or rage resulting from it are repressed, denied, or suppressed over time, it turns into resentment, hatred, enmity, and embitterment. If left unresolved, these emotions become toxic, pathological, and tend, in psychopathy, to be expressed in outwardly hostile, cruel, aggressive, vindictive, and violent behavior often motivated by the unconscious or conscious desire for retaliation, retribution, and revenge. To paraphrase Charles Manson: "The world has treated me badly, so I have the right to treat the world badly." This pithily distills the basic psychology of psychopathy. It can be understood from the standpoint of existential depth psychology, as a manifestation of what Adler (in Ansbacher & Ansbacher, 1956) called "masculine protest," consisting of "a compensatory striving for superiority (to counter-act feelings of inferiority), aggression, ambition, avarice, and envy, coupled with constant 'defiance, vengeance, and resentment" (Diamond, 1996, p. 142).

Existentially speaking, anger arises from feelings of frustration with the reality, facticity, and finitude of *existence as it truly is.* The psychopath is distinguished from most of the population by the unfortunate and fateful confluence of existential frustration and narcissistic wounding, and the inability to find ways to constructively channel the resulting feelings or anger or rage into constructive participation in the culture and creative self-expression. The clinical implication is that if psychopaths can, during the course of treatment, be helped to find new ways of dealing with their existential frustration, anger, or rage (i.e., the daimonic) in the present and future, they can conceivably alter, to some extent, the course of their own destiny despite their troubled past. It is the quality of the therapeutic relationship cultivated over time—the presence, empathy, compassion, objectivity, and acceptance of the daimonic by the therapist—that provides a safe and sacred container (*vas temenos*) in which to explore, confront, and come to terms with the psychopath's raging inner demons. As May (in Diamond, 1996) writes,

> I think there is just as much daimonic wrath in any kind of psychotherapy—except as it is avoided by the therapist. In terms of technique, those clinicians who *are* aware of the daimonic normally confront violence and rage no differently from the Freudians, Jungians, or other kinds of psychodynamically based therapists; the crucial difference is that they can get at the anger and rage more constructively, because they can recognize its valuable aspects. (pp. xxi–xxii).

It is precisely in the treatment of psychopathy and other anger-related disorders (see Diamond, 1996) that resisting the urge to suppress the daimonic and creating and cultivating a strong and enduring therapeutic alliance with the patient or client is most challenging.

Successful psychotherapy of psychopathy or APD (and, for that matter, most other mental disorders) requires that the clinician be receptive to perceiving and exploring the existential reality of frustration, anger, and rage rather than seeking to simply avoid or suppress it with psychiatric drugs, punishment, or other technical interventions. (See, for example, the experimental behavioral treatment of sociopathic teens in the prescient and disturbing 1963 novel *A Clockwork Orange* by Anthony Burgess, and director Stanley Kubrick's 1971 surreal film version of this cautionary tale.) Rather than simply being suppressed behaviorally or biochemically, anger and rage must be consciously resurrected and reconnected with the original trauma—which is not typically some single life event, but a chronic pattern of traumatizing events—if treatment is to be truly transformational. This intentional conjuring up of the patient's "demons" can be a frightening, daunting, and dangerous prospect for the clinician. All precautions must be taken to protect therapist, patient, and any potential victims, including the use of psychiatric medication or physical restraint when needed. Nevertheless, some calculated risk is always required in treatment if it is to be truly effective.

16.4.10 Evil, Creativity, and the Daimonic

The perennial problem of evil, i.e., "those attitudes and behaviors that promote excessive interpersonal aggression, cruelty, hostility, disregard for the integrity of others, self-destructiveness, psychopathology, and human misery in general" (Diamond, 1996, p. 57), is far more than a theological or philosophical quandary. It is primarily a psychological phenomenon and one of life's ultimate concerns (Frankl, 1946/1985; May, 1969; Diamond, 1996, 2018). Jung wrote extensively on the psychology of evil as originating from what he metaphorically termed the "shadow." For Jung (1961), the *shadow* was a symbol for the unacceptable, rejected, devalued, shameful, and therefore, repressed, dissociated, denied, and carefully concealed aspects of the personality and psyche, consisting partly of our most primitive, uncivilized, and destructive tendencies, but also of untapped positive, spiritual, and creative possibilities (see also Diamond, 1991, 1996, 2009a, b, c, 2018). Jung (1961) believed every human being harbors such destructive tendencies (as did the mature Freud in his theories of the *id* and *Thanatos*), but these primal psychobiological forces become even more pernicious, powerful, and potentially evil when chronically repressed.

Psychopathy is the current diagnostic construct that most closely approximates the personification of *human* evil. The psychopath in our day can be perceived as a living and breathing embodiment of evil (e.g., Charles Manson, Ted Bundy, or Adolf Hitler), and a symbolic expression of our darkest and most dangerous social impulsions and proclivities, what Jung (1961) called our "collective shadow." From this perspective, every human being harbors the inherent potentiality for psychopathic or evil behavior given the right (or wrong) circumstances. Though we all, wittingly or unwittingly, participate in evil to some extent, only a small percentage (an estimated 1–4%) of people ever become sufficiently evil to warrant being labeled psychopaths, sociopaths, or antisocial personalities, with the most severe, violent, destructive, and dangerous psychopaths comprising approximately 1% or less of the general population.

Violence is the preeminent evil of our day, and is sadly pervasive, especially in American society. While certainly not all violence is perpetrated by psychopaths, there exists a significant correlation between psychopathy and violence (Hare, 1999; Kiehl & Hoffman, 2011). If forensic clinicians care to better comprehend psychopathy, it is crucial to consider the existential, psychopathological, and societal sources of such supposedly "senseless" violence. Commenting on the existential and sociological problem of apathy, alienation, and meaninglessness in modern life, May (1972) avers that "this void is that from which the ecstasy of violence is an escape" (p. 179). Sartre (cited in May 1972) states that violence "is an organizing of one's powers to prove one's power, to establish the worth of the self" (p. 189). This existential view of violence seems significant, particularly as it pertains to the psychopath's previously noted core sense of impotence, worthlessness, victimhood, self-loathing, inadequacy, and inferiority.

Considering the immense social alienation and isolation of some psychopaths, and their inability to form close, supportive, enduring relationships, this existential analysis of the roots of violence rings especially true. Whether we speak of *instrumental* (i.e., cold, calculating, predatory violence) or *reactive* (i.e., impassioned, impulsive, affective violence) (see Meloy, 2012), violence always serves some specific purpose for the psychopath, and, therefore, holds some psychological or existential significance. Some of the psychopath's violence stems from his or her pent-up resentment, anger, and rage about having been betrayed, mistreated, and disrespected during childhood or adolescence, along with the painful frustration of not feeling recognized and valued later by society as an adult (see Diamond, 1996, 1999, 2003). From the standpoint of existential depth psychology, it is critical that psychotherapists, and especially forensic clinicians, can acknowledge the strong correlation between anger, rage, and violence in psychopathy and myriad other severe mental disorders.

Rollo May's paradoxical theory of the *daimonic* is particularly useful in more deeply comprehending the complex phenomenon of psychopathy In his controversial and more often than not misunderstood concept of the *daimonic*, May (1977), building upon Freud's (1966) seminal notion of the "id" and Jung's (1968) classic concept of the "shadow," provides a more existentially sophisticated phenomenological model of both human evil and creativity. As May (1977) explains, in his existentially informed paradigm of the daimonic, "I want to state the problem of evil in such a way that psychologists will not be able to derogate it simply as a lack of something, for example, a lack of growth or as simply immaturity, or as a process which depends always on something else, such as the doctrine of the shadow in Jungianism" (Cited in Diamond, 1996, p. 99).

For May (1969), the *daimonic* (not unlike Nietzsche's paradoxical "will to power"), is fundamentally conceived of "as an essentially undifferentiated, impersonal, and primal force of nature" (Diamond, 1996, p. 67), the "dynamic ground of existence, the primary source of vital, psychobiological energy or power" (Diamond, 1996, p. 225). May (1969) additionally describes the daimonic as "the urge in every being to affirm itself, assert itself, perpetuate and increase itself. The daimonic becomes evil when it usurps the total self without regard to the integration of the self, or to the unique forms and desires of others …" (p. 123).

May's theory of the daimonic is a radical departure and reconceptualization of traditional models from depth psychology such as the "unconscious," the "id," and the "shadow," and stresses not the deterministic forces of neurobiology and unconsciousness per se (though the influence of these must not be underestimated), but rather the individual's inescapable part in, and ultimate *responsibility* for relating to and constructively managing these dynamic psychobiological energies constructively. The daimonic can be fundamentally defined as *"any natural function which has the power to take over the whole person"* (May, 1969, p. 123). By "natural function," May refers to the powerful primal passions of love, lust, anger, rage, and the craving for power and control, as well as the primordial urge to create or destroy, which, when chronically denied, repressed, dissociated, or otherwise excluded from consciousness, can manifest in numerous mental disorders, including psychopathy. By "take over," he refers to the phenomenological fact that, when denied or repressed, the daimonic (like the "shadow" in Jung's psychology) has the intrinsic capacity to take temporary *possession* of the personality, an impressive psychological phenomenon seen, for instance, in dissociative identity disorder, and more literally depicted in Robert Louis Stevenson's *The Strange Case of Dr. Jekyll and Mr. Hyde* (1886/1964), a cautionary tale of latent psychopathy and the perennial danger of denying the daimonic. In other words, the person is subject to being "taken over" or "possessed" not by demonic entities or the devil, but by dissociated tendencies in themselves.

From the unique perspective of existential depth psychology, psychopathic violence is the ultimate *destructive* expression of the daimonic. Clinically with the daimonic, only through the acknowledgment and acceptance of his or her resentment, rage, and anger and its traumatic origins can the psychopath potentially recover from its destructive power. Much of this process depends upon the practitioner's willingness to permit the patient to experience the daimonic and remain receptive and fully present to it in the clinical setting, rather than trying to simply suppress the daimonic with psychiatric medications or evasively skirt around or mitigate it with cognitive, behavioral, or meditative techniques. As to the existential attitude taken by the therapist when working directly with such fiery and volatile emotions, May (in Diamond, 1996) remarks, "I do not believe in toning down the daimonic. This gives a sense of false comfort. The real comfort can come only in the relationship of the therapist and the client or patient" (p. xxii).

Paradoxically, like Jung's conception of the shadow, the daimonic can also be the potential source of creativity and other positive experiences such as empowerment, resolve, strength, motivation, commitment, compassion, courage, empathy, caring, love, and *eros*. As May (in Diamond, 1996) makes clear,

> the daimonic (unlike the *demonic*, which is merely destructive), is as much concerned with creativity as with negative reactions. A special characteristic of the daimonic model is that it considers both creativity on one side, and anger and rage on the other side, as coming from the same source. That is, constructiveness and destructiveness have the same source in human personality. The source is simply *human potential.* (p. xxi)

Creativity is a key element in existential depth psychology, and can play a pivotal role in the treatment of psychopathy, in part because it provides a potentially *constructive* outlet for the daimonic: "Creative endeavors can help constructively channel disturbing daimonic affects (e.g., anger, anxiety, grief) that might otherwise manifest as pathology, violence, and evil. Consequently, existential psychotherapy acknowledges and deeply respects the patient's congenital need for creative self-expression" (Diamond, 2016, p. 326). Indeed, given the predominance of destructiveness in the psychopathic personality May's (1969) definition of the *daimonic* as a power which is potentially *both creative and destructive* is crucial to the treatment process. From an existential perspective, *all* human beings possess the potentiality for good and evil. This non-dualistic existential view of human potential makes constructiveness, creativity, or even goodness a real possibility for the psychopath—at least, theoretically. Existential depth psychology seeks to assist psychopaths to discover ways of expressing the daimonic (e.g., anger or rage in particular) more productively, constructively, creatively, and prosocially.

As free and responsible beings, we can (and do) daily choose between good and evil, creativity and destructiveness, compassionate or kind and cruel or violent responses to others and the world. This existential choice or series of choices represents the fundamental decision that differentiates the primarily antisocial from prosocial person. Unfortunately, one isolated act of great creativity or kindness is never enough to negate or redeem an enduring and pervasive pattern of destructive and violent behavior. (See, for example, the fascinating and tragic case of career criminal-turned-celebrated author Jack Henry Abbott in Diamond, 1996, pp. 276–279). The genuinely creative or prosocial individual is committed and courageously struggles to consistently express the daimonic in constructive or creative rather than destructive ways (See May's 1976 book *The Courage to Create,* and Diamond, 1996). Psychologically preparing the psychopathic patient to consciously (rather than compulsively or mindlessly) choose between these two diametrically opposed but not mutually exclusive ways of being in the world—to decide to cast his or her lot toward creativity rather than destructiveness—is perhaps the ultimate aspiration in the treatment of psychopathy.

16.4.11 Mindfulness, Spirituality and Religiosity

Although religion is not necessarily the singular answer to the predicament of human existence, people everywhere throughout history have striven to discover some meaning and purpose in life, some *raison d'etre* based on those worldviews, values, or ideas they believe to be most important, essential, and sacred. "Religion," writes Rollo May (1953), is whatever the individual takes to be his [or her] ultimate concern" (p. 180). Religion can be seen as having been conceived and perpetuated to provide meaning, comfort, and succor in the face of the stark existential facts of life: evil, suffering, meaninglessness, isolation, limitation, and ultimately, death. Whether we choose some organized religious system to believe in or adopt some other philosophical, metaphysical, or scientific view of existence, we are in any case searching for answers to life's most elemental questions (e.g., What is life? Why are we born? Why do we suffer? Why must we die?). These same ultimate concerns are traditionally shared by religion, science, spirituality, and existential psychotherapy.

Are psychopaths religious? According to some research, there appears to be a negative correlation between religiosity and psychopathy (Jack et al., 2015) and positive correlation between atheism and psychopathy, with the key factor being a perceived lack of empathy in both (Lilienfeld et al., 2016). Some psychopaths seem to seek meaning and a sense of purpose and significance in both traditional and non-traditional religion, but, more often than not, they manipulatively use religion or spirituality to acquire and exercise power over others. Moreover, previously atheistic psychopaths frequently report finding religion only after being caught and incarcerated for their crimes. It is easy to take a cynical view of such supposed spiritual awakening or conversion in the psychopathic patient. However, having said that, certain psychopaths do sincerely turn to religion or spirituality as part of their rehabilitation process. The secular or religious existential therapist respects and supports this existential search for meaning, purpose, and spiritual salvation as an integral part of the psychopath's psychological growth and emotional maturation. While Eastern spiritual practices such as meditation and mindfulness have become popular with both patients and psychotherapists recently, existential therapists have long been employing similar methods in their approach. For instance, *existential awareness, discernment* (Diamond, 1996), and *mindfulness* are key concerns and clinical techniques commonly utilized in existential therapy today. These methods are consistent with existential therapy's concern with cultivating presence in the here-and-now and with the emphasis on here-and-now awareness of subjective experience (Diamond, 2016). The consistent practice of meditation or mindfulness fosters self-awareness, expanded consciousness, and an experience of *being* or *self* which transcends the Freudian notion of *ego*. From an existential perspective, the better both therapist and patient or client become at being more present and mindful in the moment, the better the chance of a positive treatment outcome (Felder et al., 2014). If the psychopath can be encouraged to be more present and mindful of the "infinitely subtle flux of feelings, impulses, sensations, and cognitions that make up his or her being from moment to moment" (Diamond, 1996, p. 231)—especially long repressed or dissociated feelings of anger, guilt, shame, compassion, and caring—the antisocial *or psychopathic* personality can potentially be slowly transformed into a more *prosocial* personality and way of being in the world.

Mindfulness, a method derived and distilled from Eastern meditative practices, is the discipline of being as *present* as possible in the moment, not only to the patient or client, but to oneself as therapist. Existential therapy places significant emphasis on *mindfulness* of the clinician as a precursor to modeling and eventually evoking this same meditative mode of awareness in the patient. In some cases, as observers, we might see the existential therapist encourage the client to practice this or some other awareness enhancing meditative method in the consulting room and at home between meetings. In addition to *presence*, there is a focus on *encounter* with, and compassion for, the client or patient's painful predicament, expressed outwardly by the practitioner's verbal and non-verbal communication, conveying an accurate and deeply caring understanding of what the person is actually feeling, thinking, and experiencing in the here-and-now. For instance, the Rogerian technique of reflective or "active listening"—succinctly paraphrasing what one hears being said and seeking confirmation of its accuracy from the client or patient—is one highly effective method of demonstrating empathy and compassion for the person's plight, and of further illuminating his or her being-in-the-world. "Religious and spiritual activities may have a significant impact on the recovery of patients with antisocial or psychopathic personality disorders (Black et al., 1995; Martens, 1977, 2003; Robins, 1996)" (Martens, 2003, p. 206). Like every psychotherapy patient, the psychopath must find some way to come to terms with the typically unfortunate specific circumstances of his or her early life, as well as with the tragic existential facts of life to which we all are subject. An existential psychotherapy that incorporates secular spirituality or religion (as does existential depth psychology) can provide a means of accomplishing this daunting task. Assisting patients in arriving at such a realistic yet accepting and appreciative attitude toward both the positive *and* negative elements in human existence can be said to be one of the ultimate concerns and aims of existential depth psychology.

16.5 Finitude, Limitation, and Existential Termination

Finally, *finitude*—the fact that human existence is inherently limited rather than infinite—is fundamental to existential thought and therapy. Thus, the effectiveness of existential treatment is generally not determined by the duration of therapy nor the frequency of sessions, but by *how well each present moment of each precious session is therapeutically utilized* (Diamond, 2016). The course of existential treatment can be brief (weeks or months) or prolonged (years or decades), but there is no presupposition regarding this matter at the outset of treatment. Nor is there a presumption that subsequent sessions will always or automatically follow the current one; this existential attitude stems in part from the recognition and acceptance of the transitory and tenuous nature of human existence and the person's intrinsic *freedom and responsibility* to *choose* –even when confined or court-mandated to attend treatment—whether to return and participate or not. Hence, each finite session—itself limited to a certain predetermined number of minutes and comprised of a beginning, middle, and ending— is, at some level, conducted deliberately as though it could be the last. Indeed, the process of psychotherapy itself is similarly conceived of as being equally finite. (And, at least in the most refractory cases, its limitations in mitigating psychopathy must be accepted.) Moreover, since, as May (1981) indicates, the purpose of existential therapy "*is to set people free*" (p. 19), this must [of necessity] inevitably include freeing them from morbid dependency on therapy or the therapist"| (Diamond, 2016, p. 339). Therapy must, like all things in life, eventually end. Separation from and loss of the therapist are not only inevitable but necessary stages in the existential treatment process, which, when avoided, might otherwise result in a state of psychological stillbirth and neurotic dependency. (See Rank (1993), who, as the first to deliberately limit the duration of psychotherapy, presaged the advent of today's time-limited brief therapies.) Acknowledging finitude and limitation in therapy can catalyze and deepen the patient's development, as the anxious anticipation that occurs leading up to and during the termination phase can sometimes precipitate the most intensive therapeutic work (Diamond, 2016). Thus, during sessions toward the conclusion of therapy we might observe a prolonged and often highly emotional conversation and exchange regarding *termination* (the cold clinical term for saying goodbye to each other, with all the powerful feelings this encounter can evoke, including sadness, grief, anger, loss, abandonment depression, panic, and separation anxiety) and its existential inescapability. How this dynamic and delicate termination phase is handled (or mis-handled) by the psychotherapist can significantly influence, for better or worse, the outcome of treatment.

16.6 Conclusion

"Existential therapy has been and remains a revolutionary force in psychological treatment" (Diamond, 2016, p. 345). Since its inception almost a century ago, many of the fundamental philosophical and methodological principles of existential therapy—such as acknowledging the need for meaning and purpose in life, working with patients in the here-and-now, focusing on process and content, and emphasizing both existential freedom and responsibility— have been subtly assimilated into mainstream theory and therapeutic practice (Diamond, 2016). However, with rare exceptions, little has been written, and certainly less researched, regarding the application of existential principles to forensic practice (see Diamond, 2005) and, more specifically, the treatment of psychopathy utilizing existential therapy. Nonetheless, as I hope to have demonstrated here, there is much to recommend it.

The psychopathic patient must find a new way of being-in-the-world, one which is not compulsively and destructively governed or blindly driven by his or her anger or rage regarding past traumatic experiences. A way of being that is not solely in opposition to or against the world, but which chooses instead to accept and productively participate in it. This calls for the courage and commitment to come to terms with the past, to make more constructive choices in the present, and to foresee and create a more meaningful and fulfilling future. It demands the adoption of a more psychological, philosophical, and possibly spiritual or religious, attitude toward existence—one that allows psychopathic patients to forgive themselves for prior evil deeds, to let go of old myths or narratives about their identity, to *accept* themselves as the imperfect, deeply flawed beings they are now, while, at the same time, choosing, step-by-step, to become more like the person they truly desire to be. Indeed, we could conclude that the awareness and experience of one's freedom to choose and decide who and how to be in the world here-and-now, coupled with an acceptance of one's personal responsibility for exercising this freedom to do so, is the *sine qua non* of any truly existential therapy.

As May (1970) indicates, at first, "the function of the therapist is to disturb homeostasis" (p. 202). This holds particularly true in the treatment of personality disorders such as psychopathy, which are, by definition, characterological, rigid, refractory, and deeply ingrained defensive patterns of cognition and behavior. In this sense, successful treatment of psychopathy or antisocial personality disorder must be prepared to confront, expose, and challenge patients' fundamental *myth* or central narrative about themselves (May 1991). For most psychopaths, that unconscious myth consists typically of having been born into and badly treated by a hostile, brutal, toxic, and rejecting environment, and, consequentially, coming to view themselves as an unworthy, unlovable, bad, or even evil being. However, especially in cases of "psychopathic narcissism," the myth also consists of a compensatory, inflated, grandiose belief about being a special, extraordinary, exceptional person to whom the usual rules of society simply do not apply. In either case, promoting and encouraging conscious awareness of this personal myth and its central part in perpetuating the psychopath's problems is the key to its potential tempering and transformation.

As with all psychotherapy patients, it is essential for the psychopath to establish a meaningful inner platform upon which to stand and from which to operate in the world, one constructed from his or her newly found values, goals, philosophy, spirituality, and sense of self. This process of inner development is a prerequisite for any significant outer change of behavior in the world. But it is fraught with real perils and potential pitfalls, and requires patience and perseverance on the part of both parties, as well as considerable courage and commitment. *Being*, especially *human* being, is always in the process of *becoming*, always in flux. As Sartre (1946/2007) suggests, human existence is defined by the fact that we choose, each moment, how to be in the world, which means that our way of being in the world is always potentially subject to some adjustment, alteration, or even radical transformation. Therefore, existentially speaking, *if we remain the same, it is because we choose to do so*.

Existential therapy cultivates the kind of relationship necessary to penetrate and potentially transform the psychopath's resistant and defensive stance toward existence—a stance or attitude in which the psychopath has, from early on, learned that *the best defense is a good offense*. The point of choosing to take an existential approach to treating psychopathy is to assist these patients in rediscovering their freedom to consciously choose how to be and behave in the world in new and more constructive ways, and to become more responsible for accepting, managing, and directing their daimonic tendencies more constructively, productively, and, even creatively. The compassionate, collaborative, supportive, professional yet personal human relationship cultivated in existential therapy provides both the structured container and catalyst for therapeutic growth and change (Diamond, 2011). Indeed, it is the nature and quality of the therapeutic relationship developed over time—the combination of presence, empathy, compassion, appropriate boundaries, objectivity, caring, and acceptance by the clinician—that provides a safe and sacred environment in which to engage in this potentially life-changing work together.

In conclusion, psychopathic defenses are extraordinarily entrenched and deeply rooted, i.e., they are, by definition, *characterological*. Nevertheless, human beings possess an ever-present possibility to change, to transcend the strictly deterministic, biologically, and instinctually motivated animalistic level of existence. The integration of existential therapy into forensic practice demands an undogmatic openness and receptivity to the perennial opportunity for *redemption*: "Redemption must always remain in our minds and hearts an ever-present (albeit sometimes highly unlikely) human potentiality" (Diamond, 2003, p. 43). No matter how far from our humanity we may have fallen, our inherent human potentiality to courageously create and redefine ourselves despite our failures, sins, and finitude, to find and fulfill our destiny, to choose between our intrinsic capacity for both evil and good, remains. Existential therapy can provide the psychopathic patient a chance to rediscover, reclaim, and consciously exercise this essential existential freedom and responsibility to choose between evil and good, destructiveness and creativity, death and life, and antisocial or prosocial attitudes and behavior. However, this radical transformation does not typically take place due to some singular, isolated decision on the part of the patient or client. Such choices must be fully committed to and consistently reasserted, both during and following treatment. For, in the final existential analysis, that basic choice or decision—and the ultimate responsibility for it —resides solely in the intrinsic and indestructible free will of the individual, and, in the end, determines his or her destiny.

References

American Psychiatric Association. (2013). *Diagnostic and statistical manual of mental disorders* (5th ed.). Author.

American Psychiatric Association. (1994). *DSM-IV: Diagnostic and Statistical Manual of Mental Disorders*. Washington, DC: American Psychiatric Press Inc.

Baskin-Sommers, A., Stuppy-Sullivan, A. M., & Buckholtz, J. W. (2016). Psychopathic individuals exhibit but do not avoid regret during counterfactual decision making. *Proceedings of the National Acadamy of Science of the United States of America, 113*, 14438–14443.

Becker, E. (1973). *The denial of death*. Free Press.

Berra, L. (2021). Existential Depression: A nonpathological and philosophical-existential approach. *Journal of Humanistic Psychology, 61*, 757–765.

Blair, R. J. R. (2003). Neurobiological basis of psychopathy. *British Journal of Psychiatry, 182*, 5–7.

Book, A., Visser, B., & Volk, A. (2015). Unpacking evil: Claiming the core of the Dark Triad. *Personality and Individual Differences, 73*, 29–38.

Camus, A. (1955). *The myth of Sisyphus & other essays* (J. O'Brien, Trans.). Librairie Gaillimard.

Cohn, H. (1999). What is existential: A response to Dr. Diamond. *Journal of the Society for Existential Analysis, 10*, 42–43.

Cleckley, H. (1941). *The mask of sanity: An attempt to clarify some issues about the so-called psychopathic personality*. Mosby.

Cooper, M. (2016). *Existential therapies* (2nd ed.). SAGE. (Original work published 2003).

Diamond, S. A. (1991). Redeeming our devils and demons. In C. Zweig & J. Abrams (Eds.), *Meeting the shadow: The hidden power of the dark side of human nature* (pp. 180–186). Tarcher/Putnam.

Diamond, S. A. (1996). *Anger, madness, and the daimonic: The psychological genesis of violence, evil, and creativity.* Foreword by Rollo May. State University of New York Press.

Diamond, S. A. (1999). Anger, madness, and the daimonic: Toward an existential depth psychology. *Existential Analysis, 10*, 27–41.

Diamond, S. A. (2003). Violence as secular evil: Forensic evaluation and treatment of violent offenders from the viewpoint of existential depth psychology. *Journal of Applied Psychoanalytic Studies, 5*, 21–45.

Diamond, S. A. (2005). Psychotherapy, evil, and the daimonic: Toward a secular spiritual psychology. In R. H. Cox, B. Ervin-Cox, & L. Hoffman (Eds.), *Spirituality and psychological health* (pp. 184–203). COSPP Press.

Diamond, S. A. (2006). Violence as secular evil: Forensic evaluation and treatment of violent offenders from the viewpoint of existential depth psychology. In T. Mason (Ed.), *Forensic psychiatry: Influences of evil* (pp. 179–206). Humana Press.

Diamond, S. A. (2009a). Existential psychotherapy. In D. Leeming, K. Madden, & S. Marlan (Eds.), *Encyclopedia of psychology and religion* (pp. 304–308). Springer.

Diamond, S. A. (2009b). Shadow. In D. Leeming, K. Madden, & S. Marlan (Eds.), *Encyclopedia of psychology and religion* (pp. 836–838). Springer.

Diamond, S. A. (2009c). Daimonic. In D. Leeming, K. Madden, & S. Marlan (Eds.), *Encyclopedia of psychology and religion* (pp. 197–200). Springer.

Diamond, S. A. (2011, March 4). Clinical despair: Science, psychotherapy, and spirituality in the treatment of depression. *Psychology Today*. Retrieved from www.psychologytoday.com/blog/evil-deeds/201103/clinical-despair-science-psychotherapy-and-spirituality-in-the-treatment-depR

Diamond, S. A. (2016). Existential therapy: Confronting life's ultimate concerns. In H. Tinsley, S. Lease, & N. Giffin Wiersma (Eds.), *Contemporary theory and practice in counseling and psychotherapy* (pp. 323–352). SAGE.

Diamond, S. A. (2018). Existential therapy and Jungian analysis: Toward an existential depth psychology. *Journal of Humanistic Psychology. OnlineFirst.*

Dolan, E. (2018). Psychopathic traits influence brain connectivity in youths with Conduct Disorder. *PsyPost*. Retrieved from https://www.psypost.org/2018/04/youths-conduct-disorder-low-levels-psychopathic-traits-less-well-connected-brains-51123

Felder, A. J., Aten, H. M., Neudeck, J. A., Shiomi-Chen, J., & Robbins, B. E. (2014). Mindfulness at the heart of existential-phenomenological and humanistic psychology: A century of contemplation and elaboration. *Humanistic Psychologist, 42*, 6–23.

Frankl, V. E. (1985). *Man's search for meaning* (rev. ed.). Washington Square Press. (Original work published 1946).

Freud, S. (1915). Thoughts for the times on war and death. In J. Strachey, A. Freud, A. Strachey, & A. Tyson (Eds.). *The standard edition of the complete psychological works of Sigmund Freud: Vol. 14*. London: Vintage.

Freud, S. (1926). Inhibitions, symptoms, and anxiety. *SE, 20*, 87–172.

Freud, S. (1929/2002). *Civilization and Its Discontents*. London: Penguin.

Freud, S. (1966). *Introductory lectures on psychoanalysis* (J. Strachey, Trans. & Ed.). Liveright Publishing Corporation. (Original work published 1936).

Frick, P. J., Lilienfeld, S. O., Ellis, M., Loney, B., & Silverthorn, P. (1999). The association between anxiety and psychopathy dimensions in children. *Journal of Abnormal Child Psychology, 27*, 383–392.

Gómez-Leal, R., Megías-Robles, A., Gutiérrez-Cobo, M. J., Cabello, R., Fernández-Abascal, E. G., & Fernández-Berrocal, P. (2019). Relationship between the Dark Triad and depressive symptoms. *Peer J, 7*, e8120. https://doi.org/10.7717/peerj.8120.

Hare, R. D. (1991). *The Hare Psychopathy Checklist-Revised*. Multi-Health Systems.

Hare, R. D. (1998). The Hare PCL-R: Some issues concerning its use and misuse. *Legal and Criminological Psychology, 3*, 101–122.

Hare, R. D. (1999). *Without conscience: The disturbing world of the psychopaths among us*. The Guilford Press.

Hedegaard, H., Curtin, S. C., & Warner, M. (2018). Suicide mortality in the United States, 1999–2017. *NCHS Data Brief, No. 330.*

Heidegger, M. (2010). *Being and time* (Rev.). SUNY Press. (Original work published 1927).
Jack, A., Friedman, J., Bovatzis, R., & Taylor, S. (2015). Why do you believe in God? Relationships between religious belief, analytic thinking, mentalizing and moral concern. *Psychiatric Annals, 45*, 195–199.
Johnson, S. (1987). *Humanizing the Narcissistic Style*. W. W. Norton & Company.
Jung, C. G. (1938). *Psychology and Religion*. New Haven: Yale University Press.
Jung, C. G. (1961). *Memories, dreams, reflections.* (R. & C. Winston, Trans. & A. Jaffe, Ed.). Pantheon Books.
Jung, C. G. (1968). *Man and his symbols*. Dell Publishing.
Jung, C. G. (1971). *Psychological Types, Collected Works, Volume 6, Princeton*, N.J.: Princeton University Press.
Kamens, S., Flanagan, E., & Robbins, B. D. (2017). Introduction to the second special issue on diagnostic alternatives. *Journal of Humanistic Psychology, 58*, 3–6.
Kamens, S., Robbins, B. D., & Flanagan, E. (2019). Introduction to the fifth special issue on diagnostic alternatives. *Journal of Humanistic Psychology, 56*, 1–6.
Karasavva, V. (2019). The fear factor: Deficits in psychopathy as an index of limbic dysregulaton. *Journal of Young Investigators, 36*, 73–80.
Karpman, B. (1948). The myth of the psychopathic personality. *The American Journal of Psychiatry, 104*, 523–534.
Kernberg, O. F. (1992). *Aggression in personality disorders and perversions*. Yale University Press.
Kiehl, K., & Hoffman, M. (2011). The criminal psychopath: History, neuroscience, treatment, and economics. *Jurimetrics, 51*, 355–397.
Kierkegaard, S. A. (1980). *The concept of anxiety: A simple psychologically orienting deliberation on the dogmatic issue of hereditary sin.* In R. Thomte, in collaboration with A. Anderson (Eds.). Princeton University Press. (Original work published 1844 in Danish, translated 1944 as *The concept of dread*).
Kohut, H. (1978). Thoughts on narcissism and narcissistic rage. In *The search for the self: Selected writings of Heinz Kohut: 1950–1978*. International University Press.
Langle, A., & Klaassen, D. (2019). Phenomenology and depth in existential psychotherapy. *Journal of Humanistic Psychology*. OnlineFirst. https://doi.org/10.1177/0022167818823281.
Lilienfeld, S. O., Latzman, R. D., Watts, A. L., Smith, S. F., & Dutton, K. (2016). Correlates of psychopathic personality traits in everyday life: Results from a large community survey. *Frontiers of Psychology, 201*. https://doi.org/10.1371/journal.pone.0149989
Lykken, D. (1995). *The antisocial personalities*. Lawrence Erlbaum Associates.
Martens, W. (2003). Spiritual psychotherapy for antisocial and psychopathic personalities: Some theoretical building blocks. *Journal of Contemporary Psychotherapy, 33*, 205–218.
Martens, W. (2014). The hidden suffering of the psychopath. *Psychiatric Times, 31*(10), 1.
May, R. (1939). *The art of counseling; how to gain and give mental health*. Nashville: Cokesbury Press.
May, R. (1953). *Man's search for himself*. New York: W. W. Norton.
May, R. (1969/2007). *Love and will*. New York : W.W. Norton.
May, R. (1970). Psychotherapy and the daimonic. In J. Campbell (Ed.), *Myths, dreams, and religion* (pp. 196–210). Society for the Arts, Religion and Contemporary Culture. Dutton.
May, R. (1972). *Power and innocence: A search for the sources of violence*. New York: W. W. Norton.
May, R. (1977). *The meaning of anxiety* (rev. ed.). Norton. (Original work published 1950 by Ronald Press Company).
May, R. (1981). *Freedom and destiny*. W W Norton & Co.
May, R. (1982). The problem of evil: An open letter to Carl Rogers. *Journal of Humanistic Psychology, 22*, 10–21.
May, R. (1983). *The discovery of being: Writings in existential psychology*. Norton.
May, R. (1991). *The cry for myth*. Norton.
May, R., Angel, E., & Ellenberger, H. F. (Eds.). (1958). *Existence: A new dimension in psychiatry and psychology*. Simon & Schuster.
Međedović, J., & Petrović, B. (2015). The Dark Tetrad: Structural properties and location in the personality space. *Journal of Individual Differences, 36*, 228–236.

Meloy, J. R. (2012). Predatory violence and psychopathy. In H. Hakkanen-Nyholm & J. Nyholm (Eds.), *Psychopathy and law*. Wiley.
Millon, T., Simonsen, E., Birket-Smith, & Davis, R. (Eds.) (1998). Psychopathy: Antisocial, criminal, and violent behavior. : The Guilford Press.
Moustakas, C. E. (1990). *Loneliness*. Simon & Schuster. (Original work published 1961).
Moustakas, C. E. (1994). *Existential psychotherapy and the interpretation of dreams*. Aronson.
Murphy, C., & Vess, J. (2003). Subtypes of psychopathy: Proposed differences between narcissistic, borderline, sadistic, and antisocial psychopaths. *Psychiatric Quarterly, 74*, 11–29.
Nietzsche, F. (2019). *The gay science: With a prelude in rhymes and an appendix of songs* (T. Common, Trans.). Anodos Books. (Original work published 1883).
Perls, F. S. (1971). *Gestalt therapy verbatim* (J. O. Stevens, Ed.). Bantam Books.
Raine, A. (1993). *The psychopathology of crime*. Academic.
Rank, O. (1936). *Will therapy* (Jesse Taft, Trans.). Knopf.
Rank, O. (1993). *The trauma of birth*. Dover Press. (Original work published 1924).
Robins, L. N. (1996). Deviant children grown up. *European Child & Adolescent Psychiatry, 5*, 44–46.
Rogers, C. (1982). Reply to Rollo May's letter to Carl Rogers. *Journal of Humanistic Psychology, 22*, 85–89.
Sandvik, A. M., et al. (2015). Psychopathy, anxiety, and resiliency—Psychological hardiness as a mediator of the psychopathy–anxiety relationship in a prison setting. *Personality and Individual Differences, 72*, 30–34.
Sartre, J.-P. (1946/2007). *Existentialism Is a Humanism*. New Haven: Yale University Press.
Sartre, J.-P. (1962). *Existential psychoanalysis*. (H. Barnes, Trans.). [Introduction by Rollo May]. Henry Regnery Company. (Original work published 1953).
Sevecke, K., Franke, S., Kosson, D., & Krischer, M. (2016). Emotional disregulation and trauma predicting psychopathy dimensions in female and male juvenile offenders. *Child and Adolescent Psychiatry and Mental Health, 10*, 43.
Skeem, J. L., Polaschek, D. L. L., Patrick, C. J., & Lilienfeld, S. O. (2011). Psychopathic personality: Bridging the gap between scientific evidence and public policy. *Psychological Science in the Public Interest, 12*, 95–162.
Spinelli, E. (2005). *The interpreted world: An introduction to phenomenological psychology* (2nd ed.). SAGE.
Tiihonen, J., Koskuvi, M., Lähteenvuo, M., Virtanen, P. L. J., Ojansuu, I., Vaurio, O., Gao, Y., Hyötyläinen, I., Puttonen, K. A., Repo-Tihonen, E., Paunio, T., Rautiainen, M.-R., Tyni, S., Koistinaho, J., & Lehtonen, S. (2020). Neurobiological roots of psychopathy. *Molecular Psychiatry, 25*, 3432–3441.
Tillich, P. (1952). *The courage to be*. Yale University Press.
Van Deurzen, E., Craig, E., Langle, A., Schneider, K., Tantam, D., & du Plock, S. (Eds.). (2019). *The Wiley world handbook of existential therapy*. Wiley-Blackwell.
Werner, K., Few, L., & Bucholz, K. (2015). Epidemiology, comorbidity, and behavioral genetics of Antisocial Personality Disorder and psychopathy. *Personality and Individual Differences, 72*, 30–34.
Winnicott, D. W. (1960). Ego distortion in terms of true and false self. In *The maturational process and the facilitating environment: Studies in the theory of emotional development* (pp. 140–157). International Universities Press.
World Health Organization. *ICD-10: The ICD-10 classification of mental and behavioural Disorders: Clinical descriptions and diagnostic guidelines*. World Health Organization.
Yalom, I. D. (1980). *Existential psychotherapy*. Basic Books.
Yalom, I. D. (1989). *Love's executioner and other tales of psychotherapy*. Harper Collins.
Yalom, I. D. (2009). *Staring at the sun: Overcoming the terror of death*. Jossey-Bass.
Yalom, I., & Josselson, R. (2013). Existential psychotherapy. In D. Wedding & R. Corsini (Eds.), *Current psychotherapies* (10th ed., pp. 265–298). Cengage.

Chapter 17
A Gestalt Therapy Perspective on Psychopathy: Bearing the Unbearable

Gianni Francesetti

Abstract The topic of psychopathy opens up many roads of inquiry—diagnostic, psychopathological, therapeutic, clinical, forensic, existential, ethical—which together outline an extremely complex landscape. The intention of this chapter is not to reduce that complexity, but rather to contribute, if possible, to highlighting it, and perhaps even to add to it. The fulcrum of this work lies in the search for a clinical dimension of meaning for psychopathic experience through a Gestalt Therapy perspective, building in particular on a fundamental construct of the approach, which is field theory. It is essential to bear firmly in mind that the search for meaning does not mean searching for justification. It means searching for a *ground*, from which a phenomenon emerges, and for *movement*, for the intentional direction the phenomenon tends to move towards. In this approach, trying to understand cannot be avoided, and it means grasping subjective experience, how it emerges, and the meaning it has. Our hope is that this exploration can give rise to potentially useful insights for clinical work.

Keywords Psychopathy · Gestalt Therapy · Field theory · Compassion · Aggression · Destructivity

> *Man does not strive to be good; the good is what it is human to strive for.*
> Perls et al., 1951, 115

> *The good bear the sensorium of the Lord on the earth. That is why they suffer as the creator suffers in the world*
> Dietrich Bonhoeffer, 2015, 25

> *The* evil *which the innocent victim feels in himself is in his executioner, but he is not sensible of the fact.*
> Simone Weil, 1952, 72

G. Francesetti (✉)
IPsiG – International Institute for Gestalt Therapy and Psychopathology, University of Torino, Turin, Italy

J. E. Vitale (ed.), *The Complexity of Psychopathy*, Dangerous Behavior in Clinical and Forensic Psychology, https://doi.org/10.1007/978-3-030-83156-1_17

17.1 Statement of Intent

The topic of psychopathy opens up many roads of inquiry—diagnostic, psychopathological, therapeutic, clinical, forensic, existential, ethical—which together outline an extremely complex landscape. The intention of this chapter is not to reduce that complexity, but rather to contribute, if possible, to highlighting it, and perhaps even to add to it. The fulcrum of this work lies in the search for a clinical dimension of meaning for psychopathic experience through a Gestalt Therapy perspective, building in particular on a fundamental construct of the approach, which is field theory. Any step towards the search for a dimension of meaning is itself a controversial move, one that cannot be taken for granted. What sense does it make to search for meaning in those folds of humanity where humanity itself seems to have ceased to exist? Is it ethical to do so? Would it not be simply better to decree that there can be no sense and meaning where the objectification of the other comes to prevail, with the potential to reach the heights of the unimaginable, of the unmentionable and unbearable, as there ends the humanity of human beings, giving way to the realm of monsters? Is evil banal (Arendt, 1963)? Are we all capable of monstrosity or is it only the work of monsters? Such questions are inevitable when entering such a terrain—a terrain where angels fear to tread (Pope, 1711)—and as such should at least be mentioned. History and daily news show us this possibility is all too real and human, touching us and demanding our attention in the way it proves constantly to occur—it is estimated that some 30,000 civilians were killed per day last century (Raine, 2014).

Here we will assume the critical position that none of us is immune to the Lucifer effect (Zimbardo, 2008). From there we will explore the issue without forgoing the search for meaning, constituent as it is to any phenomenological inquiry into psychopathology (Borgna, 1988; Stanghellini et al., 2019) and the phenomenological approach of Gestalt Therapy (Francesetti, 2015, 2019a). It is essential to bear firmly in mind that the search for meaning does not mean searching for justification. It means searching for a *ground*, from which a phenomenon emerges, and for *movement*, for the intentional direction the phenomenon tends to move towards. In this approach, trying to understand cannot be avoided, and it means grasping subjective experience, how it emerges, and the meaning it has. Only in this way can clinical work be directed above and beyond psychoeducational or pharmacological intervention. Our hope is that this exploration can give rise to potentially useful insights for clinical work. To promote greater understanding of the text, I will use as much as possible a phenomenological language, avoiding, where possible, the theoretical terminology associated strictly with Gestalt Therapy.

17.2 Psychopathy and Gestalt Therapy

Gestalt Therapy has produced rather little in the way of clinical literature on sociopathic and psychopathic disorders, although it has provided some insight for directing therapy (Bloom, 2018; Bongers, 2013; Denham-Vaughan, 2009; Djoric et al.,

2016; Francesetti, 2012; Lapides, forthcoming). Nevertheless, this approach emerged precisely from a critique of the Freudian theory of aggression and efforts to disassociate from the idea that there exists an innate destructive instinct (*Thanatos*). Humans cannot be understood abstracted from their environment and isolated from the context in which they find themselves. The concept of innate instincts is a simplification that neglects the fundamental fact that the human emerges, and is formed, in every given situation. Rather than instincts, there are possibilities and limits to creative responses in given situations.[1]

Gestalt Therapy reassesses human aggression as a creative and positive movement towards the other (*ad-graedior*, move-towards) (Perls, 1942). It is not an expression of a death instinct, but a force for reaching the other, for destructuring and being destructured, in the search for a new and creative way to encounter the other and live together (Bloom, 2013b; Salonia et al., 1996). It becomes violence when it lies outside the bounds of mutual regulation, which is all the more probable the more aggressiveness is belittled, denied, and excluded from awareness. When delegitimized, separated, and denied, it becomes an unconscious urge that is suffered, and hence cannot be regulated within the relationship.

In the foundational work of Gestalt Therapy (Perls et al., 1951), central importance is placed on analyzing the relationship between suffering, aggressiveness, therapy, and society, offering us a gateway to addressing our topic. The social context is an essential ground that cannot be ignored when making diagnostic, psychopathological, and therapeutic assessments, which can make no sense if not in the light of the relational dimension, played out on different scales, from which it takes shape. Such an approach was undoubtedly a pioneering and enlightened expression of the cultural climate prevailing in post-war New York and the radical social criticism that ensued from it. These were embodied fully by the founders of Gestalt Therapy: Laura Posner Perls and Friedrick Perls, Jewish psychoanalysts who eventually arrived in New York after fleeing Nazi Germany, and Paul Goodman, *maitre à penser* of the American youth protest movement, shaped by the Chicago School of Pragmatism, who placed into sharp focus the contradictions of America's capitalist, racist, sexist, and conformist society in the 1960s, and helped sustain its more innovative trends (Goodman, 1947, 1960). The founders caution us to beware of any definition of psychopathology that fails to consider the relationship of the individual with the community of reference. That community implicitly sets the standards of what is normal for community members and hence, subtly, for their mental health, while at the same time it contributes to shaping (pathoplasticity) and/or provoking (pathogenesis) suffering in the individual. The diagnosis of *drapetomania*, or the 'compulsive urge to escape' was formulated in the mid-1800s in the southern states of United States to stigmatize slaves that rebelled against the yoke of their masters.

[1] It is worth noting that developments in psychoanalysis in recent times have moved in much the same direction (Lackmann, 2001; Eagle, 2010).

The example is strikingly patent, now that history separates us from those times, but analogous risks still exist today.[2]

In our view, it is important to highlight the complexity of the relationship between the forces at play in the social field, which are embodied in individual behaviours and which are acted out by individuals in a circular way. Diagnostic and psychopathological frameworks always carry the risk of attributing to the individual a greater or lesser share of a social disorder which takes on shape and visibility in the individual. It is important to be aware of that risk (Lingiardi, 2018; Francesetti & Gecele, 2009). The complexity of the relationship between individual and society therefore demands particular caution when using the term 'sociopathy': "…we can speak of a conflict between the individual and society and call certain behaviour 'antisocial'. In this sense, too, we must certainly call certain mores and institutions of society "antipersonal"' (Perls et al. 1951, p. 113). Many psychopathic individuals are not in conflict with the rules and mores of society. Indeed, they can benefit from the values and gratifications of their community to experience their disorder in an ego-syntonic, and 'socio-syntonic' way. Suffice it to think of the psychopathy of people of great success in our contemporary world or of popular heroes in times of war and generalized social violence. On the other hand, individuals who act outside or against shared social norms, and thus can be defined as antisocial, may hold ethical values that are light years away from psychopathic experience. It is for these reasons that we prefer to use the term psychopathy, rather than sociopathy or *antisocial disorder* (Cleckley, 1941; Hare et al. 1991; Lingiardi and McWilliams, 2017; Meloy, 1988).

17.3 Psychopathic Experience

There is much debate over how to define the psychopathic personality and various scales have been developed and validated for identifying the condition and its severity. For a discussion of these aspects, I refer readers to the literature (Cleckey, 1941; Dazzi & Madeddu, 2009; Hare, 1980; Stone, 2006). In this chapter, we refer to psychopathic experience as a dimension of personality of greater or lesser intensity, whose functioning may be neurotic, borderline, or psychotic (Lingiardi & McWilliams, 2017). The central feature of psychopathic experience is the urge to wield power over the other by reifying her/him[3] and dominating it for one's own

[2]The DSM 5 (APA, 2013) introduced some new diagnostic categories, including *compulsive shopping disorder; compulsive sex disorder; and psychotic risk disorder*. The DSM looks at them as individual disorders, but if we consider our contemporary social field, we may ask: are individuals suffering from compulsive shopping disorder or is there a field suffering from consumerism? Are individuals suffering from compulsive sex disorder or is there a field suffering from a lack of ties and stability in relationships? Are individuals suffering from psychotic risk disorder or is there a field suffering from a lack of boundaries and ground? (Francesetti, 2013).

[3]Reification, from the Latin *res*, or *thing* + *facere,* namely *to make*: 'make into an object.'

ends. Deliberate manipulation, violence, abuse, seduction, and lying are the instruments for objectifying and dominating the other. An implicit element in wielding power and reifying is that of causing harm to the other—an element that may be more or less intentionally and consciously at the fore, in the sense that it may be the aim of the action or a side-effect in the pursuit of one's aims. Nevertheless, it is a characteristic feature of psychopathic experience. Treating the other as an object rather than a subject, and in so doing dehumanizing him, itself contains the central element of the disorder, which is to be indifferent to or to enjoy causing pain in the other (Bloom, 2013a). It is an experience that causes *une souffrance inutile*, useless suffering, something which Lévinas (1990) explored extensively starting from the horrifying and shocking incomprehensibility of the Holocaust.

There is debate as to whether or not empathetic capacity exists in psychopathic experience, but the different positions held are often the outcome of equivocal understandings of the term. Baron-Cohen in *The Science of* Evil (2011), for instance, adopts the concept of 'empathy erosion' to define psychopathy, where 'empathy' includes not only the ability to identify the experiences of the other, but also the ability to respond with a corresponding emotional state. Other authors call 'empathy' the capacity to identify the emotional states of others and 'sympathy' the capacity to respond in an affectively syntonic way (Englebert, 2019). There is a fair consensus in the literature over the fact that psychopaths are capable of grasping the affective and emotional states of the other—indeed, they excel at it to manipulate others—but they are not able to respond with an experience of sympathy and compassion towards the victim. In other words, they are able to understand what the other is feeling, what he needs, and how to motivate him, but show no authentic interest in the other, except as an object for their own ends, and feel no human and compassionate connection when faced with the pain of the other. Although psychopaths may show particular interest, care, and closeness, even emotion and feeling, they remain substantially detached and indifferent towards the other as a subject. In Buber's terms (1953), the foundational experience here is the impossibility of an authentic 'I–Thou' experience, which can nevertheless be simulated, and being condemned to experience the other as an 'It,' an object. A genuine, authentic meeting and affective connection with the other person is not possible.

One last element that is important to underscore is that psychopathic experience resembles a galaxy much more than it does a monolith. There are degrees and vast subjective differences in the experience, ranging from indifference towards the other's experience, which can lead to an affectively barren existence, even when full of strong stimuli, to criminal violence towards other people beyond the imaginable. There are people who act in a solitary fashion, completely outside the bounds of social rules, and there are others who take part in socially endorsed and rewarded actions, such as the respectfully dressed psychopaths of our own society, or executioners in situations of war or persecution.

17.4 Conditions that Foster Psychopathy

The literature and research highlight various risk factors and situations of vulnerability for the development of psychopathy. In general, they can be grouped into three classes: individual, situational and anthropological factors. These classes should be considered as complementary dimensions and not alternative categories. The specific situation of a patient can be affected by all these conditions (i.e. individual, situational and anthropological).

17.4.1 Individual Factors

Individual factors include biological conditions and individual biography. Biological conditions refer to predispositions that can foster a criminal behavior. They include genetic and epigenetic characteristics, but also hormonal and metabolic balances. Biographical conditions refer to life events and relational situations that can affect the personality's traits of the patient.

Biological Conditions Individual risk factors include genetic and biological conditions (Glenn & Raine, 2014; Rayne, 2014). According to this a line of inquiry, which finds its pioneering origins in the work of Cesare Lombroso (Gibson, 2002), there are biological predispositions that foster or lead to criminal behavior. It is risky, however, to assume that biological factors can be the cause of psychopathy if we close the door on the search for a relational meaning to the experience. Ultimately, to consider psychopaths as being biologically different from us is to reify them, which means making exactly the same move as the psychopath. Such a position, where behaviors are reduced to a specific, identifiable biological cause, has opened the gates in history to discrimination, persecution, and eugenics, based consistently on the assumption of a definitive, *a priori* knowledge of the other, where the other is not a creature (from the Latin, *a being in creation*), but an object known definitively; thus the other is reified. No longer a human in the making (as existentialism teaches us), a body which we can never determine what it will do (as Spinoza grasped), but an alien object known to us. There are many ways to objectify the Other, and one subtle way is to pretend to know her/him (Bloom, 2021). The biological data may be correlative (psychopathic experience is associated with specific neurological, hormonal, and immunity patterns, for instance), or point to predisposing factors (a certain genetic make-up raises the likelihood of psychopathic behavior), but it is very risky and scientifically wrong to treat them as simple causal mechanisms. That does not mean that all those who suffer from psychopathy can be rehabilitated or treated. It simply means that it is risky and wrong to think we can know that *a priori* on the mere basis of biological data. Biology is nothing more than a relational precipitate from the combination of two DNA chains upon conception. To understand its weight, we need to see it interact with history and the relationship. It is then that we can ask which factors of biological vulnerability may be activated in traumatic histories, or which pathways of genetic and epigenetic transmission pass on traumatic anaesthesia over the generations. In other words, biology is history—whether recent or ancient—precipitated in molecules and physiological connections.

Individual Biography In an attempt to identify individual risk factors while widening the spotlight to encompass the family and relational context, there are studies that highlight the histories of traumatic childhood development that are generally present, pervasive, and acute in psychopathic personalities (Athens, 1992; Fonagy, 1997; Kernberg, 1992; Lackmann, 2001; Meloy, 1988). This field of research suggests that relational experiences of major neglect, violence, and abuse suffered as a child cannot be processed, leading the individual to find protection in various modes of affective disconnection and inhibiting the development of a suitable capacity for emotional attunement and reflective function. The abundance of studies in this field include research on child soldiers in Sierra Leone (Ardizzi et al., 2015), where the children who had been exposed to extreme events, such as seeing the rape or murder of their parents and siblings, were then forced to torture and kill friends and acquaintances. From a neurological point of view, their chances of accessing their sadness and pain are remarkably reduced, if not impossible, whereas they have a heightened access to their anger.

The research shows how people who develop a psychopathic personality tend to have lived in a family relational field in which reifying forces were very strong. As children, many of these individuals had been treated as objects in such a traumatic way that goes beyond the ability of the child to conceive that someone who is meant to care for them can do them such harm (Fonagy & Target, 1997). That 'excess' can be tolerated by reifying and dehumanizing oneself in turn, so that the pain fades away and the relational bond maintained in a certain way. Thus, the child can anaesthetize the unbearable pain of having been treated so inhumanely, but as his pain vanishes, so does the possibility of meeting the other in that affective dimension of pain and compassion. The child soldiers of Sierra Leone are an extreme example of that process. Instead of confirming to the child his humanity, the absence of the caregiver invalidates it and becomes the absence of humanity in the child himself, through his retreat and flight from a world that is devastated, dehumanized, and unbearable (Arendt, 1958).

Every relational experience leaves behind a biological trace, while biological organization makes certain relational experiences possible. If not taken to extremes, the two perspectives, the biological and the relational, are complementary: a constitutional predisposition may favor a psychopathic type of response to a traumatic environment, while first-hand traumatic experiences can modify the functioning of the organism. Even the experiences lived by the parents or past generations can be transmitted epigenetically over time and across subsequent generations, as traumas sediment in the transgenerational memory, inscribing themselves into the flesh of each (Spagnuolo Lobb & Francesetti, 2015; Mucci, 2013).

17.4.2 Situational Factors

The situational perspective instead shines a light on the components of the context that favor or lead to psychopathic behavior. Research in this field has highlighted how a situation can bring into play psychopathic forces and lead even people who show no biological predisposition whatsoever for it, or who show elements of a personality disorder, to behave in an openly psychopathic way. Such research includes the studies by Milgram (1974) on obedience to authority and Zimbardo's Stanford Prison Experiment (Zimbardo, 2008), where in given situations—characterized by the pressures of an authority or a role, for instance, or by the dispersion of responsibility—psychopathic behaviors emerge in people who are 'normal'. This is the banality of evil described by Hannah Arendt in her coverage of Eichmann's crimes—monsters are not needed for monstrosities to be committed. If Eichmann was 'normal,' then none of us is immune to the danger of doing evil. All you need is good family men no longer fit for action on the front line to create Battalion 101, for instance, the Nazi police corps made up of reservists and charged with exterminating Polish Jews, whose crimes proved to be particularly horrendous and heinous (Browning, 2001).

17.4.3 Anthropological Factors

Finally, there is the anthropological approach (Bauman, 2011; Heidegger, 1954). First theorized by Günther Anders (1964), and developed in the work of Emanuele Severino (1998) and Umberto Galimberti (2002), such a perspective focuses on the relationship between evil and the growth of technological capacity. Anders argues there is a gap between the human capacity to produce technology (*herstellen*) and our capacity for imagination (*vorstellen*), and hence for governing the consequences. When things can technically be done, they are done—the pointless bombing of Wurzburg towards the end of the Second World War by the Allies and the atomic bombs dispatched on Hiroshima and, in particular, Nagasaki three days later[4], all occurred because we were prepared to do it and had the power to do it (Bauman, 2011). Technology amplifies the hiatus between action (power) and its consequences (destruction), rendering the destructive gesture colder, and hence easier: 'one doesn't gnash one's teeth when pressing a button… A key is a key' (Anders quoted by Bauman, 2011, p. 100).

Similar conclusions are reached by Marshall McLuhan (1964) in his analysis of the effects of technology, *regardless of the use* that is made of it. Every technological advance enhances a human organ or function—the knife enhances our teeth, the wheel our legs, eye glasses our sight, and so on. But the cost of such prosthetic enhancement is the weakening of the organ or function itself. Our teeth and our legs

[4] The justifications for the attack on Nagasaki are still debated.

are not as strong as those of our ancestors, and the habitual use of eye glasses makes the eye dependent on them, and less reactive when we take them off. The new media studied by McLuhan were radio and television, extensions of the afferent sensory nervous system that enable us to receive information in volumes previously unimaginable, while shortening both time and space. The result is that the world has become a global village, but at the cost of the torpidity of our overloaded senses. Ours is an age of narcosis—which by no coincidence shares the same root as 'narcissism': a dulling of the perception of the other. The outcome of such a sensory overexposure is flat affect and emotional detachment. Indifference. More recent technological developments go beyond that to produce a further anthropological change, as the entire world is now within our reach—quite literally, with our smartphones, the world is in our hands. That has brought us to a new quantum leap, whereby we can be present anywhere, and take action anywhere, at any time.

The growth in media presence, however, comes at the cost of reducing presence itself, which becomes disembodied in the here and now, a consequence of which is the uprooting of the present situation and the acceleration of temporality (Rosa, 2010). Diffuse presence, temporal acceleration, and the feeling of having the world within reach are all characteristics of manic experience. It is no surprise that in psychopathology we are witnessing a growth in bipolar disorders and depression, the other face of our socially manic times. The relationship here with psychopathy is also interesting, as the technological gap, desensitization, and the diffusion of presence all contribute to opening a breach with the other that can easily become indifference towards the suffering of the other. Then again, as early as the turn of the nineteenth century, Pinel called psychopathy '*manie sans délire*' (mania or insanity without delusion). The reification of the other occurs in both mania and in psychopathy, but while in the former case the subjectivity that is constituted maintains no bond with the common world, in the second case it does (Stanghellini et al., 2019). In a world that is itself manic in functioning the other can be reified without severing the bond with the common world, which is, as we said, manic. In a world oriented anthropologically in such a way that psychopathy lies not just in individuals but in entire societies, may well be a risk that should be taken seriously. The individual, situational and anthropological perspectives are thus conditions of risk that come into play in different ways and to different degrees depending on constitutional predisposition, personality, history, and biographical, historical, cultural, and micro- and macro-situations. Psychopathy, as we said, is more of a galaxy than a monolith, a universe where it is dangerous to think that complexity can be reduced in any easy way.

17.5 Searching for Meaning in What Has No Meaning: Psychopathy in the Light of Field Theory

In this section, I try to describe the psychopathic experience as a phenomenon of the field. When we apply field theory to a psychopathological phenomenon, we move our focus from the individual experience to the forces that affect the emergence of the suffering. This is considered not as an individual dysfunction, but as an emergent phenomenon that pushes in order to be transformed. From this perspective, we try to shed some new light to the psychopathic experience.

17.5.1 Some Definitions in limine

Field theory is a theoretical construct founded on the Gestalt Therapy approach, through the influence of Gestalt psychology, Kurt Lewin, and Jan Smuts (Francesetti, 2019b; Francesetti & Roubal, 2020; Parlett & Lee, 2005; Robine, 2001; Roubal & Francesetti, in press; Staemmler, 2006; Wollants, 2008). In clinical work, it is useful to bear in mind the concepts of phenomenal field, phenomenological field, and psychopathological field.[5] The phenomenal field is the horizon of phenomenal events for a given situation, the boundary within which certain phenomena tend to emerge, while others do not. For example, at a party with friends, it is easier for jokes and jests, moments of good cheer, and feelings of lightness to emerge, and time will tend to flow quickly. At a funeral wake, it is more likely that feelings of heaviness will emerge, the slowing or rarefaction of time, gloominess, and immobility. The phenomenal field is perceptible by the senses as the atmosphere of the situation, in which the forces that condition the emergence of phenomena move. With black holes, the force that bends the event horizon is gravity; with the phenomenal field, it is the intentionalities at play that bend it. In the therapeutic encounter, those forces—embodied intentionalities—move both the patient and the therapist and are co-created by them both. But in this paradigm[6]—in which the self is not a structure but a phenomenon that emerges from the situation—the forces in the phenomenal field are in motion before the subjects are differentiated and defined, for which we can say that the therapist and the patient emerge, 'are made,' within the situation and are moved by the forces in the field. The phenomenal field is *pathos*: it is suffered and not chosen (Waldenfelds, 2011). The capacity to be aware of this field, to notice the forces at play that move us, to be curious about what is happening, transforms the phenomenal field suffered—where I am *subject-to*—into a phenomenological field—where I am the *subject-of*—that is, into a field in which the space of possibilities expands and it is possible to reflect on what is happening and make choices. That passage from the phenomenal to the phenomenological is close to what Fonagy & Target (1997) describe as the capacity for reflection and mentalization. Nevertheless, from the perspective that we propose, the ability to reflect and verbalize is not only a cognitive competence, since it is combined with an embodied attunement to the sensory phenomena in motion.

[5] I refer readers to past works published for a more in-depth discussion: Francesetti, 2015, 2019a, 2019b; Francesetti and Griffero, 2019).

[6] The paradigm here is phenomenological (Wiesing, 2014), in line with studies of perception in Gestalt psychology (Francesetti, 2016), neuroscientific research on the self by Damasio (2010), and the philosophical approach of pathic aesthetics (Griffero, 2017; Böhme, 2017).

So what is a psychopathological field? It is a phenomenal field in which an absence is present, meaning an inability to be present one to the other, either because perception or emotion is dulled or restricted, or because it is not possible to be constituted as differentiated and connected subjects belonging to a common world (in which case the experience has a psychotic quality). Psychopathology can be seen as an expression of the ways one can be absent in the relationship, and therapy as a situation in which somebody—the therapist—is able to be present to those absences. The concept of field can be useful for our purposes here in this chapter, first of all to understand the emergence of psychopathic experience, and secondly to understand clinical phenomena and to guide therapy work.

17.5.2 The Psychopathic Field: The Urge to Reify

The psychopathic field is characterized by the reification of the other, by the lack of an authentic affective resonance which is essential for constituting the other as an *other-than-me*, but at the same time as an *other-like-me*. The other is thus an *it* of service to me, and not a *thou* whose dignity I acknowledge and whom I respect and sympathize with (Buber, 1923). I am deaf to the ethical call of the face of the other (Bloom, 2013a, 2021; Lévinas, 1961; Orange, 2018). We have seen how such deafness can be driven by biological dispositions, and how it is often the result of traumatic histories, but in some specific situations it can emerge, in a surprisingly easy way, in people who 'can hear clearly.'

When looking at psychopathy from the field theory perspective, what we first take into consideration is the intentionalities at play even before the subjects are differentiated. As in Pirandello's *Six Characters in Search of an Author* (1921), we can imagine how in a certain situation there can be forces that seek out bodies through which to emerge. Those forces are not, obviously, independent of the people involved and present. Quite simply, there is a level of self-emergence at which the subjects have yet to be defined, and in that undifferentiated, pre-personal level the forces at play do not yet belong to anyone, and cannot be attributed to any specific person. In the Stanford Prison Experiment, for example, reifying forces emerged in the guards not because they had psychopathic personalities, but because their role made it more likely to happen—but the forces were moving in the field as expressions of the situation. At a certain point in the experiment, the roles could have been inverted, but the result would have been the same (as history has often sadly shown, in cases where the oppressed become the oppressors once they come to power). Such a perspective can also have macro-social implications, as the general climate of a society can favor the emergence of reifying forces that then 'take hold' of the majority of people, following a Gaussian pattern of distribution. At the extremes of the curve, individual characteristics weigh in more. In the infamous Battalion 101, some were happy with the task assigned to them (most likely people with stronger psychopathic tendencies); others were more reluctant and asked not to take part in the most violent strikes (perhaps those with lower psychopathic tendencies); while the majority perpetrated the massacres of defenseless children, women, and the elderly without any particular affective involvement. The reifying forces in the situation were extreme, touching the majority of those exposed to them in different ways.

17.5.3 The Psychopathic Field in the Therapeutic Encounter: Violence Circulates and Is Circulated Even by the Therapist

Readers are referred to the literature for an in-depth description of the therapist's experiences in the clinical encounter with a psychopathic patient (McWilliams, 2011). Here we will limit our observations to how therapists often feel disgust, anger, fear, and the whole range of combinations and nuances, and the affective complexity that each specific situation entails. The outcome generally is a rejection of the patient, and the desire not to have him in therapy. A field perspective helps us to avoid considering such experiences as inappropriate or as an indicator of the therapist's lack of skill, but also as something that doesn't need any further inquiry ('who wouldn't feel repulsion towards a paedophile?'). Instead, the field perspective opens up the chance of exploring how even the therapist can be seized by the reifying forces at play in a psychopathic field. Let us look at an excerpt from a supervision session.

T.: Whenever I have to encounter S., I wish I could be elsewhere...my tummy cramps up even before setting foot in the practice. Then I see him, the indifference on his face, or his amusement as he relates all things he did to his two grandchildren, how he seduced them day after day and managed to convince them to play his 'little games,' as he calls them... how he sexually abused them just as he had abused their mother—his daughter—when she was a child.

S.: And what do you feel when you see 'the indifference on his face'?

T.: I feel contempt... I wish I could make him feel the pain his grandchildren and his daughter felt, make him feel the evil *he has done. I want to hurt him physically, smash his head in and see him suffer. That's what I wish! What a satisfaction it would be!*

Or here is another excerpt from a supervision session with a colleague who works in a prison.

T.: I'm completely shaken. My last session with R. was really disturbing. He was in a good mood, cheerful, and he proposed playing a number game that he had invented, which in the end turned out to be my birthday. I was horrified, frozen with fear. How could he have known? Was he spying on me? I felt overcome by danger and just wanted to run away as far as possible, but I felt helpless and stupid and just powerless... and I just smiled, terrified. Then I remembered that there was a guard outside the door and I calmed down, all I had to do was call out and he would come in. But for a moment it was absolutely horrifying. Talking about it now, it seems silly, there was no reason for it, but at the time it was horrible… In any case, I never want to see him again!

The therapist's experiences are obviously quite understandable and most likely we would all feel much the same way, to varying degrees and with different nuances. But we cannot close the matter with that. The therapist wished the patient would suffer, she wished she herself could make him suffer, it would be a 'satisfaction' for her—is that not a reifying movement in response to an intentionality to hurt the other? Is that not the force we said characterizes the psychopathic field? The therapist is seized by a phenomenal field in which pain needs to emerge through the other—that is the core of a psychopathic field. A pain that needs to emerge from the undifferentiated and take shape needs to be felt by the other. The first hold the psychopathic field takes on the therapist is to drive her to perpetuate it. And obviously for a good reason, as it would certainly be therapeutic for the patient to feel pain, and as a result the pain of the victim, and then a sense of guilt for it. The therapeutic act that comes from denial and aims to make the other feel the pain does nothing more than reactualize the psychopathic field.

The drive to make pain emerge through the other strikes us as a possible direction of meaning that can open up interesting roads for clinical intervention. It may be difficult to accept, but it would appear fundamental that even this dimension should be taken into consideration: that the psychopath needs the flesh of the other to make a dehumanizing pain emerge, a pain he cannot feel without using the other. A similar position is expressed by Simone Weil when she uses these words to describe her experience of the resistance to Nazism: "The innocent victim who suffers knows the truth about his executioner. The executioner does not know it. The evil which the innocent victim feels in himself is in his executioner, but this[7] cannot feel it. The innocent victim can only know the evil in the shape of suffering. That which is not felt by the criminal is his own crime. (…) It is the innocent victim who can feel hell. (…) All crime is a transference of the evil in him who acts to him who undergoes the result of the action" (Weil, 1952, pp. 122, 124). Violence is a way of making the evil present in the relational field emerge. A simple example is when a person suffers violence and the evil suffered becomes evil inflicted, that is, violence. It is only by making the evil suffered emerge that it can find another way out, an alternative way to a reifying anaesthesia that becomes violence. Only in that way can it be transformed. Psychopathic absence—the reifying of the other—is the way the pain suffered by the executioner, but which he cannot feel, comes to light.

The pain that the executioner cannot feel may be his own, the pain of his own traumatic history, a pain experienced but which he cannot face and process. Or, it may be the pain experienced by past generations and handed down relationally and biologically over the passage of generations, a pain kept alive in the traumatic stratifications of entire populations, perhaps even of the entire human race. It can also be present in the specific micro- or macro-social situation, where a reifying anaesthesia (due to reasons of role, obedience to authority, technical power or technological

[7] The executioner.

anaesthesia) makes it impossible to feel. In that sense, the psychopath is the person who brings to light a relational pain without being able to feel it himself, thus provoking it in the other. It is not possible for him to take on the pain in his own flesh, and so he uses the flesh of the other to make it emerge and exist. The core of psychopathic experience lies much deeper than empathy erosion or a lack of sympathy, which then lead, as a consequence, to the reification of the other. On the contrary, rather, the reification of the other is necessary to bring out a pain that is borne—suffered, in the sense of *su-ferre*, to bear on oneself—without being able to feel it and take it on, and cold ruthlessness is the way to make it emerge. Such a perspective can make sense of the way in which the psychopath seeks violence, which usually does not happen in any random way, but is instead planned and deliberate, driven by a *craving* to do harm. It is *intentional* violence, in the sense that it is driven by an urge that moves in a direction, towards a next. But what can be the destination of a motion that horrifies us so?

When pain is felt, in our case, by the other, the absence becomes a pain that is present, and no longer absent. And that offers the possibility of a transformative movement. On the transformation of absence into pain that we feel, Weil explains:

> The false God changes suffering into violence. The true God changes violence into suffering. (…) Patience consists in not transforming suffering into crime. That in itself is enough to transform crime into suffering. (…) Purity is absolutely invulnerable as purity, in the sense that no violence can make it less pure. It is, however, highly vulnerable in the sense that every attack of evil makes it suffer, that every sin which touches it turns in it to suffering. (…) Evil is always the destruction of tangible things in which there is the real presence of good. Evil is carried out by those who have no knowledge of this real presence. In that sense, it is true that no one is wicked voluntarily. (…) That which gives more reality to beings and things is good, that which takes it from them is evil (Weil, 1952, p. 122).

Thus, there emerges a possible meaning for what has no meaning, which is that violence is a way of making a pain present in the field exist, a pain that moves the psychopath to act, but which he cannot feel. The victim is compelled to feel and bring out the pain that the executioner cannot feel and bring into existence. The pain present in the field cannot be forgotten or evacuated. We can anaesthetize ourselves to it, but it remains there. It can be transformed into the human contact, but for that to happen it has to become present. Causing useless suffering is a possibility for a pain excluded from awareness to be transformed, to be brought to light. Evil is a passage from anaesthesia to aesthesia, from absence to presence, using the flesh of the other. Evil *is placing the pain one bears onto the flesh of the other*. The therapist is exposed to those same forces and is tempted to reject and to want to make the patient feel pain, leveraged in this by the power and knowledge of therapy. But it is only a way in which the therapist feels and suffers the phenomenal field. It is just the first step of therapy, leading to the next step of becoming aware of it and becoming curious as to what is happening, while searching for its meaning.

17.5.4 The Psychopathic Field in the Therapeutic Encounter: Compassion Springs from the Ground

What happens if the therapist notices the reifying forces moving him, but instead of acting them out slows down, is intrigued, and waits for something else to emerge from the ground? Such a stance would constitute a phronetic intervention, and not a technique or protocol that can be applied to behavior.[8] In any case, stopping and being curious in itself means differentiating oneself and slipping out of the psychopathic phenomenal field to dwell in the situation in a different way, to remain present without leaving, but also without being overwhelmed by it. To make such a shift in a field where the forces in motion can be particularly strong and can easily push one to reject the situation and flee, it is essential to anchor oneself to a strong third party—a setting that guarantees the safety of both the therapist and patient, good theory, knowledge of the psychopathic field, ongoing supervision, a clear and stable ethical benchmark, a social network that offers the therapist affective connection and personal self-confidence. There is no way a therapist can work on psychopathy without being strongly anchored to third parties that support him and the relationship, anchoring it to sufficiently secure terrain (Francesetti & Gecele, 2009).

If the therapists manage to recognize the way in which they help circulate the violence (by being seized by the reifying forces, which as we have seen can take the shape of fear, anger, and disgust) and to be intrigued and to wait, something more will emerge in the way they feel. What it is will depend—phronetically—on the therapists themselves, on the patient, and on the situation, but the direction it takes is to move the therapist to *feel pain*. That second pain is different from the first. The first is the pain of the victim, which elicits anger and disgust and which the therapist may feel personally in the form of fear. The second is pain for the patient, or the pain of the patient, a pain that he cannot feel. It is the pain that he bears without feeling it and the pain for his inability to feel pain. It is the breach in the psychopathic field that lets the healing antidote in, which is compassion. Compassion is not closeness. There is no movement towards the patient by the therapist. For any movement away from the patient (rejection and fear) or towards the patient (seduction) would be equally dangerous and should be seen as the work of the forces in the psychopathic phenomenal field. There is no admiration, fascination or justification. There is no collaboration, alliance, or complicity. There is no affection or friendship. That may all seem obvious here, but it is not so in a therapeutic relationship where it can be surprisingly easy and overwhelming to be taken in by the psychopathic game. Compassion—from the Latin *cum*, together, and *patior*, to suffer—means taking part in the suffering of the other. When that happens, the field is no longer psychopathic, it has changed. The moment in which the therapist experiences that passage, he does not feel close to the patient; indeed he may feel very distant from him in that he feels exactly how much the patient bears on himself without feeling it, and which

[8] For a discussion of clinical practice based on field theory, see Francesetti, 2019b; Francesetti and Roubal, 2020; Roubal and Francesetti, in press.

needs to be felt by somebody. The therapist is alone in that barren landscape and thus feels the boundless, unbearable solitude of the psychopath, all of which he himself cannot feel. By feeling his own helplessness and participation in such infinite suffering, the therapist sees the patient and grasps his existential core, unveiling it. In that moment, the pain which could only emerge through violence takes on shape and form as pain, wound, and solitude, the extremely distressing and fragile finitude of the human condition.

It is no coincidence that, once a therapeutic relationship is established, after a few years the psychopathic patient tends to fall into deep, major, and risky—but healthy—depression (Greenwald, 1974). Another way we can put it is that the therapist makes no move to feel compassion; he simply waits for it to take hold of him by emerging. In that touching way of being present to absence, the pain begins its transformation in the encounter, and the sign that such transformation is underway is beauty (Francesetti, 2012). When this sort of contact is made—and when it is real, that is, when it is not the fruit of manipulation by the patient, or strategy by the therapist—it marks a turning point in the therapeutic relationship, opening up a new way for pain to emerge, offering an alternative outlet to violence. However, it can take a long time for that to happen, and so it is important that the third party we spoke of remain stable and present and that the therapist find the right attitude to suffer the field, differentiating themselves and waiting, carefully, patiently, and hopefully, for the germ of compassion to bud from the ground. Field theory inverts the perspective. It is not the patient who has to change, but the therapist (Francesetti, 2019b; Francesetti & Roubal, 2020; Roubal & Francesetti, in press). In a psychopathic field, it is the therapist's compassion that opens the door to the patient's depressive and healthy pain.

17.6 A Possibility That Is Often Neglected: The Psychopathic Field Is Actualized When It Is the Victim Who Comes to Therapy

A psychopathic field can be encountered by the therapist not only when treating someone who suffers from this condition, but also when the client is the victim. Such a situation can have important clinical implications, of which here I will identify two. The first is that the therapist is subject to a vicarious trauma, in that he experiences contact with the victim traumatically, suffering a trauma in his own turn. The experiences that emerge in a reifying field can be unbearable for the therapist. When that happens, the therapist may not be able to be present to the experience and in turn will dissociate the experiences, thereby reducing his capacity to offer the patient his support and becoming himself a victim of the overwhelming forces to which he is exposed. That can give rise to personal implications, for which it is essential for the therapist to have a supervisor, tasked specifically with tracking the effects of the therapeutic situation on the therapist, to identify and manage such an eventuality.

The second clinical implication is rather less acknowledged in the literature, making it all the more important to highlight, and that is that the therapist is seized by the reifying forces of the emerging psychopathic field and circulates the violence, unwittingly retraumatizing the victim. A brief clinical example from a group therapy session can help illustrate the point.

In a group, Veronica feels deeply touched and becomes very emotional, so she asks for personal work.

'My son, now 10 years old, was sexually abused when he was 2, by a boy much older than him'

She tells me that when her son told her and her husband the games that the older boy was making him play, she was upset and started screaming, saying that it could not be true, that it was wrong, that it was impossible, and she ran away screaming and crying, leaving the child with his father. She ran to her mother and when she came back later, she was calmer but unable to speak about what happened. After two years, they decided to undergo family therapy, and it was very good for all of them. After that, for the last 6 years, nobody in the family has ever mentioned the abuse.

Now, Veronica is seized by strong emotions; she is shaking, crying. I am very touched and attuned, and I give her bodily support in order to let the feelings come out between us. She comes to a peak, her body shaken and trembling:

'I am shaken, I am scared, I feel sick, I am going to vomit'. She starts retching violently, on the verge of vomiting.

In this unbearable intensity she says *'I can't! I can't! I can't tolerate it! I can't!*

I hold her hands and immediately I feel a change in myself: I feel my body becoming stronger and stiffer and I think that she must, that it is definitely her responsibility as a mother to bear it, that she should have stayed by her child instead of running away. I feel this 'you must!' very strongly, and I become curious about it... it seems too strong, even violent... I feel the intensity and the absolute certainty at the point that I feel my reaction is out of place. I feel that my body is full of power: I know what must be done and I want to impose it. Her 'I can't' is not relevant at all.

I am surprised how strongly I am seized by these feelings. So, I wait… and I feel that I have become cold and powerful, I feel a disproportionate power over her... I realize that I am doing a kind of violence to her. I cannot accept her saying 'I can't'; she must tolerate it! I stay with this.

Something softens in my body, somewhere in my chest. I realize that I am forcing her boundaries, her limits... and this orients me to think, of course she has the right of not being able to tolerate...What would I feel if I was her? Of course, it is her right to have limitations and nobody has the right to overcome them.

And so, very simply, I say: *'no, of course you can't… you can't'*

The atmosphere and the emotions immediately change. They remain extreme, but there is no retching any more. Instead, a sobbing cry arrives, a relieving, deep, sobbing cry.

The theme of overcoming and forcing the boundaries, present in every abuse, has emerged. I embody it. By feeling it was out of place, by not re-acting, but waiting, has allowed me to feel something soft and to feel respect for her. It has oriented me. I didn't act it out, I legitimated the limit, the boundary, that in a field of abuse is crucial and transformative.

After that the emotional peak passes, she shares that this 'I can't' was always present. But it was perceived as an unbearable guilt, totally delegitimized and so it was quickly dissociated and forgotten. In any case, it was unspeakable. In both cases, of feeling and dissociating guilt, it was impossible for her to share it with her husband, because the guilt of having run away was too great. Yet it remained in her mind every day, every single day for the last nine years.

Now that the limit and the boundary is legitimated between us and in the group, everything flows. A new awareness of willing to share with her husband emerges, and she clearly realizes that they both need support, that the family sessions six years ago were good, but that there are still more issues to be processed and reprocessed, especially now that their son is entering into preadolescence.

'How do you feel Veronica?'

'I feel exhausted.... yes, really exhausted... and free'.

This example illustrates how reifying forces can seize the therapist also when it is the victim who is in therapy. The risk of retraumatisation is high, and, again, supervision is needed in order to differentiate and recognize the field's forces and the therapeutic direction.

17.7 Some Final Clinical Considerations

The field perspective we have presented here is not an alternative to the indications found in the literature for the treatment of psychopathic conditions. What we would like to do is add a further dimension of understanding, and hence of treatment, for the difficult work faced by clinicians in this field. To recap, here are some ingredients for working with psychopathic patients. In particular, we identify four elements relevant for the therapeutic process.

First Ingredient: Treatability It is important to assess the treatability of the patient (Stone, 2006). Here it should be stressed that treatability of course depends on the patients, on their awareness and motivation for therapy and on the possibility of creating a therapeutic alliance. It also depends on the therapist, on his training, supervision, and willingness to have contact with what can be rather extreme terrains of violence and reification. It is important that the therapist should be able to choose whether to take on the specific patient in therapy, otherwise they themselves will feel obliged to do therapy with the patient, just as the patient often is. It also depends on the setting, on the support that both the patient and therapist receive from institutions, the social situation, and colleagues in the professional community. A widespread belief is that such patients cannot be treated, especially when sent to therapy by court order. As Meloy (1988) writes: 'It is, in a sense, a mass retaliatory attitude where moral judgment impinges on professional assessment.

The behavioral pathology of the psychopath, to devalue and dehumanize others, becomes the concordant identification of the clinician doing to the psychopath what the clinician perceives the psychopath doing to others (pp. 325)." Treatability is therefore a key moment of assessment, which should be carried out carefully and directly by encountering the patient, and discussed with the clinical team or with a supervisor, taking into consideration a multiplicity of factors that refer not only to the patient.

The Second Ingredient: Incorruptibility Nancy McWilliams (2011) identifies a key ingredient for therapy work with psychopaths in incorruptibility: "of the therapist, the frame, and the conditions that make therapy possible (pp. 168)". We fully agree on the need for strict inflexibility on the boundaries of therapy, which must never be waived. Ultimately, that is how the third party is concretely present in therapy, providing fundamental support to the therapist. For the therapist must know that any empathy or emotional understanding that the patient might show is probably not sympathy; it is not authentic affective participation and genuine interest in the therapist. Just like any other narcissistic gratification that the therapist may feel, it is probably part of a manipulatory scheme put into act by the forces at play in every psychopathic field. Clarity and respect for boundaries support the therapist in being honest and reliable—in keeping to the contract, in being clear in their assertions, in saying what they really feel, no more, no less. And in being honest with themselves, in acknowledging their feelings of anger, indifference, fear, disgust, or even of admiration, complicity, attraction, or pleasure, and managing them as necessary for the therapeutic process. Naturally, sharing such experiences is a crucial point of therapy. But, from a field perspective, they should not be shared until they are all the therapist feels, because if seized by the field they cannot differentiate themselves. Only through differentiation can another affective and emotional ground emerge, in which the sharing of experiences can be taken into consideration (for a discussion see Francesetti, 2019b; Francesetti & Roubal, 2020; Roubal & Francesetti, in press).

The Third Ingredient: Dignity The word 'dignity' comes from the Latin *Dignus*, in turn derived from the Greek *Axios*, meaning both *worthy* and *axiom*. The etymological root of the word offers us a key insight for understanding dignity. An axiom is an assertion, an implicit truth that is self-evident, requiring no demonstration. Such is dignity. An intrinsic, humble, foundational, and inalienable value that comes from being human, it does not depend on any choice, action or quality. The equal dignity of all human beings is a historical conquest for humankind, one that cannot be taken for granted and must continuously be reaffirmed. The psychopath, by reifying the other, deprives him of his dignity. The clinician who takes on a psychopathic patient needs to rely on the support of a strong *a priori* ethic to help him acknowledge the dignity of the patient. In a psychopathic field, the pressure to deny the dignity of the other can be strong, which is why it is all the more important for the clinician to pay attention to this aspect. The acknowledgement of the other's dignity is only ever a transient conquest, and even in these clinical situations, the sense of one's dignity and the dignity of the patient will fluctuate from moment to moment. Awareness of those fluctuations and the meaning that they have in relation to what is happening in therapy are fundamental elements, because one's own sense of dignity and the dignity of the patient is a highly sensitive thermometer for the degree of psychopathy present in the field we are immersed in.

The Fourth Ingredient: Compassion Compassion is the specific element that field theory has allowed us to bring to light, as we discussed before. It arises if the conditions of treatability, incorruptibility, and dignity are all present. It is something that emerges on its own when the clinician manages to dwell in the psychopathic field while differentiating themselves at the same time and waiting, without seeking change. It can take time, a very long time, before the clinician is able to let the feeling emerge in a field that by definition has exterminated any trace of human compassion, which means that they need to be prepared for the fact that it may never happen. They wait with gentleness, that is, a specific clinical and ethical attitude (Borgna, 2019).

Being able to feel compassion is the crucial change that the clinician can evoke in such a field. It is the first step towards the possibility of feeling the patients' pain and opens the possibility for them to feel depression. Such experiences are recognized by the literature to be a turning point in the therapeutic process with psychopathic patients, but the point of therapeutic change (meaning it is not only psycho-educational) lies in the therapist's capacity to open herself to the compassion that dwells *in nuce* in the psychopathic field. Anyone can feel that what is lacking in the psychopath's actions is compassion. That lack is the empty space in which the clinician dwells carefully, patiently, exactingly, respectfully, faithfully, and perhaps even ironically. The therapist is filling compassion's empty space by their presence that waits for that feeling-- an alien in the psychopathic world. In that dwelling without any apparent action, they accomplish a fundamental act, that of lending their flesh (Marion, 2003) to feel the pain that cannot be felt and to feel the compassion that finds nobody else to come to light.

17.8 A Brief Clinical Example

Z., a patient with a psychopathic personality disorder[9] *and a successful, high-profile career in finance, came to therapy at the age of 46, after the birth of his son. His partner's pregnancy was unexpected, and unwanted, but for various reasons it was socially gratifying and hence accepted by him. Z. is the typical respectfully dressed psychopath, accustomed to using people for his professional ends, which are to make money at all costs, but secretly delighting when his profit brings a loss to a*

[9]This is a case brought for supervision and constantly followed. Here I relate it as the first-person narration of the therapist.

competitor, or even a client, providing that his hand in the affair cannot be seen. His sexual life is promiscuous, often abusive, of which his partner is more or less unaware. Lies, manipulation, seduction, and violence *all serve him for his success. But after the birth of his son, something changed. Z. began to have bouts of uncontrollable* rage, *which had led him to have physical altercations with other motorists who he would argue with on the road, to physically strike an old man who had been disrespectful towards his partner at the cinema, and to violently smash the kitchen one night when his partner had replied carelessly to him. That led him to seek therapeutic assessment to see if 'something wasn't right with his brain.' Obviously from his point of view, he was in the right to do all that he did, as it is not his fault if nearly everyone has the IQ of goldfish—they should all be exterminated for the good of humanity, but the hypocrisy of our society will not let that happen. Nevertheless, he wants to regain the self-control he had not long ago.*

Z. really is very intelligent, with a quality of thought that strikes and fascinates me. He is well-educated and his logical, scientific way of thinking is incontrovertible, able to grasp aspects of reality that I myself cannot see. His cynicism is so smooth and convincing. I cannot help but admire his qualities deeply. But I have to be careful not to take the bait of challenging him on the cultural and intelligence level, in what would be a mutual fight for dominance, while at the same time not giving in to feelings of admiration or, alternatively, disapproval and disgust. He knows all that already, admiration and disgust are what he elicits in his relationships in daily life, so he does not need to pay me to have that.

Gradually his history emerges. He does not like to talk about it and it is pointless, so he says, because he has only vague memories of it, but slowly and steadily he allows me to see the ground of his experiences. Abandoned by his drug addicted mother at the age of two years, he never knew his father and instead lived with a rather rich aunt, who never really took care of him. He was raised by nannies whom his aunt would constantly hire then dismiss, considering them beneath the dignity of the house. He was terrified of the dark and as punishment he would regularly be shut up in a lightless broom closet, or beaten with a silver candelabrum—not your ordinary wooden spoon—whenever he cried. He soon learnt to hold his tears. Z.'s existence strikes me as a crossroads of possible biological predispositions, a traumatic development, and a social condition that encourages and rewards his psychopathy. *After two years of therapy, Z. tells me how when he was seventeen years old he forced a thirteen year-old girl, a neighbour at their holiday home by the sea, to have sex with him. His aunt had hushed everything up by paying money to the young girl's parents, but then gave him a beating with the candelabrum and warned him not to be so stupid as to get caught again next time. Z. tells me all this in a clear-minded and detached way, without hint of* guilt *or acknowledgement of the suffering caused to the girl. The story horrifies me and I feel disoriented. I have an urge to shout at him, to tell him that such things are just wrong, that he is mad, to get out of here, that I never want to see his face again. But then I think that if he really is mad, then this is the right place for him to be…*

Why did I feel such a strong urge to make him go away? I realize in some part of me that there is no place for Z. to go and I have the strange, surprising feeling that he has no home, he is homeless, a child never born. An odd sadness takes hold of me, not a personal sadness or a sadness just for him, but for the horizon of misery that has opened up through him. My thoughts have no logic to them, but they elicit a strong feeling of sickness in my stomach. I let it mature, in silence. Even Z. remains silent, which is not usual for him. I feel horror for him, which is something new. Horror at not having a home, at never having had one. There was no home for him in his mother's womb, or in his father's arms. No home in the maternal house or in his aunt's. No home today as he has given up the search for his place among men, and no home here as he just makes me feeling repulsion. I do not know how, I feel it is unjustified and inappropriate, I even feel guilty for that girl for the pain I feel. But I feel a sort of suffering for him. I contain my affective resonance, it is too strong; if I let myself go it would make me cry and sob. I say nothing. I simply breathe, leaving what there is to be. Z. is watching me. I am not sure of what is going on behind those eyes, but a sort of understanding, perhaps empty of content, arises. I feel we are in the same time and place, for a moment.

The session ends without anything else of note happening, serving only to close the new chasm that has been opened and in which, perhaps, we have made a new experience of contact. The following session, Z. swaggers in and tells me how he is a fascist, that only fascists understand how the world goes. My reaction is one of desperate boredom, of the sort, 'here we go again…,' but there's something ironic in his look that keeps me alert and vigilant. He explains how the true fascist has nothing to do with the caricatures that populate history and have come to fill the newspapers in recent times. A true fascist is someone who believes in something he would be willing to give his life for; he is uncompromising, the picture of integrity. I realize that maybe he is bringing something new here, packaged in an old box, but new—the idea of being all of one piece, of not accepting compromise, of dying rather than losing one's dignity, stands in striking contrast to the seductive and lying manipulation that has characterized his life. What a novelty, and I almost missed it! He then tells me he would be ready to die for someone, that he would be ready to die for me—in all seriousness. I am left gaping and speechless. He smiles, he knows he has overstepped the mark, but he also believes that I believe his words. A great heaviness weighs on us. I try to play it down by saying, with a smile, 'Well, I never thought that one day a true fascist might save my life!' The line has the effect of lightening things up and we both laugh. But from that moment on, Z.'s depressive experiences begin to emerge, becoming ever more present, stronger, and worrying. And healthy.

17.9 The Role of Judas: A Provocative Conclusion

The reification of the other, mindless to the evil provoked, is the characteristic feature of the psychopathic field. Is it not perhaps one of the most powerful forces at play in our social field today? A society based on capital, on manic, accelerated consumption, is constantly moved by alienating forces that treat human beings as objects. Might psychopathy not be an epiphenomenon that brings to light the submerged, common, and widespread pain of not being subjects? Could what we observe in clinical experience and in the daily news perhaps be the extreme, salient, or less socio-syntonic degrees of a normal, pervasive phenomenon that is almost constituent of our social organizations? Turning the perspective on its head—by way of provocation—the picture becomes more complex. What if it were the psychopaths who identified best with the social forces of our day and were best suited to them, making them, paradoxically, the least anti-social of us all? These are all, of course, provocations, but the point is that we should never forget how the social background is always present even in individual stories and in every diagnostic and psychopathological description (Gecele, 2013). That is especially important in clinical work to understand how both we and our patients are grains of sand in which the whole world can be seen (Blake, 1863), and how the social field can support or hinder therapeutic processes. The perspective is also a necessary one if we want to avoid being seized unawares by the social field, acting out forces for whose consequences we will pay. It also helps support us in saying 'no' and breaking the confluence with social forces.

This outlook also recalls a fundamental existential question with which our founders were much concerned (Goodman, 1968; Perls, 1992), and which is the crucial question of theodicy:[10] '*unde malum*?'— or *where does* evil *come from*?. That is the question raised by Job, the innocent and righteous man from whom God took everything, wealth, children, and health (Poma, 2005). If God is good and omnipotent, why, then, should the good suffer? This is a question which belongs to all of us when we find ourselves in a state of suffering.

One possible and radical answer is that without evil there could not exist the fruits of that transformation which comes to "distil" suffering into beauty, absence into presence. Through that process, a special and unique quality of love is created which can only arise in limited beings such as our human selves. No God, precisely because of his omnipotence, could produce such love. Indeed, if a God exists, he needs us to produce it for him. The creation of love from impotent pain is only possible for a limited creature, which is constitutionally immersed in, and therefore has the possibility to distil such suffering. This vision reveals an endeavor to which all humankind contributes: the production of a unique love which we alone are able to create. And, inasmuch as we are inclined to pursue beauty, we are inevitably creative. In the words of the *Bhagavad Gita* (4:11): "Wherever they may be, men follow in my footsteps" (Francesetti, 2012).

Perhaps even Judas, and traitors like him who commit evil, have a role to play by bearing on their shoulders—suffering—the unbearable in history, so that it can come to the light and be transformed.

[10] The term theodicy, coined by Leibniz, refers to a branch of theology. Its etymological meaning derives from the Greek *théos* (god) and *díke* (justice). In other words, it treats in the "doctrine of the justice of God". Leibniz uses the term *theodicy* to refer to the doctrine of the justification of God for the evil present in creation.

References

American Psychiatric Association. (2013). *Diagnostic and statistical manual of mental disorders* (5th ed.). APA.

Anders, G. (1964). *Wir Eichmannsöhne: Offener Brief an Klaus Eichmann* [*We Sons of Eichmann. Open Letter to Klaus Eichmann*]. Beck. http://anticoncept.phpnet.us/eichmann.htm

Ardizzi, M., Martini, F., Umiltà, M. A., Evalngelista, V., Ravera, R., & Gallese, V. (2015). Impact of childhood maltreatment on the recognition of facial expressions of emotions. *PloS ONE, 10*(10), e0141732.

Arendt, H. (1958). *The human condition*. University of Chicago Press.

Arendt, H. (1963). *Eichmann in Jerusalem: A report on the banality of evil*. Penguin.

Athens, L. (1992). *The creation of dangerous violent criminals*. University of Illinois Press.

Baron-Cohen, S. (2011). *The science of evil: On empathy and the origins of cruelty*. Basic Books.

Bauman, Z. (2011). A natural history of evil. In *Collateral damages: Social inequalities in a global age*. Polity Press.

Blake, W. (1863). Auguries of innocence. In *The Pickering manuscript*. Whitefish, MT.

Bloom, D. (2013a). Situated ethics and the ethical world of Gestalt therapy. In G. Francesetti, M. Gecele, & J. Roubal (Eds.), *Gestalt Therapy in clinical practice: From psychopathology to the aesthetics of contact* (pp. 131–148). FrancoAngeli.

Bloom, D. (2013b). Reflection: In dialogue with Philip Lichtenberg's 'Exclusive and Inclusive Aggression': A window to the next resistance. *Gestalt Review, 17*, 284–289.

Bloom, D. (2018). Evil: The sight that cannot be seen; The speaking that cannot be said. In M. Spagnuolo Lobb, D. Bloom, J. Roubal, J. Zeleskov Djoric, M. Cannavò, R. La Rosa, S. Tosi, & V. Pinna (Eds.), *The aesthetic of otherness: Meeting at the boundary in a desensitized world. Proceedings*. Istituto di Gestalt HCC Publishing Co.

Bloom, D. (2021). From the Night Before Being: Contacting the Other. *Gestalt Review, 25(1), 116–142*. https://doi.org/10.5325/gestaltreview.25.1.0116

Böhme, G. (2017). *The aesthetics of atmospheres*. Routledge.

Bongers, D. (2013). Violent behaviours. In G. Francesetti, M. Gecele, & J. Roubal (Eds.), *Gestalt therapy in clinical practice: From psychopathology to the aesthetics of contact* (pp. 679–696). FrancoAngeli.

Bonhoeffer, D. (2015). *La fragilità del male. Scritti inediti*. Piemme.

Borgna, E. (1988). *I conflitti del conoscere*. Feltrinelli.

Borgna, E. (2019). *La follia che è anche in noi*. Einaudi.

Browning, C. R. (2001). *Ordinary men: Reserve Police Battalion 101 and the final solution in Poland*. Penguin.

Buber, M. (1923). *I and thou*. Touchstone.

Buber, M. (1953). The history of the dialogical principle. In *Between man and man*. Routledge and Kegan Paul.

Cleckley, H. (1941). *The mask of sanity: An attempt to clarify some issues about the so-called psychopathic personality*. Mosby.

Damasio, A. (2010). *Self comes to mind: Constructing the conscious brain*. Pantheon Books.

Dazzi, S., & Madeddu, F. (2009). *Devianza e antisocialità*. Raffaello Cortina Editore.

Denham-Vaughan, S. (2009). Ravishing beauty: In our darkest hours what will sustain us? *British Gestalt Journal, 18*, 28–29.

Djoric, J. Z., Cannavo, M., & Medjedovic, J. (2016). Emerging beauty beyond freedom: Gestalt therapy approach with offenders using CORE and CHAP instrument. In J. Roubal (Ed.), *The world of contemporary Gestalt therapy. Towards a research tradition in Gestalt therapy* (pp. 314–334). Cambridge Scholars Publishing.

Eagle, M. N. (2010). *From classical to contemporary psychoanalysis: A critique and integration*. Routledge.

Englebert, J. (2019). The psychopathology of psychopaths. In G. Stanghellini, M. Broome, A. Raballo, A. V. Fernandez, P. Fusar-Poli, & R. Rosfort (Eds.), *The Oxford handbook of phenomenological psychopathology*. Oxford University Press.
Fonagy, P. (1997). Attachment: The development of the self, and its pathology in personality disorders. In C. Maffei, J. Derksen, & H. Groen H. (Eds.), *Treatment of personality disorders* (pp. 53–68). Plenum Press.
Fonagy, P., & Target, M. (1997). Attachment and reflective function: Their role in self-organization. *Development and Psychopathology, 9*, 679–700.
Francesetti, G. (2012). Pain and beauty: From psychopathology to the aesthetics of contact. *British Gestalt Journal, 21*, 4–18.
Francesetti, G. (2013). The emergent suffering: Field perspective on psychopathology in Gestalt therapy, Chapter 6. In G. Klaren, N. Levi, & I. Vidakovic (Eds.), *Yes, we care! Social, political and culturale relationships as therapy's ground: A Gestalt perspective*. EAGT.
Francesetti, G. (2015). From individual symptoms to psychopathological fields: Towards a field perspective on clinical human suffering. *British Gestalt Journal, 24*, 5–19.
Francesetti, G. (2016). "You cry, I feel pain": The emerging, co-created self as the foundation of anthropology, psychopathology and treatment in Gestalt therapy. In J-M. Robine (Ed.), *Self: A polyphony of contemporary Gestalt therapists*. L'Exprimerie.
Francesetti, G. (2019a). *Fundamentos de psicopatología fenomenológico-gestáltica: una introducción ligera*. Los Libros del CTP. Italian Ed., 2020; Brazilian Ed., 2021; English, French, Russian and German Ed. in press.
Francesetti, G. (2019b). The field strategy in clinical practice: Towards a theory of therapeutic phronesis. In P. Brownell (Ed.), *Handbook for theory, research and practice in Gestalt therapy* (2nd ed.). Cambridge Scholars Publishing.
Francesetti, G., & Gecele, M. (2009). Gestalt therapy perspective on psychopathology and diagnosis. *British Gestalt Journal, 18*, 5–20.
Francesetti, G., & Griffero, T. (Eds.). (2019). *Psychopathology and atmospheres: Neither inside nor outside*. Cambridge Scholars Publishing.
Francesetti, G., & Roubal, J. (2020). Field theory in contemporary Gestalt therapy. Part one: Modulating the therapist's presence in clinical practice. *Gestalt Review, 24*, 113–136.
Galimberti, U. (2002). *Psiche e techne. L'uomo nell'età della tecnica*. Feltrinelli.
Gecele, M. (2013). Introduction to personality disturbances: Diagnostic and social remarks. In G. Francesetti, M. Gecele, & J. Roubal (Eds.), *Gestalt therapy in clinical practice: From psychopathology to the aesthetics of contact* (pp. 601–608). FrancoAngeli.
Gibson, M. (2002). *Born to crime: Cesare Lombroso and the origins of biological criminology*. Praeger.
Glenn, A. L., & Raine, A. (2014). *Psychopathy: An introduction to biological findings and their implications*. New York University Press.
Goodman, P. (1947). *Communitas: Means of livelihood and ways of life*. Vintage Books.
Goodman, P. (1960). *Growing up absurd: Problems of youth in the organized society*. Vintage Books.
Goodman, P. (1968). In P. D. Pursglove (1968). *Recognitions in Gestalt therapy*. Funk & Wagnalls.
Greenwald, H. (1974). *Treatment of the psychopath*. In H. Greenwald (Ed.), *Active psychotherapy* (pp. 363–377). Jason Aronson.
Griffero, T. (2017). *Quasi-things: The paradigm of atmospheres*. SUNY Press.
Hare, R. D. (1980). A research scale for the assessment of psychopathy in criminal populations. *Personality and Individual Differences, 1*, 111–120.
Hare, R. D., Hart, S. D., & Harpur, T. J. (1991). Psychopathy and the DSM-IV criteria for antisocial personality disorder. *Journal of Abnormal Psychology, 100*, 391–398.
Heidegger, M. (1954). *The question concerning technology, and other essays*. Harper Perennial Modern Thought.
Kernberg, O. (1992). *Aggression in personality disorders and perversions*. Yale University Press.
Lackmann, F. M. (2001). *Transforming aggression: Psychotherapy with the difficult-to-treat patient*. Jason Aronson.

Lapides, A. (Forthcoming). *Hate in the field: A dialogue. Alienation of otherhood.*
Lévinas, E. (1961). *Totality and infinity: An essay on exteriority* (p. 1969). Duquesne University Press.
Lévinas, E. (1990). *Alterity and transcendence*. Columbia University Press.
Lingiardi, V. (2018). *Diagnosi e destino*. Einaudi.
Lingiardi, V., & McWilliams, N. (Eds.). (2017). *Psychodynamic diagnostic manual (PDM-2)*. Guilford Press.
Marion, J.-L. (2003). *The erotic phenomenon*. University of Chicago Press.
McLuhan, M. (1964). *Understanding media: The extensions of man*. McGraw-Hill.
McWilliams, N. (2011). *Psychoanalytic diagnosis*. The Guilford Press.
Meloy, J. R. (1988). *The psychopathic mind: Origins, dynamics and treatment*. Jason Aronson.
Milgram, S. (1974). *Obedience to authority: An experimental view*. Tavistock.
Mucci, C. (2013). *Beyond individual and collective trauma: Intergenerational transmission, psychoanalytic treatment, and the dynamic of forgiveness*. Routledge.
Orange, D. M. (2018). My other's keeper: Resources for the ethical turn in psychotherapy. In M. Spagnuolo Lobb, D. Bloom, J. Roubal, J. Zeleskov Djoric, M. Cannavò, R. La Rosa, S. Tosi, & V. Pinna (Eds.), *The aesthetic of otherness: Meeting at the boundary in a desensitized world. Proceedings*. Istituto di Gestalt HCC Publishing Co.
Parlett, M., & Lee, R. G. (2005). Contemporary Gestalt therapy: Field theory. In A. L. Woldt & S. M. Toman (Eds.), *Gestalt therapy: History, theory, and practice* (pp. 41–63). Sage.
Perls, F. (1942). *Ego, hunger and aggression: A revision of Freud's theory and method* (p. 1947). G. Allen & Unwin.
Perls, L. (1992). *Living at the boundary*. Gestalt Journal Press.
Perls, F., Hefferline, R., & Goodman, P. (1951). *Gestalt therapy: Excitement and growth in the human personality.* Gestalt Journal Press, 1994.
Pirandello, L. (1921). *Six characters in search of an author and other plays* (M. Musa, Trans.). Penguin Classics, 2010.
Poma, A. (2005). *Parole vane*. Apogeo.
Pope, A. (1711). *An essay on criticism* (p. 2010). The British Library.
Raine, A. (2014). *The anatomy of violence: The biological roots of crime*. Vintage Books.
Robine, J.-M. (2001). From the field to the situation. In J.-M. Robine (Ed.), *Contact and relationship in a field perspective* (pp. 95–107). L'Exprimerie.
Rosa, H. (2010). *Alienation and acceleration: Towards a critical theory of late-modern temporality*. Aarhus University Press.
Roubal, J., & Francesetti, G. (in press). Field theory in contemporary Gestalt therapy. Part two: Paradoxical theory of change reconsidered. *Gestalt Review*.
Salonia, G., Spagnuolo Lobb, M., & Sichera, A. (1996). Prefazione. In F. Perls, R. Hefferline, & P. Goodman (Eds.), *Teoria e pratica della terapia della Gestalt. Vitalità e accrescimento nella personalità umana*. Astrolabio.
Severino, E. (1998). *Il destino della tecnica*. Rizzoli.
Spagnuolo Lobb, M., & Francesetti, G. (2015). La normalità creativa. *PNEI Rreview, 6*, 58–67.
Staemmler, F. M. (2006). A Babylonian confusion? On the uses and meanings of the term field. *British Gestalt Journal, 15*, 64–83.
Stanghellini, G., Broome, M., Raballo, A., Fernandez, A. V., Fusar-Poli, P., & Rosfort, R. (Eds.). (2019). *The Oxford handbook of phenomenological psychopathology*. Oxford University Press.
Stone, M. H. (2006). *Personality-disordered patients: Treatable and untreatable*. American Psychiatric Publishing.
Waldenfels, B. (2011). *Phenomenology of the alien: Basic concepts*. Northwestern University Press.
Weil, S. (1952). *Gravity and grace* (E. Crawford & M. von der Ruhr, Trans.). Routledge, 2002.
Wiesing, L. (2014). *The philosophy of perception: Phenomenology and image theory*. Bloomsbury.
Wollants, G. (2008). *Gestalt therapy: Therapy of the situation*. Sage.
Zimbardo, P. G. (2008). *The Lucifer effect: Understanding how good people turn evil*. Random House Trade.

Chapter 18
Group Therapy Interventions for Psychopathy: An Interpersonal Perspective

Jerry L. Jennings and Shan Jumper

Abstract This chapter revisits the research and assumptions in the field regarding psychopathy and its responsiveness to treatment from the vantage point of group therapy. The authors suggest that psychopathy is an interpersonal disorder and that group therapy is an interpersonal treatment that can be effective with severe psychopathy. Instead of segregating men who are high in psychopathy into their own groups and/or putting greater emphasis on criminogenic issues in those groups, the authors suggest that "group-centered" group therapy with healthier low or non-psychopathy peers can provide an interpersonal growth experience that can open opportunities for prosocial learning and change. The authors review the existing psychopathy research in pursuit of quality studies that are (1) specific to group therapy for a sufficient duration of time, (2) have subjects with high psychopathy, and (3) used some measure of treatment responsivity, not just recidivism alone. In addition to finding solid support for treatment effectiveness in the existing literature, new research is presented for an 8-month motivational group treatment program that focused on interpersonal relating rather than offense-related issues. A statistically significant 60% of the individuals with PCL-R scores of 30+ showed global improvements compared to just 16% of those scoring below 30. The men high in psychopathy showed a unique pattern of elevated concern with social acceptance and connection and they perceived a more positive experience of group therapeutic climate in every month of the study compared to their low psychopathy peers.

Keywords Group therapy · Psychopathy · Sex offending · Sexual abuse · Antisocial · Sociopathy · Ostracism · Attachment · Interpersonal violence · PCL-R

J. L. Jennings (✉)
Liberty Healthcare Corporation, Bala Cynwyd, PA, USA
e-mail: jerry.jennings@LibertyHealth.com

S. Jumper
IDHS Treatment and Detention Facility, Rushville, IL, USA

J. E. Vitale (ed.), *The Complexity of Psychopathy*, Dangerous Behavior in Clinical and Forensic Psychology, https://doi.org/10.1007/978-3-030-83156-1_18

18.1 Is Psychopathy Responsive to Treatment?

The problem of psychopathy poses some fundamental questions. If human evolution is grounded in the success of small, cooperative social groups, and if human nature is essentially social, what is this condition that is so quintessentially *anti*-social? What is this powerfully selfish condition that can set an individual into such frequent conflict with other people that the individual must be controlled or removed from society through punishment, banishment, and incarceration? Does psychopathy exist on a continuum of severity or are there certain individuals with such severe psychopathy that they are qualitatively different human beings? If the latter is true, what can be done with these so-called "pure psychopaths"? How can we socially integrate individuals with a disorder that seems to defy socialization? Do we give up on severe psychopathy as an untreatable condition that can only be managed? Certainly, pessimism about pure psychopathy has been posited by its share of researchers, including the first great modern expositor of the concept, Hervey Cleckley himself (1976).

There are strong opinions that treatment is either ineffective with psychopathy or that psychopathic individuals respond poorly to treatment. One rationale is that the condition of high psychopathy prevents the development of a meaningful client-therapist relationship, which is necessary for therapeutic change (Galloway & Brodsky, 2003; Harris & Rice, 2006; Skeem et al., 2002a; Wilson & Tamatea, 2013; Wong & Hare, 2005). Others have asserted that treatment can actually worsen men high in psychopathy and can increase the likelihood of recidivism, ostensibly because they use their lessons from treatment to better discern vulnerabilities in others for manipulation and exploitation (D'Silva et al., 2004; Hare et al., 2000; Harris & Rice, 2006; Looman et al., 2005; Reid & Gacono, 2000; Rice et al., 1992; Seto & Barbaree, 1999). Others point to the lack of controlled studies and methodological limitations (especially failures to operationally define psychopathy), and say there is insufficient evidence to conclude that men high in psychopathy are untreatable (Doren & Yates, 2008; Salekin, 2002; Wilson & Tamatea, 2013).

Given the negative or inconclusive results, some researchers have argued that men high in psychopathy may fare poorly in traditional treatment programs, but could respond to treatment that is more responsive to their needs (Hare, 1998; Thornton & Blud, 2007; Wong & Hare, 2009), or that subtypes of psychopathy might require different treatments (Skeem et al., 2002b). In this regard, there have been several efforts to design treatment programs specific to the needs of men high in psychopathy (Abracen et al., 2008; Harkins et al., 2013; Looman et al., 2005; Wilson & Tamatea, 2013; Wong et al., 2006). The two common presumptions among these attempts are that men high in psychopathy should be segregated from non-psychopathic peers and/or treatment should be cognitive-behavioral and focused on relevant criminogenic risk factors.

In a new effort to clarify the issue of the treatability of psychopathy, the authors reconsidered the literature from a new interpersonal perspective of group therapy. The authors attempted to identify a subset of research studies and meta-analyses that can identify something definitive about psychopathy and its responsiveness to treatment. To achieve this, the subset was limited to research that defined a sample of adult male high psychopathy subjects with PCL-R scores of 25 or greater. Next, the subset included only studies that either compared treated vs. untreated men with psychopathy or compared high vs. low psychopathy subjects who had received some sort of treatment that entailed group therapy. Therefore, the subset excluded studies that only reported or compared recidivism rates for high, medium and low psychopathy offenders and/or non-psychopathy offenders without reference to group-based treatment. The subset also excluded studies that used juveniles, females, and non-group treatments (such as electroconvulsive therapy, pharmacotherapy, individual therapy, etc.), as well as studies published before 1991. As presented in Table 18.1, the final set comprised 27 research studies/substudies, five meta-analyses, and one review that presented treatment and/or recidivism outcomes following some sort of group treatment. In addition, this final set included four studies and one meta-analysis with treatment-related information about psychopathy.

Given the authors' guiding thesis that psychopathy is an interpersonal disorder and that group therapy is an interpersonal treatment, the authors will further narrow this broad review to examine six well-designed psychopathy studies that entailed a treatment dose of at least 6 months of group treatment and included measures of group climate or group behavior. The authors will then present the results of a pilot study that suggests that men high in psychopathy are, contrary to expectations, acutely sensitive to social rejection, highly value social acceptance, and behave well in group when given the opportunity to connect with others. The chapter will conclude with a theory of why interpersonally-focused group therapy can be effective with psychopathy and recommendations for applying group therapy with this population.

18.2 The Operational Definition of Psychopathy and the "Psychopathic Sexuality Taxon"

One of the major methodological problems with the research on psychopathy has been inconsistency in its definition. There is converging evidence and general agreement that personality disorders in general, and psychopathic traits specifically, represent the extreme end of a continuum of interpersonal functioning. As summarized by Knight and King (2012), most research supports the contention that psychopathy is a dimensional trait that is best conceptualized as a continuum (Boccacini et al., 2017; Edens et al., 2006; Guay et al., 2007; Marcus et al., 2011; Walters et al., 2011). As such, there are no "psychopaths," only individuals who score above a set cut-off score of psychopathy.

Clearly the best-established measure of psychopathy is the Hare Psychopathy Checklist- Revised (PCL-R; Hare, 2003), which is internationally accepted among

Table 18.1 Treatment of psychopathy research studies

Study	Type	Treatment	N	PCL-R	Setting	Results	Measure	Sum
1 – Harkins et al. (2013)	Sex	SOST designed for PPs	N = 134 PP25 = 75	Cut = 25	SVP civil commitment facility	Hi PPs had poorer therapeutic climate than low PPs, but showed improvement over time	Group climate	Tx pos
2 – Polaschek and Ross (2010) and Ross et al. (2011)	Non	CBT, 8 mo. Intensive group, 93 sess, 7 groups over 3.5 years	N = 50 PP30 = 26	M = 19.5 PCL-SV Cut = ~30	Special unit in prison New Zealand	Both therapists & clients reported ability to form alliance regardless of PCL score. Alliance increased over time regardless of PCL. Both Hi PPs & their therapists can distinguish the work part (Goals &Tasks) from the therapeutic Bond	VRS risk WAI therapeutic alliance, motivation	Tx pos
3 – Hughes et al. (1997)	Non	CBT for MH	N = 9 PP30 = 0	Cut =? (over 30 excluded)	Secure psych hosp	Higher PCL scores made poorer therapeutic gains. Specifically Factor 1 (not F2) signif. negative correlation with global change. Net overall global positive change	Global therapeutic gains	Tx pos
4 – Olver and Wong (2009)	Sex	SOST	N = 156 PP25 =?	Cut = 25	Forensic psychiatric	Hi PPs who completed treatment & showed improvement had reduced violent & sex offending after avg. of 10 years	Recidivism, Treatment change	Tx pos
5 – Jennings and Jumper (this chapter)	Sex	Relationship. focused group ther.	N = 30 PP30 = 10 PP25 = 6	M = 24.8 Cut = 30	SVP civil commitment facility	Hi PPs made more positive ratings therapeutic climate and showed significant global progress in treatment	Group climate, tx behavior	Tx pos
6 – Hitchcock (1995)	Non	Two 12-week CBT groups, crim thinking	N = 80 PP30 = 80 40 in tx 40 no tx	Cut = 30	Prison	No difference between treatment and control, but PPs showed reduced "fragmentation" and "suggestibility" types of thinking errors	Criminal thinking	T nun

7 – Wilson and Tamatea (2013)	Non	CBT tx with intensive groups	N = 12 PP30 = 12	Cut = 30 (or high psycho-pathology)	Prison New Zealand	Believe that PP, especially Factor 1, may NOT be so "untreatable". All showed positive changes during & after tx, reduced misconducts, & exhibited stable & unstable desistance from crime – 40% went on to further intensive tx	Reduced VRS, tx behavior, desistance,	Tx pos
8 – Walton et al. (2018)	Sex	Manualized CBT in group	N = 89 PP30 = 11 PP20 to 30 = 35	M = 20.4 Cut = 30	Prison	Hi PP did NOT effect Tasks or Goals, but DID have negative effect on Bond. Hi PPs had highest therapist score on Goals & Tasks, but lowest on Bonds. Hi PPs had lowest client scores on Goals & Tasks, but medium on Bonds. No signif effect of level of PP on either client or therapist ratings on WAI nor subscales Factor 1 & 2 scores not related	Therapeutic alliance	Tx pos
9a Garrido et al. (1995)	Non	Meta-analysis A	34 studies	Some (not reported)	Prison & forensic hospital & clinic	PPs had higher recidivism than nonPPs	Recidivism	R neg
9b Garrido et al. (1995)	Non	Meta-analysis B	19 pre- & post-tx studies			Pre- and post-treatment PPs showed improvement in behavior and psych functioning	Psychological post-tx measures	Tx pos
10 – Looman et al. (2005)	Sex	7 months RTC, intensive CBT & RP SOST	N = 102 PP25 = 45	M = 22.5 Cut = 25	Prison	Hi PPs w/good tx progress reoffended at lower rate than hi PPs w/poor tx progress (58% vs 65%). Hi PPs rated as reduced risk reoffended at lower rate than those rated as unchanged (50% vs 70%). Concluded that subgroup of hi PPs may respond to intensive CBT treatment	5-year recidivism, treatment behavior, risk ratings	T pos R/SR neg

(continued)

Table 18.1 (continued)

Study	Type	Treatment	N	PCL-R	Setting	Results	Measure	Sum
11 – Guy et al. (2005)	Non	Meta-analysis	38 samples N = 5381	Yes, not reported	Prison & forensic & civil hospital	PCL scores correlated only marginally with aggression in institutional settings	Aggression & misconduct	T nun
12 – D'Silva et al. (2004)	Non	Meta-analysis	24 studies			Only 3 studies had a control of untreated PPs. 4 Hi PP showed positive response and 4 negative response to tx	Response to treatment	Tx mix
13 – Doren and Yates (2008)	Sex	Review of SO Tx	10 studies		Forensic	Shortcomings of existing research preclude a clear conclusion about "treatability"	Recidivism	Tx nun
14 – Olver et al. (2013)	Non	CBT 6–8 mo. "hi intensity" for violence reduction	N = 152 PP30 = 42	M = 26 Cut = 30	Forensic psychiatric	Positive therapeutic change negatively correlated with PCL-R, specifically Factor 1 and Affective Facet 2, suggesting Tx changes can predict recid and treatment outcome. Factor 1 correl with therapeutic change, but not Factor 2. Callous & unemotional traits (CU) are a potent responsivity issue & may be key to therapeutic responsiveness	VRS risk scores, recidivism (5 year follow-up) Therapeutic change?	Tx neg
15 – Heilbrun et al. (1998)	Non	Mental health tx	N = 218	PCL-R Cut =?	Forensic hospital	PCL-R Total score signif. correl. w/aggression & seclusion/restraint events in first 2 months and w/ post-dischg arrests for offenses against persons	Institutional adjustment, recidivism	Tx neg
16a – Hare et al. (2000)	Non	Unknown, see types below 16b,c	N = 728 PP30 = 33 PP25 = 95	M = 16.5 Cut = 30	Prison	42% of PP30 had at least one peer assault & 75% one misconduct vs 16% assault & 44% misconduct for less than 30	Institutional behavior	Info

16b – Hare et al. (2000)	Non	CBT anger mgmt & social skills	N = 268 PP30 =?	M =? Cut = 9 on PCL Factor scores	Prison	Treated hi PP Factor 1 had 86% 2-year reconvictions vs 59% for untreated hi PP Factor 1	Recidivism	R neg
16c – Hare et al. (2000)	Non	Educational & vocat. training	Same		Same	Treated hi PP Factor 1 had 50% 2-year reconvictions vs 23% for untreated hi PP Factor 1	Recidivism	R neg
17 – Ogloff et al. (1990)	Non	Therapeutic Community w/ daily 2 h large group	N = 681 PP25 = 101	M =? Cut = 25	Prison	Hi and lo PPs equal likely to participate, but hi PPs more likely to drop out of educational, vocational, & behavior programs, get fired from prison job and put in segregation. But the group that mixed hi PP and lo PP improved	Treatment & institutional behavior	Tx neg & mix
18 – Hobson et al. (2000)	Non	Therapeutic community	N = 104 PP30 =?	M = 24.1 Cut =?	Forensic	Higher PCL scores, particularly Factor 1, had disruptive behaviors in both sessions and residential wards	Treatment behavior	Tx neg
19 – Rice et al. (1992) and Harris et al. (1994b)	Sex (MH too)	Peer-run intensive TC w/"bizarre" tx methods	N = 292 146 in tx, 146 no tx	M = 19 Cut = 25	Forensic hospital	78% of treated PPs (rapists) committed serious offense vs 55% of untreated PPs (raised self-esteem, raised aggress, gave info used to exploit)	Recidivism	Tx neg
20a – Seto and Barbaree (1999)	Sex	CBT & RP SOST	N = 216 PP30 = 8 PP26 = 17	M = 16.1 Cut = 15	Prison	Hi PP rated most improved by therapist (per tx behavior) were 4X more likely to commit serious offense after avg of 32 months. Tx behavior was not related to recidivism in the initial or follow-up study	Recidivism, ratings of global chg, motiv, in-session behav, homework	Tx Neg R neg

(continued)

Table 18.1 (continued)

Study	Type	Treatment	N	PCL-R	Setting	Results	Measure	Sum
20b – Barbaree et al. (2001)	Sex	CBT & RP SOST	Same	Same	Prison	No interaction after 2 years, tx behavior not related to outcome initial or follow-up (after avg. of 62 months)	Recidivism, Tx behavior	Tx nun
21 – Tengström et al. (2000)	Non	Mental health tx	N = 121 PP26 = 32	M = 18.2 Cut = 26	Forensic hospital	66% of psychotic Hi PP had violent reconviction vs 18% for Lo PP. Factor 1 and 2 equally predictive of 2-year recidivism	Recidivism	R neg
22 – Wong et al. (2006)	Non	CBT & RP for 8 months	N = 68 PP30 and PP25 =?	M = 28.6 for treated; 28.0 for untreated	Prison	7.4 year rates and frequency of reoffending same for treated & untreated PP, but tx reduced degree of violence/severity of reoffending which shows positive "harm reduction" effect.	Recidivism	R pos
23 – Langton (2003)	Sex	CBT & RP SOST	N = 476 PP25 =?	Cut = 25	Prison	Treated PPs had more 5.9 year sex recidivism than treated nonPPs. Hi PPs rated as good response to Tx recidivated sexually at lower rate than hi PPs rated as poor response to Tx.	Recidivism, ratings & response to tx tool	R pos Tx pos
24 – Langton et al. (2006)	Sex	CBT & RP SOST	N = 476 PP30 =?	M = 15.6 Cut = 25	Prison	No diff in sex recid. for PP and nonPP after avg. of 5.9 years, but hi PP had signif. more serious non-sex offending	Recidivism	R neg
25 – Hildebrand et al. (2004)	Sex	Not CBT	N = 94 PP30 = 20 PP26 = 13	M = 22.2 Cut = 26	Forensic hospital	Treated Hi PPs had higher sex recid than treated Lo PPs	Sexual recidivism	R neg

26 – Abracen et al. (2004)	Sex	SOST Residential Tx Center	N = 142 71 in tx 71 no tx PP =?	Cut = 25	Prison	Appear no treatment effect or psychopathy did not impact treatment after about 5 years	Sex recidivism	SR nun
27 – Abracen et al. (2011)	Sex	SOST & some addictions tx	64 in tx, PP25 = 14 55 no tx, PP25 = 17	M = 18.4 Cut = 25	Prison	No diff tween treated hi PPs vs untreated hi PPs on rate of sex recid (which was lower than predicted) 9.4 years follow-up	Recidivism	SR nun
28 – Tanasichuk and Wormith (2007)	Non	Meta-analysis	21 studies			Cannot conclude treatments tried thus far are effective or ineffective with treated PPs	Recidivism, treatment behavior	Tx nun
29 – Burt et al. (2016)	Non	Community follow-up	N = 123 PP25 = 123	Cut = 25	Prison	58 offense-free PPs tended to be older when released, had better community support, and rated as lower risk	Recidivism	Info
30 – Walters (2003)	Non	Meta-analysis	42 studies	Yes	Forensic & Prison	Factor 2 correl moderately with institutional adjustment, while Factor 1 was weak correl. Less differentiation between Factor 1 & 2 on institutional adjustment	Institutional adjustment	Info
31 - Frodi, Dernevik et al. (2001)	Non	Assessed early attachment; social skills	N = 14 PP25 = ~4	PCL-SV Cut = 16	12 in prison, 2 in forensic hospital	Hi PP showed mostly Dismissive attachment style and rejecting fathers. Higher PP assoc with more violent crime, more convictions, more foster homes & more childhood physical abuse.	Attachment style – Adult Attachment Interview	Info

(continued)

Table 18.1 (continued)

Study	Type	Treatment	N	PCL-R	Setting	Results	Measure	Sum
32 – Grady et al. (2019)	Sex	Retro analysis of RTC participant characteristics	N = 109 PP25 = 34	M = 21.1 Cut = 25	Prison	Hi PP show higher rates of insecure attachment, but did not align with types. High Facet 1 correl w/Secure, low Facet 1 w/ Preoccupied, low Facet 3 w/ Insecure, low Facet 4 w/ less Preoccupied. Lo PP scored high on Dismissive. No relationship between Facets and childhood abuse	Attachment style – RSQ	Info
33 – Looman and Abracen (2006)	Sex	RTC	N = 191 PP30 =?	Cut = 25	Prison	Subgroup of hi PPs with higher item scores on F1#1 glibness, F1#2 grandiosity, F2#10 poor behavior control, & F2#14 impulsivity showed higher sex & serious recidivism	PCL-R item scores	Info
34 – Young et al. (2000)	Non	MH Tx	N = 118 PP30 = 32	PCL-R cutoff 30	Psych unit in prison	Can distinguish psychopathic Anti-Social Personality Disorder from non-psychopathic ASPD. PPs show more "pathological narcissism"	Rorschach scores	Info

Note: Coding key: *PP* psychopathy, *Hi PP* High PCL-R score, *PP30* PCL-R scores 30+, *PP25* PCL-R scores 25+
Tx treatment, *SOST* sexual offense-specific treatment, *CBT* cognitive behavioral treatment, *RP* relapse prevention, *TC* therapeutic community, *R* Recidivism, *Tx* Treatment, *Pos* positive, *Neg* negative, *Nun* mixed results or no significant differences or no apparent effect

researchers and clinicians and supported by a vast literature (Hare et al., 2000). The original PCL-R manual recommended a score of 30 as the cut-off for "high psychopathy," but the current manual offers several possible cut-off scores, including 25, 27, 30 and 33. Quinsey et al. (1998) suggest a cut-off score of 25 for "pure psychopathy." As summarized in Table 18.1, the authors identified 10 studies using a cut-off of 30, 13 studies using a cut-off of 25, and two studies using 26. The authors also included five studies that used lower cut-off scores but reported the number of subjects with scores of 25 or more. Research that did not use PCL-R scores was disregarded. For example, the Salekin (2002) meta-analysis included only four studies using the PCL-R, and Blasko and Jeglic (2016) and Mahaffey and Marcus (2006) failed to use the PCL-R at all. Similarly, the authors excluded studies of antisocial personality disorder, such as the review by Seto and Quinsey (2006), which mixed studies of antisocial personality disorder with studies of psychopathy.

The use of a high PCL-R cut-off score is important to the question of whether psychopathy exists on a continuum or whether there is a subset of individuals whose severity may rightfully constitute a discontinuous category or taxon. The theory behind the taxon is that the antisocial traits of psychopathy evolved as an alternative, reproductively viable life strategy that gained success from the fact that the great majority of humans are genetically evolved to be pro-social, that is, seeking to belong to mutually supportive, reciprocally altruistic groups (Barr & Quinsey, 2004; Harris et al., 1994a, 2001; Harris & Rice, 2006). In accordance with this theory, the broad *pro*social environment of human societies creates a paradoxical niche for a subset of decidedly *anti*social individuals, who exploit the general altruism and social acceptance of others. The essential ingredient to the adaptive survival of this hereditary anti-social subset is reproductive viability, which, in turn, is grounded in a disposition for hypersexual arousal for high mating behavior. As noted by Knight and King (2012, "if psychopaths constitute a distinct class, the possibility would exist that hypersexuality is one feature that carves that class at its joints, a marker of the divide between those who are psychopaths and the rest who are not" (p. 5).

There is abundant evidence that men high in psychopathy act impulsively, engage in promiscuous sexual behavior, and often have many short-term relationships. When applied in combination with their propensity for deception, manipulation, and superficial charm, high psychopathy men can be very effective in preying upon the good intentions, unguardedness, and vulnerabilities of potential victims, while being unencumbered by feelings of guilt or remorse. Driven by a higher level of hypersexuality, they use anti-social tactics to create opportunities for sex with more partners. Thus, impulsive hypersexuality may be the hallmark of a "pure psychopathy" taxon.

Knight and King (2012) assert that the empirical support for a psychopathy taxon is limited to a single series of three studies: In the first study, Harris et al. (1994a) analyzed the PCL-R scores for 653 serious offenders from a maximum security forensic psychiatric facility and found that Factor 2 scores (i.e., socially deviant lifestyle) denoted a distinct class of offenders, but that Factor 1 (interpersonal and affective characteristics) showed no evidence of personality disturbance.

Subsequently, Skilling et al. (2002) followed up the same sample and replicated the same result of a Factor 2-focused taxon. A third study by Harris et al. (2007) also found a distinct category of sex offenders who were distinguished by this combination of psychopathic features and a history of promiscuous and coercive sexual behavior.

18.3 Why the Sex Offense-Specific Treatment Field Is Important to the Study of Psychopathy

The theory of the psychopathic hypersexuality taxon leads us to the field of sex offense-specific treatment (SOST), which has expanded greatly in the past 30 years (Jennings & Deming, 2016). There are four reasons that the field of SOST is important to the study of psychopathy. First, there is a large body of research that shows significant numbers of sex offenders are high in psychopathy. Whereas Hare (1998) estimates that the rate of psychopathy in the general population is about 1%, the rate of psychopathy among sex offenders is estimated to be 10–15% for child molesters and 40–50% for rapists and those who offend against both adults and youth (Hare, 1999). Observed rates of psychopathy in samples from sexually violent predator (SVP) civil commitment programs in the United States are extremely high. In their study of five state SVP programs, Jumper et al. (2012) found that 38% of a sample of 229 SVPs in the Illinois program had PCL-R scores exceeding 30 and mean score of 25.8. By comparison, 30% of a national composite sample of 1481 SVPs from California, Texas, Minnesota, and Wisconsin had PCL-R scores exceeding 30 and a mean score of 24.2.

Second, research and assessments in the SOST field frequently use the Hare PCL-R, which facilitates comparisons and aggregation of psychopathy data for analysis. The PCL-R has become the second most commonly used risk assessment measure for sexual offending used by forensic psychologists, second only to the Static-99 (Boccaccini et al., 2017). The reason is that the PCL-R is an excellent measure of psychopathic traits, which are strongly correlated with general offending. Even though the PCL-R is only moderately correlated with sex offending (Hanson & Morton-Bourgeon, 2005; Hawes et al., 2013), the PCL-R still provides "relatively good predictive validity with respect to sexual offenses, particularly when combined with measures of sexual deviance" (Hare, 2003, p. 154). The PCL-R has also contributed to decisions to civilly commit "sexually violent predators" (SVPs) in the United States.

Third, one of the most frequent reasons that men with psychopathy will receive group treatment is because they have been mandated to attend sex offense-specific treatment. This means that mandated SOST programs and treatment centers for civilly committed SVPs may be one of the largest sources of sizeable numbers of high psychopathy subjects for study. It also means that many of the available studies of the treatment responsivity of psychopathy entail sex offense-specific treatment.

Indeed, as shown in Table 18.1, the authors' subset includes 15 studies of psychopathy treatment focused on sex offenders compared to 14 studies of non-sexual offenders. This majority of sex offender studies means that conclusions about the treatment responsivity of men with psychopathy will be heavily influenced by their responsivity to sex offense-specific treatment.

Finally, the research literature suggests a strong relation between psychopathy, sexual deviance and reoffending. Based on their meta-analysis of 20 studies using the PCL-R and 5,239 subjects, Hawes et al. (2013) showed that sex offenders with both high levels of psychopathy and sexual deviance are three times more likely to reoffend than other sex offenders. They also found that PCL-R Factor 2 scores are much stronger predictors of sexual reoffending (d = .44) than Factor 1 scores (d = .17) and Total PCL-R scores (d = .36). A subset of five studies that used PCL-R Facet subscale scores found that Facet 2b (Antisocial Behavior) was correlated with sexual recidivism (d = .40) while the other three Facet scores were not (d = .01 to .09).

The Hawes et al. (2013) meta-analysis points to the importance of PCL-R Factor 2 and Facet 2b to the question of psychopathy and its responsiveness to treatment. Moreover, these findings are consistent with the research series conducted by Harris et al. (1994a), which identified Factor 2 as the key element to a taxonic category of pure psychopathy. Factor 1 consists of *Facet 1a – Interpersonal Characteristics* (e.g., glibness, grandiosity, manipulative, superficiality) and *Facet 1b – Deficient Affective Characteristics* (e.g., lack of remorse, lack of empathy, failure to accept responsibility, callousness). Factor 2 consists of *Facet 2a – Impulsive Lifestyle* (e.g., irresponsibility, impulsivity, stimulation seeking) and *Facet 2b – Antisocial Behavior* (e.g., poor behavioral control, history of juvenile delinquency, criminal versatility).

While Hawes et al. (2013) points to Factor 2 as the strongest predictor of recidivism, the authors' review found that most studies which reported on PCL-R Factor scores and *treatment responsiveness* (rather than recidivism alone) showed no clear cut pattern as follows:

Factor 1 has a negative impact on treatment responsiveness: Olver et al. (2013) found that Factor 1 (Personality) and Facet 1b (Affective Deficiency) were negatively correlated with therapeutic change, suggesting that callous and unemotional traits may be barriers to responsivity. Similarly, Hobson et al. (2000) found that men with higher PCL scores (particularly higher Factor 1 scores) showed poor adjustment to treatment. Hughes et al. (1997) also found that Factor 1 had a significant negative correlation with global positive change in cognitive behavioral treatment (CBT). Finally, Hare et al. (2000) found that treated men with psychopathy and high Factor 1 scores had significantly more recidivism than untreated men with psychopathy.

Factor 2 has a negative impact on treatment responsiveness: One meta-analysis of 42 studies by Walters (2003) suggested that Factor 2 had a stronger negative impact on treatment responsiveness. This meta-analysis found that Factor 2 correlated moderately well with institutional adjustment in prison and forensic hospitals, but Factor 1 was only weakly correlated.

Factors 1 and 2 have equal, mixed or nil impact on treatment responsiveness: Looman and Abracen (2006) identified a subgroup of high psychopathy prisoners with especially high rates of sexual and non-sexual recidivism who displayed a unique constellation of four elevated PCL-R item scores: Factor 1 items of Glibness and Grandiosity and Factor 2 items of Poor Behavior Control and Impulsivity. Alternatively, Tengstrom et al. (2000) showed *both* Factor 1 and 2 were equally predictive of 2-year recidivism for the mental health treatment of 121 criminal offenders with schizophrenia, while Walton et al. (2018) found that *neither* Factor 1 nor Factor 2 was related to client or therapist ratings of therapeutic alliance.

18.4 What Is the Nature of the Treatment Given to Men with Psychopathy?

As previously noted, the authors' review of available high psychopathy research found that most of the studies entailed sex offense-specific treatment (SOST). In practice, this means that the treatment received was nearly always CBT-oriented and was largely delivered in the form of structured psychoeducational groups, which are typically organized into a curriculum of treatment topics/targets that are presumed to reduce sexual recidivism. Some common topics include cognitive distortions, offending patterns, deviant arousal, social skills, and victim empathy. The authors' review identified 13 studies using this type of CBT-oriented treatment with high psychopathy sex offenders, and two studies that used other types of SOST (Hildebrand #25 and Jennings #5; Table 18.1).

The authors identified a second set of treatment studies for high psychopathy that were also group-based but were *not* focused on sex offense-specific treatment. Four were in forensic hospital settings and focused on mental health issues, with the first three using CBT (Hughes #3, Heilbrun #15, Olver #14, Tengstrom #21). Four programs were in prison settings and focused on mental health and related issues as follows: Polaschek #2 used CBT for mental health; Hare #16b,c used CBT for anger management and social skills; Hitchcock #6 used CBT groups for criminal thinking; and Wilson #7 used CBT with "intensive groups."

A third type of treatment that has been used with high psychopathy individuals is the Therapeutic Community (TC) model. The most frequently cited study applied an intensive TC model to a population of men with psychopathy and other mentally disordered offenders, which they believed would be appropriate for men high in psychopathy (Rice et al., 1992; Harris et al., 1994b). Based in a secure forensic hospital, this mental health TC program operated for 10 years and mixed patients high in psychopathy with the other forensic patients. Using a matched-sample design, the authors conducted a retrospective study and found that 78% of the 146 treated patients with psychopathy committed new serious offenses compared to 55% of the 146 untreated patients with psychopathy (untreated men were incarcerated in prison rather than hospitalized). Those with psychopathy showed more problem behaviors in the TC but were just as likely as non-psychopathic patients to achieve positions of trust and early recommendations for release. Although treatment helped the non-psychopathic patients to behave in prosocial and noncriminal ways, the researchers speculated that treatment for the patients with psychopathy emboldened them to manipulate and exploit others.

It is notable that this TC study is routinely cited as evidence that treatment can worsen men with psychopathy. On closer examination, however, the viability of the treatment used in this study is questionable:

> Though considered innovative at the time, [this TC program] simply seems bizarre by contemporary standards. The treatment program was peer oriented with little input from the professional staff. Offenders were encouraged to act as therapists and were largely responsible for the day-to-day operation of the program. Techniques used included marathon group therapy (*up to 80 hours in length*) and nude encounter groups. (Looman et al., 2005, p. 552, italics added).

Three other studies of TC treatment with men with psychopathy were focused on substance abuse rehabilitation. Ogloff et al. #17 (1990) found that men with psychopathy in a prison TC were less motivated than non-psychopathic peers, while Hobson et al. #18 (2000) found that forensic patients with higher PCL scores (particularly higher Factor 1 scores) showed poor adjustment to treatment. A fourth TC study by Richards et al. (2003) also found that patients with higher PCL-R scores displayed poorer treatment behavior, but this study was excluded because the subjects were female and none scored over 30 on the PCL-R.

18.4.1 Differences Found When Outcome Is Measured as Recidivism vs. Treatment Responsivity

At the broadest level, studies of psychopathy treatment effectiveness can be divided into those that focused entirely or primarily on recidivism and those that focused more on measures of treatment behavior and/or progress. The studies that focused on recidivism nearly always showed that subjects with high psychopathy recidivated at higher rates than those with low psychopathy as follows: Four studies and one meta-analysis showed that those higher in psychopathy had more general recidivism (Seto #20a, Hare #16b,c, Langton #24, Tengstrom #21, Garrido #9a); one study showed more general and sexual recidivism (Looman #10); one study showed more sexual recidivism (Hildebrand #25); and two studies showed no difference in sexual recidivism (Seto #20b, Abracen #27). Only one study showed that high psychopathy men had less general and less sexual recidivism (Olver #4); and one study showed reduced sexual recidivism (Langton #23). By ignoring the Seto #20b study, which negated the results of the earlier Seto #20a study using the same sample, the authors derive a final tally of six studies and one meta-analysis showing that treated men with psychopathy have higher rates of recidivism, two showing no difference, and two showing reduced recidivism (see Table 18.2).

Table 18.2 Summary tally of high psychopathy treatment studies

Primary measure of improvement	Positive	Neutral/Mixed	Negative
Recidivism	2 studies	2 studies	6 studies, 1 MA
Treatment responsivity	7 studies, 1 MA	4 studies, 4 MAs	4 studies
Both combined	9 studies, 1 MA	6 studies, 4 MAs	9 studies

In contrast, the studies that measured treatment-related variables demonstrate more optimistic results. The primary measures of treatment improvement as summarized in Table 18.1 are variable and include the following:

- Therapist ratings of global improvement (#3, #5, #20a);
- Ratings of participation and appropriate behavior in group (#23);
- Therapist and client ratings of therapeutic climate/alliance (#1, #2, #5, #8);
- Reduced thinking errors (#6, #22);
- Ratings of positive behavior in treatment (#4, #7, #10, #14);
- Engagement in vocational, educational and positive behavior programs (#16b,c, #17);
- Institutional adjustment and misconduct (#11, #15, #16a, #17, #18, #30);
- Attachment deficits (#5, #31, #32); and
- Meta-analytic global ratings of post-treatment improvement (#9b, #12, #9b, #28)

The results of the authors' review found seven studies and one meta-analysis (Garrido #9b) that showed a positive treatment effect for high psychopathy (Harkins #1, Polaschek #2, Hughes #3, Olver #4, Jennings #5, Wilson #7, Walton #8). Eight studies showed mixed positive and negative changes or no clear treatment-related effect, of which four were research studies (Hitchcock #6, Looman #10, Ogloff #17, Seto/Barbaree #20b) and four were meta-analyses (Guy #11, D'Silva #12, Doren #13, Tanasichuk #28). Finally, four studies showed a negative treatment effect (Olver #14, Heilbrun #15, Hare #16bc, Hobson #18). The review excluded Seto #20a because the result was negated by Seto #20b using the same sample and excluded Rice #19 as a treatment not worthy of consideration. In short, there is plenty of support for the treatability of psychopathy.

18.4.2 Selected Studies That Speak Specifically to Treatment Responsiveness in Group Therapy

Based on the authors' review, six psychopathy research studies stand out for closer examination because they meet five criteria. Each study (1) focused specifically on group therapy, (2) consisted of at least 6 months of group treatment, (3) included a measure of treatment responsivity, (4) applied a solid methodology, and (5) used a PCL-R cut-off of 25 or more for high psychopathy. The measures of treatment responsivity varied among the six studies as detailed below. Two studies used the same measure of therapeutic alliance (Walton et al., 2018; Polaschek & Ross, 2010/2011), one used a measure of group therapeutic climate (Harkins et al., 2013), and three used various measures of treatment behavior ratings (Langton, 2003; Looman et al., 2005; Wilson & Tamatea, 2013).

The impact of psychopathy on therapeutic alliance: Walton et al. (2018) were the first to study the therapeutic alliance of sex offenders with elevated psychopathy. They studied 19 consecutive treatment cohorts over a 3-year period. The prison-based SOST program entailed 24–30 months of weekly group therapy in a manualized CBT format that covered seven modules. The 89 clients rated the quality of their therapy relationship with both a primary and secondary therapist, and vice versa, using the Working Alliance Inventory (WAI). The 36-item WAI has three subscales: Therapeutic **Bond** – "I appreciate my therapist as a person"; **Task** agreement – "My therapist and I agree about steps to be taken to improve my situation"; and **Goals** agreement – "I have doubts about what we are trying to accomplish in counseling."

The clients were assigned to three comparison groups based on PCL-R scores. Eleven men were high in psychopathy (score > 30), 34 were moderate (score 20–30), and 44 were low (score < 20). Walton et al. (2018) found no differences between high, moderate and low groups on either the clients' or the therapists' average total WAI score, nor for the Task and Goals subscales. They did, however, find that the high psychopathy group had significantly lower scores on the Bond subscale. They concluded that high psychopathy does not affect the clients' perception of Tasks or Goals within the therapeutic relationship, but can have a negative impact on the client-therapist Bond. They theorized that men with high psychopathy may not "feel" the Bond of connection to their group therapists but they can still reach agreement with their therapists regarding the Goals and Tasks of the group therapy work.

The results from the study by Walton et al. (2018) align with those from two earlier studies of non-sex offending prisoners by Polaschek and Ross (2010) and Ross et al. (2011), which also used the WAI. Using a subject sample of 50 prisoners (26 with PCL-SV equivalent scores of 30 or more), they found that **both clients and their therapists reported the ability to form a therapeutic alliance regardless of the severity of psychopathy** and that the perceived alliance increased over time, also regardless of severity. Like Walton et al. (2018), these researchers found that high psychopathy clients and their therapists could distinguish the Goals and Tasks aspects of therapy from the therapeutic Bond.

Impact of psychopathy on group therapeutic climate: Harkins et al. (2013) tested whether the therapeutic climate of sex offense-specific treatment groups in a program designed for high psychopathy could make a positive impact on the treatment-interfering characteristics of the condition (e.g., arrogance, deception, shallow affect). Using a population of 75 SVPs who were high in psychopathy in Wisconsin's secure civil commitment center, they created four treatment tracks based on PCL-R scores and IQ: one track for PCL-R scores above 25 and average IQ; one for PCL-R scores below 25 and average IQ; one for PCL-R scores above 25 and low IQ; and one for PCL-R scores below 25 and low IQ.

The high PCL-R treatment track addressed the same four criminogenic need areas as the low PCL-R track, which were deviant sexual interest, distorted attitudes, socio-affective functioning, and self-management. But Harkins et al. (2013) modified the high psychopathy track to specifically address psychopathy as a treatment responsivity factor. The therapists in this track did not push for self-disclosure of offending behavior, eliminated interventions designed to develop victim empathy, and used rewards for prosocial behavior that would appeal to the group members' self-interest.

Both the group leader and group members completed the Group Environment Scale (GES) at the beginning of treatment and again after 8 months. The GES is a 90-item self-report scale with 10 subscales measuring different aspects of group climate and functioning. This study found significant improvements with the high psychopathy group as shown by higher levels of Cohesion, Task Orientation, Order/Organization, and reduced levels of Anger/Aggression. By comparison, the low psychopathy group showed only a positive reduction in Anger/Aggression and a worsening in Expressiveness. Even though the therapeutic climate was rated less positively by clients and therapists in the high psychopathy treatment track, Harkins et al. (2013) concluded that the overall climate was generally acceptable throughout treatment.

Psychopathy *and treatment behavior ratings*: Wilson and Tamatea (2013) studied the effectiveness of a specialized CBT rehabilitative treatment program, which used intensive group therapy, for a group of high psychopathy prisoners. They followed the progress of 12 men with PCL-R scores of 30 or more who participated in up to 11 months of treatment in this High-Risk Personality Programme. All 12 showed positive changes during and after treatment including reduced misconducts and successful desistance from crime after release.

Similarly, Looman et al. (2005) conducted a study of 45 high psychopathy prisoners with PCL-R scores of 25 or more who participated in a 7-month residential sex offense-specific treatment program using CBT and relapse prevention. The program offered both group and individual therapy and targeted denial and minimization, development of an offence chain, victim awareness/empathy, and relapse prevention planning. The psychologist responsible for each client's treatment gave a yes/no opinion as to whether the client's risk had been reduced through his participation in treatment. The global risk reduction rating was based on actuarial tools, individual performance on treatment tasks, in-group behavior, behavior in the residential unit, and behavior in off-unit activities, such as recreation and hobby craft. Ultimately, the psychologists opined that risk was reduced for 68% and not reduced for 32% of the 118 men with high psychopathy. Looman et al. (2005) found that high psychopathy men with good treatment progress reoffended at a lower rate (58%) than high psychopathy men with poor treatment performance (70%) and concluded that there may be a subset of high psychopathy subjects that may respond well to intensive CBT-based treatment.

Finally, Langton (2003) also studied the association between ratings of treatment responsivity and recidivism. Incarcerated sex offenders were assigned to four groups based on high and low PCL-R scores (cut-off = 25) and high and low ratings on treatment responsiveness. Independent raters applied a Response to Treatment tool to the post-treatment reports of 444 men. The 8-item tool included a "conduct in group" subscale composed of attendance, group participation, homework completion, and appropriate behavior in group, as well as four treatment target items. Langton (2003) did survival analyses for a period of 5.9 years using sexual recidivism as the dependent variable. This study found a significant interaction effect in which treated high psychopathy sex offenders who were rated as having responded more positively to treatment recidivated sexually at a lower rate than treated high psychopathy sexual offenders who were rated as having responded poorly to treatment.

18.5 New Pilot Study of Interpersonal Group Treatment of Psychopathy

Based on the focused review of these six well-designed group treatment studies, it is clear that looking at measures of treatment responsiveness (rather than recidivism alone) yields a decidedly more optimistic view of psychopathy and its treatability. To add to this optimism, the author offer the results of a small pilot study that explored the use of relationship-focused group therapy with civilly committed "sexually violent predators" (SVPs). The original impetus for conducting this pilot study was not related to psychopathy. It was planned as an alternative approach to engage and motivate a large subset of men who had stopped making progress in their long-term, secure residential, sex offense-specific treatment. As a collective group, the men had been incarcerated and/or institutionalized for many years – even decades for some. Poor responsivity was reflected in lack of motivation to engage meaningfully in the main sex offense-specific treatment program, which was predominantly cognitive-behavioral with a focus on Self-Regulation and the Good Lives Model. Poor motivation might take the form of disruptive behavior in groups, failure to perform assignments, reluctance to self-examine, hostility, silence or minimal participation in groups, denial and minimization, unwillingness to discuss offense behavior, and "just going through the motions."

Since so many of these individuals appeared to have serious problems with interpersonal relations, it was decided to set aside the usual focus on sex offending behavior and criminogenic issues and focus instead on creating opportunities to experience positive interpersonal relating in a cohesive group. The group sessions were unstructured in the sense of having no psychoeducational curriculum, assignments, or planned discussion topics. Instead, the primary focus was to encourage and facilitate positive personal interactions with peers in a safe and supportive group environment by applying the empirically based principles of effective general group therapy (Burlingame et al., 2011; Yalom & Leszcz, 2020).

The specific model and methodology for the new group program was "group-centered" group therapy designed for sex offenders (Sawyer & Jennings, 2014,

2016) and the clinicians received training in the method prior to launching the pilot project. This group methodology is best understood as contrasted with the "spokes-of-the-wheel" approach that is common in CBT-oriented offender-specific psycho-educational group treatment (Jennings & Sawyer, 2003). This common problem occurs when the therapist knowingly or unknowingly focuses attention on one group member at a time because the therapist's priority is to "teach" concepts (e.g., cognitive distortions, relapse prevention, etc.) and assure that homework assignments are being completed. In effect, this approach produces a series of one-to-one educational encounters between the therapist and individual members, which stifles interaction, prevents the development of direct personal connections with one another, and hinders natural tendencies for social bonding (group cohesion). In addition to inducing boredom and lethargy as the members "wait" for their turn, the "spokes" approach can increase defensiveness by creating a "hot seat" and causes members to be self-absorbed as they attend to their singular relationship with the therapist rather than to their peers.

In contrast to the "spokes" approach, the guiding principle of group-centered group is that most interventions should be directed toward interactions and relationships occurring in the group in the present moment. Thus, the group therapist can apply any given individual's specific issue (e.g., hypermasculinity, loneliness, self-denigration) into a sharable issue that can engage and benefit multiple group members here-and-now, while promoting further interpersonal relating and social connection. Since the authors were applying a motivational framework model called "Barriers to Change" (Burrowes & Needs, 2009), the five groups were called "Power to Change" groups. It was hypothesized that the negative interpersonal attitudes and attachment deficits of these residents could be a common barrier to change that prevented meaningful engagement in treatment. If this barrier could be reduced using interpersonally-focused group therapy, the individual would be better motivated to return to the regular sex offense-specific treatment program (Jennings et al., 2021).

For the purpose of writing this chapter, the authors returned to the original sample data from the interpersonal group therapy initiative above (Jennings et al., 2021) and retroactively analyzed the results in terms of high and low psychopathy. Out of 50 original subjects, the authors were able to create a new sub-sample of 30 individuals who had PCL-R scores. The average PCL-R score for the sub-sample was 24.8, with a SD of 6.64. Using the highest PCL-R cut-off score of 30, the authors created two comparison groups: The "high psychopathy" group consisted of ten residents with a PCL-R score of 30+ with a mean of 32.2 and SD of 2.14. The "non-psychopathy" group consisted of 20 residents with PCL-R scores below 30, with a mean of 21.1 and SD of 4.78.

18.5.1 Measures and Procedure

The original sample of 50 men (which included the 30 men in the subsample) were assigned to one of five therapy groups that all began at the same time. As shown in Table 18.3, all five groups had a mix of high and low psychopathy members, but

Table 18.3 Impact of high psychopathy on the five groups

Group	# of members with PCL-R ≥30	Avg PCL-R of members high in psychopathy	Avg PCL-R of all group members	# of grads[a] with high psychopathy & low psychopathy (improved)	Group climate ratings	Group therapist alignment
Red	3	34.5	26.6	2 of 3 high 1 of 4 low	Medium 3.1	Poor r = .24
Purple	3	30.2	25.3	1 of 3 high 1 of 4 low	Medium 3.3	Medium r = .49
Blue	1	33.0	21.1	1 of 1 high 0 of 6 low	Worst 2.7	Worst r = .13
Green	1	34.7	28.4	1 of 1 high 0 of 1 low	Best 4.4	Good r = .64
Orange	2	30.0	25.7	1 of 2 high 1 of 4 low	Best 4.3	Best r = .86
Total				6 of 10 high 3 of 19 low		

[a]Since PCL-R scores were not available for all subjects, the actual total number of group members in each group was larger those shown

there was an unequal distribution of high psychopathy members across groups, ranging from one to three per group. Each group had two co-therapists and up to ten members. All clinicians had a master's or doctoral degree in mental health. To minimize therapist bias, the five groups were arranged to contain a mix of members from different treatment teams. The men had free choice to volunteer to complete a set of questionnaires on an anonymous basis once a month over the course of the project.

There were three primary measures of treatment change or responsivity as follows:

1. ***Recommendation for "graduation."*** Each pair of group therapists, in conjunction with the clinicians on the client's designated treatment team, conjointly assessed the progress of their respective group members and, when applicable, they made a determination that an individual was ready to "graduate" from the interpersonally-focused group in order to reenter the main treatment program. The recommendation for graduation was a global assessment of treatment progress based on the quality of the individual's participation and prosocial behavior in the therapy group, but also considered the individual's behavior in the residential milieu. Thus, a positive assessment of treatment progress could be attenuated based on contradictory evidence of anti-social behavior occurring outside the group in the residential environment.
2. ***Pre- and post-treatment attachment.*** Based on research showing that attachment styles can directly impact both the quality of the therapeutic relationship and perceptions of the therapeutic climate (Sawyer & Jennings, 2016), it was hypothesized that insecure attachment may be a common barrier to engaging in and benefiting from treatment. The authors used the 17-item, self-report

Relationship Style Questionnaire (RSQ) as the measure of secure/insecure attachment (Griffin & Bartholomew, 1994). The participants completed the RSQ at the beginning of the study and 8 months later. Item scores were summed into four subscales that correspond to four attachment styles: Secure, Dismissive/Avoidant, Fearful/Avoidant, and Preoccupied/Anxious. Of the 30 men in the PCL-R subsample, 21 completed the pre- and post-treatment RSQ, and nine declined. Three of the 10 men high in psychopathy declined.

3. ***Monthly ratings of group therapeutic climate.*** Once each month, the participants evaluated the therapeutic climate of their respective groups by completing the Group Climate Questionnaire (GCQ). The GCQ is the most commonly used measure of group process in the group psychotherapy literature (Johnson et al., 2006). With just 12 items, the GCQ has the advantage of ease of administration. Item scores are averaged to yield three subscale scores corresponding to three dimensions of group climate: *Engagement* is the extent to which members feel connected to each other and actively participate in group process. It is roughly equivalent to cohesion, which is considered the foremost therapeutic factor in group therapy (Yalom & Leszcz, 2020; Burlingame et al., 2018). *Conflict* is the degree of conflict, hostility, and tension in the group. *Avoidance* is the degree to which the group members avoid looking at important issues, both personally and interpersonally. A total of 28 of the 30 subjects in the subsample completed the monthly GCQ during the 8 months. All 10 of the men high in psychopathy completed the GCQ. The co-therapists also rated their groups each month using the GCQ, which was used to assess the degree of alignment between the ratings of the co-therapists and their group members.

18.5.2 Results and Discussion

Graduation By the time of the final administration of the RSQ in the eighth month, a total of 13 men were "graduated" from their respective Power to Change groups and returned to the regular SOST treatment program while the others continued as needed in the interpersonally-focused groups. Of the ten high psychopathy men with scores of 30+, 60% were graduated, compared to just 16% of the 19 men with scores below 30. A chi square analysis showed a significant difference in rate of graduation (X^2 (1, N = 21) = 4.947, p < .05).

Attachment Styles Statistical tests were performed for the four Relationship Style Questionnaire (RSQ) subscale scores and 17 item scores. There were no significant differences between the high psychopathy and low psychopathy men for any item or subscale for either the pre-test or post-test RSQ scores. But there were significant changes in pre-test to post-test for both the low and high psychopathy men for the specific items shown in Table 18.4. The men high in psychopathy showed improvements in three item scores from pre-test to post-test, which were statistically significant or approaching significance: item #4 – reduced worry of being hurt by getting

Table 18.4 RSQ attachment measure

	High Psychopathy		Non-Psychopathy	
	Pre	Post	Pre	Post
4. I worry that I will be hurt if I allow myself to become too close to others.	3.4 sd 1.1	2.0 sd 1.4	3.2 sd 1.4	3.0 sd 1.3
7. I worry about being alone.	2.9 sd 1.5	2.4 sd 1.6	3.8 sd 1.4	1.8 sd 0.8
11. I worry that others don't value me as much as I value them.	3.4 sd 1.1	2.1 sd 0.9	2.3 sd 1.2	2.2 sd 0.8
17. I worry about having others not accept me.	4.0 sd 1.0	2.6 sd 1.5	3.8 sd 1.3	1.9 sd 1.1
Secure Subscale (composed of Items 3, 7, 8, 10, 17)	15.6 sd 2.9	12.4 sd 4.8	15.2 sd 3.2	10.8 sd 3.5

too close to others (p. < .050), #11 – reduced worry of not being valued by others (p. < .050), and #17 – reduced worry about not being accepted by others (p. < .062). The men who were low in psychopathy also showed significant improvement in item #17 (p. < .0005), as well as improvement in item #7 – reduced worry about being alone (p. < .0002). The non-psychopathic men also showed significant improvement on the composite secure attachment subscale (p. < .005), which includes both items #7 and #17.

It is interesting that the men high in psychopathy showed sharp reductions in worrying about getting hurt by becoming too close and worrying about not being valued by others, while the non-psychopathic men showed no change in these items. At the same time, the high psychopathy men and non-psychopathic men shared the same sharp reduction in worry about not being accepted by others. Perhaps the fear of social rejection for non-psychopathic men is driven more by fear of being alone, while the fear of rejection for the men high in psychopathy (who are probably well-accustomed to being alone) is fueled more by fear of being devalued or hurt emotionally by others.

To explore further the potential differences in sensitivity to social evaluation/rejection between the two groups and their response to treatment, the authors selected a subset of RSQ items that seemed most applicable to social acceptance. As shown in the Fig. 18.1 profiles below, the high psychopathy men showed the largest reductions in worry about getting hurt by others (#4), being under-valued by others (#11), gaining acceptance (#17), being alone (#7), and discomfort with closeness (#14). The non-psychopathic men also showed significant reductions in worry about being alone (#7) and gaining acceptance (#17), but showed little change on the other socially sensitive items.

Perceptions of the Group Experience To further explore the issue of differing sensitivity to social acceptance, the authors analyzed differences in how the men perceived the therapeutic climate of the relationship-focused groups. Statistical tests were performed for the three Group Climate Questionnaire subscale scores and 12

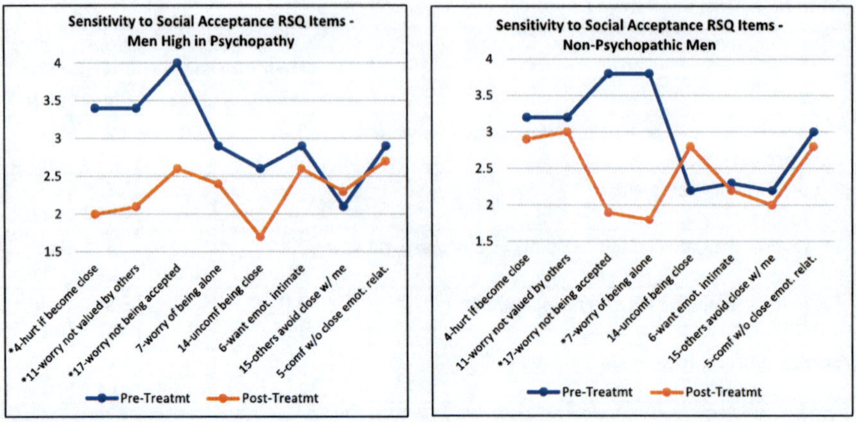

Fig. 18.1 Comparative profiles of high psychopathy and non-psychopathy men on RSQ

GCQ item scores. Only item #3 (avoidance of important issues) showed a statistically significant difference during the fifth month. Nevertheless, despite the lack of statistically significant differences for any individual GCQ items, the high psychopathy group reported more positive perceptions of the group experience on every subscale and 11 of 12 item scores for every month of the treatment period. These results are presented in Table 18.5.

As shown in Fig. 18.1, the men high in psychopathy perceived more liking and caring among group members, less friction and anger, less withdrawal and distancing, less tension and anxiety, and more revelation of sensitive personal feelings. The one item in which the men high in psychopathy had a more negative perception of therapeutic climate was confrontation and challenging among group members, which seems consistent with the RSQ pattern of being sensitive to social acceptance/rejection.

18.6 Conclusion and Recommendations

In seeking a more definitive answer to the question of the treatability of psychopathy, the authors attempted to identify a subset of research studies and meta-analyses that could best speak to the issue. The authors found that when effectiveness is measured in terms of recidivism alone, the research suggests that men with high psychopathy respond poorly to treatment. However, when effectiveness is measured in terms of treatment responsivity variables, the research suggests that men high in psychopathy can respond quite well to treatment. To gain a closer view, the authors identified a short-list of six well-designed studies in which subjects high in psychopathy received intensive group treatment of at least 7 months in duration and

Table 18.5 Number of months in which high-psychopathy or low-psychopathy rated group climate as better

	High Psychopathy Rated as Better	Low-Psychopathy Rated as Better	Equal ratings
Engagement subscale			
1. The members liked and cared about each other.	5	0	3
2. The members tried to understand why they do the things they do, tried to reason it out.	6	2	0
4. The members felt what was happening was important and there was a sense of participation.	4	3	1
8. The members challenged and confronted each other in their efforts to sort things out.	2	6	0
11. The members revealed sensitive personal information or feelings.	8	0	0
Conflict subscale			
6. There was friction and anger between the members	7	1	0
7. The members were distant and withdrawn from each other.	7	1	0
10. The members rejected and distrusted each other.	5	2	1
12. The members appeared tense and anxious.	7	0	1
Avoidance subscale			
3. The members avoided looking at important issues going on between themselves.	4	3	1
5. The members depended upon the group leader(s) for direction.	5	3	0
9. The members appeared to do things the way they thought would be acceptable to the group.	5	3	0

that used some measure of treatment responsivity (with or without a recidivism measure). This shortlist showed that high psychopathy men and their group therapists can form an effective therapeutic alliance, high psychopathy groups can develop adequate levels of group cohesion and positive therapeutic climate, and high psychopathy subjects with positive ratings of treatment behavior had lower recidivism that those rated poorly.

In turn, the authors' own small pilot study suggested that, contrary to expectations, high psychopathy men appeared to be sensitive to interpersonal acceptance and connection. The high psychopathy men consistently viewed their group therapy experience as more positive than their non-psychopathic peers in every month of the eight-month treatment from beginning to end. Most surprisingly, the authors found that a significantly greater number of high psychopathy men were judged by the group therapists to have excelled in the interpersonal-focused group treatment as compared to their non-psychopathic peers. The first and most obvious explanation for these surprising results would be that the high psychopathy men "excelled" in detecting what the group therapists expected of them, rather than in making genuine improvements in prosocial attitudes. The socially desired behavior was, in essence, to participate in group in a polite, respectful manner that appeared cooperative and helpful to others and seemed emotionally sincere. The reward for displaying socially cooperative behavior was the opportunity to "graduate" from the motivational group in order to re-enter the main sex offense-specific treatment program, which is the route leading to eventual release. While this reward was the same for both the high psychopathy and non-psychopathic men, it could be that those high in psychopathy were more skilled at figuring out what was expected of them and then displayed those behaviors to achieve their goal of gaining release more quickly.

A retrospective study of psychopathy, attachment, and childhood abuse by Grady et al. (2019) may support this idea of "faking good." Using the same RSQ self-report measure of attachment, they found that the men high in psychopathy (PCL-R > 25) did not align with any one of the three types of insecure attachment, while the non-psychopathic men were predominantly Dismissive/Avoidant in type.[1] Instead, Grady et al. (2019) unexpectedly found that men with high scores on the Interpersonal Facet 1a of Factor 1 scored higher on the Secure type of attachment. Since Facet 1a includes features like superficiality and manipulativeness, it could reflect the idea that the men with psychopathy were faking good.

A related Facet 1a explanation is that the high psychopathy men behaved well and expressed positive views of the group treatment experience simply for the presumed psychopathic thrill or satisfaction of tricking and manipulating the group leaders. This could be true, but it seems unlikely that this could have been rewarding enough to sustain the prosocial pattern in their monthly GCQ ratings of group climate for eight consecutive months. It also seems unlikely that the high psychopathy men could discern and fake the social desirability of their self-ratings of secure/insecure attachment on the RSQ at the outset of the pilot and then fake an improvement on their initial self-ratings 8 months later.

In the interest of new approaches to psychopathy, what if we consider the results of this pilot study as reflective of an authentic prosocial change in behavior rather than as faking good? What if men high in psychopathy really are acutely sensitive to social rejection, desire social acceptance, and respond well when they have an opportunity to experience social acceptance? And, if men high in psychopathy truly

[1] To help elucidate how the features of the Dismissive attachment style type relate to the psychopathy facets, Sawyer and Jennings (2016, p. 121) summarize the type as follows: "Dismissing adults desire a high level of independence and self-sufficiency. They downplay the importance of relationships and avoid attachment. They have an overinflated view of self and a critical or poor view of others. They are emotionally constricted and suppress feelings and deal with perceived rejections by further distancing themselves or disparaging the other."

value acceptance, why do they repeatedly act in ways that result in rejection, punishment, and harm to others?

With due caution, the authors considered an admittedly radical theory that draws upon research on the powerful impact of social exclusion and ostracism, such as bullying (Baumeister & Leary, 1995; Williams & Nida, 2011). This growing body of research consistently demonstrates that just two to three minutes of relatively innocuous ostracism in a social psychology lab, such as being ignored or excluded in a silly Cyberball game, will produce surprisingly intense feelings of sadness and anger. Williams and Nida (2011) assert that ostracism is experienced in three stages. In the "*immediate*" stage, the exclusion/rejection is physically felt as emotional pain and threatens four essential needs: belonging, self-esteem, control and meaning. In the next stage of "*coping*," the ostracized person tries to recover or improve their inclusionary status. As long as re-inclusion is perceived as possible, the ostracized person will be highly attentive to social information and will strive for re-inclusion, which, when successful, will fortify feelings of belonging, self-worth, meaningfulness, and perceived control over the future. When re-inclusion is thwarted or perceived as unlikely, however, the person experiences sadness and pain and, if the ostracism continues, he or she will become "*depleted in their coping capacity*", the third stage, and descend into alienation, depression, helplessness and unworthiness.

While most people will withdraw and shut down in the third stage of depletion, the ostracism researchers identify a subset of individuals who respond to continuing ostracism by taking anti-social actions to regain a sense of control and self-worth. These individuals lash out with aggression or take actions that force others to notice their existence. Consistent with this, Leary et al. (2003) found that 13 of 15 school shooters had been targets of ostracism. Although anti-social actions will usually fail to gain inclusion (and contribute to further ostracism), these actions provide a way for the person to reestablish control over the social environment (i.e., a sense of self-efficacy). In effect, the ostracized person avoids or lessens the expected pain of rejection by taking control through a "preemptive strike" against the anticipated social rejection. With repeated experiences of ostracism, the aggression and antisocial behavior becomes habituated, and the individual may even self-ostracize to prevent further rejection at the hands of others.

The authors wonder if it is possible that some persons high in psychopathy may belong to this subgroup of third stage victims who respond to ostracism with aggression and hostility rather than depletion and withdrawal. According to the ostracism theorists, the individual uses hostility and trickery to maintain a sense of self-worth and self-efficacy in the face of social rejection and helplessness. In other words, if a youth experiences repeated episodes of rejection, ostracism, abuse, victimization, and humiliation (and if he also lacks caretakers and friends who can counter these hurts with acceptance and inclusion), the youth may find less pain and greater self-efficacy in living an antisocial lifestyle that, paradoxically, rejects and abuses others and society at large.

By applying ostracism theory to psychopathy, it is possible to reconceptualize the classic characteristics of psychopathy in terms of a learned developmental response to ostracism. The characteristics of callousness, coldness, emotionlessness, and glibness can be seen as a long-term effect of suppressing emotions to cope with or avoid the pain of exclusion. The hostility, cunning, exploitation, and even impulsivity, can be seen as a learned readiness to strike first against a world of expected social rejection or as a way to forcibly gain inclusion. The psychopathic readiness to hurt and reject others (before they can hurt and reject him) can explain the characteristic lack of remorse and lack of empathy for victims. The absence of long-term goals, impulsivity, and need for stimulation can be seen as efforts to escape from the interminable boredom, emptiness, and loneliness of a habitual life of exclusion and aloneness. The characteristics of parasitic lifestyle, sexual promiscuity, and exploitative behavior can be seen as misguided efforts to gain some semblance of acceptance and belonging and to satisfy the innate human need for tangible physical touch – even if that touch is secured through force or deception. The characteristic of grandiosity can be explained as a mask of self-esteem for a loner who has failed in gaining praise or acceptance.

If third stage ostracism and exclusion have the potential power to transform a particular subset of youth into adults with high psychopathy, the authors suggest that social acceptance and inclusion should have some counter-veiling power that can be used to mediate or rehabilitate psychopathy. The authors believe that group therapy is the precise modality that, when delivered in a relationship-focused fashion, can provide an authentic experience of belonging, acceptance, and positive emotions that can, in itself, strengthen pro-social attitudes and promote positive interpersonal behavior and self-esteem (i.e., reduce anti-social behavior). In short, it is suggested that an effective therapeutic application of social inclusion – through the modality of relationship-focused group therapy – could or should be a primary target of treatment for high psychopathy.

In light of the authors' research review on responsiveness to group treatment and the results of the pilot study, the following recommendations are proposed for group therapy with men who are high in psychopathy:

1. ***Mix men high in* psychopathy *with non-psychopathic peers:*** One of the basic tenets of group therapy is to have a heterogeneous mix of individuals in the group (if they share a common level of intelligence and functioning). The group should have a mix of traits and personalities, such as introverted and extroverted, high energy and low energy, talkative and reticent, old and young, new members and long-standing members.

Similarly, the authors suggest that it may be more effective to mix high psychopathy men with non-psychopathic men in a treatment group for several reasons. First, men high in psychopathy need exposure to non-psychopathic peers who are already capable of positive interpersonal relating. They need to observe their healthier peers as role-models for how men can bond and relate positively to each other. They need to see how their non-psychopathic peers support each other and resolve differences, and how they help each other and accept help from each other. Second, men high in psychopathy need to observe and experience what it is like to be part of a living social group that can provide acceptance, nonjudgement, and support. If the group is composed entirely of men with high psychopathy, the members are denied an opportunity to experience and feel, first-hand, what it is like to be amongst others in a cohesive, accepting social group.

Third, the therapy group needs to have a core membership with enough health and cohesion to tolerate the inevitable disruptive or inappropriate behavior of a high psychopathy member – *without* responding with exclusion, rejection or ostracism. By keeping the door open to continued inclusion, the person high in psychopathy can have the new experience of a "second chance" at belonging. The inclusion and acceptance offered by the group motivates the individual with psychopathy to learn and try different behaviors that yield more feelings of self-worth and belonging. Such a therapeutic experience is nearly impossible if the group is composed entirely of mutually guarded, hostile, and distrustful men who share a common expectation of social ostracism and a readiness to act out.

2. ***Allow time for the development of cohesion:*** All groups go through distinct stages of development. Groups begin with reticence and apprehension and require a higher degree of guidance from the group leader (Sawyer & Jennings, 2016). In the beginning, conflict is generally low and avoidance of emotional issues is high. But this changes as the members build trust in the safety of the group and feel increasingly safe from social attack or rejection. Group cohesion, the all-important glue of belonging and acceptance, takes time to develop but typically shows a steady increase over time. As cohesion and trust build, the members are more willing to take risks in disclosing deeper feelings and emotional material and can handle higher levels of conflict and emotional intensity (and with decreasing guidance from the group leader).

The research shows that psychopathic subjects are quite capable of forming a therapeutic alliance and developing group cohesion. It may take longer to form the group bond and the bond may not be as strong as in non-psychopathic groups but cohesion can be achieved and maintained with high psychopathy. It just takes more time, greater patience, and careful attention to reinforcing cohesion in the group.

3. ***Maintain safety and protect members from confrontation*****:** As detailed in their comprehensive review of group therapy with men who sexually offend, Jennings and Deming (2016) found that confrontation is ineffective, if not counter-therapeutic. Confrontation is strongly negatively correlated with the effectiveness of treatment groups and is universally disliked and rejected by the clients themselves. The use of confrontation in front of peers can heighten fears of public humiliation and social rejection and harms the group therapeutic climate. Perhaps this need to be safe from personal attack and ostracism may be foremost for men high in psychopathy. The group therapist needs to be proactive in both stopping potential aggression and confrontation and in taking action to restore the sense of safety and acceptance in the group.
4. ***Relationship focus before problem focus*****:** In a recent meta-analysis of decades of group therapy research, Burlingame et al. (2018) concluded that (1) groups that intentionally *emphasize cohesion* as a therapeutic strategy are more effective than ones that neglect or ignore it, and (2) groups that *emphasize greater interaction* among group members are more effective than groups that focus on solving

problems. These two factors may be especially important for high psychopathy subjects in two major respects. First, as noted, the men with high psychopathy need and can benefit highly from the group experience of social cohesion, belonging, acceptance, and positive interactions. Second, if group treatment is *exclusively* focused on offending behavior (through CBT interventions such as challenging offense-supportive beliefs, correcting thinking errors, creating offense cycles, and planning relapse prevention), the individual is forced to see himself and expose himself in terms of his worst and most shameful traits and acts. For the person high in psychopathy, this process confirms that he only gets attention for being bad, hopeless, vile, and deserving of ostracism.

Alternatively, if the group can focus *first* on providing a group experience of acceptance and belonging (before concentrating CBT on offense behavior), the high psychopathy individual has a unique opportunity to discover, express, and be rewarded by society (the group) for his good traits and capacity for good deeds. The group can be a therapeutic experience that can build self-esteem (rather than bravado and grandiosity) and bolster a greater degree of interpersonal trust and mutuality. In turn, this will hopefully better enable the high psychopathy individual to participate honestly and meaningfully in the offense-specific work of treatment.

References

Abracen, J., Looman, J., & Langton, C. (2008). Treatment of sexual offenders with psychopathic traits: Recent research developments and clinical implications. *Trauma, Violence & Abuse, 9*(3), 144–166.

Abracen, J., Looman, J., Ferguson, M., Harkins, L., & Mailloux, D. (2011). Recidivism among treated sexual offenders and comparison subjects: Recent outcome data from the Regional Treatment Centre (Ontario) high-intensity Sex Offender Treatment Programme. *Journal of Sexual Aggression, 17*(2), 142–152.

Barbaree, H., Seto, M., Langton, C., & Peacock, E. (2001). Evaluating the predictive accuracy of six risk assessment instruments for adult sex offenders. *Criminal Justice and Behavior, 28*(4), 490–521.

Barr, K., & Quinsey, V. (2004). Is psychopathy a pathology or a life strategy? Implications for social policy. In C. Crawford & C. Salmon (Eds.), *Evolutionary psychology, public policy, and personal decisions* (pp. 293–317). Erlbaum.

Baumeister, R., & Leary, M. (1995). The need to belong: Desire for interpersonal attachments as a fundamental human motivation. *Psychological Bulletin, 117*(3), 497–529.

Blasko, B., & Jeglic, E. (2016). Sexual offenders' perceptions of the client-therapist relationship: The role of risk. *Sexual Abuse, 28*(4), 271–290.

Boccaccini, M., Chevalier, C., Murrie, D., & Varela, J. (2017). Psychopathy Checklist-Revised use and reporting practices in sexually violent predator evaluations. *Sexual Abuse, 29*(6), 592–614.

Burlingame, G., McClendon, D., & Yang, C. (2018). Cohesion in group therapy: A meta-analysis. *Psychotherapy, 55*(4), 384–398.

Burrowes, N., & Needs, A. (2009). Time to contemplate change? A framework for assessing readiness to change with offenders. *Aggression and Violent Behavior, 14*(1), 39–49.

Burt, G., Olver, M., & Wong, S. (2016). Investigating characteristics of the nonrecidivating psychopathic offender. *Criminal Justice and Behavior, 43*(12), 1741–1760.

Cleckley, H. (1976). *The mask of sanity*. Mosby.
D'Silva, K., Duggan, C., & McCarthy, L. (2004). Does treatment really make psychopaths worse? A review of the evidence. *Journal of Personality Disorders, 18*(2), 163–177.
Doren, D., & Yates, P. (2008). Effectiveness of sex offender treatment for psychopathic sexual offenders. *International Journal of Offender Therapy and Comparative Criminology, 52*(2), 234–245.
Edens, J., Marcus, D., Lilienfeld, S., & Poythress, N. (2006). Psychopathic, not psychopath: Taxometric evidence for the dimensional structure of psychopathy. *Journal of Abnormal Psychology, 115*(1), 131–144.
Frodi, A., Dernevik, M., Sepa, A., Philipson, J., & Bragesjo, M. (2001). Current attachment representations of incarcerated offenders varying in degree of psychopathy. *Attachment & Human Development, 3*(3), 269–283.
Galloway, V., & Brodsky, S. (2003). Caring less, doing more: The role of therapeutic detachment with volatile and unmotivated clients. *American Journal of Psychotherapy, 57*(1), 32–38.
Garrido, V., Esteban, C., & Molero, C. (1995). The effectiveness in the treatment of psychopathy: A metaanalysis. *Issues in Criminological and Legal Psychology, 24*, 57–59.
Grady, M., Looman, J., & Abracen, J. (2019). Childhood abuse, attachment, and psychopathy among individuals who commit sexual offenses. *Sexual Addiction and Compulsivity, 26*(1), 1–26.
Griffin, D., & Bartholomew, K. (1994). The metaphysics of measurement: The case of adult attachment. In K. Bartholomew & D. Perlman (Eds.), *Advances in personal relationships: Attachment processes in adult relationships (Vol. 5)* (pp. 17–52). Jessica Kingsley.
Guay, J., Ruscio, J., Knight, R., & Hare, R. (2007). A taxometric analysis of the latent structure of psychopathy: Evidence for dimensionality. *Journal of Abnormal Psychology, 116*(4), 701–716.
Guy, L., Edens, J., Anthony, C., & Douglas, K. (2005). Does psychopathy predict institutional misconduct among adults? A meta-analytic investigation. *Journal of Consulting and Clinical Psychology, 73*(6), 1056–1064.
Hanson, R., & Morton-Bourgon, K. (2005). The characteristics of persistent sexual offenders: A meta-analysis of recidivism studies. *Journal of Consulting and Clinical Psychology, 73*(6), 1154–1163.
Hare, R. (1999). *Without conscience: The disturbing world of the psychopaths among us*. Guilford Press.
Hare, R. (2003). *The Psychopathy Checklist-Revised* (2nd ed.). Multi-Health Systems.
Hare, R., Clark, D., Grann, M., & Thornton, D. (2000). Psychopathy and the predictive validity of the PCL-R: An international perspective. *Behavioral Sciences & the Law, 18*, 623–645.
Harkins, L., Beech, A., & Thornton, D. (2013). The influence of risk and psychopathy on the therapeutic climate in sex offender treatment. *Sexual Abuse, 25*(2), 103–122.
Harris, G., & Rice, M. (2006). Treatment of psychopathy. In C. Patrick (Ed.), *Handbook of psychopathy* (pp. 555–572). Guilford.
Harris, G., Rice, M., & Cormier, C. (1994a). Psychopaths: Is a therapeutic community therapeutic? *Therapeutic Communities, 15*, 283–299.
Harris, G., Rice, M., & Quinsey, V. (1994b). Psychopathy as a taxon: Evidence that psychopaths are a discrete class. *Journal of Consulting and Clinical Psychology, 62*, 387–397.
Harris, G., Skilling, T., & Rice, M. (2001). The construct of psychopathy. In M. Tonry (Ed.), *Crime and justice: An annual review of research* (pp. 197–264). University of Chicago Press.
Harris, G., Rice, M., Hilton, N., Lalumiere, M., & Quinsey, V. (2007). Coercive and precocious sexuality as a fundamental aspect of psychopathy. *Journal of Personality Disorders, 21*(1), 1–27.
Hawes, S., Boccaccini, M., & Murrie, D. (2013). Psychopathy and the combination of psychopathy and sexual deviance as predictors of sexual recidivism: Meta-analytic findings using the Psychopathy Checklist-Revised. *Psychological Assessment, 25*(1), 233–243.
Heilbrun, K., Hart, S., Hare, R., Gustafson, D., Nunez, C., & White, A. (1998). Inpatient and post-discharge aggression in mentally disordered offenders: The role of psychopathy. *Journal of Interpersonal Violence, 13*(4), 514–527.

Hildebrand, M., deRuiter, C., & de Vogel, V. (2004). Psychopathy and sexual deviance in treated rapists: Association with sexual and non-sexual recidivism. *Sexual Abuse, 16*(1), 1–24.

Hitchcock, G. (1995). *Efficacy of cognitive group therapy with incarcerated psychopaths*. Unpublished dissertation.

Hobson, J., Shine, J., & Roberts, R. (2000). How do psychopaths behave in a prison therapeutic community? *Psychology, Crime and Law, 6*(2), 139–154.

Hughes, G., Hogue, T., Hollin, C., & Champion, H. (1997). First-stage evaluation of a treatment programme for personality disordered offenders. *Journal of Forensic Psychiatry, 8*(3), 515–527.

Jennings, J., & Deming, A. (2016). Review of the empirical and clinical support for group therapy specific to sexual abusers. *Sexual Abuse, 29*(8), 731–764.

Jennings, J., Jumper, S., & Baglio, C. (2021). Using relationship-focused group therapy to target insecure attachment as a barrier to sex offense-specific treatment: A pilot study. *Open Journal of Social Sciences, 9*, 386–408. Special issue: Violence and Abuse.

Jennings, J., & Sawyer, S. (2003). Principles and techniques for maximizing the effectiveness of group therapy with sex offenders. *Sexual Abuse, 15*(4), 251–267.

Johnson, J., Pulsipher, D., Ferrin, S., Burlingame, G., Davies, R., & Gleave, R. (2006). Measuring group processes: A comparison of the GCQ and CCI. *Group Dynamics: Theory, Research, and Practice, 10*(2), 136–145.

Jumper, S., Babula, M., & Casbon, T. (2012). Diagnostic profiles of civilly committed sexual offenders in Illinois and other reporting jurisdictions: What we know so far. *International Journal of Offender Therapy and Comparative Criminology, 56*(6), 838–855.

Knight, R., & King, M. (2012). Typologies for child molesters: The generation of a new structural model. In B. Schwartz (Ed.), *The sexual offender* (pp. *7*:1–32). Civic Research Institute.

Langton, C. (2003). *Contrasting approaches to risk assessment with adult male sexual offenders: An evaluation of recidivism prediction schemes and the utility of supplementary clinical information for enhancing predictive accuracy*. Dissertation Abstracts International: Section B: The Sciences and Engineering, 64(4-B), 1907.

Langton, C., Barbaree, H., Harkins, L., & Peacock, E. (2006). Sex offenders' response to treatment and its association with recidivism as a function of psychopathy. *Sexual Abuse, 18*(1), 99–120.

Leary, M., Kowalski, R., & Smith, L. (2003). Case studies of the school shootings. *Aggressive Behavior, 29*(3), 202–214.

Looman, J., Abracen, J., Serin, R., & Marquis, P. (2005). Psychopathy, treatment change, and recidivism in high-risk, high-need sexual offenders. *Journal of Interpersonal Violence, 20*(5), 549–568.

Mahaffey, K., & Marcus, D. (2006). Interpersonal perception of psychopathy: A social relations analysis. *Journal of Social and Clinical Psychology, 25*(1), 53–74.

Marcus, D., Sanford, G., Edens, J., Knight, R., & Walters, G. (2011). Taxometrics and evolutionary theory: The case of the psychopathic sexuality taxon. *Scientific Review of Mental Health Practice, 8*(1), 6–16.

Ogloff, J., Wong, S., & Greenwood, A. (1990). Treating criminal psychopaths in a therapeutic community program. *Behavioral Sciences & the Law, 8*, 81–90.

Olver, M., & Wong, S. (2009). Therapeutic responses of psychopathic sexual offenders: Treatment attrition, therapeutic change, and long-term recidivism. *Journal of Consulting and Clinical Psychology, 77*(2), 328–336.

Olver, M., Lewis, K., & Wong, S. (2013). Risk reduction treatment of high-risk psychopathic offenders: The relationship of psychopathy and treatment change to violent recidivism. *Personality Disorders: Theory, Research, and Treatment, 4*(2), 160.

Polaschek, D., & Ross, E. (2010). Do early therapeutic alliance, motivation, and stages of change predict therapy change for high-risk, psychopathic violent prisoners? *Criminal Behaviour and Mental Health, 20*(2), 100–111.

Quinsey, V., Harris, G., Rice, M., & Cormier, C. (2006/1998). *Violent offenders: Appraising and managing risk* (2nd ed.). American Psychological Assoc.

Reid, W., & Gacono, C. (2000). Treatment of antisocial personality, psychopathy, and other characterologic antisocial syndromes. *Behavioral Sciences & the Law, 18*(5), 647–662.

Rice, M., Harris, G., & Cormier, C. (1992). An evaluation of a maximum security therapeutic community for psychopaths and other mentally disordered offenders. *Law and Human Behavior, 16*(4), 399–412.

Richards, H., Casey, J., & Lucente, S. (2003). Psychopathy and treatment response in incarcerated female substance abusers. *Criminal Justice and Behavior, 30*(2), 251–276.

Ross, E., Polaschek, D., & Wilson, M. (2011). Shifting perspectives: A confirmatory factor analysis of the Working Alliance Inventory (short form) with high-risk violent offenders. *International Journal of Offender Therapy and Comparative Criminology, 55*(8), 1308–1323.

Salekin, R. (2002). Psychopathy and therapeutic pessimism: Clinical lore or clinical reality? *Clinical Psychology Review, 22*, 79–112.

Sawyer, S., & Jennings, J. (2014). Facilitating group-centered treatment groups for sex offenders. In M. Carich & S. Mussack (Eds.), *The Safer Society handbook of sexual abuser assessment and treatment* (pp. 125–150). Safer Society Press.

Sawyer, S., & Jennings, J. (2016). *Group therapy with sexual abusers: Engaging the full potential of the group experience*. Safer Society Press.

Seto, M., & Barbaree, H. (1999). Psychopathy, treatment behavior, and sex offender recidivism. *Journal of Interpersonal Violence, 14*, 1235–1248.

Seto, M., & Quinsey, V. (2006). Toward the future: Translating basic research into prevention and treatment strategies. In C. Patrick (Ed.), *Handbook of psychopathy* (pp. 589–601). Guilford.

Skeem, J., Monahan, J., & Mulvey, E. (2002a). Psychopathy, treatment involvement, and subsequent violence among civil psychiatric patients. *Law and Human Behavior, 26*, 577–603.

Skeem, J., Poythress, N., Edens, J., Lilienfeld, S., & Cale, E. (2002b). Psychopathic personality or personalities? Exploring potential variants of psychopathy and their implications for risk assessment. *Aggression and Violent Behavior, 8*, 513–546.

Skilling, T., Harris, G., Rice, M., & Quinsey, V. (2002). Identifying persistently antisocial offenders using the Hare Psychopathy Checklist and DSM antisocial personality disorder criteria. *Psychological Assessment, 14*(1), 27.

Tanasichuk, C., & Wormith, J. (2007). *Does treatment makes psychopaths worse? A meta-analytic review*. Paper delivered at the North American Criminal Justice and Correctional Psychology Conference, Ottawa, Canada.

Tengström, A., Grann, M., Långström, N., & Kullgren, G. (2000). Psychopathy (PCL-R) as a predictor of violent recidivism among criminal offenders with schizophrenia. *Law and Human Behavior, 24*(1), 45–58.

Thornton, D., & Blud, L. (2007). The influence of psychopathic traits on response to treatment. In H. Herve & J. Yuille (Eds.), *The psychopath: Theory, research, and practice* (pp. 505–539). Routledge.

Walters, G. (2003). Predicting institutional adjustment and the Psychopathy Checklist factor scores: A meta-analysis. *Law and Human Behavior, 27*, 541–558.

Walters, G., Marcus, D., Edens, J., Knight, R., & Sanford, G. (2011). In search of the psychopathic sexuality taxon: Indicator size does matter. *Behavioral Sciences & the Law, 29*(1), 23–39.

Walton, A., Jeglic, E., & Blasko, B. (2018). The role of psychopathic traits in the development of the therapeutic alliance among sexual offenders. *Sexual Abuse, 30*(3), 211–229.

Williams, K., & Nida, S. (2011). Ostracism: Consequences and coping. *Current Directions in Psychological Science, 20*(2), 71–75.

Wilson, N., & Tamatea, A. (2013). Challenging the "urban myth" of psychopathy untreatability: The High-Risk Personality Programme. *Psychology, Crime & Law, 19*(5–6), 493–510.

Wong, S., & Hare, R. (2005). *Program guidelines for the institutional treatment of violent psychopaths*. Multi-Health Systems.

Wong, S., Witte, T., Gordon, A., Gu, D., & Lewis, K. (2006). *Can a treatment program designed primarily for violent risk reduction reduce recidivism in psychopaths?* Presented at the annual meeting of the Canadian Psychological Association, Calgary, AB.

Yalom, I., & Leszcz, M. (2020). *The theory and practice of group psychotherapy* (6th ed.). Basic Books.

Young, M., Justice, J., Erdberg, P., & Gacono, C. (2000). The incarcerated psychopath in psychiatric treatment: Management or treatment. In C. Gacono (Ed.), *The clinical and forensic assessment of psychopathy* (pp. 313–331). Lawrence Erlbaum.

Chapter 19
Family Therapy Interventions for Psychopathy

Vilas Sawrikar, David J. Hawes, and Mark R. Dadds

Abstract Research into developmental aspects of antisocial behaviour and psychopathy has made strong progress in recent decades. The findings most notably informed by growing evidence regarding callous-unemotional (CU) traits suggest that the neurodevelopmental abnormalities associated with psychopathy emerge early in life, and are shaped by genetics, biology, and environmental factors. In line with this, initial trials of intervention programs for antisocial youth with CU traits have begun to show the potential for family-based interventions to reduce antisocial behaviour as well as CU traits when delivered early in life. Importantly, this research also suggests family interventions may need to be adapted to meet the unique needs of high CU youth. This chapter reviews current best approaches to adapting family interventions for antisocial youth with CU traits. We further argue that it is timely to examine the integration of current theories of antisocial behaviour with emerging scientific frameworks for personalizing clinical intervention. Three core issues are discussed in accordance with scientific frameworks for personalizing interventions relevant to adapting family interventions for high CU youth: (i) research supporting family interventions as an evidence supported treatment for antisocial behaviour as the primary problem (ii) research supporting family-based interventions as the best model of intervention for antisocial youth with CU traits, and (iii) putative treatment strategies that may be integrated or adapted for family interventions such that programs are tailored to the unique developmental aspects of antisocial behaviour among high CU youth. An evaluation of promising best-treatment approach(es) is discussed as well as future directions for research.

Keywords Antisocial behaviour · Callous-unemotional traits · Psychopathy · Family interventions · Parenting · Personalizing interventions

V. Sawrikar (✉)
The University of Edinburgh, Edinburgh, UK
e-mail: vilas.sawrikar@ed.ac.uk

D. J. Hawes · M. R. Dadds
The University of Sydney, Sydney, NSW, Australia

J. E. Vitale (ed.), *The Complexity of Psychopathy*, Dangerous Behavior in Clinical and Forensic Psychology, https://doi.org/10.1007/978-3-030-83156-1_19

19.1 Introduction

Research into developmental aspects of antisocial behavior has made strong progress in recent decades, with findings indicating that the neurodevelopmental abnormalities associated with psychopathy emerge early in life, and are shaped by genetics, biology, and environmental factors (Frick & Viding, 2009; Larsson et al., 2008; Viding et al., 2005). In line with this, recent clinical research has been guided by the assumption that interventions for individuals with psychopathic features stand the best chance of producing significant and durable effects when delivered early in life (Salekin et al., 2010). Moreover, there has been a growing recognition that existing interventions may need to be adapted to meet the unique needs of such individuals.

Recent efforts to develop such interventions for children and adolescents have been informed most notably by the growing evidence regarding callous-unemotional (CU) traits. In contrary to conceptualization of psychopathy in adults (e.g., Hare, 1993), research examining CU traits among youth have not historically focused on the antisocial behavior, but rather the affective (e.g., lack of empathy; lack of guilt; shallow emotions) and interpersonal (e.g., callous use of others for own gain) characteristics of the individual (Frick et al., 2014b). There is now much evidence that CU traits are characteristic of youth with conduct problems who follow particularly severe and chronic trajectories towards delinquency (Frick & White, 2008; Viding & Kimonis, 2018). Research has shown that youth diagnosed with conduct problems and co-occurring CU traits demonstrate more severe, and more instrumental patterns of aggression and antisocial behavior with higher rates of offending, incarceration, and recidivism compared to antisocial youth without CU traits (Frick et al., 2003; Lynam, 1998; Särndal et al., 2003). However, despite the grim picture that may at times appear to emerge from evidence regarding the prognosis of youth with CU traits, research demonstrating positive responses to early intervention among this subgroup has grown considerably in recent years. Reviews of intervention programs for youth with CU traits have begun to show the potential for family-based interventions to reduce conduct problems as well as CU traits when delivered early in life (Frick et al., 2014b; Hawes et al., 2014; Salekin et al., 2010). These findings are important as they challenge the therapeutic pessimism that has overshadowed the treatment of individuals with psychopathic traits historically (Salekin et al., 2010).

Compared to established evidence-based interventions for conduct problems, those designed for youth with conduct problems and CU traits remain very much in the preliminary stages of development. Research focused on such innovations has occurred against a background of growing interest in stratified medicine concerned with identifying neurobiological indices to guide the selection of treatments for specific diagnoses (Insel et al., 2010; National Research Council, 2011). The aim of tailoring psychosocial treatments for putative sub-populations within diagnostic groups has also emerged as a major theme within the 'science of personalizing interventions' in efforts to identify and disseminate empirically supported therapies

(ESTs) for the diversity of youth referred to treatment (Kennedy et al., 2017; Ng & Weisz, 2016). Growing recognition of the heterogeneity in mental health disorders has led to growing interest into methods of personalizing interventions that preserves the tenets of ESTs while it being delivered in a way that considers individual client characteristics that may impact outcomes. Several key stages of personalizing interventions are emphasized, including methods of assessment and selecting, adapting, and delivering treatments according to the evidence for achieving better outcomes for samples with similar patient characteristics. Overall, frameworks for personalizing interventions add another contextual layer to be used in conjunction with models of psychopathology to conduct research and translate evidence that can inform each stage of personalizing interventions. The most commonly evaluated approach with youths has been concerned in large part with developing approaches to the adaptation of existing ESTs for subgroups at risk for poor treatment outcomes (Ng & Weisz, 2016). As will be discussed, however, clinical research focused on adapting existing ESTs to meet the unique needs of youth with conduct problems and CU traits has only recently begun to emerge. The science of personalizing interventions is used here as a translational research framework to synthesize evidence gathered from evaluating models of antisocial behavior into putative strategies for delivering ESTs tailored for youth with conduct problems and CU traits.

As presented in this chapter, emerging evidence supports early intervention for youth with CU traits that is family-based and focuses primarily on parenting practices. We further argue that it is timely to examine the integration of current theories of antisocial behavior with emerging scientific frameworks for personalizing clinical intervention. This chapter is organized according to the three core issues outlined by Ng and Weisz (2016) in their scientific framework for personalizing clinical interventions specific to treatment selection and planning – the stage relevant for adapting interventions. The first of these concerns relate to identifying ESTs for the primary problem. We therefore commence with an overview of family interventions as the current EST for when conduct problems is the primary presenting problem in treatment. The second issue concerns prioritizing treatments associated with good/better outcomes for samples similar to the patient identified; in this case, when youth are diagnosed with conduct problems and CU traits. Accordingly, we address the question of what is the current best-treatment approach(es) for youth with CU traits. We emphasize the theory and research findings suggesting family-based treatments represent the best model of intervention for high CU youth. The third issue pertains to identifying treatment strategies suggested for the type of characteristics the patient has. Here, we consider putative treatment strategies that may be integrated or adapted for family interventions to address the unique risk characteristics associated with CU traits. This last section is split into reviewing the current literature which conceptualizes therapeutic targets for high CU youth, followed by a discussion on putative strategies in tailoring aspects of family intervention based on this research. For the purpose of the review, family interventions will refer to any treatment in which parents/caregivers are actively involved or play an active role as the behavioral change agent in improving child behavior. Thus, even interventions that are predominantly delivered to the child individually, but with just some parent sessions, will still be included.

19.2 Existing Interventions for Youth Conduct Problems

Reviews of psychosocial interventions for conduct problems have emphasized that the most effective treatments presently available are family-based (Comer et al., 2013; Eyberg et al., 2008; Kaminski & Claussen, 2017; Michelson et al., 2013). Meta-analytic reviews have found that the effects following family-based interventions are moderate post-treatment (Lundahl et al., 2006; Maughan et al., 2005; Mingebach et al., 2018; Sanders et al., 2014), while youth of parents who participated in family-based interventions are known to be better adjusted than approximately 80% of youth whose parents did not (Serketich & Dumas, 1996). Further, studies examining follow-up outcomes suggest two-thirds of cases remain in the nonclinical range 1-year after treatment with ongoing benefits for social and emotional adjustment a decade after treatment completion (Beauchaine et al., 2005; Kaminski & Claussen, 2017; Webster-Stratton et al., 2011). Moreover, the importance of family-based intervention for conduct problems has been supported for youth across a range of developmental stages. For instance, the gold-standard treatment for conduct problems in early- to middle-childhood is Parent Management Training (PMT) based on social learning theory (Comer et al., 2013), while interventions targeted toward preadolescent and adolescent youth are known to be most effective when they include a parent-focused component, either alone or in combination with other components (e.g., Epstein et al., 2015). Indeed, the translation of family-based models of conduct problems into widely-disseminated evidence-based interventions can be considered one of the most noteworthy achievements of the mental health sciences to date. The field has also seen growing interest in scaling up these family-based interventions as part of a continuum of evidence-based psychological services in youth mental health to meet the needs of communities at large (e.g., The Psychological Therapies "Matrix"; NHS, 2015).

Conduct problems are hypothesized to develop from, and be maintained by, risk mechanisms embedded in the various contexts and social relationships that make up the ecology of the developing child, the most important of which is the family. Operant conditioning and social learning theory (e.g., Bandura, 1977) has been particularly influential in this regard, allowing behavioral scientists to conceptualize family interactions that reinforce and maintain persistent patterns of antisocial behavior (Patterson, 1982). The family interactional process described by Patterson (1982) that later came to be known as 'coercion theory' proposes that environmental contributions to conduct problems operate through mechanisms within moment-to-moment parent-child interactions. Patterson (1982) described coercive parent-child interactions as 'reinforcement traps'. Here, child problem behaviors are negatively reinforced when child escalatory behaviors successfully extinguish a parent's effort to manage the child, while parent capitulations are negatively reinforced by the removal of child escalatory behavior. Because parents trapped in such cycles tend to also be less attentive to positive behaviors and avoid unnecessary interactions with the child, positive reinforcement for desirable behaviors also decreases. The net effect of this is to implicitly reinforce disruptive and aggressive child behavior and encourage the use of such behavior in future social interactions.

PMT is one of the most prominent examples of an evidence-based intervention model based on social learning theory (e.g., Dishion et al., 2016). It typically consists of a set of procedures and skills teaching parents to interact differently with their children to 'break' the proverbial reinforcement traps. Programs based on coercion theory assume that reductions in conduct problems are achieved by shutting down and replacing escalating cycles of coercion with parent-child contingencies that promote healthy and effective behavior. Components are designed to improve the quality of parent-child relationships, increase reinforcement for positive behaviors, and teach discipline strategies in which calm and consistent consequences are used to set limits on negative behavior. For example, parents are commonly supported to implement brief 'time-out' sequences for younger children (below 8 years old) and logical consequences (i.e., response cost) for older children, as part of behavior correction techniques used during escalating, coercive interactions (Brestan & Eyberg, 1998). Widely evaluated programs based on social learning theory include the Parent Management Training Oregon Model (PMTO; Forgatch & Patterson, 2010); Triple P—Positive Parenting Program (Sanders, 2012); Helping the Noncompliant Child (McMahon & Forehand, 2003); Incredible Years (IY; Webster-Stratton & Reid, 2003); and Parent-Child Interaction Therapy (PCIT; Brinkmeyer & Eyberg, 2003; McNeil & Hembree-Kigin, 2010). Programs are delivered either in individual or group format, and have been adapted for eHealth (e.g., Sanders et al., 2012). Programs also use different methods of skills coaching (video-feedback - IY or live coaching - PCIT), while others have combined PMT with child therapy to achieve clinical objectives (e.g., Kazdin, 2003).

The delivery of evidence-based interventions for conduct problems can be disrupted or hindered by a range of factors, and the importance of using theory-driven strategies to manage such disruptions has received growing attention in the clinical literature (Scott & Dadds, 2009). For instance, parents of youth with conduct problems are known to experience poor mental health and distress themselves, as well as higher rates of marital discord and family dissatisfaction, all of which can contribute to poor treatment outcomes (Griest & Forehand, 1983). Conduct problems can also be associated with dysfunctional power hierarchies between parent and child subsystems that perpetuate and maintain the function of the antisocial behavior, as well as interfering with parents' capacity to enforce consistent age-appropriate limits. Furthermore, parents of youth with conduct problems may develop problematic attributions and feelings about their child which can undermine how well parents adhere to and implement the prescribed parenting strategies commonly found in PMT programs (Dadds et al., 2003; Slep & O'Leary, 1998). Various PMT programs based on social learning theory have therefore incorporated additional treatment components to target domains beyond child behavior, or integrated additional theoretical principles to guide treatment delivery with complex cases.

One example of this is Integrated Family Intervention (IFI; Dadds & Hawes, 2006), a manualized intervention program with social learning theory at its core, which draws also on attachment theory, cognitive theory, and structural family systems theory to overcome the common barriers that multi-stressed families often experience when attempting to change parenting practices and home-based routines. These theoretical principles, as well as additional treatment components, are used to address factors that often play an important indirect role in maintaining complex presentations of conduct problems. These factors may include insecure parent-child attachment dynamics, dysfunctional power hierarchies in the family structure, marital discord, problematic parental attributions, and the impact of parental distress on treatment progress. The integration of behavioral-attachment conceptualizations of conduct problems can help to explain some problematic child behaviors that operant principles cannot, such as why some children seem driven to elicit potentially harmful attention from parents (Dadds & Hawes, 2006; Greenberg et al., 1993). Parents are supported to implement strategies in ways that are sensitive to, and capitalize on, parent-child attachment processes. For instance, parents' use of reinforcement strategies emphasizes caregiver proximity, while parents are supported to use limit-setting strategies in ways that do not inadvertently threaten attachment security. The flexible structure of IFI allows practitioners to deliver core PMT components while choosing also from various cognitive-behavioral modules to augment therapy based on their clinical formulation of a case.

Multicomponent approaches that draw upon PMT skills alongside other components focused on parents, other family members, peers, or the child, have received particularly strong support in the treatment of conduct problems in late childhood and adolescence (Garland et al., 2008). Functional Family Therapy (FFT) is one such intervention that combines social learning and systemic theory (Sexton & Alexander, 1999). It focuses on the behavioral-contextual influence of family interactions in the development and maintenance of antisocial behaviors, and frames such behavior in relation to its function in disrupting the organization and structure of family systems (Alexander & Barton, 1995; Alexander & Parsons, 1982; Minuchin, 1967). From such a perspective, antisocial behavior is seen resulting from a lack of reciprocal reinforcement of clear, meaningful communication within the family system (Alexander, 1973; Alexander & Barton, 1995). Specific aspects of the family system that might be addressed include (i) subsystem boundaries and dysfunctional parent-child coalitions, in order to unify parental systems and increase consistency in limit-setting; (ii) power hierarchies, in order to re-position the parental subsystem above the child subsystem; and (iii) the functional purpose of antisocial behavior, in order to reduce its system-maintaining qualities. FFT also emphasizes a contextual approach to processes affecting therapy, such as client motivation, therapist skills, training and supervision, and multiple agency systems that surround families and therapists (Alexander & Robbins, 2011). Research has shown that FFT is effective in reducing adolescent delinquency, recidivism, and substance abuse, as well as improving overall family functioning (Alexander & Sexton, 2002; Kazdin, 1997; Sexton & Alexander, 2003; Sexton & Turner, 2010).

Multisystemic Therapy (MST) also incorporates PMT skills alongside an expanded range of components that target the multiple, interconnected systems occupied by adolescents (individual, family, and extrafamilial systems), to reduce antisocial behavior. MST emphasizes behavior change in the youth's natural environment, capitalizing on the child capacities to achieve clinical outcomes (Henggeler et al., 2009). In addition to parent-focused components, MST includes components for peer intervention, school intervention, and individual-oriented interventions (e.g., cognitive-behavior therapy for comorbid mental health issues). Importantly, this intervention posits that improved caregiver and family functioning is central to maximizing improvements in antisocial behavior (Huey et al., 2000). MST is considered 'well-established' for adolescents, with efficacy studies showing positive treatment effects in the treatment of criminal behavior, substance abuse, emotional disturbance, and reducing recidivism and out-of-home placement (Borduin et al., 1990; Henggeler et al., 1986, 1992, 2002). At the same time, however, mixed findings regarding the effectiveness of MST in various countries have raised questions regarding the transportability of the intervention model across geographic and cultural boundaries (Fonagy et al., 2018).

In summary, family-based interventions represent the most effective form of treatment for child and adolescent conduct problems currently available, and the overall weight of available evidence supports programs based on behavioral versus non-behavioral underpinnings (Kaminski & Claussen, 2017). At the same time, there is noteworthy diversity in how evidence-based interventions for conduct problems deliver treatment components and incorporate theoretical perspectives on child development and family systems, and the extent to which they also directly target the youth's own competencies (e.g., self-regulation, social skills). Importantly, the broad scope of such interventions can be seen to present a range of possibilities for work concerned with personalizing treatment for specific subgroups of children.

19.3 The Importance of Family-Based Interventions for Youth with Psychopathic Traits

Despite ongoing questions regarding the therapeutic needs of youth with CU traits, it has been proposed that family-based interventions represent the best starting point in treatment planning for such individuals (Hawes et al., 2014; Salekin et al., 2010). One might argue that if psychopathy manifests itself as a set of personality traits arising from heritable neurobiological characteristics, clinical approaches that focus on social-ecological risk mechanisms seem counterintuitive for such youth. As will be discussed, however, several lines of research have provided compelling support for a family-based approach.

First, the most effective interventions presently available for conduct problems among youth with CU traits are family-based interventions (e.g., PMT). Among the key support for adapting existing family-based interventions are results indicating that although the effectiveness of such treatment appears to be reduced among such youth, clinically significant gains are nonetheless often still observed. A review by Hawes et al. (2014) examining the impact of CU traits on family-based interventions found that children with conduct problems and co-occurring CU traits often demonstrated significant pre- to post-treatment improvements in conduct problems, albeit to a lesser extent than for youth without CU traits. These findings are more consistent when interventions are behavioral in nature and comprise PMT components (Waller et al., 2013). The current evidence therefore supports behavioral family interventions as a class of therapy that can be considered beneficial for reducing conduct problems among youth with CU traits, but also highlights that high CU traits identify a clinical phenotype of antisocial youth whose needs are not completely met by current best-practice treatments.

Second, family-based interventions have the best evidence base for producing change in CU traits; particularly those programs based on social-learning theory (Hawes et al., 2014). Several studies investigating the effects of PMT on child CU traits have now reported pre- to post-treatment changes in levels of CU traits among young children with conduct problems (Hawes & Dadds, 2007; Kolko et al., 2009; McDonald et al., 2011; Somech & Elizur, 2012). Tests of mediation in this research suggested that reductions in CU traits were partially accounted for by changes in harsh, inconsistent, and ineffective parenting, highlighting the importance of targeting parenting behaviors among high CU youth (Elizur et al., 2017; McDonald et al., 2011). Comparatively, programs specifically targeting youth using individual-oriented therapy have not been found to show similar reductions in CU traits (Wilkinson et al., 2016). This may reflect that individual-oriented therapy is commonly reserved for youth at older ages, when antisocial behavior and emotion-related deficits are perhaps more entrenched. Indeed, evidence that CU traits respond to family-based interventions during adolescence is at present limited and mixed (Butler et al., 2011; Manders et al., 2013). A possible interpretation is that early childhood may represent a developmentally sensitive 'window' during which time targeted changes to parenting practices are able to re-direct trajectories of at-risk youth toward healthy neurodevelopment.

Finally, current developmental models of psychopathy predict that environmental contexts serve to potentiate the expression of biological vulnerabilities associated with the risk for psychopathy (Dishion & Patterson, 2006). These models propose that key risk factors associated with psychopathy such as temperament, social-cognitive style, and intelligence, are partly environmentally-formed biosocial traits, and that neural substrates implicated in these dispositional characteristics are shaped through multiple repeated interactions within the family and broader social contexts across development (Dishion & Patterson, 2006; Lewis, 2000). This has important implications for translational work concerned with designing interventions for youth with CU traits. First, it highlights the importance of understanding how parenting and family processes contribute to expressions of CU traits over time (Willoughby et al., 2013). Second, and most importantly, it serves to provide ways of thinking about how to create environments for potentiating change in neurobiological substrates underlying psychopathy. Elsewhere in the literature, interventions for young children who have a traumatic brain injury (TBI) are relevant to this point. Successful interventions for youth with TBI are implemented through intensive and persistent behavioral training in the child's rearing environment (Ylvisaker et al., 2005). Greater neuroplasticity in children is hypothesized to support re-organization of brain circuitry from sustained intervention (Slifer & Amari, 2009). Likewise, neuro-circuitry abnormalities associated with CU traits may be amenable to change from intensive behavioral interventions that target the family environment. Indeed, as Salekin et al. (2010) argue, despite common disorders such as depression and anxiety having heritable aspects and documented brain anomalies, it is widely recognized nonetheless that recovery from these disorders is possible following behavioral therapy.

19.4 Conceptualizing Therapeutic Targets for Youth with Psychopathic Traits

The research reviewed suggests that antisocial youth, even those with early signs of CU traits, can benefit from early intervention programs based on PMT (Salekin et al., 2010). It is likely that change mechanisms implicated in these family-based interventions overlap with those implicated in child and adolescent CU traits. However, evidence of reduced treatment response among youth with CU traits following such intervention raises questions of how family-based interventions could be adapted to optimize outcomes for these young people. Logically, there has been growing interest in the extent to which mechanisms targeted in family-based intervention for child conduct problems map onto those that account for the problems of children with CU traits (Salekin et al., 2010).

Notably, it is hypothesized that the development of antisocial behavior among youth with high CU traits is characterized by unique neuropathology, that is somewhat distinct from that implicated in the antisocial behavior of youth without CU traits (Salekin & Lochman, 2008). Particular attention has been given to the emotional deficits associated with CU traits as potential mechanisms that may disrupt healthy development by interfering with learning processes that rely on being able to form associations between disadvantageous behavior and negative affective states (Anderson & Kiehl, 2014). Further, a second pathway has been proposed that emphasizes the role of dispositional characteristics associated with CU traits (e.g., fearlessness, insensitivity to punishment, low responsiveness to distress cues) in interfering with the development of moral reasoning, empathy, and in turn, prosocial behavior (Frick et al., 2014a; Frick & Viding, 2009; Frick & White, 2008). It has been hypothesized that high CU youth have impairments in integrating emotional information and empathic reasoning into monitoring and governing behavior, making it difficult to socialize adaptive behavior in this putative subgroup (Blair & Mitchell, 2009; Kiehl, 2006).

Investigations from cognitive neuroscience have implicated functional differences in brain regions involved in the processing of emotional cues, reinforcement learning, and emotion regulation (e.g., amygdala, ventromedial, prefrontal, orbitofrontal cortex, and caudate; Jones et al., 2009; Sebastian et al., 2016). Of interest has been the differentiated functional and neural connectivity in limbic and prefrontal regions, as well as anterior cingulate cortices responsible for emotion recognition, decisions making, moral processing, and empathy (Blair, 2005; De Brito et al.,

2009). Findings have generally correlated CU traits with hypo-amygdala responsiveness to emotionally salient cues (Anderson & Kiehl, 2014). For boys, CU traits have also been linked to low cortisol levels, a marker of stress reactivity to stimuli, which may lead to diminished avoidance of aversive cues (Loney et al., 2006). As such, high CU youth may have difficulty forming stimulus-punishment associations for learning adaptive behavior. Further, research from behavioral genetics have suggested polymorphisms affect the functional integrity of the amygdala and medial frontal cortex, predisposing individuals to reduced emotional and amygdala responsiveness (Blair, 2008a). Findings from such research is consistent with theory that youth with CU traits are associated with atypical neurodevelopment in brain regions and systems important for integrating emotional information into higher order cognitive processes affecting forms of emotional learning, stimulus-reinforcement learning, and moral socialization (Blair, 2008b; Kiehl, 2006).

Research examining social cognition and the processing of emotional cues has also pointed to differential risk pathways towards conduct problems among youth with high versus low CU traits. One of the most consistent findings here has been that high CU youth show poorer recognition of, and less responsiveness to, emotional states in others, with particularly pronounced difficulties in recognizing expressions of fear and distress (Dawel et al., 2012; Kimonis et al., 2006; Marsh & Blair, 2008). Researchers have accordingly proposed that CU traits are associated with "fear blindness", a generalized deficit in processing displays of fear. There is also evidence to indicate that this may be accounted for by reduced attention to the eyes of others and emotionally salient cues in the environment (Blair, 2005; Dadds et al., 2006; Muñoz, 2009; Stevens et al., 2001). Dadds and colleagues (Dadds et al., 2006; Dadds et al., 2008; Dadds et al., 2011) showed that CU traits were associated with reduced frequency and duration of children's eye gaze toward the eye region of adult faces. These results were found in eye-tracking research while participants watched images of adult emotional faces, as well as in observational studies involving the coding of parent-child interactions during emotionally engaging tasks (e.g., 'love' scenario). Dadds et al. (2014) posited that a child's lack of eye contact with attachment figures may prevent them from benefiting from the critical parent-child exchanges early in development that establish the foundations of emotion understanding, conscience, and empathy.

Research has also supported the view that CU traits are associated with diminished development of cognitive and affective empathy (Frick et al., 2014a). A number of studies have shown that CU traits are uniquely associated with deficits in affective empathy, independent of conduct problem severity (Anastassiou-Hadjicharalambous & Warden, 2008; Dadds et al., 2009; Jones et al., 2010; Pasalich et al., 2014; Schwenck et al., 2012). Aspects of cognitive empathy, such as perspective-taking skills (e.g., Hoffman, 1994) may also be impaired in youth with CU traits and are thought to play an important role in the differences seen in affective empathy. For instance, Lui et al. (2016) showed that associations between CU traits and affective empathy were partially mediated by the youth's ability for affective perspective taking. Furthermore, deficient capacities in perspective taking skills have been found to be associated with other emotion related difficulties such as knowledge of causes of emotions among high CU youth (O'Kearney et al., 2017). The capacity to take cognitive and affective perspectives is also considered crucial to inhibiting aggressive behavior (e.g., Feshbach, 1984), adding further support to the view that developmental pathways toward conduct problems among youth with high CU traits may relate largely to dispositional child characteristics.

Elsewhere in the literature a somewhat parallel body of research has examined the relationship between parenting and conduct problems in the context of high versus low levels of CU traits. Findings from these studies suggest the development of conduct problems among youth with high CU traits are less proximally associated with negative parenting practices typically targeted in family interventions such as coercive and harsh/inconsistent discipline (Oxford et al., 2003; Wootton et al., 1997). Some research has suggested that time-out may be less effective in reducing conduct problems among high CU youth than those without CU traits (Hawes & Dadds, 2005), while other research has shown that it may actually induce escalations of conduct among youth with CU traits (Haas et al., 2011). It has been proposed that these patterns of findings support the theoretical assumption that the capacity to inhibit behavior in the presence of punishment cues is limited in youth with CU traits, making socializing through punishment less effective (Dadds & Salmon, 2003). This hypothesis has been supported by studies showing that youth with CU traits are less likely to modify behavior in response to punishment (e.g., Blair et al., 2001). We note that reward-based strategies have been proposed to be more effective for reducing conduct problems given higher reward-orientation in high CU youth (Bayliss et al., 2010; Hawes & Dadds, 2005). While differential sensitivity to punishment-reward has not always been found (e.g., Ortiz et al., 2018), related evidence on the whole supports the view that somewhat distinct reward-related processes are involved in the development of conduct problems among youth with high versus low CU traits.

Interestingly, it is a lack of parental warmth/involvement rather than exposure to negative parenting that appears to be most proximal to the development and maintenance of conduct problems among high-CU youth (Kochanska et al., 2013; Kroneman et al., 2011; O'Connor et al., 2016; Pasalich et al., 2011; Waller et al., 2013). Indeed, the quality of attachment security and related processes (e.g., parental warmth, responsiveness) may be of relevance to interventions for these youth. For instance, studies have shown that attachment problems at age four prospectively predict CU features at age fifteen (Sonuga-Barke et al., 2010), and that increased exposure to parental warmth/involvement predicts decreasing levels of CU traits over time (Pardini et al., 2007; Pasalich et al., 2016). In our own research at the Child Behavior Research Clinic, Pasalich et al. (2012) used the Manchester Child Attachment Story Task to examine parent-child attachment relationships among referred youth with high versus low CU traits. It was found that youth with higher levels of CU traits were more likely to have disorganized representations of parent-child attachment relationships. High CU youth appeared to have a general lack of organization and coherence in attachment schemas, which is consistent with theory proposing that such youth have impairments in attending to emotional cues from attachment figures, which may in turn interfere with the processing of attachment-related information (Dadds et al., 2014; Fonagy, 2003). Taken together, these findings suggest that the inclusion of intervention components that target parent-child attachment dynamics may potentially enhance the treatment outcomes of youth with CU traits.

In sum, there is growing evidence that risk processes involved in the development of antisocial behavior and CU traits are somewhat distinct from those have been described for antisocial youth without these traits. Abnormalities in brain structure and function, particularly those related to integrating emotional responses and moral reasoning in higher-order processes, likely adversely impact on capacities to learn and establish pro-social behavior among high CU youth. Although these findings may suggest that the types of conduct problems and family dynamics associated with CU traits are to some extent child-driven, the risk pathways followed by these children are nonetheless understood to involve complex interactions between multilevel systems (e.g., gene x environment). From this perspective, interpersonal processes involving parenting, attachment, and empathic communication during parent-child exchanges could potentially be exploited to remediate deficits in neurobiology and cognition, as discussed in the following section.

19.5 Progress in Adapting Family Interventions for Youth with Psychopathic Traits

Evidence of poorer outcomes from family-based interventions among youth with CU traits has spurred growing interest in developing precise clinical approaches that match the phenotypical characteristics of youth with high CU traits. Available evidence regarding the neuropathological correlates associated with CU traits has the potential to inform such work by outlining the deviations from healthy development that may account for reduced treatment responses to established family-based interventions. Such accounts provide some basic organizing principles for approaching such intervention and progress in this work to date reflect three emerging themes.

The first theme in adapting family interventions focuses on CU traits' association with a punishment insensitive learning style and higher reward-driven behavior (Bayliss et al., 2010; Miller et al., 2014). In this context, researchers have sought to modify reinforcement procedures, hypothesizing that behavior among high CU youth could be improved through enhancing reward-oriented strategies (e.g., dynamic and individualized token economies) while minimizing the emphasis on punishment and discipline-related procedures (e.g., time-out). Initial pilot studies provided early positive results with findings indicating that negative behavior (e.g., aggression, teasing, stealing) among youth with CU traits ($n = 11$) was lowest when discipline-related procedures were de-emphasized (Miller et al., 2014). Waschbusch et al. (2020) extended this work while conducting a larger evaluation of modified reinforcement procedures within a behavior therapy program that included individual- and parent-focused components in a 7-week summer-program for youth with ADHD and co-occurring ODD/CD (n = 46). Using a within-group design, Waschbusch et al. (2020) evaluated the comparative effects between the standard approach versus behavioral approaches which de-emphasized punishment, emphasized reward techniques, and combined low-punishment and high-reward strategies. However, there was no evidence that modifying reinforcement procedures was superior compared to the standard approach in terms of outcomes in social play behavior and disruptive behavior problems.

These latter findings converge with research suggesting that differential responsivity to punishment-reward in youth with high CU traits may not be as robust as expected. Ortiz et al. (2018) conducted an experimental test of whether CU traits in children 3–8 years of age are associated with differential response to reward versus punishment components of parenting interventions for conduct problems. Neither type nor dosage of modified parent training components moderated relations between CU traits and treatment response. We note that similar outcomes were found in a clinical study involving individual therapy coaching skills development in self-control and problem-solving techniques (Byrd et al., 2018). Overall, these findings appear to suggest that treatment personalization focused on modifying reinforcement procedures alone may not be an optimal approach when used for youth with CU traits. Furthermore, several researchers have highlighted theoretical reasons for including established evidence-based discipline components for this subgroup. Youth with high levels of CU traits are known to experience harsher and critical parenting behaviors (Salihovic et al., 2012), which in turn are related to the development of CU traits (Pardini et al., 2007). Thus, choosing to modify or de-emphasize components teaching parents non-forceful punishment strategies may in fact be a disservice to these families given that such components represents an important ingredient for reducing conduct problems and promoting healthy child development (Dadds & Tully, 2019; Patterson et al., 2002). Waschbusch et al. (2020) suggested from their results that reducing the magnitude of punishment, while at the same time increasing its likelihood, may be a better approach in deterring antisocial behavior for high CU youth, a hypothesis that requires testing in future clinical studies.

The second emerging theme relates to improving the emotional quality of the parent-child relationship in order to buffer against the emergence and amplification of CU traits among at-risk youth. This theme reflects research showing that the development of conduct problems and antisocial behaviors among youth with high levels of CU traits may be more proximally associated with low parental warmth and sensitivity than harsh and inconsistent discipline practices (e.g., Kroneman et al., 2011; Pasalich et al., 2011). Further, parental warmth, positive expressiveness, sensitivity, and a responsive parenting style, are all implicated in the development of healthy capacities for empathy and prosocial behavior, and may represent protective processes among youth with early behavioral indicators of CU traits (Waller & Hyde, 2018; Wright et al., 2018; Zhou et al., 2002). Studies have found that children with elevated CU traits who were exposed to higher levels of warm and responsive parenting are less likely to develop conduct problems and CU traits over time (Pardini et al., 2007; Waller et al., 2014; Wright et al., 2018). These findings are consistent with models implicating attachment security in the development of conscience, empathy, and emotional intelligence (Davidov & Grusec, 2006; Kochanska, 1997). No clinical studies have explicitly tested the direct effects of targeting attachment security on treatment outcomes. As discussed below, however, attachment theory has been used to inform two studies of interventions incorporating adjunctive components targeting emotion processing deficits associated with CU traits (cf. Dadds et al., 2019; Kimonis et al., 2019).

The third emerging theme relates to treatment components designed to target the deficits in emotion processing and responses to emotional stimuli exhibited by youth with CU traits (Frick et al., 2014b; Marsh & Blair, 2008). A key question has been whether youth with high CU traits can be trained to overcome their apparent fear blindness. Early experimental work showed that deficits in the recognition of fear cues among children with CU traits could be temporarily corrected by directing these children to focus on the eye regions of faces when viewing emotional stimuli (Dadds et al., 2006). These early findings were translated into a targeted intervention for youth with high CU traits that consisted of a computer-based emotion recognition training program (ERT) as an adjunct to IFI (Dadds et al., 2012). Participants (age 6–16 years) with clinic-referred conduct problems were randomized to standard IFI versus IFI plus an ERT component. The ERT component was based on the Mindreading program developed to coach children with autism to identify and interpret emotional expressions (Baron-Cohen et al., 2004). It was delivered through four child and parent–child sessions involving computerized modules and weekly homework of parent–child emotion-focused games. Results indicated that CU traits moderated outcomes such that youth with high CU traits responded less well to standard IFI, while the combination of IFI and ERT produced significant improvements in affective empathy and conduct problems for youth with high CU traits.

Despite the significant findings, key predictions regarding mechanisms of change were not supported. Specifically, Dadds et al. (2012) hypothesized that improvements in conduct problems during treatment would be explained by changes in emotion recognition and affective empathy, but this was not supported by mediation analyses. As such, Dadds et al. (2012) speculated that the ERT component, which embedded intensive emotion-focused activities in parent-child protocols, may have translated into therapeutic gains by inadvertently improving emotion-related qualities in participants' parent-child relationship. In turn, it was proposed that clinical strategies for increasing emotional engagement in the parent-child relationship (e.g., parental warmth and sensitivity) may have the potential to remediating core deficits associated with CU traits (Hawes et al., 2014).

This potential direction was explored in a recent proof-of-concept study that drew on these emerging themes, to enhance therapeutic gains in conduct problems, as well as reductions in CU traits, among young children (aged 3–8 years) with high levels of CU traits (Dadds et al., 2019). Families were randomized to two active treatment conditions, comprising (1) IFI plus an adjunctive emotional engagement component, versus (2) IFI plus an adjunctive child centered play component (e.g., evidence-based strategies for engaging children in parent-child play that is child-led and developmentally appropriate). In this study, emotional engagement was operationalized in terms of reciprocal eye contact and targeted through a component involving parent-focused skills-training and structured in vivo parent child interactions, designed to be delivered in conjunction with IFI. The aim was to improve the child's attention to emotional salient cues, as well as the quality of the parent-child relationship, by promoting emotionally engaging parent-child interactions and reciprocal shared eye contact during routine activities (e.g., reading, storytelling, and casual conversation). Improvements in emotional engagement was predicted to translate into enhanced treatment outcomes via three key mechanisms; it was proposed that (i) improvements in the quality of the parent-child relationship instigated by shared eye contact would act as a motivating reward for child prosocial behavior, (ii) improvements in child's attention and response to emotional content of parental communication would help to remediate emotional processing deficits and improve child cooperation, and (iii) eye contact would activate neuropeptide networks (e.g., oxytocin) and neural connectivity to aid normative development of emotion processing in higher order circuitry. Positive changes in these mechanisms were hypothesized to increase attention to salient emotional stimuli during parent-child interactions and normalize neurodevelopment for integrating emotional information into higher-order processes (Dadds et al., 2019).

Dadds et al. (2019) found that emotional engagement was associated with short-term improvements in children's reciprocated eye gaze; however, this was not maintained at the 3-month follow-up. Contrary to expectations, there was no difference in outcomes in conduct problems between the two treatment conditions and, while there were reductions in CU traits, the final levels of CU traits were still in the borderline high range. Notably, the study remains the only trial to date in which a randomized control design has been used to evaluate the specific effects of parent-child emotional engagement on parent training outcomes. Also unique to this study were inclusion criteria requiring child participants to have high as well as stable levels of CU traits, based on screening across two pre-treatment time points. As such, while an adjunctive component targeting emotional engagement did not enhance the treatment outcomes of these participants, it is also possible that such a screening approach resulted in a sample of youth whose CU traits were particularly treatment resistant. Further, Dadds et al. (2019) speculated that deficits in eye gaze may have a particularly stubborn set-point that is established early in development. While temporary improvements may be possible to achieve through brief intervention, sustained changes may therefore be much harder to produce.

Such considerations regarding the intensity and developmental timing of treatment may be particularly important to consider when adapting family-based interventions for youth with CU traits. As already noted, in other clinical fields such as youth TBI, successful interventions have been characterized by higher intensity of behavioral training delivered to children at relatively early ages. One study that reflects such an approach is Kimonis et al.'s (2019) preliminary evaluation of an enhanced parenting intervention program (PCIT-CU) targeted to children aged 3-to-6 years. As highlighted by Kimonis et al. (2019), critical milestones in moral development and emotion recognition primarily occur prior to age 6. Again, this intervention involves adjunctive components based on each of the three emerging themes of personalization presented here. Adjunctive components were aimed at promoting greater attachment security and modifying reinforcement procedures to accommodate for a punishment insensitive learning style. Additionally, the emotion-processing needs of children with CU traits were targeted with a Coaching and Rewarding Emotional Skills (CARES) adjunctive module. Using a single-group intervention design, Kimonis et al. (2019) found that the enhanced intervention was associated with reductions in conduct problems and CU traits, as well as improvements in empathy in the range of medium and large effect sizes post-treatment. Importantly, these changes were sustained at the 3-month follow-up assessment. While the sample was not screened for high-stable CU traits, or randomized to different treatment conditions, the results provide preliminary support for this targeted intervention.

19.6 Conclusions and Future Directions

In summary, an emerging body of clinical research has begun to investigate novel adaptations to current best-practice family interventions, with the aim of better addressing the cognitive-emotional deficits that characterize youth with CU traits. A strength of this work has been an emphasis on theory-driven design, with these adaptations based largely on the translation of current developmental models of risk pathways toward antisocial behavior and psychopathy. To date, this research has provided little evidence that adaptations to reinforcement procedures alone are likely to enhance the treatment gains of these young people. On the other hand, the most rigorous research to examine such adaptations has provided support for the combination of PMT and emotion recognition training (ERT) (Dadds et al., 2012). Questions regarding the change mechanisms in this intervention nonetheless need to be answered, including those related to the role of child-focused cognitive remediation versus emotion-related processes in the parent-child relationship.

Moreover, apparent mixed findings from recent research has highlighted further considerations for such research (e.g., developmental timing of treatment delivery; sampling of children based on severity versus stability of CU traits). Future research would benefit from an agenda that reflects consensus in the field regarding these questions and issues.

Clearly more clinical research is needed given the paucity of evidence for optimizing treatment outcomes in this population. For instance, no studies to our knowledge have yet evaluated whether components improving empathy by targeting the youth's ability for affective perspective-taking can optimize outcomes. Additionally, we note that greater methodological rigor in clinical research will be required to adequately evaluate adapted versions of established interventions. The gold standard method for evaluating whether adjunctive components enhance treatment outcomes is the randomized control trial (RCTs), however, the use of such a design in research investigating adapted interventions for youth with CU traits has been particularly limited (e.g., Dadds et al., 2012, 2019). Thus, future RCT research is need in which adapted treatments are pitted against standard family-based programs to examine the incremental benefits of modifying such programs. The use of RCT designs to test putative change mechanisms also stands to elucidate the ingredients necessary for achieving optimal outcomes for subgroups of antisocial youth such as those with CU traits (Kazdin, 2007, 2009). Trials that incorporate long-term follow-up and the assessment of adaptive changes in behavior and brain circuitry would be particularly valuable (Anderson & Kiehl, 2014; Caldwell et al., 2012).

It is likely that future progress in adapting family-based intervention for youth with CU traits will be reliant on further advances in models of the risk processes that drive the development of CU traits and related conduct problems. A recent review of the literature highlighted that significant gaps remain in such models (Viding & Kimonis, 2018). Trajectories towards psychopathy are likely characterized by interactions across multiple systems leading to multiplicative risk processes toward atypical neurodevelopment. Recognition of the potential for parenting behaviors and attachment systems to influence the emergence and maintenance of CU traits in low- versus high-trait anxiety children is one example of multilevel processes that may be important to incorporate into future treatment planning (e.g., Pardini et al., 2007). Kimonis and colleagues have shown variants of psychopathic traits based on differences in anxious/emotional responding and maltreatment histories appear to be associated with distinct etiological pathways to psychopathy (Kimonis et al., 2012, 2017). Thus, research mapping family-based mechanisms (e.g., parenting practices, attachment) onto psychopathy variants and treatment outcomes may be particularly fruitful.

Finally, future advances in this field may come from work investigating synergies between behavioral and biochemical interventions ('biobehavioural treatments'; Dadds & Rhodes, 2008). A potential candidate for such purposes is neuropeptide oxytocin, which researchers have proposed may aid affiliative bonding and remediate emotional attentional deficits in clinical populations (Domes et al., 2007). While clinical research on biobehavioral treatments for youth with CU traits has yet to be published, intervention research in children with autism has provided some preliminary data to suggest that intranasal oxytocin can improve emotion recognition during an emotion processing task (Guastella et al., 2015). Given that the type of social, emotional, and empathic difficulties exhibited by children with autism share similar phenomenology to those associated with CU traits (Hawes et al., 2013), future research investigating similar approaches for youth with CU traits would appear justified. Such approaches may target key oxytocin systems contributing to dysfunction associated with poor attention to and recognition of emotions, as well as deficiencies in affiliative/prosocial behavior (e.g., Cecil et al., 2014; Dadds et al., 2014).

As presented in this chapter, evidence supports adapting established family-based interventions for antisocial behavior to better meet the needs of youth with CU traits, and clinical work based on this aim should be informed by the broader science of personalizing interventions that has emerged in recent years. Our review has highlighted three key themes concerning progress in theory-driven adaptations of this kind related to (i) the expansion and modification of evidence-based reinforcement components, (ii) the formulation of emotion-related treatment targets in the parent-child relationship, and (iii) the role of youth-focused components targeting deficits in emotion processing and social cognition. An agenda for future research based on these themes is well worth pursuing and may play an important role in shifting clinical views about psychopathy from those of pessimism to those of hope.

References

Alexander, J. F. (1973). Defensive and supportive communications in normal and deviant families. *Journal of Consulting and Clinical Psychology, 40*(2), 223–231.

Alexander, J. F., & Barton, C. (1995). Family therapy research. In R. H. Mikesell, D.-D. Lusterman, & S. H. McDaniel (Eds.), *Integrating family therapy: Handbook of family psychology and systems theory* (pp. 199–215). American Psychological Association.

Alexander, J. F., & Parsons, B. V. (1982). *Functional family therapy*. Brooks/Cole Publishing Company.

Alexander, J. F., & Robbins, M. S. (2011). Functional family therapy. In *Clinical handbook of assessing and treating conduct problems in youth* (pp. 245–271). Springer.

Alexander, J. F., & Sexton, T. L. (2002). Functional family therapy: A model for treating high-risk, acting-out youth. In *Comprehensive handbook of psychotherapy: Integrative/Eclectic* (Vol. 4, pp. 111–132). Wiley.

Anastassiou-Hadjicharalambous, X., & Warden, D. (2008). Physiologically-indexed and self-perceived affective empathy in conduct-disordered children high and low on callous-unemotional traits. *Child Psychiatry and Human Development, 39*(4), 503–517.

Anderson, N. E., & Kiehl, K. A. (2014). Psychopathy: Developmental perspectives and their implications for treatment. *Restorative Neurology and Neuroscience, 32*(1), 103–117.

Bandura, A. (1977). Self-efficacy: Toward a unifying theory of behavioral change. *Psychological Review, 84*(2), 191–215.

Baron-Cohen, S., Golan, O., Wheelwright, S., & Hill, J. J. (2004). *Mind reading: The inter- active guide to emotions*. Jessica Kingsley Limited.

Bayliss, C. M., Miller, A. K., & Henderson, C. E. (2010). Psychopathy development and implications for early intervention. *Journal of Cognitive Psychotherapy, 24*(2), 71–80.

Beauchaine, T. P., Webster-Stratton, C., & Reid, M. J. (2005). Mediators, moderators, and predictors of 1-year outcomes among children treated for early-onset conduct problems: A latent growth curve analysis. *Journal of Consulting and Clinical Psychology, 73*(3), 371–388.

Blair, R. J. R. (2005). Responding to the emotions of others: Dissociating forms of empathy through the study of typical and psychiatric populations. *Consciousness and Cognition, 14*(4), 698–718.

Blair, R. J. R. (2008a). Fine cuts of empathy and the amygdala: Dissociable deficits in psychopathy and autism. *The Quarterly Journal of Experimental Psychology, 61*(1), 157–170.

Blair, R. J. R. (2008b). The amygdala and ventromedial prefrontal cortex: Functional contributions and dysfunction in psychopathy. *Philosophical Transactions of the Royal Society of London B: Biological Sciences, 363*(1503), 2557–2565.

Blair, R. J. R., & Mitchell, D. G. V. (2009). Psychopathy, attention and emotion. *Psychological Medicine, 39*(4), 543–555.

Blair, R. J. R., Colledge, E., & Mitchell, D. G. V. (2001). Somatic markers and response reversal: Is there orbitofrontal cortex dysfunction in boys with psychopathic tendencies? *Journal of Abnormal Child Psychology, 29*(6), 499–511.

Borduin, C. M., Henggeler, S. W., Blaske, D. M., & Stein, R. J. (1990). Multisystemic treatment of adolescent sexual offenders. *International Journal of Offender Therapy and Comparative Criminology, 34*(2), 105–113.

Brestan, E. V., & Eyberg, S. M. (1998). Effective psychosocial treatments of conduct-disordered children and adolescents: 29 years, 82 studies, and 5,272 kids. *Journal of Clinical Child Psychology, 27*(2), 180–189. https://doi.org/10.1207/s15374424jccp2702_5

Brinkmeyer, M. Y., & Eyberg, S. M. (2003). Parent-child interaction therapy for oppositional children. In A. E. Kazdin & J. R. Weisz (Eds.), *Evidence-based psychotherapies for children and adolescents* (pp. 204–223). Guilford Press.

Butler, S., Baruch, G., Hickey, N., & Fonagy, P. (2011). A randomized controlled trial of multisystemic therapy and a statutory therapeutic intervention for young offenders. *Journal of the American Academy of Child & Adolescent Psychiatry, 50*(12), 1220–1235.

Byrd, A. L., Hawes, S. W., Burke, J. D., Loeber, R., & Pardini, D. A. (2018). Boys with conduct problems and callous-unemotional traits: Neural response to reward and punishment and associations with treatment response. *Developmental Cognitive Neuroscience, 30*, 51–59.

Caldwell, M. F., McCormick, D., Wolfe, J., & Umstead, D. (2012). Treatment-related changes in psychopathy features and behavior in adolescent offenders. *Criminal Justice and Behavior, 39*(2), 144–155.

Cecil, C. A. M., Lysenko, L. J., Jaffee, S. R., Pingault, J.-B., Smith, R. G., Relton, C. L., Woodward, G., McArdle, W., Mill, J., & Barker, E. D. (2014). Environmental risk, oxytocin receptor gene (OXTR) methylation and youth callous-unemotional traits: A 13-year longitudinal study. *Molecular Psychiatry, 19*(10), 1071–1077.

Comer, J. S., Chow, C., Chan, P. T., Cooper-Vince, C., & Wilson, L. A. S. (2013). Psychosocial treatment efficacy for disruptive behavior problems in very young children: A meta-analytic examination. *Journal of the American Academy of Child & Adolescent Psychiatry, 52*(1), 26–36.

Dadds, M. R., & Hawes, D. J. (2006). *Integrated family intervention for child conduct problems: A behaviour-attachment-systems intervention for parents*. Australian Academic Press.

Dadds, M. R., & Rhodes, T. (2008). Aggression in young children with concurrent callous–unemotional traits: Can the neurosciences inform progress and innovation in treatment approaches? *Philosophical Transactions of the Royal Society B: Biological Sciences, 363*(1503), 2567–2576.

Dadds, M. R., & Salmon, K. (2003). Punishment insensitivity and parenting: Temperament and learning as interacting risks for antisocial behavior. *Clinical Child and Family Psychology Review, 6*(2), 69–86.

Dadds, M. R., & Tully, L. A. (2019). What is it to discipline a child: What should it be? A reanalysis of time-out from the perspective of child mental health, attachment, and trauma. *American Psychologist, 74*, 794–808.

Dadds, M. R., Mullins, M. J., McAllister, R. A., & Atkinson, E. (2003). Attributions, affect, and behavior in abuse-risk mothers: A laboratory study. *Child Abuse & Neglect, 27*(1), 21–45.

Dadds, M. R., Perry, Y., Hawes, D. J., Merz, S., Riddell, A. C., Haines, D. J., … Abeygunawardane, A. I. (2006). Attention to the eyes and fear-recognition deficits in child psychopathy. *The British Journal of Psychiatry, 189*(3), 280–281. Retrieved from http://bjp.rcpsych.org/content/bjprcpsych/189/3/280.full.pdf

Dadds, M. R., El Masry, Y., Wimalaweera, S., & Guastella, A. J. (2008). Reduced eye gaze explains "fear blindness" in childhood psychopathic traits. *Journal of the American Academy of Child & Adolescent Psychiatry, 47*(4), 455–463.

Dadds, M. R., Hawes, D. J., Frost, A. D. J., Vassallo, S., Bunn, P., Hunter, K., & Merz, S. (2009). Learning to 'talk the talk': The relationship of psychopathic traits to deficits in empathy across childhood. *Journal of Child Psychology and Psychiatry, 50*(5), 599–606. Retrieved from https://doi.org/10.1111/j.1469-7610.2008.02058.x.

Dadds, M. R., Jambrak, J., Pasalich, D., Hawes, D. J., & Brennan, J. (2011). Impaired attention to the eyes of attachment figures and the developmental origins of psychopathy. *Journal of Child Psychology and Psychiatry, 52*(3), 238–245.

Dadds, M. R., Cauchi, A. J., Wimalaweera, S., Hawes, D. J., & Brennan, J. (2012). Outcomes, moderators, and mediators of empathic-emotion recognition training for complex conduct problems in childhood. *Psychiatry Research, 199*(3), 201–207.

Dadds, M. R., Allen, J. L., McGregor, K., Woolgar, M., Viding, E., & Scott, S. (2014). Callous-unemotional traits in children and mechanisms of impaired eye contact during expressions of love: A treatment target? *Journal of Child Psychology and Psychiatry, 55*(7), 771–780.

Dadds, M. R., English, T., Wimalaweera, S., Schollar-Root, O., & Hawes, D. J. (2019). Can reciprocated parent–child eye gaze and emotional engagement enhance treatment for children with conduct problems and callous-unemotional traits: A proof-of-concept trial. *Journal of Child Psychology and Psychiatry, 60*(6), 676–685.

Davidov, M., & Grusec, J. E. (2006). Untangling the links of parental responsiveness to distress and warmth to child outcomes. *Child Development, 77*(1), 44–58.

Dawel, A., O'Kearney, R., McKone, E., & Palermo, R. (2012). Not just fear and sadness: Meta-analytic evidence of pervasive emotion recognition deficits for facial and vocal expressions in psychopathy. *Neuroscience & Biobehavioral Reviews, 36*(10), 2288–2304.

De Brito, S. A., Mechelli, A., Wilke, M., Laurens, K. R., Jones, A. P., Barker, G. J., Hodgins, S., & Viding, E. (2009). Size matters: Increased grey matter in boys with conduct problems and callous–unemotional traits. *Brain, 132*(4), 843–852.

Dishion, T. J., & Patterson, G. R. (2006). The development and ecology of antisocial behavior in children and adolescents. In D. Cicchetti & D. J. Cohens (Eds.), *Developmental psychopathology, Vol 3: Risk disorder and adaptation*. Wiley.

Dishion, T., Forgatch, M., Chamberlain, P., & Pelham, W. E. (2016). The Oregon model of behavior family therapy: From intervention design to promoting large-scale system change. *Behavior Therapy, 47*(6), 812–837.

Domes, G., Heinrichs, M., Gläscher, J., Büchel, C., Braus, D. F., & Herpertz, S. C. (2007). Oxytocin attenuates amygdala responses to emotional faces regardless of valence. *Biological Psychiatry, 62*(10), 1187–1190.

Elizur, Y., Somech, L. Y., & Vinokur, A. D. (2017). Effects of parent training on callous-unemotional traits, effortful control, and conduct problems: Mediation by parenting. *Journal of Abnormal Child Psychology, 45*(1), 15–26.

Epstein, R., Fonnesbeck, C., Williamson, E., Kuhn, T., Lindegren, M. L., Rizzone, K., Krishnaswami, S., Sathe, N., Ficzere, C. H., Ness, G. L., Wright, G. W., Raj, M., Potter, S., & McPheeters, M. (2015). *Psychosocial and pharmacologic interventions for disruptive behavior in children and adolescents*. Rockville, Agency for Healthcare Research and Quality (US). Retrieved from Comparative Effectiveness Reviews website: https://www.ncbi.nlm.nih.gov/books/NBK327222/

Eyberg, S. M., Nelson, M. M., & Boggs, S. R. (2008). Evidence-based psychosocial treatments for children and adolescents with disruptive behavior. *Journal of Clinical Child & Adolescent Psychology, 37*(1), 215–237.

Feshbach, N. D. (1984). Empathy, empathy training and the regulation of aggression in elementary school children. In *Aggression in children and youth* (pp. 192–208). Springer.

Fonagy, P. (2003). Towards a developmental understanding of violence. *The British Journal of Psychiatry, 183*(3), 190–192.

Fonagy, P., Butler, S., Cottrell, D., Scott, S., Pilling, S., Eisler, I., Fuggle, P., Kraam, A., Byford, S., Wason, J., Ellison, R., Simes, E., Ganguli, P., Allison, E., & Goodyer, I. M. (2018). Multisystemic therapy versus management as usual in the treatment of adolescent antisocial behaviour (START): A pragmatic, randomised controlled, superiority trial. *The Lancet Psychiatry, 5*(2), 119–133.

Forgatch, M. S., & Patterson, G. R. (2010). Parent management training—Oregon model: An intervention for antisocial behavior in children and adolescents. In J. R. Weisz & A. E. Kazdin (Eds.), *Evidence-based psychotherapies for children and adolescents* (pp. 159–177). The Guilford Press.

Frick, P. J., & Viding, E. (2009). Antisocial behavior from a developmental psychopathology perspective. *Development and Psychopathology, 21*(4), 1111–1131.

Frick, P. J., & White, S. F. (2008). Research review: The importance of callous-unemotional traits for developmental models of aggressive and antisocial behavior. *Journal of Child Psychology and Psychiatry, 49*(4), 359–375.

Frick, P. J., Cornell, A. H., Barry, C. T., Bodin, S. D., & Dane, H. E. (2003). Callous-unemotional traits and conduct problems in the prediction of conduct problem severity, aggression, and self-report of delinquency. *Journal of Abnormal Child Psychology, 31*(4), 457–470. https://doi.org/10.1023/A:1023899703866

Frick, P. J., Ray, J. V., Thornton, L. C., & Kahn, R. E. (2014a). Annual research review: A developmental psychopathology approach to understanding callous-unemotional traits in children and adolescents with serious conduct problems. *Journal of Child Psychology and Psychiatry, 55*(6), 532–548.

Frick, P. J., Ray, J. V., Thornton, L. C., & Kahn, R. E. (2014b). Can callous-unemotional traits enhance the understanding, diagnosis, and treatment of serious conduct problems in children and adolescents? A comprehensive review. *Psychological Bulletin, 140*(1), 1–57.

Garland, A. F., Hawley, K. M., Brookman-Frazee, L., & Hurlburt, M. S. (2008). Identifying common elements of evidence-based psychosocial treatments for children's disruptive behavior problems. *Journal of the American Academy of Child & Adolescent Psychiatry, 47*(5), 505–514.

Greenberg, M. T., Speltz, M. L., & Deklyen, M. (1993). The role of attachment in the early development of disruptive behavior problems. *Development and Psychopathology, 5*(1–2), 191–213.

Griest, D. L., & Forehand, R. (1983). How can I get any parent training done with all these other problems going on? The role of family variables in child behavioral therapy. *Child & Family Behavior Therapy, 4*(1), 73–80.

Guastella, A. J., Gray, K. M., Rinehart, N. J., Alvares, G. A., Tonge, B. J., Hickie, I. B., Keating, C. M., Cacciotti-Saija, C., & Einfeld, S. L. (2015). The effects of a course of intranasal oxytocin on social behaviors in youth diagnosed with autism spectrum disorders: A randomized controlled trial. *Journal of Child Psychology and Psychiatry, 56*(4), 444–452.

Haas, S. M., Waschbusch, D. A., Pelham, W. E., King, S., Andrade, B. F., & Carrey, N. J. (2011). Treatment response in CP/ADHD children with callous/unemotional traits. *Journal of Abnormal Child Psychology, 39*(4), 541–552.

Hare, R. D. (1993). *Without conscience: The disturbing world of the psychopaths among us*. The Guildford Press. New York: Pocket Books.

Hawes, D. J., & Dadds, M. R. (2005). The treatment of conduct problems in children with callous-unemotional traits. *Journal of Consulting and Clinical Psychology, 73*(4), 737.

Hawes, D. J., & Dadds, M. R. (2007). Stability and malleability of callous-unemotional traits during treatment for childhood conduct problems. *Journal of Clinical Child and Adolescent Psychology, 36*(3), 347–355.

Hawes, D. J., Dadds, M. R., Brennan, J., Rhodes, T., & Cauchi, A. (2013). Revisiting the treatment of conduct problems in children with callous-unemotional traits. *Australian & New Zealand Journal of Psychiatry, 47*(7), 646–653.

Hawes, D. J., Price, M. J., & Dadds, M. R. (2014). Callous-unemotional traits and the treatment of conduct problems in childhood and adolescence: A comprehensive review. *Clinical Child and Family Psychology Review, 17*(3), 248–267. https://doi.org/10.1007/s10567-014-0167-1

Henggeler, S. W., Rodick, J. D., Borduin, C. M., Hanson, C. L., Watson, S. M., & Urey, J. R. (1986). Multisystemic treatment of juvenile offenders: Effects on adolescent behavior and family interaction. *Developmental Psychology, 22*(1), 132–141.

Henggeler, S. W., Melton, G. B., & Smith, L. A. (1992). Family preservation using multisystemic therapy: An effective alternative to incarcerating serious juvenile offenders. *Journal of Consulting and Clinical Psychology, 60*(6), 953–961.

Henggeler, S. W., Clingempeel, W. G., Brondino, M. J., & Pickrel, S. G. (2002). Four-year follow-up of multisystemic therapy with substance-abusing and substance-dependent juvenile offenders. *Journal of the American Academy of Child & Adolescent Psychiatry, 41*(7), 868–874.

Henggeler, S. W., Schoenwald, S. K., Borduin, C. M., Rowland, M. D., & Cunningham, P. B. (2009). *Multisystemic therapy for antisocial behavior in children and adolescents*. Guilford Press.

Hoffman, M. L. (1994). The contribution of empathy to justice and moral judgment. *Reaching Out: Caring, Altruism, and Prosocial Behavior, 7*, 161–194.

Huey, S. J., Henggeler, S. W., Brondino, M. J., & Pickrel, S. G. (2000). Mechanisms of change in multisystemic therapy: Reducing delinquent behavior through therapist adherence and improved family and peer functioning. *Journal of Consulting and Clinical Psychology, 68*(3), 451–467.

Insel, T., Cuthbert, B., Garvey, M., Heinssen, R., Pine, D. S., Quinn, K., Sanislow, C., & Wang, P. (2010). Research domain criteria (RDoC): Toward a new classification framework for research on mental disorders. *The American Journal of Psychiatry, 167*(7), 748–751.

Jones, A. P., Laurens, K. R., Herba, C. M., Barker, G. J., & Viding, E. (2009). Amygdala hypoactivity to fearful faces in boys with conduct problems and callous-unemotional traits. *American Journal of Psychiatry, 166*(1), 95–102.

Jones, A. P., Happé, F. G. E., Gilbert, F., Burnett, S., & Viding, E. (2010). Feeling, caring, knowing: Different types of empathy deficit in boys with psychopathic tendencies and autism spectrum disorder. *Journal of Child Psychology and Psychiatry, 51*(11), 1188–1197.

Kaminski, J. W., & Claussen, A. H. (2017). Evidence base update for psychosocial treatments for disruptive behaviors in children. *Journal of Clinical Child & Adolescent Psychology, 46*(4), 477–499. https://doi.org/10.1080/15374416.2017.1310044

Kazdin, A. E. (1997). Practitioner review: Psychosocial treatments for conduct disorder in children. *Journal of Child Psychology and Psychiatry, 38*(2), 161–178.

Kazdin, A. E. (2003). Problem-solving skills training and parent management training for conduct disorder. In A. E. Kazdin & J. R. Weisz (Eds.), *Evidence-based psychotherapies for children and adolescents* (pp. 241–262). The Guilford Press.

Kazdin, A. E. (2007). Mediators and mechanisms of change in psychotherapy research. *Annual Review of Clinical Psychology, 3*, 1–27.

Kazdin, A. E. (2009). Understanding how and why psychotherapy leads to change. *Psychotherapy Research, 19*(4–5), 418–428.

Kennedy, E. M. M., French, L., & Roberts, C. (2017). Personalised interventions for subgroups of children with conduct problems. *The Cochrane Database of Systematic Reviews, 2017*(8), CD012746.

Kiehl, K. A. (2006). A cognitive neuroscience perspective on psychopathy: Evidence for paralimbic system dysfunction. *Psychiatry Research, 142*(2–3), 107–128.

Kimonis, E. R., Frick, P. J., Fazekas, H., & Loney, B. R. (2006). Psychopathy, aggression, and the processing of emotional stimuli in non-referred girls and boys. *Behavioral Sciences & the Law, 24*(1), 21–37.

Kimonis, E. R., Frick, P. J., Cauffman, E., Goldweber, A., & Skeem, J. (2012). Primary and secondary variants of juvenile psychopathy differ in emotional processing. *Development and Psychopathology, 24*(3), 1091–1103.

Kimonis, E. R., Fanti, K. A., Goulter, N., & Hall, J. (2017). Affective startle potentiation differentiates primary and secondary variants of juvenile psychopathy. *Development and Psychopathology, 29*(4), 1149–1160.

Kimonis, E. R., Fleming, G., Briggs, N., Brouwer-French, L., Frick, P. J., Hawes, D. J., Bagner, D. M., Thomas, R., & Dadds, M. (2019). Parent-child interaction therapy adapted for preschoolers with callous-unemotional traits: An open trial pilot study. *Journal of Clinical Child & Adolescent Psychology, 48*(sup1), S347–S361.

Kochanska, G. (1997). Multiple pathways to conscience for children with different temperaments: From toddlerhood to age 5. *Developmental Psychology, 33*(2), 228–240.

Kochanska, G., Kim, S., Boldt, L. J., & Yoon, J. E. (2013). Children's callous-unemotional traits moderate links between their positive relationships with parents at preschool age and externalizing behavior problems at early school age. *Journal of Child Psychology and Psychiatry, 54*(11), 1251–1260.

Kolko, D. J., Dorn, L. D., Bukstein, O. G., Pardini, D., Holden, E. A., & Hart, J. (2009). Community vs. clinic-based modular treatment of children with early-onset ODD or CD: A clinical trial with 3-year follow-up. *Journal of Abnormal Child Psychology, 37*(5), 591–609.

Kroneman, L. M., Hipwell, A. E., Loeber, R., Koot, H. M., & Pardini, D. A. (2011). Contextual risk factors as predictors of disruptive behavior disorder trajectories in girls: The moderating effect of callous-unemotional features. *Journal of Child Psychology and Psychiatry, 52*(2), 167–175.

Larsson, H., Viding, E., & Plomin, R. (2008). Callous—Unemotional traits and antisocial behavior: Genetic, environmental, and early parenting characteristics. *Criminal Justice and Behavior, 35*(2), 197–211.

Lewis, M. D. (2000). The promise of dynamic systems approaches for an integrated account of human development. *Child Development, 71*(1), 36–43.

Loney, B. R., Butler, M. A., Lima, E. N., Counts, C. A., & Eckel, L. A. (2006). The relation between salivary cortisol, callous-unemotional traits, and conduct problems in an adolescent non-referred sample. *Journal of Child Psychology and Psychiatry, 47*(1), 30–36.

Lui, J. H. L., Barry, C. T., & Sacco, D. F. (2016). Callous-unemotional traits and empathy deficits: Mediating effects of affective perspective-taking and facial emotion recognition. *Cognition and Emotion, 30*(6), 1049–1062.

Lundahl, B., Risser, H. J., & Lovejoy, M. C. (2006). A meta-analysis of parent training: Moderators and follow-up effects. *Clinical Psychology Review, 26*(1), 86–104. Retrieved from http://ac.els-cdn.com/S0272735805001169/1-s2.0-S0272735805001169-main.pdf?_tid=12c9dac6-f3ec-11e6-ae07-00000aacb35f&acdnat=1487210773_561238a647184f485d67351f502d132e

Lynam, D. R. (1998). Early identification of the fledgling psychopath: Locating the psychopathic child in the current nomenclature. *Journal of Abnormal Psychology, 107*(4), 566. Retrieved from http://ovidsp.tx.ovid.com/ovftpdfs/FPDDNCGCMHCJEL00/fs046/ovft/live/gv023/00004468/00004468-199811000-00003.pdf

Manders, W. A., Deković, M., Asscher, J. J., van der Laan, P. H., & Prins, P. J. M. (2013). Psychopathy as predictor and moderator of multisystemic therapy outcomes among adolescents treated for antisocial behavior. *Journal of Abnormal Child Psychology, 41*(7), 1121–1132.

Marsh, A. A., & Blair, R. J. R. (2008). Deficits in facial affect recognition among antisocial populations: A meta-analysis. *Neuroscience & Biobehavioral Reviews, 32*(3), 454–465.

Maughan, D. R., Christiansen, E., Jenson, W. R., Olympia, D., & Clark, E. (2005). Behavioral parent training as a treatment for externalizing behaviors and disruptive behavior disorders: A meta-analysis. *School Psychology Review, 34*(3), 267–286.

McDonald, R., Dodson, M. C., Rosenfield, D., & Jouriles, E. N. (2011). Effects of a parenting intervention on features of psychopathy in children. *Journal of Abnormal Child Psychology, 39*(7), 1013–1023.

McMahon, R. J., & Forehand, R. (2003). *Helping the noncompliant child: A clinician's guide to effective parent training*. Guilford.

McNeil, C. B., & Hembree-Kigin, T. L. (2010). *Parent-child interaction therapy*. Springer Science & Business Media.

Michelson, D., Davenport, C., Dretzke, J., Barlow, J., & Day, C. (2013). Do evidence-based interventions work when tested in the "real world?" A systematic review and meta-analysis of parent management training for the treatment of child disruptive behavior. *Clinical Child and Family Psychology Review, 16*(1), 18–34.

Miller, N. V., Haas, S. M., Waschbusch, D. A., Willoughby, M. T., Helseth, S. A., Crum, K. I., Coles, E. K., & Pelham, W. E., Jr. (2014). Behavior therapy and callous-unemotional traits: Effects of a pilot study examining modified behavioral contingencies on child behavior. *Behavior Therapy, 45*(5), 606–618.

Mingebach, T., Kamp-Becker, I., Christiansen, H., & Weber, L. (2018). Meta-meta-analysis on the effectiveness of parent-based interventions for the treatment of child externalizing behavior problems. *PLoS One, 13*(9), e0202855.

Minuchin, S. (1967). *Families of the slums: An exploration of their structure and treatment*. Basic Books.

Muñoz, L. C. (2009). Callous-unemotional traits are related to combined deficits in recognizing afraid faces and body poses. *Journal of the American Academy of Child & Adolescent Psychiatry, 48*(5), 554–562.

National Research Council. (2011). *Toward precision medicine: Building a knowledge network for biomedical research and a new taxonomy of disease*. National Academies Press.

Ng, M. Y., & Weisz, J. R. (2016). Annual research review: Building a science of personalized intervention for youth mental health. *Journal of Child Psychology and Psychiatry, 57*(3), 216–236.

NHS. (2015). *The matrix (2015) a guide to delivering evidence-based psychological therapies in Scotland*. NHS.

O'Connor, T. G., Humayun, S., Briskman, J. A., & Scott, S. (2016). Sensitivity to parenting in adolescents with callous/unemotional traits: Observational and experimental findings. *Journal of Abnormal Psychology, 125*(4), 502–513.

O'Kearney, R., Salmon, K., Liwag, M., Fortune, C.-A., & Dawel, A. (2017). Emotional abilities in children with oppositional defiant disorder (ODD): Impairments in perspective-taking and understanding mixed emotions are associated with high callous–unemotional traits. *Child Psychiatry & Human Development, 48*(2), 346–357.

Ortiz, C., Hawes, D. J., Lorber, M., Lazer, S., & Brotman, L. M. (2018). Are callous-unemotional traits associated with differential response to reward versus punishment components of parent-training? A randomized trial. *Evidence-Based Practice in Child and Adolescent Mental Health, 3*(3), 164–177.

Oxford, M., Cavell, T. A., & Hughes, J. N. (2003). Callous/unemotional traits moderate the relation between ineffective parenting and child externalizing problems: A partial replication and extension. *Journal of Clinical Child and Adolescent Psychology, 32*(4), 577–585.

Pardini, D. A., Lochman, J. E., & Powell, N. (2007). The development of callous-unemotional traits and antisocial behavior in children: Are there shared and/or unique predictors? *Journal of Clinical Child and Adolescent Psychology, 36*(3), 319–333.

Pasalich, D. S., Dadds, M. R., Hawes, D. J., & Brennan, J. (2011). Do callous-unemotional traits moderate the relative importance of parental coercion versus warmth in child conduct problems? An observational study. *Journal of Child Psychology and Psychiatry, 52*(12), 1308–1315.

Pasalich, D. S., Dadds, M. R., Hawes, D. J., & Brennan, J. (2012). Attachment and callous-unemotional traits in children with early-onset conduct problems. *Journal of Child Psychology and Psychiatry, 53*(8), 838–845.

Pasalich, D. S., Dadds, M. R., & Hawes, D. J. (2014). Cognitive and affective empathy in children with conduct problems: Additive and interactive effects of callous–unemotional traits and autism spectrum disorders symptoms. *Psychiatry Research, 219*(3), 625–630.

Pasalich, D. S., Witkiewitz, K., McMahon, R. J., Pinderhughes, E. E., & Group, C. P. P. R. (2016). Indirect effects of the Fast Track intervention on conduct disorder symptoms and callous-unemotional traits: Distinct pathways involving discipline and warmth. *Journal of Abnormal Child Psychology, 44*(3), 587–597.

Patterson, G. R. (1982). *Coercive family process* (Vol. 3). Castalia Publishing Company.

Patterson, G. R., Reid, J. B., & Eddy, J. M. (2002). A brief history of the Oregon model. In J. B. Reid, G. R. Patterson, & J. Snyder (Eds.), *Antisocial behavior in children and adolescents: A developmental analysis and model for intervention* (pp. 3–20). American Psychological Association.

Salekin, R. T., & Lochman, J. E. (2008). Child and adolescent psychopathy: The search for protective factors. *Criminal Justice and Behavior, 35*(2), 159–172.

Salekin, R. T., Worley, C., & Grimes, R. D. (2010). Treatment of psychopathy: A review and brief introduction to the mental model mpproach for psychopathy. *Behavioral Sciences & the Law, 28*(2), 235–266.

Salihovic, S., Kerr, M., Özdemir, M., & Pakalniskiene, V. (2012). Directions of effects between adolescent psychopathic traits and parental behavior. *Journal of Abnormal Child Psychology, 40*(6), 957–969.

Sanders, M. R. (2012). Development, evaluation, and multinational dissemination of the triple P-positive parenting program. *Annual Review of Clinical Psychology, 8*, 345–379.

Sanders, M. R., Baker, S., & Turner, K. M. T. (2012). A randomized controlled trial evaluating the efficacy of triple P online with parents of children with early-onset conduct problems. *Behaviour Research and Therapy, 50*(11), 675–684.

Sanders, M. R., Kirby, J. N., Tellegen, C. L., & Day, J. J. (2014). The triple P-positive parenting program: A systematic review and meta-analysis of a multi-level system of parenting support. *Clinical Psychology Review, 34*(4), 337–357.

Särndal, C.-E., Swensson, B., & Wretman, J. (2003). *Model assisted survey sampling*. Springer.

Schwenck, C., Mergenthaler, J., Keller, K., Zech, J., Salehi, S., Taurines, R., Romanos, M., Schecklmann, M., Schneider, W., Warnke, A., & Freitag, C. M. (2012). Empathy in children with autism and conduct disorder: Group-specific profiles and developmental aspects. *Journal of Child Psychology and Psychiatry, 53*(6), 651–659.

Scott, S., & Dadds, M. R. (2009). Practitioner review: When parent training doesn't work: Theory-driven clinical strategies. *Journal of Child Psychology and Psychiatry, 50*(12), 1441–1450. https://doi.org/10.1111/j.1469-7610.2009.02161.x

Sebastian, C. L., De Brito, S. A., McCrory, E. J., Hyde, Z. H., Lockwood, P. L., Cecil, C. A. M., & Viding, E. (2016). Grey matter volumes in children with conduct problems and varying levels of callous-unemotional traits. *Journal of Abnormal Child Psychology, 44*(4), 639–649.

Serketich, W. J., & Dumas, J. E. (1996). The effectiveness of behavioral parent training to modify antisocial behavior in children: A meta-analysis. *Behavior Therapy, 27*(2), 171–186.

Sexton, T. L., & Alexander, J. F. (1999). *Functional family therapy: Principles of clinical intervention, assessment, and implementation*. RCH Enterprises.

Sexton, T. L., & Alexander, J. F. (2003). Functional family therapy: A mature clinical model for working with at-risk adolescents and their families. In T. L. Sexton, G. R. Weeks, & M. S. Robbins (Eds.), *Handbook of family therapy: The science and practice of working with families and couples* (pp. 323–348). Brunner-Routledge.

Sexton, T., & Turner, C. W. (2010). The effectiveness of functional family therapy for youth with behavioral problems in a community practice setting. *Journal of Family Psychology, 24*(3), 339–348.

Slep, A. M. S., & O'Leary, S. G. (1998). The effects of maternal attributions on parenting: An experimental analysis. *Journal of Family Psychology, 12*(2), 234–243.

Slifer, K. J., & Amari, A. (2009). Behavior management for children and adolescents with acquired brain injury. *Developmental Disabilities Research Reviews, 15*(2), 144–151.

Somech, L. Y., & Elizur, Y. (2012). Promoting self-regulation and cooperation in pre-kindergarten children with conduct problems: A randomized controlled trial. *Journal of the American Academy of Child & Adolescent Psychiatry, 51*(4), 412–422.

Sonuga-Barke, E. J., Schlotz, W., & Kreppner, J. (2010). Differentiating developmental trajectories for conduct, emotion, and peer problems following early deprivation. *Monographs of the Society for Research in Child Development, 75*(1), 102–124.

Stevens, D., Charman, T., & Blair, R. J. R. (2001). Recognition of emotion in facial expressions and vocal tones in children with psychopathic tendencies. *The Journal of Genetic Psychology, 162*(2), 201–211.

Viding, E., & Kimonis, E. R. (2018). Callous–unemotional traits. In C. J. Patrick (Ed.), *Handbook of psychopathy* (2nd ed., pp. 144–164). The Guilford Press.

Viding, E., Blair, R. J. R., Moffitt, T. E., & Plomin, R. (2005). Evidence for substantial genetic risk for psychopathy in 7-year-olds. *Journal of Child Psychology and Psychiatry, 46*(6), 592–597.

Waller, R., & Hyde, L. W. (2018). Callous-unemotional behaviors in early childhood: The development of empathy and prosociality gone awry. *Current Opinion in Psychology, 20*, 11–16.

Waller, R., Gardner, F., & Hyde, L. W. (2013). What are the associations between parenting, callous–unemotional traits, and antisocial behavior in youth? A systematic review of evidence. *Clinical Psychology Review, 33*(4), 593–608.

Waller, R., Gardner, F., Viding, E., Shaw, D. S., Dishion, T. J., Wilson, M. N., & Hyde, L. W. (2014). Bidirectional associations between parental warmth, callous unemotional behavior, and behavior problems in high-risk preschoolers. *Journal of Abnormal Child Psychology, 42*(8), 1275–1285.

Waschbusch, D. A., Willoughby, M. T., Haas, S. M., Ridenour, T., Helseth, S., Crum, K. I., Altszuler, A. R., Ross, J. M., Coles, E. K., & Pelham, W. E. (2020). Effects of behavioral treatment modified to fit children with conduct problems and callous-unemotional (CU) traits. *Journal of Clinical Child & Adolescent Psychology, 49*(5), 639–650.

Webster-Stratton, C., & Reid, M. J. (2003). The incredible years parents, teachers and children training series: A multifaceted treatment approach for young children with conduct problems. In A. E. Kazdin & J. R. Weisz (Eds.), *Evidence-based psychotherapies for children and adolescents* (pp. 224–240). Guilford Press.

Webster-Stratton, C., Rinaldi, J., & Reid, J. M. (2011). Long-term outcomes of incredible years parenting program: Predictors of adolescent adjustment. *Child and Adolescent Mental Health, 16*(1), 38–46. https://doi.org/10.1111/j.1475-3588.2010.00576.x

Wilkinson, S., Waller, R., & Viding, E. (2016). Practitioner review: Involving young people with callous unemotional traits in treatment–does it work? A systematic review. *Journal of Child Psychology and Psychiatry, 57*(5), 552–565.

Willoughby, M. T., Mills-Koonce, R., Propper, C. B., & Waschbusch, D. A. (2013). Observed parenting behaviors interact with a polymorphism of the brain-derived neurotrophic factor gene to predict the emergence of oppositional defiant and callous–unemotional behaviors at age 3 years. *Development and Psychopathology, 25*(4pt1), 903–917.

Wootton, J. M., Frick, P. J., Shelton, K. K., & Silverthorn, P. (1997). Ineffective parenting and childhood conduct problems: The moderating role of callous-unemotional traits. *Journal of Consulting and Clinical Psychology, 65*(2), 301–308. Retrieved from http://graphics.tx.ovid.com/ovftpdfs/FPDDNCIBADIBJG00/fs046/ovft/live/gv023/00004730/00004730-199704000-00012.pdf

Wright, M. F., Wachs, S., & Harper, B. D. (2018). The moderation of empathy in the longitudinal association between witnessing cyberbullying, depression, and anxiety. *Cyberpsychology: Journal of Psychosocial Research on Cyberspace, 12*(4), 6.

Ylvisaker, M., Turkstra, L. S., & Coelho, C. (2005). Behavioral and social interventions for individuals with traumatic brain injury: A summary of the research with clinical implications. *Seminars in Speech and Language, 26*(04), 256–267.

Zhou, Q., Eisenberg, N., Losoya, S. H., Fabes, R. A., Reiser, M., Guthrie, I. K., Murphy, B. C., Cumberland, A. J., & Shepard, S. A. (2002). The relations of parental warmth and positive expressiveness to children's empathy-related responding and social functioning: A longitudinal study. *Child Development, 73*(3), 893–915.

Chapter 20
Neuropsychological Considerations in Psychopathy

Katy Drorit Gaines

Abstract Psychopathy is considered a serious mental health syndrome. Comprehensive scientific examination is necessary in the understanding, classification, and treatment of psychopathy. Neuropsychology as a field has provided theoretical explanations for psychopathy and neuropsychological assessments are highly instrumental in providing a neuropsychological profile consistent with psychopathy. This chapter will provide an overview of neuroscientific findings related to the mental health understanding of psychopathy and how these contributions have impacted the neuropsychological assessment of the syndrome.

Keywords Neuropsychology · Psychopathy · Assessment · Emotion · PCL-R · Legal considerations

20.1 Introduction

Psychopathy is considered a serious mental health syndrome. Comprehensive scientific examination is necessary in the understanding, classification, and treatment of psychopathy. Neuropsychology as a field has provided theoretical explanations for psychopathy and neuropsychological assessments are highly instrumental in providing a neuropsychological profile consistent with psychopathy. This chapter will provide an overview of neuroscientific findings related to the mental health understanding of psychopathy and how these contributions have impacted the neuropsychological assessment of the syndrome.

K. D. Gaines (✉)
Neuro Health, Inc., Beverly Hills, CA, USA
e-mail: drgaines@neurohealthmed.com

J. E. Vitale (ed.), *The Complexity of Psychopathy*, Dangerous Behavior in Clinical and Forensic Psychology, https://doi.org/10.1007/978-3-030-83156-1_20

20.1.1 Neuropsychological Assessments

Comprehensive neuropsychological assessments are designed to evaluate a wide range of human functions - thought, behavior, emotion, and cognition. Those aspects break down into sub-functions that occur as neurological processes take place neurochemically and metabolically in neuropathways that connect various regions of the brain. Through assessments, these sub-functions are identified and described, bringing about a full picture of the person's thoughts, behaviors, emotions, and cognitive abilities. This complex microanalysis and macroanalysis of human data, in the context of understanding how neurobiological processes impact neurcognitive functions that then are expressed in the psychology of a person, is where neuropsychology resides and provides great value to the understanding of human beings.

Historically, neuropsychology progressed from theory-testing methodologies into the rapid development of hundreds of standardized neuropsychological instruments and procedures that were successfully designed to identify sub-functions, measure their level of functionality, and correlate these sub-functions with regions of the brain. These meaningful correlations utilize structural imaging techniques, such as functional Magnetic Resonance Imaging (fMRI) and others that detect electrical or metabolic activity, such as Electroencephalography (EEG) and Positron Emission Tomography (PET). Standardized neuropsychological measures are continuously and rigorously examined for validity and reliability, and often have been normed using thousands of participants. This is an area that continues to develop; many of the measures have been normed accounting for level of education, and some provide ethnic-sensitive norms. A vast majority of the instruments are developed and normed in English, and their conversion to other languages has continued to occur in recent decades.

Neuropsychological examination provides a numerical table that represents the "neuropsychological profile" of the individual. This profile taps into functions such as intelligence, memory, executive functions, fine motor and sensory abilities, attention and concentration, and language. It can also provide insight to the level of effort and motivation of the person at the time of examination, as well as premorbid functioning; it divides functions into visuospatial and verbal domains. Finally, psychological assessment instruments, such as depression, anxiety, and hopelessness scales, personality testing measurements, structured and semi-structured diagnostic interviews that correlate with the Diagnostic and Statistical Manual of Mental Disorders, Fifth Edition (DSM-5; American Psychiatric Association, 2013), interviews, meticulous medical records review, and direct observation are also used to establish the neuropsychological profile. The profile is then compared to neuropsychological profiles that have been developed based on extensive data collected from individuals diagnosed with the respective disorder. This pertains as well to the neuropsychological assessment of psychopathy, in which interpretation of the profile of the tested individual is compared to the data-based profile of psychopathy.

20.1.2 Psychopathy: Definition

Psychopathy can be described as a complex developmental syndrome that is characterized by the constellation of significant emotional deficits, behavioral disturbances, and marked risk for aggression and violence (Hare, 2003). While several cognitive, emotional, and behavioral features of psychopathy overlap with those of Antisocial Personality Disorder (ASPD), psychopathy and ASPD are not interchangeable. The diagnostic criteria for ASPD require social and behavioral deficits. While psychopathy shares with ASPD similar social and behavioral deficits, it also requires unique emotional deficits that are central in the identification of the disorder and are often associated with higher risk of aggression and violence (Hare, 2003). It is estimated that only about a third of all individuals who are diagnosed with ASPD also meet the criteria for psychopathy (Hart & Hare, 1996).

20.1.3 Understanding Neurodevelopment

Most fundamentally, we are first to understand that as the brain changes and develops, so do the relationships between the various areas of the brain and their interactions (Luria, 1980). While early scientists attempted to map the brain into localized regions responsible for specific functions, it was later discovered that most functions of the brain occur in processes that utilize various areas and often depend on primary and secondary functions. As development occurs, disruptions in the primary and secondary sensory processes may influence the later development of higher cortical functions and complex systems. Early age disruptions prevent the development of complex functions needed in adulthood, leaving a more pronounced impact as compared to the same disruptions occurring in adulthood, once complex neuronal networks matured (see Gaines & Soper, 2018, for a review).

While the adult brain shows a nearly complete development by the mid to late 20's, the neurodevelopmental processes that take place in childhood are profound over the span of development (Rourke et al., 1986), with critical neuroanatomical changes that underline cognitive and emotional processes necessary for the mature brain. Neurogenesis of synaptic blooming and pruning suggests that in the healthy and developing brain, development occurs in critical and sensitive periods, wherein the construction, enhancement, and consolidation of neuronal connections occurs. These unique periods are often referred to as "Windows of Opportunities" (National Research Council (US) and Institute of Medicine (US) Committee on Integrating the Science of Early Childhood Development, 2000; Thompson & Nelson, 2001). They are referred to as "windows," since they are considered optimum times when the brain is ready and in a state of optimal capacity to receive the learning that should occur in the specific areas of development (sensory, motor, language, etc.). While learning occurs throughout the lifespan via experiences (Greenough et al.,

1987), learning during these windows of opportunity occurs at an incredible rate, through exposure to experiences that trigger and stimulate learning and growth.

Significant learning takes place during the stages of neurodevelopment. Luria's model of the developmental stages of executive functions is based on phases of higher cortical maturation (Horton, 1987; Luria, 1963, 1966, 1969, 1973). He proposed five stages in the functional development of the brain, a development that relies on interactions the person has with the sensorial, emotional, physical, and interpersonal environment. Each stage provides milestones in arousal, sensory, and motor development, allowing for the young brain to recognize, comprehend, and appreciate the basic natures of perceived objects and their symbolic representations. The fourth and fifth stages of development are instrumental in cognitive processes in which we see differences between the normal and psychopathic brain. The fourth stage is associated with the posterior tertiary areas, especially the parietal lobes. During this stage, sensorial abilities are formed, such as integration of information across sensory modalities, reasoning that is symbolic and abstract, and comprehension of a perspective other than their own with a fuller appreciation for the social environment. This critical stage can be considered the first of higher cortical functioning, occurring as the brain becomes more efficient, at around the ages of 6 and 7. The fifth and final stage, which continues into adolescence and early adulthood, involves completion of the development of the frontal regions, specifically the prefrontal areas. During this period, the brain develops the ability to engage in, complete, and successfully execute complex mental activities, such as complex problem solving, abstract reasoning, intentional and working memory, and monitoring, evaluation, and regulation of behavior (Gaines & Soper, 2018).

20.2 Neurodevelopmental Aspects of Psychopathy

The prefrontal areas of the brain and what is considered the limbic system are most associated with identified abnormalities in the psychopathic brain (Blair, 2013; Blair & Zhang, 2020; Contreras-Rodríguez et al., 2015; Kiehl et al., 2001). To understand their significance, we must appreciate that the prefrontal areas receive a variety of emotional, sensory, and memory-related information, and organize the received data to make judgments and decisions, and produce adaptive motor and emotive responses. Impact to the prefrontal area (traumatic or degenerative) may temporarily or permanently disrupt or alter the executive process at various conjunctions, from encoding and retrieval to planning and organization, which may result in poor decision-making, emotional dysfunction, behavioral dysregulation, attention and concentration problems, disinhibition and other disturbances (Gaines et al., 2016). Neuropsychological abnormalities may vary in terms of quantity and quality, depending on the nature of the neurocognitive disruptions and the period in which they occur in developmental stages.

The field of neuropsychology recognizes that neurodevelopmental processes and related milestones must take place for normal neurodevelopment to occur, and that those processes impact emotional, behavioral, cognitive, and social abilities. Distinct anatomical markers associated with the psychopathic brain strongly suggest that psychopathy is characterized by neurodevelopment disruptions (Boccardi et al., 2011; Frick, 1998; Kiehl et al., 2001; Korponay et al., 2017; Ly et al., 2012; Obradović et al., 2007; Philippi et al., 2015; Pujol et al., 2019). For individuals with psychopathy, learning and reinforcement are disrupted (Blair & Mitchell, 2009; Lindner et al., 2018). The process of reinforcement learning is marked with dysfunction in the amygdala and the process of representation of reinforcement value is marked with dysfunction in the ventromedial frontal cortex. Top-down attentional control impacts the emotional responsiveness to emotional stimuli, another function of the amygdala, and is associated with areas such as the lateral frontal, dorsomedial, and parietal cortices (Blair & Mitchell, 2009; Mitchell et al., 2007; Pessoa & Ungerleider, 2004).

Psychopathic traits are present in the early years of life and tend to remain moderately or highly stable throughout the lifespan (López-Romero et al., 2014), supporting the position that psychopathy is a developmental disorder. While antisocial traits can stem from environmental and neurobiological factors, psychopathy is uniquely characterized by severe emotional deficits that tend to be highly resistant to positive social and environment impact (Lynam et al., 2007; Munoz & Frick, 2007). Traditional therapeutic methods have proven ineffective while therapies that focus on treating neuropsychological deficits during the neurodevelopmental years show promise (Anderson & Kiehl, 2014). The nature of these emotional deficits results in a person highly divorced from typical human needs to bond, relate, and feel compassion, and instead presents with goal-directed, self-serving behavior, who thrives on the manipulation and exploitation of others and exhibits a high propensity toward violence. As a result, psychopathic individuals are three times more likely to re-offend, and four times more likely to re-offend using violence, when compared to offenders with low psychopathic traits (Hemphill et al., 1998). The two main neuropsychological dysfunctions observed in individuals with psychopathy are attentional (Newman et al., 2007) and emotional processing (Blair, 1995; Frick & Viding, 2009).

20.2.1 Neuroscience and Psychopathy

Brain imaging studies identify distinct structural deficits associated with various disorders and syndromes. As a result, neuropsychological evaluations often support diagnostic impressions with imaging data that supports or explains functional deficits in the measured cognitive areas. Affective deficits, which are identified in measures such as the Psychopathy Checklist-Revised (PCL-R; Hare, 2003) and collateral review of the person's history, correlate with fMRI studies that find deficits in the input of limbic structures, specifically the amygdala, prefrontal cortex, and the hippocampus. For example, Kiehl et al. (2001) found significant affective abnormalities associated with psychopathy. Using fMRI analyses, neuronal activity during performance on an affective memory task was compared for psychopathic criminals, non-psychopathic criminals, and non-criminal control participants. Results detected significantly less affect-related activity in the limbic areas of the brain: amygdala and hippocampal formation, parahippocampal gyrus, ventral striatum, and in the anterior and posterior cingulate gyri for psychopathic criminals. Although useful for supporting diagnostic impressions, it is important to note that analyses of imaging data are not required in order to provide diagnostic impressions in neuropsychological assessments.

20.2.2 Structural and Functional Brain Abnormalities

The last decade has seen a significant increase in brain imaging studies of psychopathy. Areas associated with emotive processing, such as the limbic system, are found to show abnormalities in the psychopathic brain. Current research supports the hypothesis that psychopathic traits are associated with abnormalities in the amygdala, orbital frontal cortex, and extended paralimbic structures (predominantly the anterior and posterior cingulate cortex and the superior temporal gyrus; Kiehl et al., 2001). Moreover, lesions in anatomical areas that are associated with psychopathy were found with individuals who displayed psychopathic symptoms (Boccardi et al., 2011). Another established model of psychopathy focuses on learning; it hypothesizes that psychopathic individuals suffer from associative learning dysfunction associated with selective amygdala and orbitofrontal cortex abnormalities (Motzkin et al., 2011; Rothemund et al., 2012). Associative learning is essential in normal socialization (Blair, 2003). Although the etiology of these brain abnormalities is unknown, clinical findings support that suggests that the associated affective deficits are present in the early years of life (Frick, 1998). Moreover, longitudinal studies have found high year-to-year stability of psychopathic traits in at-risk males ages 8–16 (Obradovic et al., 2007). This further supports the hypothesis that psychopathy is a developmental condition with strong genetic loading.

Psychopathic individuals struggle to conceptualize abstract ideas, a function associated with the right hemisphere (Bottini & Corcoran, 1994). Several studies have detected abnormalities in volume, cortical thickness, and activation in the right hemisphere for individuals with psychopathy (Kiehl et al., 2004; Korponay et al., 2017; Ly et al., 2012). In a study by Kiehl et al. (2004), psychopathic individuals, as compared with controls, showed poorer behavioral performance for processing abstract words on a lexical decision block when concrete words and pseudowords or abstract words and pseudowords were introduced. Processing of old stimuli showed activation in the interior cingulate, bilateral fusiform gyrus, left middle temporal gyrus, right posterior superior temporal gyrus, and left and right inferior frontal gyrus. While differentiation between the processing of abstract and concrete stimuli occurred in the right anterior temporal gyrus and supporting cortex, the study showed that the brains of psychopathic individuals failed to show such differentiation when processing the two types of words.

Cortical thickness is often evaluated as a measure of the normal brain, and neurobiological abnormalities of the cortical thickness is often associated with various psychiatric disorders. Psychopathic inmates, when compared with non-psychopathic inmates, exhibited a significantly thinner cortex in the left and right precentral gyri, the left and right anterior temporal cortices, the left insula, dorsal anterior cingulate cortex, and the right inferior frontal gyrus. This data controlled for differences in IQ, age, and substance abuse history (Ly et al., 2012).

Current understanding of neuropsychological processes is enhanced by identifying their occurrence in neuronal networks. Broadening the understanding of neuronal networks' pathology associated with psychopathy, Philippi et al. (2015) investigated psychopathy and the connectivity of several networks using fMRI with 142 adult male prison inmates. Regression analyses related network connectivity to overall psychopathy, PCL-R Factor 1 (interpersonal/affective traits), Factor 2 (lifestyle/antisocial traits), and the four PCL-R facets (interpersonal, affective, lifestyle, and antisocial). Default mode network, frontoparietal network, and cingulo-opercular networks were analyzed, along with two comparison primary sensory networks, the visual and auditory. Each Factor was uniquely associated with a pattern of functional connectivity within three primary cortical networks. Reduced functional connectivity was associated with Factor 1, while heightened functional connectivity was associated with Factor 2. The overall score of psychopathy was specifically associated with reduced functional connectivity between the dorsal anterior cingulate cortex and the lateral parietal cortex.

A sample of 124 adult male prison inmates participated in a multimodal neuroimaging study of prefrontal cortex volume and functional connectivity in psychopathy (Korponay et al., 2017). Volumetric analyses found significant correlations between volume size and the severity of psychopathy in prefrontal subregions when using an assessment of resting-state functional connectivity. Overall psychopathy severity and Factor 2 scores were associated with larger volume in the prefrontal subregion, specifically in the medial orbitofrontal cortex and dorsolateral prefrontal cortex. Functional connectivity between several areas of the prefrontal cortex was also positively correlated with Factor 2 scores.

Imaging studies detect structural abnormalities in the limbic system, supporting the theory of psychopathy as an emotional disorder. In their review of neuroimaging findings relevant to conduct disorder and psychopathy, Blair and Zhang (2020) noted that the severity of psychopathy is positively associated with extent of cavum septum pellucidum, suggesting disruption neurodevelopmentally within the limbic regions. They clarify the association between conduct disorder and particularly callous-unemotional traits and white matter tract abnormalities even if it remains less transparent exactly which tracts are disrupted. Inconsistencies in direction of emotionality and reward responsiveness require further studies. Thus far, data supports the position that callous-unemotional traits/psychopathy represent a neurodevelopmental disorder in the early stages of development and is associated with compromised emotional (limbic) functioning.

Anatomical alterations in psychopathy involve primarily two interconnected systems: a ventral system connecting the anterior temporal lobe to anterior and ventral frontal areas, and a dorsal system that connects the medial frontal lobe to the posterior cingulate cortex/precuneus complex and, in turn, to medial structures of the temporal lobe (Pujol et al., 2019). Emotional flow breakdown is hypothesized by the authors to occur in the ventral and dorsal systems, whereby emotion is integrated anomalously into cognition in the psychopathic brain when moral challenge is present. Some suggested theoretical frameworks such as somatic markers and mirror neurons explain the empathy deficits psychopathic individuals exhibit (Alcázar-Córcoles et al., 2008), although these have yet to be fully investigated.

The overall significance of the available structural and functional findings of abnormalities in brain areas that involve the limbic system and executive regions is that they provide support to both the emotional and attentional theories of psychopathy. In addition to research studies focusing on differences between the brains of individuals with Antisocial Personality Disorder and individuals with psychopathy, recent data has shifted to also examine structural and functional differences between successful and unsuccessful psychopaths, as will be discussed later in this chapter.

20.3 Psychopathy: Attentional Deficits

The response modulation hypothesis proposed attentional deficits in the psychopathic brain (Newman et al., 2007). According to this hypothesis, emotional deficits are a result of another process that takes place – a heightened top-down attentional control that prevents emotional content from being processed. Physical information that is goal-directed becomes primary, supersedes abstract secondary information such as affective information, and prevents that information from being processed, thereby blocking the abstract information from passing through the limbic neuropathways and arriving at the amygdala (Newman et al., 1997, 2007). In other words, visual information as primary information is immediately prioritized and secondary information blocked. Inability to process two different sets of information creates a bottleneck blocked with primary, goal-directed information. While the response modulation hypothesis has existed for more than two decades, Blair (2013) lists areas of concern that question the theory in its current form, including that the studies were inconsistent with general findings on attentional manipulation and that fear-potentiated startle (FPS) studies support some aspect of the theory but not others.

20.4 Psychopathy: Emotional Deficits

Psychopathy is also understood as a disorder characterized predominantly by profound deficits in emotional processing: reduced autonomic response to the pain and distress of others, reduced recognition of certain emotional expressions associated with happiness, sadness, and fear (while intact for anger and disgust), reduced aversive conditioning, and significant difficulties with reinforcement-based decision making (Blair, 2013). Early arguments hypothesized that in psychopathic individuals the reward mechanism is intact while the punishment mechanism is impaired (Blair, 1995; Fowles, 1988; Hare, 1975). However, it was later found that psychopathic individuals may not display within-normal reward mechanisms in particular scenarios, such as reward that follows a punishment (Budhani et al., 2006), suggesting that decision-making processes were more complex with psychopathic individuals, making predictability more challenging.

Other disorders are characterized by emotional deficits, including ASPD and developmental disorders such as autism spectrum disorder. To allow for clear differential diagnosis, one needs to detect a disorder-specific profile. For example, individuals diagnosed with ASPD often suffer from impaired executive functioning, while individuals with autism show impairment in Theory of Mind. Both executive functioning and Theory of Mind are intact in psychopathic individuals (Blair, 2013; Blair et al., 1996; Morgan & Lilienfield, 2000).

Emotion-based perspectives link emotional deficits primarily to alterations in amygdala-ventromedial frontal circuits. However, as Blair (2013) argues, these models alone cannot explain why individuals with psychopathy can regularly benefit from emotional information when it becomes the focus of attention and why they are resistant to interference from nonaffective contextual cues. Anatomical changes and differences in functional connectivity may provide an explanation for this pattern. Subjects with psychopathy showed gray matter reduction involving prefrontal cortex, paralimbic, and limbic structures (Contreras-Rodríguez et al., 2015; Korponay et al., 2017; Philippi et al., 2015; Pujol et al., 2019). Using seed-based connectivity mapping technique, Contreras-Rodríguez et al. (2015) found that participants with psychopathy had reduced functional connectivity between limbic-paralimbic structures and prefrontal areas, along with heightened connectivity within the dorsal lobe. Moreover, heightened connectivity at the medial-dorsal frontal cortex and anatomical changes converged. Abnormalities in the topological makeup of the neuronal network disrupt the integration of neuronal networks, which results in continually impaired learning and integration of information in the psychopathic brain (a process referred to as the Impaired Integration Theory [IIT]; Espinoza et al., 2018). Specific topological abnormalities consistent with IIT were identified with measured psychopathic traits in males and females (Lindner et al., 2018). Overall, each representative theory may provide an explanation to some but not all psychopathic traits.

20.5 Diagnostic Considerations

Neuropsychological assessment evaluates the cognitive, emotional, and behavioral presentation of the individual, thereby identifying strengths and weaknesses that provide a neuropsychological profile. The profile then allows the clinician to identify diagnostic criteria. The same process occurs in the neuropsychological assessment of psychopathy. Because psychopathic individuals have a psychological profile of antisocial traits, damage to society, violence, and involvement with the criminal system, neuropsychological assessment for this disorder mostly occurs in a forensic setting. While individuals may be identified with the disorder in a clinical setting, it is rare (Hare, 2003). A neuropsychological assessment identifies the profile of psychopathy using the presence of certain features in the interpersonal, affective, behavioral, and life-style domains, based on standardized administered instruments, observation, structural and semi-structural interviews, and collateral information. The clinician may identify certain features that may be present both in antisocial and psychopathic profiles. Not all individuals who are antisocial are also psychopathic, and vice versa. Neuropsychological assessments and brain imaging techniques have demonstrated that individuals with ASPD suffer from attention deficits, impulsivity, cognitive inflexibility, and inappropriate processing of contextual cues in the environment, all of which increase their chances of making poor behavioral choices (Fitzgerald & Demakis, 2007). The neuropsychological profile of individuals with psychopathy may display some similarities to the profile of ASPD, in addition to the interpersonal, affective, and behavioral markers of psychopathy. Those markers are divided into interpersonal features (grandiose thinking, deception, dominance, superficiality, and manipulation), affective traits (a person who is shallow, unable to form strong emotional bonds with others, and displays lack empathy, guilt, or remorse), and behavioral and lifestyle aspects (irresponsible and impulsive behavior, and a tendency to ignore or violate social conventions and morals).

20.5.1 Antisocial Personality Disorder, Psychopathy, and the DSM-5

The DSM-5 diagnostic criteria for ASPD requires that the person shows disregard for and violation of others' rights since age 15, as indicated by the presence of at least three features demonstrating failure to comply with laws and social norms and criminal behavior, lying, conning, deceiving, and manipulating others for pleasure or profit, poor planning or impulsivity, irritability and aggression, blatantly disregarding the safety of others and self, irresponsibility in various commitments such as work, finances, and family, lack of remorse for actions that harmed or resulted in the mistreatment of others, and rationalizing to avoid accountability (American Psychiatric Association, 2013). In addition, the person needs to be at least 18 years of age at the time of diagnosis, have a history that is consistent with conduct disorder prior to the age of 15, and his/her antisocial behavior does not occur exclusively during the course of bipolar disorder or schizophrenia. Psychopathy is not described as independent disorder, but rather it is mentioned in a separate section: Emerging Measures and Models. In this section, the DSM-5 recognizes the shortcomings of the current model, such as the overlap of traits between the various personality disorders, and proposes an alternative model of assessing personality disorders in specific domains. ASPD is described by a moderate or greater impairment in at least two aspects of personality functioning: identity, self direction, empathy, and intimacy, in addition to the presence of at least six pathological personality traits within the following two domains: Antagonism: manipulativeness, callousness, deceitfulness, and hostility, and Disinhibition: risk-taking, impulsivity, and irresponsibility. When aspects that are unique to psychopathy are identified, psychopathy can be added as a specifier under this model: Low levels of anxiousness or stress immunity (Affectivity Domain), withdrawal (Detachment Domain), and high levels of attention-seeking and bold lifestyle (Antagonism Domain) (APA, 2013). While many ASPD features may be present in a psychopathic individual, psychopathy adds unique factors to the psychological profile. Experts attempt to describe these unique factors and look at their etiology using pathology theory modalities (emotional versus attentional), diagnostic criteria (PCL-R and the DSM-5) and taxonomies, all of which add features to the personality disorder.

20.5.2 Neuropsychological Profiles of Psychopathy Versus Antisocial Personality Disorder

Early challenges in the study of psychopathy and neuropsychological dysfunction involved lack of uniformity in the diagnostic criteria for psychopathy, lack of clear differentiation from ASPD, the usage of tests that are considered dorsolateral, and less advanced brain imaging techniques (Jurado & Junqué, 1996). In the last decade, as the PCL-R has become the "gold standard" assessment instrument of psychopathy and imaging techniques have improved, an increasing number of studies have demonstrated higher uniformity in the assessment of psychopathy, allowing for greater comparison in study results.

Individuals with ASPD show impaired inhibitory control, impaired decision-making, and venturesomeness on the Eysenck Questionnaire when compared to controls (Chamberlain et al., 2016). Other factors correlated with ASPD, such as history of illegal behavior, pathological gambling, unemployment, and drug use. Jurado and Junqué (1996) have argued that differentiation between orbital and dorsolateral prefrontal systems should be considered when researching neuropsychological deficits in psychopathy, and hypothesized that both ASPD and psychopathy will be associated with orbitoventral dysfunction.

Psychopathic traits were assessed using the PCL-R and compared with abnormalities in microstructural integrity of white-matter tracts using Diffusion-weighted MRI index of white-matter integrity (Fractional Anisotropy) in 15 male offenders with impulse control problems and 10 without. In impulsive offenders, Factor 1 (interpersonal-affective) traits were negatively correlated with index results of white-matter integrity in the anterior and posterior temporal lobe and orbitofrontal area. Additionally, elevations on the affective traits were associated with lower index results of white-matter integrity in the right temporal lobe (Vermeij et al., 2018). Hoppenbrouwers et al. (2013) were able to associate white matter abnormalities with specific neurocognitive networks with the two major factors of psychopathy using fractional anisotropy when psychopathic offenders compared to healthy controls. Those were detected in three main white matter clusters, representing two major networks: a striato-thalamo-frontal and an amygdalo-prefrontal. The antisocial component of the PCL-R correlated with deficits in the striato-thalamo-frontal network while the interpersonal/affective correlated with white matter deficits in the orbitofrontal cortex and frontal pole.

20.6 Neuropsychological Assessment

It is critical to administer a comprehensive neuropsychological battery of tests in the forensic assessment of psychopathy and conduct a thorough review of collateral information, such as medical records, legal records, prior mental health or psychological evaluations, and interviews. Identification of developmental disorders, history of acquired or traumatic brain injuries, seizure disorders, and severe mental illness may explain emotional deficits and executive dysfunction not attributable to psychopathy. A comprehensive neuropsychological battery includes standardized measures that examine effort, sensory-motor functioning, language and memory, executive functions, visuospatial and verbal abilities, intellectual functioning, mental control, attention, and concentration, and processing speed. Personality measures and structured/semi-structured clinical interviews that identify DSM-IV disorders are also used.

20.6.1 The Psychopathy Checklist-Revised (PCL-R)

The instruments developed by Hare and colleagues (e.g., PCL-R, PCL: SV, PCL: YV) attempt to measure a distinct cluster of personality traits and socially deviant behaviors which fall into four facets: interpersonal, affective, lifestyle and antisocial. With several decades of research providing empirical support, the PCL-R (Hare, 1991, 2003) is the most widely regarded measure of psychopathy and is considered the "gold standard" in the field (Acheson, 2005). It is a 20-item rating scale that utilizes case history information, a semi-structured interview, and specific scoring criteria to rate each item in terms of severity using 0, 1, and 2, as it applies to the evaluated person. Scores can range from 0 to 40, reflecting a greater level of pathological traits as the value increases. A cutoff score of 30 is recommended to be used in identifying significant psychopathy (Hare, 2003). Standardized administration includes both interview and file review, while non-standardized administration can be comprised of file review only, when interviewing the person is not possible.

The PCL-R is designed to address the clinical construct of psychopathy and has been found to be an effective tool in predicting recidivism, risk of violence, and treatment outcome (Beszterczey et al., 2013). It covers four main domains: Interpersonal, Affective, Lifestyle, and Antisocial. Interpersonal and Affective load Factor 1 and Lifestyle and Antisocial load Factor 2. There are 18 traits that are divided into the four domains, and two traits that contribute to the total score but do not load into either of the Factors (Item 11: Promiscuous Sexual Behavior, and Item 17: Many Short Term Martial Relationships). Factor 1 encompasses the interpersonal domain (i.e., glibness-superficial charm, grandiose sense of self-worth, pathological lying, and conning-manipulative tendencies), and the affective domain (i.e., lack of remorse or guilt, shallow affect, callous-lack of empathy, and failure to accept responsibility). Factor 2 encompasses antisocial lifestyle (i.e., need for stimulation, parasitic lifestyle, lack of realistic long-term goals, impulsivity, and irresponsibility), and antisocial behavior (i.e., poor behavioral controls, early behavioral problems, juvenile delinquency, revocation of conditional release, and criminal versatility). Another type of analysis of the PCL-R proposes a 3-factor model in which 13 selected items fall into the three categories of interpersonal, affective, and lifestyle (Cooke & Michie, 2001). These 13 items are selected based on the arguments that some items in the PCL-R are more associated with antisocial tendencies than psychopathy, and that the 13 items selected are predominately associated with psychopathy (Cooke & Michie, 2001). While the model seems to have value (Cooke et al., 2005), literature is divided on the statistical and empirical support to the model (Hare & Neumann, 2008; Neumann et al., 2007).

While some studies have examined a lower cutoff (such as 25), IRT analyses and meta-analysis have demonstrated that using the cutoff of 30 captures similar levels of psychopathology across gender (male-female), some ethnic differences (such as Caucasian and African-American), and populations (offenders and patients) (Bolt et al., 2004, 2007; Cooke et al., 2001, 2005; Skeem et al., 2004). Hare (2003) reports that about 15% of male offenders and 10% of female offenders meet the cutoff of 30 on the PCL-R. It is of note that there is variation of scores on individual items among gender and ethnic differences on the PCL-R (Hare & Neumann, 2009).

20.6.2 Error Reduction and Rater Bias

While studies show that the PCL-R has high internal consistency and reliability (Storey et al., 2016), using a single instrument in neuropsychological evaluations to determine the presence of a disorder is considered insufficient and must be avoided. This becomes particularly relevant in forensic assessments where diagnostic determination often carries serious legal implications, and in clinical settings where treatment determinations are made. Standardized administration for arriving at the score is critical, and attention to biases and tendencies in interview style must be implemented to avoid over-rating or under-rating. Psychopathy is often fascinating to the general public but also to clinicians, and the desire to identify, along with a curiosity to examine, a person with psychopathy can possibly skew an examiner to overrate toward psychopathy. This can be a greater problem with inexperienced examiners. A comprehensive and detailed review of collateral material and historical data must be conducted and examined against the results of the PCL-R administration. Inconsistencies must be identified and examined, with investigation into the possible reasons for the inconsistencies and attempt at resolving those must be made and discussed in the final assessment report. The experienced examiner will also account for error in measurement (Hare, 2003) and be able to justify item scoring.

It is important to recognize that various items in the PCL-R are symptoms of other psychiatric disorders, and therefore the process of differentiation and ruling out other disorders is essential for diagnostic accuracy and is expected to be addressed in a comprehensive, thoughtfully constructed neuropsychological report. For example, impulsivity is found in individuals suffering from Attention Deficit Hyperactivity Disorder, juvenile delinquency is a marker for Antisocial Personality Disorder, grandiose sense of self-worth is an aspect of Narcissistic Personality Disorder, and shallow affect can be found in individuals suffering from psychosis.

It has been reported that rater bias is found in clinicians involved in adversarial proceedings (Murrie et al., 2008) and that error in measurement should be accounted for in final analysis (Hare, 2003). Given these concerns, the following steps are recommended to increase diagnosis accuracy:

1. Familiarize yourself with the PCL-R, how to use it, interpret it, understand error in measurement, and know the limitation of this instrument;
2. Administer precisely as guided in the professional administration manual (if variations occurred, acknowledge those and provide relevant commentary in your final analyses);
3. Score exactly as instructed, provide detailed description of the interview notes and justification in scoring, and be prepared to be asked about it as necessary;
4. While some neuropsychological instruments can be administered with a non-standardized (but justified) administration and/or scoring, it is not recommended to do so with the PCL-R, as errors and biases can easily occur and implications in adjudication and treatment can be detrimental when diagnosis is inaccurate;
5. Analysis and assessment of PCL-R results must be carefully compared to other sources of data and examined against them for accuracy and reliability;
6. Error in measurement must be taken into account in the final analysis.

An added complexity to the PCL-R is the correlations identified between the factors. Statistical techniques remove the effects of one factor over the other to isolate the association of a factor and an outcome variable. However, the removal of correlates detecting psychopathy in the factors compromises the ability to identify what remains to be analyzed and arguably the ability to detect psychopathy as it is used in the factors (Lynam et al., 2006). While the Factor 1 and Factor 2 factors in the PCL-R are highly correlated, it is the combination of high scores on both factors that research has found to be highly predictive of violent behavior, and using only one factor compromises the predictive value of the instrument (Hare & Neumann, 2009; Harpur & Hare, 1991; Walsh & Kosson, 2008).

20.6.3 Derivatives of the PCL-R

The Hare Psychopathy Checklist: Screening Version (PCL- SV; Hart et al., 1995) and the Hare Psychopathy Checklist: Youth Version (PCL-YV; Forth et al., 2003) are scoring scales derived from the PCL-R, using a select set of items. The PCL-SV consists of 12 items which are scored in a similar manner to the PCL-R (i.e., a 3 point scale of 0,1, and 2). The instrument is designed to be used as a screening tool for psychopathology. Collection of information during interview and from collateral sources is often less detailed, but its structure and empirical support are similar to that of the PCL-R. It has been found to be predictive of violence and aggression in forensic and clinical settings (Dahle, 2006; Doyle et al., 2002; Edens et al., 2006; Hare, 2003; Tengström, 2001). Scores at or above the cutoff score of 18 on the PCL- SV (which are equivalent to scores of 30 or above on the PCL-R) have been found in less than 1% of a large community sample (Neumann & Hare, 2008).

The PCL-YV is a modified version of the PCL-R intended to be administered to adolescents. It is comprised of 20 items that translate into 3 or 4 factors, and is supported by similar correlations and psychometric properties to the PCL-R. Theoretical support, but also suggested guidance to the appropriate usage of psychopathy in youth, stems predominantly from the developmental perspective (Frick, 2007; Frick & Marsee, 2006). Adolescents are not fully developed neurologically and psychologically until the mid-20's, rendering many traits malleable to change, influence, developmental processes and individual differences in rate of maturation. Some traits that are considered by the PCL-R may be within behaviors expected in adolescence. Other concerns relate to giving the serious diagnosis of psychopathy to a minor, and the legal, social, and treatment-related implications of doing so (Kolbe, 2007). It is also important to recognize that the PCL-YV may be a predictor for ASPD. Therefore, differential effects of the PCL-YV factors needs to be examined in addition to total scores (Book et al., 2006). When identifying psychopathy in adolescents, psychopathic traits need to be present consistently, over time, in various social and contextual circumstances (Hare & Neumann, 2009).

20.6.4 Self-report Instruments

There is an increased use of self-reported questionnaires in the assessment of psychopathy in both adults and adolescents. Measures include the Antisocial Process Screening Device (Frick & Hare, 2001), the Child Psychopathy Scale (CPS; Lynam & Gudonis, 2005), the Psychopathic Personality Inventory (PPI; Lilienfeld & Andrews 1996), the Youth Psychopathic Personality Inventory (YPI; Andershed et al., 2002), and the Self-Report Psychopathy Scale (SRP-II; Williams et al., 2007). These can be rated by parents, teachers, or the individual about themselves.

Self-reported questionnaires have been found to be informative in research settings (Gordts et al., 2017; Miller et al., 2008). However, it has been suggested that these instruments are limited in the insight they can provide in the affective and interpersonal domains, are only moderately correlated with the PCL instruments, and are subject to impression management (Blair, 2013; Hare & Neumann, 2009). These limitations become meaningful in clinical and forensic evaluations, in which diagnosis has legal and treatment implications.

20.7 Successful Versus Unsuccessful Psychopathy

Psychopathy is a rarity. In the general population, its prevalence is estimated at 1%. In the business world, about 3.5% (Gao & Raine, 2010). It is significantly more common in incarcerated or antisocial individuals, although certainly not all who are incarcerated or antisocial are psychopathic. Successful psychopaths are ones who managed to avoid conviction, while unsuccessful psychopaths have been or are currently incarcerated (Lilienfeld et al., 2015). It is hypothesized that successful psychopaths manage to avoid incarceration because they are aware of the need to control their antisocial and psychopathic urges and are better able to inhibit them (Gao & Raine, 2010). Inhibition of urges and behaviors is considered an executive function of the frontal lobe. Imaging data seems to support this theory of more intact executive functions in the brains of successful psychopaths as opposed to the brain of unsuccessful psychopaths. Structural differences have been detected between the two types of psychopaths. In the prefrontal cortex, unsuccessful psychopaths exhibit reduction in grey matter and volume thickness, features that were not detected with the successful psychopaths. Both successful and unsuccessful psychopaths show bilateral volume reduction at the amygdala (Raine et al., 2004; Yang et al., 2010). An exaggerated structural hippocampal asymmetry (right over left) in the anterior region was identified in the brains of the unsuccessful psychopaths relative to both the brains of the successful psychopaths and the controls (Raine et al., 2004). In unsuccessful psychopaths, poor contextual fear conditioning, affect dysregulation, and insensitivity to predictive cues may be the outcome of underlying neurodevelopmental abnormalities that manifest in atypical asymmetries in the anterior hippocampus.

Given the supportive data, the neurobiological model hypothesizes that successful psychopaths have normal or amplified neurobiological functioning that explains their normal or even superior cognitive functioning, and that this state allows them to achieve their goals using covert and non-violent methods while controlling impulsivity and aggression (Gao & Raine, 2010). The neurobiology of unsuccessful psychopaths, on the other hand, supported by neuropsychological findings, identifies structural and functional impairments and autonomic nervous system dysfunction that underlie neuropsychological deficits in the emotional, cognitive, and behavioral domains and likely result in criminal behavior and violence.

Successful psychopaths may have superior executive functioning not only over unsuccessful psychopaths but the general population (Gao & Raine, 2010; Lilienfeld et al., 2015). Intact executive functioning allows the successful psychopath to learn and make rational decisions, even in areas that are affect-based, at least as long as the affective demand is rather superficial and does not require intense and complex emotive processes such as empathy and interpersonal dynamics. Executive dysfunction is detected in neuropsychological testing when administering structured and unstructured measures of executive functioning, associated scientifically with the frontal lobe (e.g., Fine & Delis, 2011; Melrose et al., 2013; Park et al., 2020).

Ishikawa et al. (2001) used neuropsychological measures to compare successful and unsuccessful psychopaths. Their study found that successful psychopaths demonstrated superior performance on the Wisconsin Card Sorting Test (WCST) and heightened cardiovascular stress reactivity when compared with the unsuccessful and controls. Interestingly, the successful psychopaths also reported greater parental absence. Abnormal parent-child relationship, such as absence, instability, and other attachment-related disruptions compromises the necessary neuropsychological development of affect regulation and empathy (Panfile & Laible, 2012; Waters et al., 2010). It has been long hypothesized that psychopathy is found in conjunction with poor empathy, emotional dysregulation and insecure attachment (Donahue et al., 2014; Mack et al., 2011; Mikulincer & Shaver, 2007). A disturbed parent-child relationship contributes to significant impairments in the sense of self and others and interpersonal dynamics into adulthood (Mack et al., 2011).

Successful psychopaths may engage in behaviors that border on being illegal or exploit legal loopholes. They tend to manipulate and hurt others in non-criminal ways that are nevertheless considered immoral, unethical, immoral, or irresponsible. Lack of moral conscience and self-centered goals and action to satisfy those goals with a lack of regard to their negative impact on others and the use of violence to achieve them is common. Further research is necessary to investigate the impact of neurodevelopment on the differentiation between successful and unsuccessful psychopaths.

20.8 Legal Considerations in Neuropsychological Assessment of Psychopathy

As clinical and research data continue to emerge in the area of psychopathy as a diagnosis and its utility as a predictive tool for positive prognosis and risk of recidivism, neuropsychological and psychological assessments, which utilize standardized measures such as the PCL-R and its derivatives, has become essential to the courts (de Boer et al., 2008; Walsh & Walsh, 2006). Forensic assessors are able to opine on the significance of such assessments and have made assessment procedures pertinent in addressing forensic referral questions (Archer et al., 2006; Lally, 2003). The experienced examiner evaluates two aspects of criminal behavior: what inhibits harmful behavior and what promotes it. Psychopathic personality traits, some of which are shared with ASPD, are associated with increased risk in committing crimes (Hare et al., 2000; Porter & Porter, 2007). For example, empathy, fear of punishment, sense of guilt, and close bonds inhibit harmful behaviors, while impulsivity, need for power and control, grandiosity, and aggression promote harmful behaviors. Psychopathy is one of the most generalized risk factors for recidivism in the criminal system, making the evaluation of psychopathy and the use of the PCL-R essential in risk assessments (Hare & Neumann, 2009).

As robust evidence of deficits in specific yet intricate neuronal networks that are associated with psychopathy emerge, the debate regarding the legal responsibility psychopathic individuals have over their criminal behavior becomes more relevant. If deficits in human aspects such as morality, empathy, and inhibition of aggression are the results of a damaged brain, how do free choice and intent factor into culpability? Crime causation is impacted greatly by psychopathology, as ample research identifies a host of psychopathologies that are considered risk factors to crime (Schlesinger, 2007). It has been argued that psychopathy should correlate significantly with specific rational incapacities across contexts for deficiencies to grant partial or complete criminal exculpation, and that the available neuropsychological data do not support the position that psychopaths have such general exculpatory incapacities (Jurjako & Malatesti, 2018). Others conclude that psychopaths are likely not fully responsible for their actions but nevertheless civil commitment would still be warranted (Fox et al., 2013). Others caution against changing legal treatment of crimes committed by psychopathic individuals until clarity on diagnosis, etiology, and link to criminality is achieved (Gonzalez-Tapia et al., 2017). Undoubtedly, the argument of causation and culpability in the legal system and the impact of neurobiology on choice in behavior is critical in its social implications and should be considered carefully, with scientific claims thoughtfully examined to avoid substantial harm.

Expert bias tendencies to over diagnose psychopathy in the forensic system must be recognized and should be mitigated with greater training of forensic assessors, use of multiple psychological instruments to determine diagnosis, and increased theoretical and professional clarity on the diagnostic requirement and diagnostic procedures. Diagnosis of psychopathy in youth raises several and serious concerns, as evidence shows that assessors may not consider developmental changes and acknowledge them in their report to the court (Viljoen et al., 2010). The diagnosis of psychopathy is considered severe and rare, with the expectation of it to be persistent and untreatable in therapy. Labeling an adolescent with the disorder may set them up for a life where legal sanctions to their crimes will be maximized and consideration of mitigating factors minimized. Review of legal cases involving psychopathy as evidence presented in adolescent criminal cases suggested that the findings of psychopathy were influential, even when judges generally did not directly refer to it in making the final legal decisions (Viljoen et al., 2010). It also found that the presence of psychopathy diagnosis in these cases implied poor prognosis in therapy (difficult or impossible to treat) and that the lack of psychopathy served as support to positive prognosis in therapy and more lenient sanctions (Viljoen et al., 2010)

While the combination of psychopathic traits, such as the need to exercise control over others, egocentric focus, and lack of empathy is shown to increase the risk for the victimization of others in an aggressive and violent manner (Hare, 2003; Meloy, 2002; Porter & Woodworth, 2006; Woodworth & Porter, 2002), the current definition of psychopathy does not include violence (Peterson & Brown, 2015), partly since not all psychopaths become violent. Risk assessments in nature are the science of probability, not determination - they aim to predict the chance an event will occur in the future. Risk assessment instruments have demonstrated usefulness (Harris & Rice 2007; Monahan et al., 2001). Actuarial risk instruments are based on static historical factors and empirical data, while structured clinical assessments provide procedures that include structured clinical decisions based on specific criteria. Both methods of risk assessment have been found to perform about equally well (Hare & Neumann, 2009).

In sum, comprehensive e neuropsychological assessments provide value in diagnostic determination, prediction of recidivism, and the formulation of a treatment plan using standardized measures and clinical judgement.

20.9 Neuropsychological Research: Frontiers

Future research may examine the relevance of further establishing the contribution of early life stress to abnormalities in the limbic system and specific to a learned blockage of emotional self-exposure. The role of genetic factors, and those factors with early life stress are yet to be examined. Inconsistencies in direction of emotionality and reward responsiveness require clarification. A common genetic factor is suggested to account for substantial variance in psychopathy domains (Larsson et al., 2006; Viding et al., 2007), and multiple studies suggest that personality traits are transmitted from father-to-offspring by genetics (Beaver et al., 2011; Blair, 2003). The potential role of androgenic hormones in the development of cortical anomalies is another area that is actively researched. Neuroendocrine markers of psychopathic traits, such as testosterone and cortisol, have been identified (Glenn, 2009; Welker et al., 2014), and their impact on neurodevelopment has yet to be understood.

Studies using neuropsychological instruments have examined ASPD traits and psychopathic traits and differentiation of performance on measures across various domains have been meaningful in identifying profiles between ASPD and psychopathy, and between successful and unsuccessful psychopathy. However, it is necessary to gain insight into the neuropsychological profile over neurodevelopment, and investigate the possible presence of mitigating and exacerbating factors to psychopathy-related deficits.

References

Acheson, S. K. (2005). Review of the Hare psychopathy checklist—Revised. In R. A. Spies & B. S. Plake (Eds.), *The sixteenth mental measurements yearbook* (2nd ed., pp. 429–431). Buros Institute of Mental Measurements.

Alcázar-Córcoles, M. A., Verdejo-García, A., & Bouso-Saiz, J. C. (2008). La neuropsicología forense ante el reto de la relación entre cognición y emoción en la psicopatía [forensic neuropsychology at the challenge of the relationship between cognition and emotion in psychopathy]. *Revista de Neurologia, 47*, 607–612.

American Psychiatric Association. (2013). *Diagnostic and statistical manual of mental disorders* (5th ed.). APA.

Andershed, H., Kerr, M., & Stattin, H. (2002). Psychopathic traits in non-referred youths: A new assessment tool. In E. Blauw & L. Sheridan (Eds.), *Psychopaths: Current international perspectives* (pp. 131–158). Elsevier.

Anderson, N. E., & Kiehl, K. A. (2014). Psychopathy: Developmental perspectives and their implications for treatment. *Restorative Neurology and Neuroscience, 32*, 103–117. https://doi.org/10.3233/RNN-139001

Archer, R. P., Buffington-Vollum, J. K., Stredny, R. V., & Handel, R. W. (2006). A survey of psychological test use patterns among forensic psychologists. *Journal of Personality Assessment, 87*, 84–94.

Beaver, K. M., Rowland, M. W., Schwartz, J. A., & Nedelec, J. L. (2011). The genetic origins of psychopathic personality traits in adult males and females: Results from an adoption-based study. *Journal of Criminal Justice, 39*, 426–432. https://doi.org/10.1016/j.jcrimjus.2011.07.002

Beszterczey, S., Nestor, P. G., Shirai, A., & Harding, S. (2013). Neuropsychology of decision making and psychopathy in high-risk ex-offenders. *Neuropsychology, 27*, 491–497. https://doi.org/10.1037/a0033162. PMID: 23876121.

Blair, R. J. R. (1995). A cognitive developmental approach to morality: Investigating the psychopath. *Cognition, 57*, 1–29.

Blair, R. J. R. (2003). Neurobiological basis of psychopathy. *British Journal of Psychiatry, 182*, 5–7.

Blair, R. J. R. (2013). Psychopathy: Cognitive and neural dysfunction. *Dialogues in Clinical Neuroscience, 15*, 181–190.

Blair, R. J. R., & Mitchell, D. G. (2009). Psychopathy, attention and emotion. *Psychological Medicine, 3*, 543–555.

Blair, R. J. R., & Zhang, R. (2020). Recent neuro-imaging findings with respect to conduct disorder, callous-unemotional traits and psychopathy. *Current Opinion in Psychiatry, 33*, 45–50.

Blair, R. J. R., Sellars, C., Strickland, I., Clark, F., Williams, A., Smith, M., & Jones, L. (1996). Theory of mind in the psychopath. *Journal of Forensic Psychiatry, 7*, 15–25.

Boccardi, M., Frisoni, G. B., Hare, R. D., Cavedo, E., Najt, P., Pievani, M., et. al. (2011). Cortex and amygdala morphology in psychopathy. *Psychiatry Research, 193*(2), 85–292.

Bolt, D. M., Hare, R. D., Vitale, J. E., & Newman, J. P. (2004). A multigroup item response theory analysis of the psychopathy checklist—Revised. *Psychological Assessment, 16*, 155–168.

Bolt, D. M., Hare, R. D., & Neumann, C. S. (2007). Score metric equivalence of the Psychopathy Checklist-Revised (PCL-R) across criminal offenders in North America and the United Kingdom: A critique of Cooke, Michie, Hart, and Clark (2005) and new analyses. *Assessment, 14*, 44–56.

Book, A., Clark, H., Forth, A. E., & Hare, R. D. (2006). The psychopathy checklist-revised and the psychopathy checklist: Youth version. In R. Archer (Ed.), *Forensic uses of clinical assessment instruments* (pp. 147–179). Lawrence Erlbaum Associates.

Bottini, G., & Corcoran, R. (1994). The role of the right hemisphere in the interpretation of figurative aspects of language: A positron emission tomography activation study. *Brain, 117*, 1241–1253.

Budhani, S., Richell, R. A., & Blair, R. J. (2006). Impaired reversal but intact acquisition: Probabilistic response reversal deficits in adult individuals with psychopathy. *Journal of Abnormal Psychology, 115*, 552–558.

Chamberlain, S. R., Derbyshire, K. L., Leppink, E. W., & Grant, J. E. (2016). Neurocognitive deficits associated with antisocial personality disorder in non-treatment-seeking young adults. *The Journal of the American Academy of Psychiatry and the Law, 44*, 218–225.

Contreras-Rodríguez, O., Pujol, J., Batalla, I., Harrison, B. J., Soriano-Mas, C., Deus, J., López-Solà, M., Macià, D., Pera, V., Hernández-Ribas, R., Pifarré, J., Menchón, J. M., & Cardoner, N. (2015). Functional connectivity bias in the prefrontal cortex of psychopaths. *Biological Psychiatry, 78*, 647–655.

Cooke, D. J., & Michie, C. (2001). Refining the construct of psychopathy: Towards a hierarchical model. *Psychological Assessment, 13*, 171–188.

Cooke, D. J., Kosson, D. S., & Michie, C. (2001). Psychopathy and ethnicity: Structural, item, and test generalizability of the psychopathy checklist—Revised (PCL-R) in Caucasian and African American participants. *Psychological Assessment, 13*, 531–542.

Cooke, D. J., Michie, C., Hart, S. D., & Clark, D. (2005). Assessing psychopathy in the UK: Concerns about cross-cultural generalisability. *British Journal of Psychiatry, 186*, 335–341.

Dahle, K. P. (2006). Strengths and limitations of actuarial prediction of criminal reoffence in a German prison sample: A comparative study of LSI-R, HCR-20 and PCL-R. *International Journal of Law and Psychiatry, 29*, 431–442.

de Boer, J., Whyte, S., & Maden, T. (2008). Compulsory treatment of dangerous offenders with severe personality disorders: A comparison of the English DSPD and Dutch TBS systems. *Journal of Forensic Psychiatry and Psychology, 19*, 148–163.

Donahue, J. J., McClure, K. S., & Moon, S. M. (2014). The relationship between emotion regulation difficulties and psychopathic personality characteristics. *Personality Disorders: Theory, Research, and Treatment, 5*(2), 186–194.

Doyle, M., Dolan, M., & McGovern, J. (2002). The validity of north American risk assessment tools in predicting in-patient violent behaviour in England. *Legal Criminological Psychology, 7*, 141–154.

Edens, J. F., Skeem, J. L., & Douglas, K. S. (2006). Incremental validity analyses of the violence risk appraisal guide and the psychopathy checklist: Screening version in a civil psychiatric sample. *Assessment, 13*, 368–374.

Espinoza, F. A., Vergara, V. M., Reyes, D., Anderson, N. E., Harenski, C. L., Decety, J., Rachakonda, S., Damaraju, E., Rashid, B., Miller, R. L., Koenigs, M., Kosson, D. S., Harenski, K., Kiehl, K. A., & Calhoun, V. D. (2018). Aberrant functional network connectivity in psychopathy from a large (N = 985) forensic sample. *Human Brain Mapping, 39*, 2624–2634. https://doi.org/10.1002/hbm.24028

Fine, E. M., & Delis, D. C. (2011). Delis–Kaplan executive functioning system. In J. S. Kreutzer, J. DeLuca, & B. Caplan (Eds.), *Encyclopedia of clinical neuropsychology*. Springer. https://doi.org/10.1007/978-0-387-79948-3_1539

Fitzgerald, K. L., & Demakis, G. J. (2007). The neuropsychology of antisocial personality disorder. *Disease-A-Month: DM, 53*, 177–183. https://doi.org/10.1016/j.disamonth.2007.04.010

Forth, A., Kosson, D., & Hare, R. (2003). *The Hare psychopathy checklist: Youth version, technical manual*. Multi-Health Systems, Inc.

Fowles, D. C. (1988). Psychophysiology and psychopathy: A motivational approach. *Psychophysiology, 25*, 373–391.

Fox, A., Kvaran, T., & Fontaine, R. (2013). Psychopathy and culpability: How responsible is the psychopath for criminal wrongdoing? *Law & Social Inquiry, 38*, 1–26.

Frick, P. J. (1998). Callous-unemotional traits and conduct problems: Applying the two-factor model of psychopathy to children. In: D. J. Cooke, A. E. Forth, & R. D. Hare (Eds.), *Psychopathy: Theory, Research, and Implications for Society* (pp. 161–188). Kluwer Academic Publishers.

Frick, P. J. (2007). Using the construct of psychopathy to understand antisocial and violent youth. In H. Hervé & J. C. Yuille (Eds.), *The psychopath: Theory, research, and practice* (pp. 343–367). Lawrence Erlbaum Associates.

Frick, P. J., & Hare, R. D. (2001). *The antisocial process screening device*. Multi-Health Systems.

Frick, P. J., & Marsee, M. A. (2006). Psychopathy and developmental pathways to antisocial behavior in youth. In C. J. Patrick (Ed.), *Handbook of psychopathy* (pp. 353–374). Guilford Press.

Frick, P. J., & Viding, E. (2009). Antisocial behavior from a developmental psychopathology perspective. *Development and Psychopathology, 21*, 1111–1131.

Gaines, K. D., & Soper, H. V. (2018). Neuropsychological assessment of executive functions following pediatric traumatic brain injury. *Applied Neuropsychology: Child, 7*, 31–43.

Gaines, K. D., Soper, H. V., & Berenji, G. R. (2016). Executive functioning of combat mild traumatic brain injury. *Applied Neuropsychology: Adult, 23*, 115–124. https://doi.org/10.1080/23279095.2015.1012762

Gao, Y., & Raine, A. (2010). Successful and unsuccessful psychopaths: a neurobiological model. *Behavioral Sciences & the Law, 28*, 194–210.

Glenn, A. L. (2009). Neuroendocrine markers of psychopathy. In M. S. Ritsner (Ed.), *The handbook of neuropsychiatric biomarkers, endophenotypes and genes* (pp. 59–70). Springer. https://doi.org/10.1007/978-1-4020-9838-3_5

Gonzalez-Tapia, M. I., Obsuth, I., & Heeds, R. (2017). A new legal treatment for psychopaths? Perplexities for legal thinkers. *International Journal of Law and Psychiatry, 54*, 46–60.

Gordts, S., Uzieblo, K., Neumann, C., Van den Bussche, E., & Rossi, G. (2017). Validity of the self-report psychopathy scales (SRP-III full and short versions) in a community sample. *Assessment, 24*, 308–325.

Greenough, W. T., Black, J. E., & Wallace, W. S. (1987). Experience and brain development. *Child Development, 58*, 539–559.

Hare, R. D. (1975). Psychopathy. In P. H. Venables & M. J. Christie (Eds.), *Research in psychophysiology* (pp. 325–348). Wiley.

Hare, R. D. (1991). *The Hare psychopathy checklist—Revised*. Multi-Health Systems.

Hare, R. D. (2003). *The Hare psychopathy checklist—Revised* (2nd ed.). Multi-Health Systems.

Hare, R. D., & Neumann, C. S. (2008). Psychopathy as a clinical and empirical construct. *Annual Review of Clinical Psychology, 4*, 217–246.

Hare, R. D., & Neumann, C. S. (2009). Psychopathy: Assessment and forensic implications. *The Canadian Journal of Psychiatry, 54*, 791–802.

Hare, R. D., Clark, D., Grann, M., & Thornton, D. (2000). Psychopathy and the predictive validity of the PCL-R: An international perspective. *Behavioral Sciences & the Law, 18*, 623–645.

Harpur, T. J., & Hare, R. D. (1991). *Psychopathy and violent behaviour: two factors are better than one*. Paper presented at the 99th annual meeting of the American Psychological Association, San Francisco (CA).

Harris, G., & Rice, M. (2007). Characterizing the value of actuarial violence risk assessment. *Criminal Justice and Behavior, 34*, 1638–1656.

Hart, S. D., & Hare, R. D. (1996). Psychopathy and antisocial personality disorder. *Current Opinion in Psychiatry, 9*, 129–132.

Hart, S. D., Cox, D. N., & Hare, R. D. (1995). *Manual for the Hare psychopathy checklist: Screening version (PCL:SV)*. Multi-Health Systems.

Hemphill, J. F., Hare, R. D., & Wong, S. (1998). Psychopathy and recidivism: A review. *Legal and Criminological Psychology, 3*, 139–170.

Hoppenbrouwers, S. S., Nazeri, A., de Jesus, D. R., Stirpe, T., Felsky, D., Schutter, D. J., Daskalakis, Z. J., & Voineskos, A. N. (2013). White matter deficits in psychopathic offenders and correlation with factor structure. *PLoS One, 8*, e72375. https://doi.org/10.1371/journal.pone.0072375

Horton, A. M., Jr. (1987). Luria's contributions to clinical and behavioral neuropsychology. *Neuropsychology, 1*, 39–44.

Ishikawa, S. S., Raine, A., Lencz, T., Bihrle, S., & Lacasse, L. (2001). Autonomic stress reactivity and executive functions in successful and unsuccessful criminal psychopaths from the community. *Journal of Abnormal Psychology, 110*, 423–432.

Jurado, M. A., & Junqué, C. (1996). Psicopatía y neuropsicología del córtex prefrontal [Psychopathy and neuropsychology of the prefrontal cortex]. *Actas luso-espanolas de neurologia, psiquiatria y ciencias afines, 24*, 148–155.

Jurjako, M., & Malatesti, L. (2018). Neuropsychology and the criminal responsibility of psychopaths: Reconsidering the evidence. *Erkenntnis, 83*, 1003–1025. https://doi.org/10.1007/s10670-017-9924-0

Kiehl, K. A., Smith, A. M., Hare, R. D., Mendrek, A., Forster, B. B., Brink, J., & Liddle, P. F. (2001). Limbic abnormalities in affective processing by criminal psychopaths as revealed by functional magnetic resonance imaging. *Biological Psychiatry, 50*, 677–684.

Kiehl, K. A., Smith, A. M., Mendrek, A., Forster, B. B., Hare, R. D., & Liddle, P. F. (2004). Temporal lobe abnormalities in semantic processing by criminal psychopaths as revealed by functional magnetic resonance imaging. *Psychiatry Research, 130*, 27–42.

Kolbe, V. L. (2007). A cloudy crystal ball: Concerns regarding the use of juvenile psychopathy scores in judicial waiver hearings. *Developments in Mental Health Law, 26*, 10.

Korponay, C., Pujara, M., Deming, P., Philippi, C., Decety, J., Kosson, D. S., Kiehl, K. A., & Koenigs, M. (2017). Impulsive-antisocial psychopathic traits linked to increased volume and functional connectivity within prefrontal cortex. *Social Cognitive and Affective Neuroscience, 12*, 1169–1178.

Lally, S. J. (2003). What tests are acceptable for use in forensic evaluations? A survey of experts. *Professional Psychology: Research and Practice, 34*, 491–498.

Larsson, H., Andershed, H., & Lichtenstein, P. (2006). A genetic factor explains most of the variation in the psychopathic personality. *Journal of Abnormal Psychology, 115*, 221–230. https://doi.org/10.1037/0021-843X.115.2.221

Lilienfeld, S. O., Watts, A. L., & Smith, S. F. (2015). Successful psychopathy: A scientific status report. *Current Directions in Psychological Science, 24*, 298–303.

Lindner, P., Flodin, P., Budhiraja, M., Savic, I., Jokinen, J., Tiihonen, J., & Hodgins, S. (2018). Associations of psychopathic traits with local and global brain network topology in young adult women. *Biological Psychiatry: Cognitive Neuroscience and Neuroimaging, 3*, 1003–1012.

López-Romero, L., Romero, E., & Villar, P. (2014). Assessing the stability of psychopathic traits: Adolescent outcomes in a six-year follow-up. *The Spanish Journal of Psychology, 17*, E97. https://doi.org/10.1017/sjp.2014.93

Luria, A. R. (1963). *Restoration of function after brain injury*. Macmillan.

Luria, A. R. (1966). *Higher cortical functioning in man*. Basic Books.

Luria, A. R. (1969). Cerebral organization of conscious acts: A frontal lobe function. In *Invited address to the 19th international congress of psychology*, London, England.

Luria, A. R. (1973). *The working brain*. Basic Books.

Luria, A. R. (1980). *Higher cortical functions*. Basic Books.

Ly, M., Motzkin, J. C., Philippi, C. L., Kirk, G. R., Newman, J. P., Kiehl, K. A., & Koenigs, M. (2012). Cortical thinning in psychopathy. *The American Journal of Psychiatry, 169*, 743–749.

Lynam, D. R., & Gudonis, L. (2005). The development of psychopathy. *Annual Review of Clinical Psychology, 1*, 381–407.

Lynam, D. R., Hoyle, R. H., & Newman, J. P. (2006). The perils of partialling: Cautionary tales from aggression and psychopathy. *Assessment, 13*, 328–341.

Lynam, D. R., Caspi, A., Moffitt, T. E., Loeber, R., & Stouthamer-Loeber, M. (2007). Longitudinal evidence that psychopathy scores in early adolescence predict adult psychopathy. *Journal of Abnormal Psychology, 116*, 155–165.

Mack, T. D., Hackney, A. A., & Pyle, M. (2011). The relationship between psychopathic traits and attachment behavior in a non-clinical population. *Personality and Individual Differences, 51*(5), 584–588. ISSN 0191-8869.

Meloy, J. R. (2002). The "polymorphously perverse" psychopath: Understanding a strong empirical relationship. *Bulletin of the Menninger Clinic, 66*, 273–290.

Melrose, R. J., Harwood, D., Khoo, T., Mandelkern, M., & Sultzer, D. L. (2013). Association between cerebral metabolism and Rey-Osterrieth complex figure test performance in Alzheimer's disease. *Journal of Clinical and Experimental Neuropsychology, 35*, 246–258.

Mikulincer, M., & Shaver, P. R. (2007). A behavioral systems perspective on the psychodynamics of attachment and sexuality. In D. Diamond, S. J. Blatt, & J. D. Lichtenberg (Eds.), *Attachment and sexuality* (pp. 51–78). The Analytic Press/Taylor & Francis Group.

Miller, J. D., Gaughan, E. T., & Pryor, L. R. (2008). The Levenson self-report psychopathy scale: An examination of the personality traits and disorders associated with the LSRP factors. *Assessment, 15*, 450–463.

Mitchell, D. G., Nakic, M., Fridberg, D., Kamel, N., Pine, D. S., & Blair, R. J. R. (2007). The impact of processing load on emotion. *NeuroImage, 34*, 1299–1309.

Monahan, J., Steadman, H., Silver, E., Appelbaum, P., Robbins, P., Mulvey, E., Roth, L., Grisso, T., & Banks, S. (2001). *Rethinking risk assessment: The MacArthur study of mental disorder and violence*. Oxford University Press.

Morgan, A. B., & Lilienfield, S. O. (2000). A meta-analytic review of the relation between antisocial behavior and neuropsychological measures of executive function. *Clinical Psychology Review, 20*, 113–136.

Motzkin, J. C., Newman, J. P., Kiehl, K. A., & Koenigs, M. (2011). Reduced prefrontal connectivity in psychopathy. *Journal of Neuroscience, 31*, 17348–17357.

Munoz, L. C., & Frick, P. J. (2007). The reliability, stability, and predictive utility of the self-report version of the antisocial process screening device. *Scandinavian Journal of Psychology, 48*, 299–312.

Murrie, D. C., Boccaccini, M. T., Johnson, J. T., & Janke, C. (2008). Does interrater (dis)agreement on psychopathy checklist score in sexually violent predator trials suggest partisan allegiance in forensic evaluations? *Law and Human Behavior, 32*, 352–362.

National Research Council (US) and Institute of Medicine (US) Committee on Integrating the Science of Early Childhood Development. (2000). In J. P. Shonkoff & D. A. Phillips (Eds.), *From neurons to neighborhoods: The science of early childhood development*. National Academies Press.

Neumann, C. S., & Hare, R. D. (2008). Psychopathic traits in a large community sample: Links to violence, alcohol use, and intelligence. *Journal of Consulting and Clinical Psychology, 76*, 893–899.

Neumann, C. S., Hare, R. D., & Newman, J. P. (2007). The super-ordinate nature of the psychopathy checklist-revised. *Journal of Personality Disorders, 21*, 102–117.

Newman, J. P., Schmitt, W. A., & Voss, W. D. (1997). The impact of motivationally neutral cues on psychopathic individuals: Assessing the generality of the response modulation hypothesis. *Journal of Abnormal Psychology, 106*, 563–575.

Newman, J. P., Brinkley, C. A., Lorenz, A. R., Hiatt, K. D., & MacCoon, D. G. (2007). Psychopathy as psychopathology: Hare's essential contributions. In H. Herve & J. C. Yuille (Eds.), *The psychopath: Theory, research, and practice* (pp. 173–206). Lawrence Erlbaum Associates.

Obradović, J., Pardini, D. A., Long, J. D., & Loeber, R. (2007). Measuring interpersonal callousness in boys from childhood to adolescence: An examination of longitudinal invariance and temporal stability. *Journal of Clinical Child and Adolescent Psychology, 36*, 276–292.

Panfile, T. M., & Laible, D. J. (2012). Attachment security and child's empathy: The mediating role of emotion regulation. *Merrill-Palmer Quarterly, 58*(1), 1–21.

Park, S. Y., Byun, B. H., Kim, B. I., Lim, S. M., Ko, I. O., Lee, K. C., Kim, K. M., Kim, Y. K., Lee, J.-Y., Bu, S. H., Kim, J. H., Chi, D. Y., & Ha, J. H. (2020). The correlation of neuropsychological evaluation with 11C-PiB and 18F-FC119S amyloid PET in mild cognitive impairment and Alzheimer disease. *Medicine, 99*, e19620. https://doi.org/10.1097/MD.0000000000019620

Pessoa, L., & Ungerleider, L. G. (2004). Neuroimaging studies of attention and the processing of emotion-laden stimuli. *Progress in Brain Research, 144*, 171–182.

Peterson, J. K., & Brown, J. (2015). Psychopathy in the criminal justice system. *College of liberal arts all faculty scholarship*. Paper 7. https://digitalcommons.hamline.edu/cla_faculty/7

Philippi, C. L., Pujara, M. S., Motzkin, J. C., Newman, J. P., Kiehl, K. A., & Koenigs, M. (2015). Altered resting-state functional connectivity in cortical networks in psychopathy. *The Journal of Neuroscience, 35*, 6068–6078.

Porter, S., & Porter, S. (2007). Psychopathy and violent crime. In H. Herve & J. C. Yuille (Eds.), *The psychopath: Theory, research, and practice* (pp. 287–300). Lawrence Erlbaum Associates.
Porter, S., & Woodworth, M. (2006). Psychopathy and aggression. In C. J. Patrick (Ed.), *Handbook of psychopathy* (pp. 481–494). Guilford Press.
Pujol, J., Harrison, B. J., Contreras-Rodriguez, O., & Cardoner, N. (2019). The contribution of brain imaging to the understanding of psychopathy. *Psychological Medicine, 49*, 20–31.
Raine, A., Ishikawa, S. S., Arce, E., Lencz, T., Knuth, K. H., Bihrle, S., LaCasse, L., & Colletti, P. (2004). Hippocampal structural asymmetry in unsuccessful psychopaths. *Biological Psychiatry, 55*, 185–191.
Rothemund, Y., Ziegler, S., Hermann, C., Gruesser, S. M., Foell, J., Patrick, C. J., & Flor, H. (2012). Fear conditioning in psychopaths: Event-related potentials and peripheral measures. *Biological Psychology, 90*, 50–59.
Rourke, B. P., Fisk, J. L., & Strang, J. D. (1986). *Neuropsychological assessment of children: A treatment-oriented approach*. Guilford Press.
Schlesinger, L. B. (2007). *Explorations in criminal psychopathology: Clinical syndromes with forensic implications* (2nd ed.). Charles C. Thomas Publisher, Ltd.
Skeem, J. L., Edens, J. F., Camp, J., & Colwell, C. H. (2004). Are there ethnic differences in levels of psychopathy? A meta-analysis. *Law and Human Behavior, 28*, 505–527.
Storey, J. E., Hart, S. D., Cooke, D. J., & Michie, C. (2016). Psychometric properties of the Hare psychopathy checklist-revised (PCL-R) in a representative sample of Canadian federal offenders. *Law and Human Behavior, 40*, 136–146.
Tengström, A. (2001). Long-term predictive validity of historical factors in two risk assessment instruments in a group of violent offenders with schizophrenia. *Nordic Journal of Psychiatry, 55*, 243–249.
Thompson, R. A., & Nelson, C. A. (2001). Developmental science and the media: Early brain development. *American Psychologist, 56*, 5–15.
Vermeij, A., Kempes, M. M., Cima, M. J., Mars, R. B., & Brazil, I. A. (2018). Affective traits of psychopathy are linked to white-matter abnormalities in impulsive male offenders. *Neuropsychology, 32*, 735–745.
Viding, E., Frick, P. J., & Plomin, R. (2007). Etiology of the relationship between callous-unemotional traits and conduct problems in childhood. *British Journal of Psychiatry: Supplement, 49*, S33–S38.
Viljoen, J., MacDougall, E., Gagnon, N., & Douglas, K. (2010). Psychopathy evidence in legal proceedings involving adolescent offenders. *Psychology, Public Policy, and Law, 16*, 254–283.
Walsh, Z., & Kosson, D. S. (2008). Psychopathy and violence: The importance of factor level interactions. *Psychological Assessment, 20*, 114–120.
Walsh, T., & Walsh, Z. (2006). The evidentiary introduction of psychopathy checklist-revised assessed psychopathy in US courts: Extent and appropriateness. *Law and Human Behavior, 30*, 493–507.
Waters, S., Virmani, E., Thompson, R., Meyer, S., Raikes, H., & Jochem, R. (2010). Emotion regulation and attachment: Unpacking two constructs and their association. *Journal of Psychopathology and Behavioral Assessment, 32*, 37–47. https://doi.org/10.1007/s10862-009-9163-z
Welker, K. M., Lozoya, E., Campbell, J. A., Neumann, C. S., & Carré, J. M. (2014). Testosterone, cortisol, and psychopathic traits in men and women. *Physiology & Behavior, 129*, 230–236.
Williams, K. M., Paulhus, D. L., & Hare, R. D. (2007). Capturing the four-factor structure of psychopathy in college students via self-report. *Journal of Personality Assessment, 88*, 205–219.
Woodworth, M., & Porter, S. (2002). In cold blood: Characteristics of criminal homicides as a function of psychopathy. *Journal of Abnormal Psychology, 111*, 436–445.
Yang, Y., Raine, A., Colletti, P., Toga, A. W., & Narr K. L. (2010). Morphological alterations in prefrontal cortex and amygdala in unsuccessful psychopaths. *Journal of Abnormal Psychology, 119*(3), 546–554. [PubMed: 20677843]

Chapter 21
Criminal Justice Responses to Psychopathy

Devon L. L. Polaschek

Abstract Psychopathy is an intriguing, complex and popular concept, with relevance to multiple parts of the criminal justice system. The extent and nature of its relevance depends in turn on how psychopathy is defined and understood, both by those assessing it, and those who use such assessments for decision-making. This chapter considers key definitional issues, before examining psychopathy's relevance to the criminal justice system, including to risk assessment and recidivism prediction, and treatment prognosis. The chapter concludes with a discussion of some of the ethical and practical issues that are emerging as research on the PCL scales continues to grow, alongside the development of newer purpose-designed measures, and finally closes with some points about psychopathy as a personality disorder.

Keywords Psychopathy · PCL-R · Criminal justice · Risk assessment · Crime · Ethical considerations

21.1 Introduction

Psychopathy is an intriguing, complex and popular concept, with relevance to multiple parts of the criminal justice system. The extent and nature of its relevance depends in turn on how psychopathy is defined and understood, both by those assessing it, and those who use such assessments for decision-making. This chapter considers key definitional issues, before examining psychopathy's relevance to the criminal justice system, including to risk assessment and recidivism prediction, and treatment prognosis. The chapter concludes with a discussion of some of the ethical and practical issues that are emerging as research on the PCL scales continues to grow, alongside the development of newer purpose-designed measures, and finally closes with some points about psychopathy as a personality disorder.

D. L. L. Polaschek (✉)
Te Whare Wānanga o Waikato The University of Waikato, Hamilton, New Zealand
e-mail: polascde@waikato.ac.nz

J. E. Vitale (ed.), *The Complexity of Psychopathy*, Dangerous Behavior in Clinical and Forensic Psychology, https://doi.org/10.1007/978-3-030-83156-1_21

21.2 Defining Psychopathy

Psychopathy's modern history is usually anchored with reference to the work of Cleckley, who was intrigued by the way that people high in psychopathy could present—at least initially—in a positive, well-adjusted manner, while also clearly being psychologically maladjusted (Cleckley, 1988). The introduction of the first of Hare's Psychopathy Checklists in the 1980s[1] represented a major step forward in providing clear diagnostic criteria that have been welcomed and widely adopted, but also represented a significant departure from Cleckley's views. Lively debate continues on whether the nomological net (i.e., the concepts of interest) for psychopathy should include adaptive features such as those noted by Cleckley, or be limited to a more narrowly antisocial range of symptoms. According to one school of thought, these more adaptive features, typically referred to today under the labels "boldness" or "fearless dominance" are not only needed to be true to the complexity of Cleckley's early conceptualization of psychopathy, but also may help to explain inconsistent characteristics within and across people with psychopathy and to clarify relationships with key correlates of psychopathy (e.g., deficits in experiences of fear). They also have value for understanding psychopathy's relationship to maladaptive behavior, including offending, and therefore are relevant to the criminal justice system.

Patrick et al. (2009) proposed a Triarchic Model of Psychopathy, intended to capture the range of historic and contemporary conceptualizations. They proposed that psychopathy should be understood as the interaction between the construct of Disinhibition (i.e., externalizing psychopathology)—which is not unique to people high in psychopathy (Poythress et al., 2010a, b)—and one or both of Meanness, and Boldness (also referred to as Fearless Dominance, see the Psychopathic Personality Inventory-Revised; PPI-R; Lilienfeld & Widows, 2005). Disinhibition is associated with a variety of behavioral and emotional problems, including stress sensitivity, proneness to negative emotionality, a short-term focus on acting without sufficient affective or urge regulation, and socially deviant behavior (e.g., drug abuse; Patrick et al., 2012). Although common in people with offending histories, its relationship with negative emotionality, anxiety, and affective reactivity contradicts conceptualizations of what is known as primary psychopathy (i.e., coldblooded, calculating, affectively stable if shallow; Lilienfeld et al., 2012).

Boldness captures positive, potentially adaptive aspects of psychopathy such as resilience to stress, rapid recovery from threat, social poise and self-confidence (Patrick et al., 2009), and persuasiveness and dominance (Patrick & Drislane, 2015). It does not follow that everything about Boldness is positive. For example, Boldness has been found to be related to low Agreeableness from the Five Factor Model of

[1] Throughout the chapter "PCL" refers to one or more of the following: the Psychopathy Checklist Revised (PCL-R; [Hare, 1991; 2nd Edition: Hare, 2003]), the Psychopathy Checklist: Youth Version (PCL:YV; Forth et al. (2003)), the Psychopathy Checklist: Screening Version (PCL:SV; Hart et al. (1994)).

personality (Poy et al., 2014) and, in offenders, to self-absorbed exploitativeness, and feelings of superiority over others (Stanley et al., 2013). PPI-R Fearless Dominance predicted proactive aggression in a prisoner sample (Cima & Raine, 2009).

Finally, Meanness variously encompasses a willingness to predate on, exploit, and abuse others, with corresponding low empathy, dismissive orientation to attachment, and excitement seeking. Patrick et al. (2009) propose that Meanness and Boldness may be phenotypic expressions of a common underlying fearless genotype. The genotype's expression diverges in response to additional etiological components (e.g., parenting style, child abuse history; Moffitt et al., 1996; Odgers et al., 2008).

Lilienfeld et al. (2016) suggested we view psychopathy "as a compound trait, that is a *configuration* of largely uncorrelated attributes that combine to forge an interpersonally malignant condition…rather than a classical syndrome, that is, a constellation of signs and symptoms that covary across individuals" (p. 1174). Defining psychopathy in this non-unitary way helps to capture some of the variability in people who are high on disinhibition (Poythress et al., 2010a, b), and may accommodate people with high scores on the one of the Psychopathy Checklists who also show high negative emotionality (Sissons & Polaschek, 2018), and lack prominent characteristics of boldness (Daly, 2017). It facilitates the investigation of claims that psychopathy can be found in all walks of life (Neumann & Hare, 2008), in contrast to very low rates of psychopathy found in community samples using the PCL scales (e.g., < 1%, Coid et al., 2009; see also Hare, 2003; Neumann & Hare, 2008; Salekin et al., 2001). The argument that Boldness or Fearless Dominance—which are not strongly captured within the Psychopathy Checklists—should be regarded as peripheral or irrelevant to psychopathy because of minimal correlations with other factors is not necessarily a conceptual problem (Lilienfeld et al., 2012). Fearless Dominance on its own is not psychopathy, but neither is Disinhibition or Meanness (Lynam & Miller, 2019). Psychopathy arguably resides within people rather than measures; rather than existing as separate entities within people, components interact with each other to create a distinct personality style and behavior patterns. Boldness with disinhibition may be a very problematic combination when boldness alone is not.

Why is how we define psychopathy important? Because different definitions have fundamentally different purposes. Including Fearless Dominant or Boldness attributes in combination with dysfunctional characteristics associated with Disinhibition matches better the clinical descriptions of psychopathy, and psychopathy, as a type of personality disorder or psychopathology, is first a clinical, not criminological, construct.

The main alternative view of psychopathy, prevalent throughout the criminal justice system, is that it is simply a high score on one of the Psychopathy Checklists: most often the PCL-R. This problem of conflating measures with constructs is unusually prominent in this literature (Skeem et al., 2011). The PCL-R items and scoring have not been updated since publication 30 years ago (Hare, 1991; but see updated technical manual; Hare, 2003), which is also unusual for a psychometric instrument. Nevertheless, the PCL-R's dominance of research on psychopathy is profound, with between 900 and 1000 new research articles appearing in Google Scholar each of the last 5 years. Consequently, the PCL-R is often treated as if it *is* psychopathy rather than the most popular measure of it. Research with other measures is growing. Already, there is sufficient empirical evidence to show that different measurement scales—for instance, the PCL measures, and the Psychopathic Personality Inventory (PPI-R; Copestake et al., 2011; Hughes et al., 2013)—are not interchangeable in how they operationalize the construct and in their relationships with other variables. But most alternative scales are self-report, and it is unlikely that they will be accorded the status of a more comprehensive, clinician-rated instrument for important decisions. It is thus very important when talking about psychopathy to be clear about the definition and measure in use.

The PPI-R, along with the more recent Triarchic Psychopathy Measure (Patrick, 2010), can depict a more extroverted, less neurotic psychopathy, when compared to the meaner, more emotionally variable, more criminal characterization associated with the PCL-R (Skeem et al., 2011). Cleckley's psychopaths, based on recent systematic ratings of 15 of his case studies, were almost all judged to have low anxiety, with three-quarters also rated as relatively fearless. Few were particularly "callous, physically aggressive, or cruel" (Crego & Widiger, 2016, p. 84). Although the development of the PCL-R began with Cleckley's work as a starting point, the focus on measurement of criminals, the use of criminal behavior as evidence of criteria, and the absence of criteria that related to social adeptness and stress immunity have contributed to a meaner, and sometimes more distressed and neurotic portrayal of psychopathy. It is important to bear this picture in mind since it is the typical picture for a person with psychopathy in the criminal justice system.

Interestingly, even when psychopathy is defined as a high PCL-R score, it is still neither a unitary nor homogeneous disorder. The psychometric development of the 4 facets within the PCL-R has been valuable in this regard. There is a growing body of work calling for, or showing, the value of PCL-psychopathy analyses at the factor and facet level (Hare, 2016). More evidence is accumulating of divergent relationships between facets and external correlates, and even co-operative suppressor effects (Hicks et al., 2017). The PCL scales do not readily separate out high scoring people with and without significant negative emotionality, neuroticism, and anxiety. As a result, people with similar scores present quite variably in clinical correctional settings (Sissons & Polaschek, 2018), and require distinct strategies for engaging and motivating them to remain in treatment. It remains to be seen whether this facet-based research will add value to the use of the PCL scales in criminal justice work by better explaining meaningful variability between people. It may help to resolve confusing claims about people with high psychopathy scores being calculating yet impulsive, emotionally detached and shallow, yet filled with rage and bent on revenge (DeLisi, 2016).

Because this chapter is about the criminal justice system, much of the rest of it will focus on psychopathy as it is captured in higher scores on one of the PCL measures, which I refer to as *PCL-psychopathy* for clarity. I also use the term PCL to refer to any one or all of the PCL measures. We turn now to some important applications of PCL-psychopathy assessments to the criminal justice system.

21.3 PCL-Psychopathy as a Predictor of Risk of Recidivism

Even though psychopathy is a disorder of personality and the PCL-R was not designed to be a risk assessment measure (Hare, 2016), the main use of PCL-psychopathy assessment in the criminal justice system is to make judgements about future risk of crime, and in particular, it is the most often used measure of violence risk (alongside the HCR-20; Hurducas et al., 2014). In North America, "a formal assessment of psychopathy is an important component of a comprehensive psychological risk assessment" (Olver & Wong, 2019, p. 666); a view that is consistent with apparent growth in its use in addressing legal questions over the last decade (DeMatteo et al., 2016).

Risk assessment is an essential task in the criminal justice system, as in many other arenas. It informs decisions from the point of arrest through to release from custody or sentence discharge, or post-custody civil commitment. It can affect whether a person is remanded in custody or on bail, the level of institutional security, prison visiting conditions, home and work release program eligibility, and community sentencing conditions. In countries such as the US, it may also affect whether a young person is tried as an adult, and whether the death penalty is imposed.

Many studies have examined the predictive validity of PCL-psychopathy for any new reconviction, for sexual or violent recidivism, and for in-custody behavioral infractions. Olver and Wong (2019) identified 13 meta-analyses of this research. The largest of these comprises 19 studies with over 15,000 people. It found that Factor 1 scores are "a relatively weak and inconsistent predictor of recidivism" (Leistico et al., 2008, p. 668), with Factor 2 typically more predictive, and sometimes significantly more so. Other meta-analyses have found a similar pattern (Hawes et al., 2013; Hemphill et al., 1998; Salekin et al., 1996; Singh et al., 2011; Yang et al., 2010).

PCL Factor 1 best represents the core personality traits of psychopathy, while Factor 2 represents behavioral or social deviance aspects that are common among offenders (i.e., not unique to psychopathy). These findings suggest that the predictive accuracy of the PCL scales is driven largely by items that are not unique to psychopathy, meaning the success of the PCL scales as risk instruments comes mainly from their ability to capture predictive characteristics that are shared with (other) purpose-built static risk assessment measures. Studies that compare the PCL measures with other types of risk assessment find that for general recidivism, they perform about equivalently to risk assessment measures (Kroner et al., 2005; Olver et al., 2009).

The PCL-R has shown predictive validity with institutional infractions, both violent and non-violent. Again, most often Factor 2 has been found to be more predictive; But for institutional behavior Factor 1 has also demonstrated predictive validity (Guy et al., 2005; Leistico et al., 2008; Walters, 2003). Overall, the results suggest that PCL Factor 1 can be predictive of some behaviors or outcomes that are psycholegally relevant. However, how and when these associations are relevant to deciding psycho-legal matters requires more research.

Some quite strong claims have been made about the importance of psychopathy in the prediction of violence (e.g., Hare, 2003; Reidy et al., 2013). Several studies have compared the predictive performance of the PCL scales against other measures, including newer instruments designed specifically for the assessment of violence risk. Singh et al. (2011) compared nine risk assessment instruments across nearly 26,000 participants, based on studies published since the mid-1990s. The PCL-R had the lowest predictive validity (Median AUC = .66), with violence-specific instruments generally yielding better results. Unfortunately, these authors did not break down results for the PCL-R by factors or facets. The authors concluded that there were "substantial differences between the predictive validity of these tools" (Singh et al., 2011, p. 509). A second meta-analysis by Yang et al. (2010) compared nine scales on the prediction of violence, based on 28 research reports published in the decade from 1999, and again found approximately equal and moderate predictive validity across the instruments. The exception was PCL-R Factor 1, which performed no better than chance.

The final aspect of risk prediction is whether PCL-psychopathy predicts "psychopathic" violence, a term used by some writers to refer to any violence committed by people with high PCL-psychopathy scores (Reidy et al., 2013; Walsh, 1999), and by others to indicate a type of violence distinct to high levels of psychopathy (see Hare, 2003, for a review). Such a term could be taken by lay people to convey that there is something especially "psychopathic" (e.g., unusually "coldblooded") about this violence (Hare, 1996). In research that has set out to test this idea, instrumental violence—a form of violence in which the behavior is directed toward utilitarian goals, may appear planned, and is usually not substantially driven by emotional dysregulation—is seen as a proxy for this potentially unique form of psychopathic violence. For example, Woodworth and Porter (2002) predicted and found that most of the homicides committed by a sample of male prisoners with PCL-R scores over 29 were primarily instrumental. However, half of the non-psychopaths also committed primarily instrumental homicides, suggesting instrumental homicides were not that distinctive to high-PCL scorers. A recent meta-analysis concluded that there was a lack of support for the idea that psychopathy was associated with instrumental more than reactive violence (Blais et al., 2014).

More recent research has continued to confirm that future violence, including serious violence in the first 90 days after release from prison, aggressive prison infractions, and future violence convictions, is predicted best by PCL-R Factor 2, rather than Factor 1 (Camp et al., 2013; Kennealy et al., 2010). Given an apparent lack of evidence (a) that there is a unique type of violence associated with psychopathy, and (b) that violence is predicted better by the less distinctively psychopathic Factor 2, a narrower definition of "psychopathic violence" and more convincing empirical evidence are needed to avoid giving the impression that a psychopathy assessment can provide more useful information about future violence than can a specific risk measure for violence.

The predictive ability of the PCL-R with sexual offending has been examined separately from crime and other types of violence. A recent comprehensive meta-analysis showed that PCL-R total scores, Factor 2 scores, and antisocial facet scores predicted sexual reconviction moderately strongly, whereas Factor 1, its facets and the lifestyle facet of Factor 2 were all non-significant predictors (Hawes et al., 2013). Importantly, the Hawes meta-analysis also found a large increase in the likelihood of sexual recidivism in men with high levels of both sexual deviance and psychopathy.

To summarize, PCL-psychopathy scores have predictive validity with regard to new convictions—violent and any—and institutional behavior. However, as there is limited evidence that Factor 1 scores make a statistically meaningful contribution over Factor 2 and its facets in the prediction of violence and crime, there is no case for arguing that psychopathy makes a unique contribution over risk assessments that do not also set out to diagnose psychopathy (see Skeem et al., 2011, for a more detailed review). Nevertheless, some scholars have interpreted findings that PCL-psychopathy is a moderate predictor of crime to suggest that psychopathy is the mental disorder that *causes* criminal propensity. I consider this idea next.

21.4 Does Psychopathy Explain Crime and Violence?

While in the clinical forensic literature considerable debate is ongoing about how best to understand the definition and measurement of psychopathy and its relationship to criminal propensity, on a somewhat parallel track, developmental and lifestyle criminology (DLC) theories have developed, along with important longitudinal studies that test aspects of these theories (Farrington, 2015). These theories explicitly capture individual heterogeneity in the sources of criminal propensity by measuring and investigating longitudinally the contribution of a wide range of variables from the person and their environment to long term criminal propensity (Farrington, 2003).

Farrington (2005), a leading researcher in this area, concluded "there needs to be more integration of the psychopathy literature and the main stream literature on delinquency and crime" (p. 494). This is a fruitful idea, and Farrington and colleagues have pursued it, particularly with reference to understanding child and adolescent psychopathy, and its development (e.g., Farrington et al., 2010). Research from the Dunedin longitudinal study (Moffitt et al., 1996; Moffitt et al., 2002) on early-onset, chronic offenders—or life-course-persistent (LCP) offenders as Moffitt (1993) termed them—entering adulthood also refers to the development of psychopathic personality characteristics, but used the term interchangeably with antisocial personality disorder.

Fox et al. (2015) recently outlined some ways in which they saw psychopathy as being useful in DLC theories, although their definition of psychopathy was also not entirely clear.[2] They argued that incorporating psychopathy into DLC theories might

[2] Fox et al. (2015; p. 276) referred to "the original psychopathy clinical construct", but appeared to mean PCL-psychopathy scores rather than Cleckley's original work.

account for some part of the unexplained variance in research findings based on these theories. For example, they suggested that "there is clear opportunity to integrate psychopathy into Moffitt's taxonomy, particularly in the describing the origins and behaviors of LCP offenders" (p. 284). This is a more problematic form of DLC-psychopathy integration, because it would appear to be at more risk of tautology. Research currently traces the origins of LCP offending at least back to birth, making it difficult to see how psychopathy, a disorder that at best is not diagnosable until later in childhood at the earliest, could be causal in the LCP pathway. Furthermore, diagnosing psychopathy without predictor-criterion contamination is also problematic when it becomes a causal factor in development, rather than the result of other causal processes.

DeLisi (2016) has gone farther, to propose psychopathy as a theory in its own right; as a "unified theory of crime". DeLisi (2019) suggested that psychopathy had exceptional explanatory power with regard to antisocial behavior from childhood onwards, despite the tautology issue described above. More recently, he wrote "Perhaps rivalled by no criminological theory but self-control theory (Gottfredson & Hirschi, 1990), the theory of psychopathy provides the instantiation of the antisocial person" (2019, p. 5). Yet DeLisi (2016) also recognized that psychopathy is "multifaceted" and described it as a "syndrome". While DeLisi has marshalled and critiqued an impressive array of relevant research showing overlap between features of psychopathy and risk factors for crime, it is notable that much of what he reviews is as much concerned with the ongoing efforts to understand what psychopathy is, as it is with how psychopathy can explain crime.

Walters (2004) has critiqued the idea of psychopathy as a general theory of crime, mainly based on the PCL-R. He noted that while it was a parsimonious and fruitful concept, it was otherwise weak on epistemic criteria for evaluating a good theory. However, he did not rule out the value of psychopathy as a part of the development of an effective theory of crime. Even though it may not be particularly helpful in deciphering the mysteries of crime, the psychopathy concept can be of assistance in identifying the qualities of a good general theory of crime by its own omissions and limitations (Walters, 2004).

Psychopathy is not in itself a theory. It is a concept, or construct, or diagnosis. Correctly labelling someone as having the essential characteristics of a concept or construct, or as meeting diagnostic criteria for a particular mental disorder does not automatically clarify etiology. For psychopathy to be a theory, at a minimum labelling someone as psychopathic needs to confer some form of explanatory advantage with regard to the etiology of crime over not labelling them. But the etiology of psychopathy itself remains unclear (Auty, 2019; Farrington, 2018), as is usually the case with syndromes. At this stage, multiple etiological pathways are likely, given the range of putative mechanisms under investigation (see Patrick, 2018). It is difficult to see how a disorder with no clear etiology can serve to explain phenomena as complex and variable as crime commission and criminal career trajectories.

21.5 Psychopathy and Treatability

In Cleckley's time, there were no empirically validated psychological treatments that were effective in reducing either psychopathic personality characteristics, or even the tendency toward antisocial behavior, leading Cleckley (1988) and his contemporaries to a pessimistic view of treatability. Treatments used were predominantly unstructured insight-oriented talking therapies (Salekin, 2002), and would also not have been effective in reducing criminal risk in offenders more generally (Polaschek, 2014; Polaschek & Daly, 2013), given what is now known about what works and does not work in the treatment of recidivism risk (Bonta & Andrews, 2016). If a number of people do not respond to an offered treatment by progressing as expected, the treatment itself may be subject to scrutiny. If people with certain characteristics in common seem not to respond to *any* of our best attempts at effective treatment, then the clients themselves can become the object of our scrutiny; They may be judged untreatable. Nevertheless, an individual's treatability or amenability to treatment is best understood in interaction with the effectiveness of the available treatments.

21.6 Reducing Recidivism Risk Through Treatment

In recent years, progress has been made with regard to how we think about the treatability of psychopathy by asking the question in a slightly different way: to what extent can the criminal propensity of people who score highly on PCL-psychopathy be altered through treatment? In order to address this question, we first need to understand what works to alter criminal recidivism risk more generally in offenders, before applying this understanding to people in treatment who have high PCL-psychopathy. The relevant research first examines whether treatment appears to reduce their expected recidivism, and second, whether they respond to treatment by making as much behavioural change as people who have lower PCL-psychopathy scores.

21.6.1 Risk-Reducing Interventions for Offenders

A growing body of scientific evidence over 40 years serves to guide decisions about the types of services and interventions that reduce recidivism in a number of criminal justice systems. Often referred to as the "what works" research (Craig et al., 2013), and organized into a variety of principles that form the spokes of an umbrella framework known as the Risk-Need-Responsivity (RNR) model, these studies and their associated meta-analyses guide assessment and intervention with people engaged in repetitive criminal behavior (Polaschek, 2020). Although highly psychological in nature, the approach differs considerably from conventional clinical psychology, given the limited role for diagnosis and treatment of mental disorders in the reduction of criminal risk (Bonta et al., 2014). Consequently, the factors associated with ongoing offending are much better understood than previously, leading to more confidence about treatability of entrenched criminality. Cognitive–behavioral group-based interventions that focus on these factors have become popular, but many other types of interventions have also shown effectiveness (Bonta & Andrews, 2016; McGuire, 2002).

The most important components of this approach are that (a) the impact of tertiary prevention (i.e., reducing crime in identified criminals) will be maximized if we reserve treatment resources and human service for those who are at higher risk of recidivism, and then provide them with relatively intensive assistance (the *risk* principle); (b) the majority of time in intervention is directed at reducing the influence of potentially changeable correlates of recidivism: particularly such factors as antisocial peers and beliefs, antisocial temperamental factors such as emotional volatility and impulsivity, alcohol and drug use, poor school, work, and family functioning and aimless use of leisure/recreation time (the *need* principle); (c) maximizing the use of behavioral and social learning principles that are effective in influencing people to make change (the *general* part of the responsivity principle, and (d) providing interventions and services that fit with what engages the person best in change, and minimize obstacles to their engagement such as difficulties with cognitive functioning, mental illness, and language or hearing impairments (the *specific* part of the responsivity principle; Bonta & Andrews, 2016).

Of these first three core RNR principles (Risk, Need, Responsivity), the number that a program adheres to is associated with the size of recidivism reductions it achieves. The impact on crime for services addressing all three principles is modest but important, with reported effect sizes ranging from 0.15 to 0.34 (Andrews & Bonta, 2010). An effect size of .15 indicates that 15 people per 100 whose reconviction was predicted were not reconvicted. For example, if 57.5% of untreated offenders were reconvicted during follow-up, the corresponding rate for treated offenders would be 42.5%: a relative reduction in this example of more than 25%.

Other important findings that are sometimes overlooked have to do with implementation integrity and staffing characteristics. Programs are more likely to lead to a reduction in recidivism if staff are trained and supervised in their practice, and if there is a documented manual for the intervention. Staff behavior is also predictive of recidivism reduction. Staff selected for their relationship skills (warm, empathic, collaborative, able to use humor effectively), and staff who show the timely and regular use of reinforcement to shape desired behavior, and occasional disapproval for undesirable behavior, who teach program participants relevant skills, use authority effectively, and engage in advocacy and brokerage are also associated with risk-reducing interventions (Bonta & Andrews, 2016). In this approach, when offenders in treatment behave in ways that challenge engagement and change – and if higher-risk clients have been chosen, they usually will – effective therapists endeavor to work *with* the difficult characteristics (e.g., lack of attention or interest, hostility, poor compliance) rather than taking them as indicators that the client is not suitable for treatment. This tendency to regard treatment-disrupting behavior as expected and not insurmountable is important because a number of these same characteristics that disrupt the process of treatment also contribute to offense risk, making them more prominent in the very clients who are the highest priority for treatment, according to the risk principle (see also Skeem & Polaschek, 2020).

21.6.2 Treatment, PCL-Psychopathy and Recidivism Outcomes

This evidence on how to reduce criminal risk in people with the most extensive criminal histories becomes relevant to psychopathy because the very clients that the risk principle directs us to prioritize for treatment almost inevitably have high PCL-psychopathy scores. This is what we would expect given that the PCL-R predicts recidivism. For example, in New Zealand, intensive intervention programs housed in dedicated prison units are provided for men with an estimated likelihood of returning to prison of 70% or higher within 5 years, and with conviction histories on average of around 40 convictions including 5 for violence. Repeated quasi-experimental evaluations of these programs show that they are effective in reducing recidivism (e.g., Polaschek, 2011; Polaschek et al., 2005; Polaschek et al., 2016). Previous research established that the average score for attendees at one of these units was around the cut-off for psychopathy (18 on the PCL:SV; Daly, 2017). PCL:SV scores were also found to be unrelated to violent reconviction ($r = .05$; Polaschek, 2008). In other words, these programs routinely work with people with significant psychopathic features to achieve improvements in crime-related behavior.

Wong et al. (2012) matched a treatment sample of offenders with PCL–R scores greater than 25 who undertook and completed the Aggressive Behavior Control (ABC) program in the Regional Psychiatric Centre (RPC) in Saskatoon, Saskatchewan (see Wong & Gordon, 2013, for a full description of the treatment model) with a matched no-treatment control group. PCL–R total scores were matched, along with Factor 1 and Factor 2 scores, age of first conviction, and ethnicity. However, matched pairs could only be established for 32 of over 500 original cases, and the mean follow-up time was not reported. On 11 distinct recidivism outcomes, no significant differences were found, with a rate of any reconviction of 94% for each group, and statistically equivalent violent reconviction proportions (81.3% treated, 84.4% matched untreated). Most of the mean results favored the treatment group, but considerable within-group variability was evident. In additional analyses based on sentence length indices, treated men had better outcomes than the comparisons for all 7, with 3 attaining statistical significance: longest sentence given during the follow-up, the longest aggregated sentence given, and the sum of aggregate sentences given (Wong et al., 2012). Overall, this study lacked statistical power, providing at best, tentative evidence of improved outcomes for treated participants.

Two other quasi-experimental studies suggest that treatment can reduce the risk of criminal behavior in PCL- high-scoring people. The first was a study of civil psychiatric patients released into the community which found that high PCL-psychopathy people who attended fewer than six sessions of "psychiatric treatment as usual" (mostly psychotherapy and medication) were 3.5 times more likely to commit a violent act in the following 10 weeks than those who attended more than six sessions. PCL-R score did not moderate the effect of treatment. The extent to which services would align with the RNR model discussed earlier is not clear.

The second was a rigorous study evaluating the effects of a unique program: the Mendota Juvenile Treatment Center (MJTC) in Madison, Wisconsin. The MJTC operates as a secure hospital for the most difficult youth offenders in the state (Caldwell & Van Rybroek, 2005). The diverse team of specialists provides individualized interventions to youth in residence according to need, including "tutoring and educational services, group and individual counselling, psychopharmacological interventions, and family therapy" (Caldwell & van Rybroek, 2013, p. 574). While in the center, the day-to-day behavior of residents is monitored by trained ward staff and others (Caldwell et al., 2007). Within this program, adolescents earn privileges following relatively short periods of improved behavior; effectively it is a well-implemented contingency management program that provides incentives for compliance with unit operations and engagement in treatment (Caldwell et al., 2007). Behavioral ratings are also indicators of progress on criminal behavior-related treatment goals and have served as a dependent variable in MJTC research.

A propensity score-matched sample of comparison youth referred from two secure correctional facilities to the MJTC for assessment, stabilization, and then return to the original facility was compared on recidivism outcomes with a sample retained at the MJTC for treatment because of poor adjustment at the original facility. Matching for likelihood of retention for treatment was determined using 21 assessment variables. The two samples were equivalent on PCL:YV scores (means were 32.8 and 32.6 for the treatment and comparison youths respectively). Over a mean of 53 months of community follow-up, there were clear differences in favor of the treated boys. Comparison group members had more than twice as many new charges for offenses, twice the rate of felony arrests, and more than three times as many violent convictions (Caldwell et al., 2006b). Furthermore, PCL: YV scores were unrelated to outcome, suggesting that the differences resulted from some form of behavior change that was more prognostic than the scores for psychopathy.

It is encouraging that studies suggest that effective treatment to reduce criminal risk may be possible in people with high PCL-psychopathy, but the evidence remains scant. Given the importance of this issue to decision-making in the criminal justice system, more investment in research to evaluate programs running in other jurisdictions, more experimental programs (e.g., Kemp & Baskin-Sommers, 2019), and randomized controlled trials of standardized programs are needed (Hecht et al., 2018).

21.6.3 PCL-Psychopathy and Change in Treatment

Measures of progress in treatment need to be predictive of recidivism if they are to represent a test of the Need principle: the assertion that working to change changeable risk factors in treatment (also known as criminogenic needs in the RNR model), variable risk factors (Polaschek & Skeem, 2018), and dynamic risk factors (Wong & Gordon, 2006) will lead to changes in expected vs. actual recidivism. Two studies have linked change in treatment for people with high psychopathy scores to recidivism. This research has used either the Violence Risk Scale (VRS; Wong & Gordon, 2016) or the Violence Risk Scale: Sex Offender version (VRS: SO; Wong et al., 2003). These scales contain multiple items based on putatively changeable risk factors (e.g., criminal peers, impulsivity, sexual compulsivity, interpersonal aggression, emotional control, substance abuse linked to offending), and are rated by clinicians or other staff working with the client, based on as wide a range of information as possible on the person's behavior and its function. Distinctive to these measures is that change is derived from progress between measurement occasions on a modified version of the Transtheoretical Model of Change (Prochaska et al., 1992), applied to each risk factor with a score high enough to warrant attention in treatment. Unlike most instruments which are fully re-administered at each measurement time, here the amount of movement between stages on a scale from Precontemplation to Maintenance is subtracted from the overall score to indicate treatment progress and reduced recidivism risk (Wong & Gordon, 2016).

In an intensive high-risk sex offender program at the Saskatchewan Regional Psychiatric Centre in Canada, high PCL-R-scoring men were assessed over the course of treatment to have made measurable progress on the VRS- SO's risk-related treatment targets (Olver & Wong, 2009). More risk-reducing change was associated with a reduction in the likelihood of being reconvicted of sexual and violent offenses. A second study from this research group focused on serious high-risk violent offenders (PCL-R $M = 26$). Paralleling results from the earlier study of sex offenders, the more that these predominantly psychopathic offenders changed in VRS risk factors over treatment, the less likely they were to be reconvicted for violent offenses (Lewis et al., 2013). Using the same sample, Olver et al. (2013) found that the amount of change on the VRS for these high-risk violent offenders was correlated significantly with three of the four facets of the PCL–R (range − .15 to −.26, ns correlation for Lifestyle facet). But when both factors were analyzed together, only Factor 1 and the affective facet of Factor 1 (when all four facets were analyzed together) uniquely contributed to the prediction of VRS change.

These two studies tentatively suggest that high PCL-scoring people with a propensity toward serious crime and an extensive criminal history can make changes in a way that is similar to others on a scale like the VRS. Improvement was linked statistically to actual reductions in serious criminal outcomes, supporting both the Risk and Need principles. One obvious limitation of these studies is that there is no untreated comparison group; we therefore cannot be certain the change is a consequence of program attendance. But there is indirect evidence that reduced recidivism can be linked to the program itself in two outcome evaluations with untreated comparison groups included (Olver & Wong, 2013; Wong et al., 2012), although the untreated group was not assessed for change in VRS risk factors, so the nature and volume of change in each group remains unknown.

Even if they can change, are people with higher levels of psychopathy more resistant to change? Do psychopathic characteristics relate to how much change is made? A similar question is implicit in Bonta and Andrews' (2016) Risk principle: that although we should direct our best resources toward our higher risk cases, it will take more intensive effort all around to see the benefits of doing so. It might therefore follow that higher psychopathy may reduce the amount of change people make. Several studies address this issue.

A recent study with a similar population in New Zealand – high-risk psychopathic and violent offenders in a prison treatment program – found no evidence that PCL-psychopathy was related to change: non-significant correlations were obtained between the PCL: SV total score, or any of the four facets or two factors, and VRS-rated change (*r*s. -02 to .13; Daly et al., 2017). However, the amount of change made in this program was lower than in the Canadian study (NZ mean VRS change = 3.8 *sd* = 2.6; vs. 4. 7, *sd* = 3.0; Olver et al., 2013). An alternative explanation for the divergent findings is that the Daly study used field ratings—dynamic risk data were collected prospectively by multiple therapists using interview and file information—whereas in Olver et al. (2013), dynamic risk data were collected retrospectively, mainly by one author using archival file information only. Sewell and Olver (2018) conducted similar analyses with treated sex offenders from the Clearwater program at the same Canadian facility. Based on PCL-R scores, they obtained correlations with VRS: SO change ranging from −.19 (Affective facet) and − .12 (Interpersonal facet) to −.04 and .04 for the Lifestyle and Antisocial facets respectively, with only the Lifestyle facet uniquely predictive in multivariate predictive analyses with all 4 facets.

So, there is a mixed picture of the relationship between PCL-psychopathy and treatment change. More investigation is needed, especially of how the individual factors and facets are associated with both "treatment-interfering" behavior and change (Thornton & Blud, 2007; Wong, 2013; Wong & Hare, 2005). Relatedly, both Olver et al. (2013) and Sewell and Olver (2018) provide evidence that even among those with high PCL scores, there is important variation in who benefits from treatment that we do not yet understand. In both of these studies, there were high-PCL treatment completers whose recidivism outcomes were similar, or even perhaps better than some low-PCL-scoring completers, in cases where the high scorers were rated as having made more than the median amount of change. That people with high PCL-R scores can make change in treatment that reduces their recidivism should be all the stimulus we need to continue researching this important area.

21.7 Treatability of Psychopathy

It is important to distinguish the treatment of psychopathy as a personality disorder from enhancing desistance and reducing criminal orientation of people who currently score highly on PCL-psychopathy. The treatment focus for the personality disorder assumes that characteristics typical of Factor 1 of the PCL measures may also be targeted for change, and therefore more directly linked to criminal risk. By contrast, it is common in the criminal justice field to regard the reduction of recidivism in people with high PCL-R scores as being the treatment of psychopathy and even to center treatment recommendations around the psychometric structure of the PCL. For example, Wong et al. (2012) proposed that PCL factor 1 items are indicators of treatment-challenging behavior and should be monitored and managed, while Factor 2 items are targeted through risk-reducing treatment. This is certainly a useful rubric. Treating people with high PCL scores to reduce their risk of recidivism should have the most effect on Factor 2, but for clarity, it may be useful not to refer to this work as the treatment of psychopathy since it is neither seeks to, nor probably achieves, change on the characteristics most typical of psychopathy.

There is clear evidence to support the effectiveness of the approach proposed by Wong et al. (2012), but studies of whether core psychopathy symptoms (e.g., grandiosity, meanness, superficiality) can be reduced in treatment are difficult to find. Studies included in Salekin's (2002) review of therapy for psychopathy used inconsistent or undocumented diagnostic criteria, and evaluated effectiveness across a wide range of symptoms and other outcomes. A more recent review also did not identify any studies that purported to have altered symptoms of psychopathy per se (Salekin et al., 2010). The predominance of diagnosis based on the PCL-psychopathy scales—which are not suited to capturing symptom *change*—and the dearth of recent studies that purport to treat the personality disorder of psychopathy means that successful psychopathy treatments have not yet been identified[3] (Hecht et al., 2018).

The related research literature on symptom amelioration or attenuation and improvements in psychosocial functioning of the DSM-IV Cluster B personality disorders also remains sparse. There is some evidence for positive treatment effects, based on measures of symptom reduction and psychosocial functioning (e.g., Bartak et al., 2011; Vermote et al., 2010) but few controlled studies. Although gains can be demonstrated, effective treatment is expensive, intensive, and requires considerable staff training and skill (Bateman et al., 2015). This is a similar picture to the treatment of psychopathy.

[3] In New Zealand, correctional practice with the PCL:SV has been described as a potential model for training and use (R. D. Hare, personal communication with D. Riley, 31 October 2003). After a 3-day training workshop, registered (i.e., licensed) psychologists complete a number of assessments that include PCL:SVs under supervision (i.e., they are reviewed by the primary trainer and feedback is given). All PCL assessments that go to court are also reviewed by the trainer (N. Wilson) and this been the practice now for over 20 years. The use of an evidence recording sheet enables the reviewer to evaluate both the quality of the information recorded and the accuracy of the resulting scoring.

21.8 Specific Psycho-Legal Uses of the PCL-Psychopathy Measures

That measures of psychopathy—particularly the PCL scales—serve the dual purpose of both identifying or screening for the clinical disorder of psychopathy and providing a risk estimate for various outcomes of relevance to the criminal justice system likely accounts for their popularity with mental health clinicians undertaking assessments in criminal and civil cases with adults or young people. The use of the PCL scales in US psycho-legal contexts has been growing for some time (DeMatteo et al., 2010). Use has most often been in support of the prosecution side, or the court itself. Use is also growing in Europe (DeMatteo et al., 2019). By contrast, in New Zealand, PCL-psychopathy is seldom used in civil or criminal determinations (N. J. Wilson, personal communication, 21 October 2019).

Much of the research on psycho-legal uses comes from the US (DeMatteo et al., 2014), where the PCL measures are in use in a range of contexts to assist decision-makers, including "sexually violent predator (SVP) commitment, juvenile transfer decisions [e.g., to adult court], capital sentencing, general sentencing, mental state at the time of the offense, and determination of future dangerousness [e.g.., parole]" (DeMatteo et al., 2016, p. 207), as well as response to treatment that might reduce risk (Viljoen et al., 2010). Various pieces of legislation or policy actually require its use (e.g., for SVP commitment in Texas; DeMatteo et al., 2014).

There are several important issues to consider in using a PCL scale to assess and provide expert testimony. In addition to establishing whether the assessment results have predictive validity in the particular setting (i.e., its probative value), it is also important to consider whether its use, and the resulting perceptions of the offender as psychopathic or not, will result in biased decisions, because of stereotypes or stigma associated with the term (Edens et al., 2018). DeMatteo et al. (2016) have reviewed several more common uses of PCL-psychopathy evidence, weighing the empirical support for use in the particular context against the potential for prejudice to be introduced, and reached some conclusions about whether the evidence then meets standards for admissibility- a question they suggest is rarely asked. Collectively, the main uses of the PCL involve decisions about whether to detain people for longer periods, or in harsher conditions, or to execute them. Implicitly or explicitly, these types of deliberations assume that the people under consideration will also be unlikely to respond to treatment or otherwise reduce their dangerousness in the foreseeable future (Edens et al., 2018). We review each of these most common contexts for PCL use in the next sections.

21.8.1 Transfer of Young People to Adult Court for Trial

DeMatteo et al. (2016) suggest that the process by which juvenile court judges decide to retain young people in their own court or transfer them to adult court (i.e., judicial transfer) is the most relevant to admissibility issues because it relies on the judge's discretion in how to apply rules of evidence. Of the various factors that judges evaluate to make such decisions, risk assessment and treatment amenability are the most relevant in regard to the use of the PCL scales (DeMatteo et al., 2016). The first use but not the second is supported by evidence.

The PCL:YV predicts recidivism of any type, and violent recidivism with small to moderate effects, but has been found to be a non-significant predictor of sexual recidivism in young people (Olver et al., 2009). Studies of treatment amenability are fewer, but as with adults, tend to show that youth will be more challenging to treat if they have high PCL:YV scores (Polaschek & Skeem, 2018; Viljoen et al., 2010). However, the positive results from the Mendota Juvenile Treatment Center research (Caldwell et al., 2006a) suggest that it is too soon to conclude that these youth do not respond to treatment.

21.8.2 Death-Penalty-Related Sentencing

In some countries and jurisdictions, the death penalty is available as a sentencing option, particularly for some forms of homicide ("capital cases"). DeMatteo et al. (2016) report that the PCL-R has been used both by the prosecution as evidence that the alleged offender has been malingering in a proposed insanity defense, and in sentencing, for judgements about future dangerousness. But few studies have examined the relationship between malingering and PCL-psychopathy, although DeMatteo et al. (2016) concluded there was sufficient evidence to support its use to refute the defense of insanity. Although psychopathy may increase the likelihood of malingering, it does not serve to definitively diagnose it. Other relevant evidence concerning the possibility that psychopathy is incompatible with mental disorder has seldom been discussed.

With regard to assessment of dangerousness, future danger to others is considered an aggravating factor for capital sentencing in some US states (DeMatteo et al., 2016). The PCL-R has been used for these assessments, notwithstanding the lack of clarity about what constitutes "dangerousness", and the wider issues associated with its use for violence assessments noted above.

21.8.3 Civil Detention Through Designation as a Sexually Violent Predator

DeMatteo et al. (2014) found that these types of hearings represented the most frequent use of the PCL scales in legal proceedings. Although treatability is supposed to be an important component of these determinations, the main focus is typically "dangerousness" (Olver, 2019). DeMatteo et al. (2016) concluded, after reviewing the evidence from 3 studies, that the PCL could validly be used to predict long term sexual recidivism. The case for its use with short-term sexual recidivism (<10 years) was judged less compelling, suggesting it should not be used for this purpose. Olver (2019) also notes that it is a much more modest predictor than for other types of recidivism, but notes that it becomes relevant in risk assessment when high PCL-psychopathy scores co-exist with documented sexual deviance (see also Hawes et al., 2013).

21.8.4 Assessment of Treatment Amenability

In the literature on using PCL measures to assess treatment amenability, the purpose of such assessments is usually opaque. Is it being used to make judgements about whether a person's assessed dangerousness will be able to be reduced through engagement in treatment? If so, there is no evidence at this point that PCL-psychopathy scores are useful for this purpose. For instance, people with high PCL scores can reduce their risk of recidivism in response to treatment. In fact, the research reviewed earlier suggests that those with higher scores should be prioritized by criminal justice systems for treatments that are intended to reduce recidivism risk.

On the other hand, there is tentative evidence that although people with high PCL scores can respond to treatment by making as much change as those with low scores, on average, higher scoring people are more challenging to work with and make less change than people with lower scores. In other words, this "averaged" result conceals heterogeneity in treatment response among high-PCL-scoring people (Lewis et al., 2013; Sewell & Olver, 2018). But even if this research is replicated successfully, there is still no current method of determining which high scorers may or may not respond. There is no valid way of making these determinations at the point of sentencing. As Edens et al. (2018) suggest, at this stage "the degree to which psychopathy is in fact amenable to intervention remains an area of open inquiry" (p. 738).

21.8.5 Other Uses in Other Jurisdictions

It is likely that the PCL-psychopathy scales have been used in almost any circumstance where some form of risk assessment is needed, because of their predictive relationship to recidivism. For example, the PCL-R may be used in parole decisions (e.g., in California where its inclusion in assessment is now required for parole consideration; Guy et al., 2015). In Canada, New Zealand and Australia, the PCL scales, among other instruments, may be used to provide relevant evidence for a variety of decisions based on legislation that allows for extended containment (e.g., longer sentences; indefinite sentences) for those deemed "too risky" (Edens et al., 2018; Glazebrook, 2010). Canada has "Dangerous Offender" legislation that allows for the indeterminate sentencing of people judged to be threatening to community safety in respect of violent or sexual behavior. The United Kingdom wrote it into the requirements for admission to a Dangerous and Severe Personality Disorder program (Kirkpatrick et al., 2010).

New Zealand has one of the highest imprisonment rates in the western world, higher than Western Europe, Australia, England and Wales, and much of Eastern Europe. Although international comparisons are methodologically challenging, New Zealand has been estimated to have the highest per capita imprisonment rate for sexual and violent offences (combined) of 33 countries (Boomen, 2018). These figures suggest there is no shortage of serious offenders coming through the criminal justice system. Yet New Zealand's uses for the PCL scales are quite different from the practices captured in US case law (e.g., DeMatteo et al., 2014). New Zealand no longer has the death penalty and there is also little incentive to use the PCL scales to make a case to transfer young people into adult court since all homicide cases are already referred there, and all other offences are tried in youth courts. All NZ Department of Corrections psychologists are trained in the use of the PCL-R and PCL:SV, and are typically one of two health assessors (the other is independent) in cases before the court for (a) Preventive Detention, an indefinite custodial sentence, with the potential for life parole, that may be imposed on a person who has just been convicted of a qualifying sexual or violent offence and where there is judged to be a significant, ongoing risk of reoffending; (b) Extended Supervision Orders, where a person finishing a finite prison sentence who is considered to be at high risk of sexual offending, or at very high risk of violent offending, can be subject to 10 years of formal supervision of varying intensity and restrictiveness to monitor and manage the person's long term risk to the community; and (c) Public Protection Orders (PPOs; [Public Safety (Public Protection Orders) Act 2014]), which are civil detention orders imposed by the Courts on people who are concluding a finite prison sentence, and are considered too high risk to manage on an Extended Supervision Order because of imminence and seriousness of violent or sexual offending risk. PPOs may be applied for either in the last 6 months of the prison sentence, or in the community for someone in the most intensive form of Extended Supervision Order, typically, on 24-h person-to-person monitoring.

New Zealand uses the PCL-R and PCL:SV typically as one of several instruments to provide a comprehensive basis for risk estimation. It is relatively rarely used for at least three reasons: (1) because of the availability of a more informative, New Zealand-based and therefore better validated automated actuarial assessment instrument (the RoC*RoI; Bakker et al., 1999); (2) because PCL assessments are time consuming, and (3) because New Zealand has largely avoided adopting the term "psychopath" in judicial and board decision-making, so that the diagnosis of psychopathy is not a salient part of such decisions. Even hearings with the most serious consequences (e.g., Public Protection Orders) only infrequently feature expert defense evidence that includes a PCL-R assessment, which means "most [Corrections] assessments go relatively unchallenged" (N. J. Wilson, personal communication, 21 October 2019). A PCL assessment may be used for high- or very high-risk sexual offenders, based on the research on the apparent synergistic effects of sexual deviance and psychopathy (J. Smith, personal communication, 8 November, 2019), and this use has been accepted in the NZ courts (Glazebrook, 2010).

21.9 Field Reliability and Validity

Use of the PCL scales for any decisions about a person's future rest on the assumption that the scales can be scored reliably. Data in the PCL manuals suggest that the PCL-R *can* be rated relatively consistently by two independent raters (Hare, 2003), which is a notable achievement for any measure that is based on extensive clinical material, and therefore requires more training and subjective judgement than simple static items such as "age at first conviction". But just because an instrument *can* be rated reliably does not mean that it will be in all circumstances, and of course inter-rater reliability doesn't mean by inference that absolute scores obtained are credible; some PCL assessors reliably give higher scores than others to those they are assessing (Boccaccini et al., 2008).

Ratings made in routine practice have become a recent focus of concern. It is not entirely clear what "routine practice" actually is, but it is likely to differ from the more rigorous procedures used in research in several important ways. First, there will usually only be one rater, or if more than one assessment is undertaken, it is unlikely that the assessors will confer to develop a more reliable score. Second, practices for evaluating and documenting the volume and quality of evidence collected for scoring are unknown and likely to be highly variable. Third, the training, skill, and experience of the assessor will be variable, as will the use of supervision or any ongoing quality assurance process. Fourth, in routine practice, the assessor will be undertaking an assessment for a specific purpose that may introduce conscious or unconscious biases into the assessment. Research investigating the reliability of "real world" ratings has grown in the last decade, and recent reviews note that there is substantial variability in reliability (DeMatteo et al., 2019; Edens et al., 2018), with poorer results in a range that is unacceptable for use (see also Edens et al., 2015; Jeandarme et al., 2017).

Furthermore, rating differences have been noted to be related to the perspective of counsel (i.e., prosecution vs. defense; Murrie et al., 2008; Murrie et al., 2009). Using experimental manipulations, these apparent allegiance effects have been shown to exist even when clinicians are randomly assigned to work with the "prosecution" or "defense" (Murrie et al., 2013). This experiment by Murrie et al. (2013) suggests that one source of error comes from clinicians' temporary allegiance to the side that retains the expert. Interestingly, the effect sizes for the difference between those "working" for the prosecution and defense in this experiment were similar in magnitude to those found in the Murrie et al. (2009) field study of actual practice.

Murrie et al. (2013) also examined whether there is error between raters in the opposite direction to what would be expected given the allocated allegiances (i.e., where scores were higher for those working for the defense than for those on the prosecution side). Large differences in the opposite direction were still well above what would be predicted, but not nearly as often as for allegiance-consistent differences. They found no evidence of more enduring personal differences in the two groups (defense vs. prosecution) based on opinion ratings of support for SVP-type policies, nor estimates of the typical PCL-R score for a sex offender with an adult or with a child victim, leaving open to future research a deeper understanding of what causes such effects.

Boccaccini et al. (2008) estimated that allegiance-based error accounted for about 20% of the variance in scores. But there are other potential sources of apparent bias, though only a few studies to date have examined these (Jeandarme et al., 2017). For example, the appearance of assessor allegiance effects may result from lawyers retaining those they perceive to be sympathetic to their side based on the assessor's previous work, or only taking forward assessments by those experts who provide the most favorable scores.

Other studies that include court- or board-appointed as well as defense and prosecution-retained experts provide evidence that differences are found even when allegiance should be to the triers of fact themselves (Edens et al., 2015; see also Lloyd et al., 2010). These results suggest other important sources of bias. One that Boccaccini et al.'s (2008) study suggested that can be separated from allegiance-based error comes from potentially stable scoring differences between evaluators. They reported this source as accounting for perhaps 30% of the variance in scores, which is not too far behind the 45% they attributed to differences between offenders themselves. In other words, these figures are based on differences between evaluators working for the same counsel, even though all were ostensibly employed by the court itself. One study found that more Agreeable assessors (assessed on the Neo-PI-R; Costa & McCrae, 1992) gave lower scores (Miller et al., 2011). Other pertinent findings come from a study that found that more experienced assessors produced lower scores (Murrie et al., 2013), and another that found that more experienced assessors' scores may be more predictive of reoffending (Boccaccini, 2017).

A few studies have examined relationships between score patterns and other types of contextual factors. Using determinations of "not guilty by reason of insanity" for patients residing in prisons or hospitals in Belgium, Jeandarme et al. (2017) hypothesized both that overall reliability would be lower than in the PCL-R manual, and that there would be systematic differences based on whether the person was assessed in prison or hospital. They expected that prison assessment scores might be lower—because lower scores facilitate transfers to hospital—and hospital scores would be higher because hospital staff are less experienced with psychopathic patients or because they have better patient alliances.

Scores from prisons were lower than those completed in hospital when compared for the same person. Jeandarme et al. (2017) also found considerable evidence of scoring unreliability, with almost half of scores having differences of more than two Standard Errors of Measurement (i.e., differing by more than 6 points on the PCL-R). Interestingly, predictive validity was also poor in this study, with Factor 1 and total PCL-R scores predicting neither general nor violent recidivism. Factor 2 scores predicted general recidivism and predicted violent recidivism when hospital and prison samples were combined.

Factor 1 scores, crucial to the diagnosis of psychopathy as a personality disorder, have been found to have poorer field reliability than Factor 2 scores (Miller et al., 2012). Miller et al. (2012) found that Facet 2 scores were also significantly less reliable than Facet 4, while Sturup et al. (2014) found Facet 4 was very reliable, compared to the other 3 facets. There are numerous reasons for why this pattern of findings might occur, including that the qualities of Factor 1 are harder to score with file data, or that information about them may be more likely to be missing and may vary more across interviews. Again, it is an area worthy of ongoing research.

Taken together, this emerging body of research should reduce confidence in current field use of the PCL scales. If practitioners are to continue to offer assessments based on these measures to those making any important decisions about another person's life, it is imperative that some forms of accreditation and quality assurance processes are developed and then tested for reliability and validity.

21.10 Generalizability Across Nations and Ethnicities

Given the preponderance of North American research on PCL-psychopathy, the extent to which findings apply across other jurisdictions and to other ethnicities is another factor in determining the PCL scales' suitability for psycho-legal use. If there are variations across nations and cultures, it becomes particularly important to validate the instrument in the culture in which it is to be used (Hare, 2003), rather than relying on generalizing from other research with an unknown relationship to the culture in question. There are at least two layers of relevant issues. First, do measures perform similarly across nations? For larger countries, within-nation variability may also be important. Not only do states or other smaller geographical units within large countries differ in their ethnic histories and composition, but they may also have different criminal justice systems: another potential source of variation in predictive accuracy.

Second, within nations there are complex ethnic differences that may have a bearing on the properties of PCL assessments. A third set of issues remains largely unaddressed but limits understanding of the first two- to what extent are findings of similarity or difference within or across nations influenced by the cultural capabilities and biases of the assessor? We turn now to research on these issues.

21.10.1 Comparability Across Nations in Mean Scores, Factor Structures, and Recidivism Prediction

Before examining whether there are differences in scores between racial and ethnic minorities and dominant groups, we need first to examine comparisons across nations. Much of this research is from countries that have European-originating (i.e., North American "white") majorities. There is a tendency to assume all "whites" are equivalent, regardless of nationality, but research suggests otherwise. As far back as the mid-1990s, Cooke (1998) had accumulated data from 16 studies of various nations in Europe with lower scores than in North American standardization samples. Although it is possible these results reflect some form of sampling bias, Cooke (1998) also suggested that they may indicate a reduced prevalence of psychopathy in these countries, or that the outward expression of PCL-psychopathy was somehow different in Europe. Cooke (1995) had already found in a study of prison violence in Scotland that using a cut off of 30 on the PCL-R resulted in only 3% of Scottish prisoners meeting criteria compared to 28% of North American prisoners (Hare, 1991), with mean scores of 13.8 vs. 23.6 respectively. Further analyses with these adult male prisoner samples found high congruence between Factor 1 and Factor 2, with similar amounts of variance explained across each sample, and similar internal reliability. Differences also did not appear to be due to under-rating in the UK (Cooke, 1998). Lastly, Cooke (1998) used Item Response Theory to compare the two sets of scores and concluded that in Scotland, some items (callous/lack of empathy, glibness/superficial charm) only become observable when the person being rated has a higher level of the underlying trait. Overall, regression analyses suggested a score of 25 in Scottish prisoners was equivalent to the 30 cut off in North America (Cooke, 1998). An explanation provided for these differences was that aspects of Scottish socialization may dampen down the overt expression of some Factor 1 qualities. However, the authors also suggested that reduced prevalence may be due to selective migration to bigger urban areas outside of Scotland (Cooke & Michie, 1999).

Since the completion of Cooke's work 20 years ago, there has been considerable expansion in the range of research outside of North America, allowing for more to be said about both national and ethnic differences. Research has continued to find that in non-North American samples, mean scores for prisoners are significantly lower. For example, 17 prisoner samples (n = 3063) yielded a mean of 18.1 (SD = 8.4; Fanti et al., 2018) compared to 22.1 (sd = 7.9) for North American prisoners (n = 5408; from Hare, 2003); a moderate effect size (d = .49). However, closer inspection reveals that lower scores come from British, Portuguese, German and Belgian samples, with those from Brazil, Finland, Norway and Spain being comparable to the US and Canada. Fanti et al. (2018) conclude there is insufficient consistent evidence to suggest that scores outside of North America should be adjusted. They speculate that differences in how prison and health systems identify and respond to mental disorder may be as important as (other) differences in culture (Fanti et al., 2018). Lower PCL scores may be found in systems where mentally disordered offenders are siphoned off into specialist forensic psychiatric facilities; a point previously made by Sullivan and Kosson (2006).

When first published, the PCL-R was described as having a correlated 2-factor structure, while more recently both 3-factor (with antisocial/criminal behavior removed; Cooke et al., 2001; Cooke & Michie, 2001) and 4-factor solutions (i.e. also called "facets"; e.g., Hare, 2003) have been tested and met satisfactory psychometric standards with North American samples, with high internal reliability and similar items loading on each factor across solutions. Samples from a range of European nations have also been used to test for generalizability of factor structure. In reviewing these findings, Fanti et al. (2018) concluded that there was evidence for "weak invariance for the PCL-R factor structure across cultures", but the evidence was "limited and somewhat inconsistent" (p. 537), which may in part be due to underpowered samples. More research in nations outside of Europe is also needed on this point.

Finally, investigations into recidivism prediction and relationships to criminal career characteristics suggest that PCL scale performance is broadly comparable across nations, based on adult prisoners, and less often, on forensic psychiatric patients. Studies from individual nations (e.g., Norway, Spain the UK, the Netherlands, Germany) suggest the PCL-R yields similar results to US research with few exceptions (Fanti et al., 2018).

21.10.2 Comparisons Across Ethnicities Within Nations

Turning now to distinct ethnicities within nations, a number of studies have compared African-American and European-American samples (e.g., Cooke et al., 2001). Fewer studies have examined other ethnicities either within North America, or within other nations where the PCL-psychopathy scales are used for determining psycho-legal outcomes. In western nations, some non-European ethnicities and indigenous people are much more prevalent in criminal justice systems than they are in the nation itself, and may also constitute a significant proportion of prisoners. For example, indigenous Australians—constituting a little over 3% of that nation's population—have been reported to be the world's most imprisoned people, at a 2015 per capita rate of 1356, higher than imprisoned African Americans, and twice the rate of NZ Māori (Anthony, 2017, June 6). If instruments are to be used to make decisions about overrepresented non-European and indigenous people, it is even more important that the instruments are at least as valid for these uses, and that their relative performance is well understood. One important aspect of relative performance is calibration. For example, a scale may be equally accurate in predicting recidivism for two ethnicities, while at the same time, rates of recidivism associated with a specific score may be much lower for one ethnicity than the other. This is the pattern of findings reported by Olver et al. (2018a, b), who, even though they found that relationships between PCL-R scores and recidivism were similar in strength for both indigenous and non-indigenous people, when they investigated predictive invariance at specific cut offs, higher rates of recidivism were found for indigenous people. This study, which combined four samples (total n = 1163) of adult men completing federal custodial sentences, found statistically significant differences on Factor 2, the Lifestyle and Antisocial Facets, and total PCL-R scores, with indigenous men scoring more highly, while non-indigenous men scored higher on the Interpersonal facet.

Research across cultures that suggests that the PCL scales can be used with people from a variety of countries has led to assumptions that they are also safe to use with populations on which they have not been specifically tested or designed. In the absence of specific validation studies, concern has been raised that these instruments may not be safe for use with indigenous peoples (Haag et al., 2016; Shepherd, 2016; Tamatea, 2017). To some extent, the concerns vary with the types of items and how they are scored, as well as with how the overall results are used. For example, imagine a static-item based risk assessment that is based entirely on criminal history "facts" and has been validated and calibrated with the particular population. Arguably such a measure carries somewhat less risk of mis-rating by individual assessors than one with items that require gathering and scoring clinical and social information, provided it is not then further subjectively interpreted (e.g., overridden by clinical intuition or by other scale scores that allow more room for subjectivity; Gardner et al., 2018). And such scales, when used actuarially, still implicitly support biases in criminal justice processing for ethnic minorities and indigenous people since they are calibrated on a system that may have these biases built into it (Eckhouse et al., 2019).

But instruments such as the PCL-R that require considerable interpretation of behavior, both recorded by others in files and from interviews conducted by assessors who vary in specific cultural competence may provide much more scope for biases in the scoring process that can be hard to detect. It is entirely plausible that the evidence that African-Americans are perceived by Americans of European origin as "more violent, aggressive and worthy of punishment than Whites" (Skeem et al., 2004, p. 509) may play a role in such an assessment. It is equally plausible outside of North America that a recent European immigrant to one country from another may have quite a different perception of the "aggressiveness" of a local indigenous person than one who grew up beside such people. Such a perception might result in giving a higher score than would otherwise be the case, leading to a higher estimate of risk.

The picture gets even more complicated if the understanding of the PCL-R is that it is capturing a personality disorder that causes crime. Relationships between culture, personality characteristics and their expression across settings are likely to be relevant to the scoring of PCL-psychopathy but, again, are very difficult to detect. Furthermore, research suggesting that there may be ethnic differences in correlates of psychopathy (e.g., processing of information in experimental tasks) also suggest the need for caution in understanding how ethnicity may affect PCL-scoring and what scores mean (see Fanti et al., 2018, for a review). The research suggests caution in the use of the PCL scales outside of North America, and especially with non-Europeans, unless validated with the population in question.

21.11 Potential for Stigmatization and Prejudiced Decision Making

I argued earlier that the assessment of psychopathy is not and should not be considered to be concordant with the assessment of risk. Justification for the preferential use of psychopathy measures for risk assessment requires firstly that the validity and reliability of PCL scales in risk estimation be established. It also necessitates that the choice of the PCL does not significantly distort the decision-maker's perception of the risk posed by the assessee, because of their own perception of risk deriving from the psychopathy label and assumed characteristics. In other words, a client who is assessed using the PCL-R should not be seen as more risky than an equivalent client assessed with another risk measure, simply because the first client's risk measure is also used to diagnose psychopathy.

The DeMatteo et al. (2016) review described earlier that considered both the usefulness and relevance of information on PCL-psychopathy for the trier of fact, also reached conclusions about whether the *label* of "psychopath" had been demonstrated to be prejudicial in the same context. DeMatteo et al. (2016) concluded, perhaps surprisingly, that there was no evidence that youth transfer decisions or sexually violent predator decisions were associated with a concerning level of prejudice in fact triers. In contrast, psychopathy labelling was associated with a greater likelihood of jurors perceiving a death penalty-eligible defendant as dangerous, and as suitable for the death penalty.

Research on the association between the label of "psychopath" and resulting decisions is addressing one type of labelling: specific labelling effects. A second type, however, is criterion effects (or "trait-related" effects), which are those resulting from the presence of particular symptoms of the disorder (e.g., callousness; Murrie et al. (2005), cited in DeMatteo et al., 2019). For example, Chauhan et al. (2007) used vignettes to show that undergraduate students thought the presence of typical Factor 1 traits was associated with greater dangerousness in youths, while clinicians saw the label of psychopathy itself to indicate less treatment amenability, and law students and judges showed no effects for either labels or traits.

A recent meta-analysis of 10 jury simulation studies may have gone some way to clarifying the importance of traits vs. labels. Kelley et al. (2019) observed that the confusing results in previous research may have been due to a failure to distinguish whether jurors' perceptions of the level of psychopathy pertaining to a particular defendant were due to the influence of mental health experts telling jurors about the defendant's level of PCL-psychopathy (the label) or to other sources of information that caused jurors to infer psychopathy in the defendant. Kelley et al. (2019) reasoned that weak differences between a control condition (i.e., no expert evidence on psychopathy provided) and a condition in which an expert gave evidence on psychopathy in some studies may have been due not to a lack of expert credibility, but to control jurors forming the view that the defendant was psychopathic on the basis of the other information they were given about the case. Using the affective and interpersonal characteristics that lay people rate as prototypical of psychopathy, they found that juror ratings of defendants as evil and dangerous were significantly related to perceptions of psychopathy, and these same perceptions predicted recommendations for capital sentences and for longer sentences. For the most part, it did not matter whether there was an expert providing evidence of psychopathy or not. There was also no effect on treatment amenability whether expert evidence was given or not.

Recall that the research reviewed earlier in this chapter—particularly research comparing the factors and facets of the PCL measures—indicates that these same affective and interpersonal characteristics of psychopathy are less related, and in some cases unrelated, to criminal risk. In other words, jurors use these less relevant characteristics of psychopathy to form perceptions of greater evil and dangerousness in a defendant, and to recommend or confer harsher sentences. These findings suggest that perceptions of psychopathy, whether generated by expert evidence, or other information, are themselves prejudicial for defendants.

In actual court processes, the picture may be even more complicated. There is some evidence that clinical evaluators themselves may be subject to similar prejudicial ideas. For example, in an experiment in which 108 doctoral-qualified forensic assessors completed PCL-Rs on up to 4 hypothetical cases, believing they were completing a genuine assessment in a sex offender civil commitment process, Gardner et al. (2018) found that Factor 1 accounted for 3 times as much variance in predicting clinicians' risk judgements as Factor 2. Relatedly, the Chauhan et al. (2007) study found that clinicians saw the label of psychopathy itself to indicate less treatment amenability. In juvenile justice, clinicians' perceptions of treatment amenability appeared to be less influenced by perceptions of psychopathic traits, but in young people with little history of antisocial behavior, a label of psychopathy was associated with increased risk ratings (Rocket et al., 2007).

This small collection of studies suggests, again, that further research will be important in order to understand the full effects of perceptions of psychopathy on risk judgements made by clinicians, including whether they affect PCL-psychopathy scoring itself. As with allegiance effects, if clinicians' perceptions of the client are another source of bias in their assessments, we need to know, and understand in turn whether these biases influence decision-makers' perceptions of dangerousness, treatment amenability, and other important applications.

21.12 Ethical and Practical Issues and Implications

These final sections of the chapter consider the ethical and practical issues and implications of the use of PCL measures and the construct of psychopathy in the criminal justice system, and, where possible, consider some solutions. It appears that, when they hear the term "psychopath" applied to someone, lay people, and no small number of professionals—judges, lawyers, probation officers, even health professionals—envision movie psychopaths or notorious serial killers. Even when we avoid labels and talk only about specific psychopathic traits, such as glib and superficial, lacking remorse, callous and so on, it appears that decision-makers overrate the probative value of these features and may choose more severe options as a result.

Although the taxonomic description of someone as a psychopath (rather than as highly or moderately psychopathic) based on a PCL-psychopathy score may make dichotomous legal decisions seem more straightforward, it does not make them more accurate. In the words of Edens et al. (2018), "a diagnosis of psychopathy should not be equated with a designation of 'dangerousness', nor should it foster any particular level of confidence regarding dichotomous predictions of violence for a specific offender" (p. 738). In other words, it is rather difficult as experts to use measures of psychopathy in psycho-legal contexts and have control over the "message", specifically the creation of an accurate perception of what the resulting information about psychopathy adds and does not add for decision-makers. This problem then raises the question: is it ethical for an assessor to continue using an instrument once it has been shown that the results may be subject to significant misinterpretation by people making major decisions about the life of the evaluated person?

Alongside this problem, several other concerns are becoming more evident as research accumulates. Growing research evidence for a lack of reliability in field scoring of the PCL-R poses a clear ethical concern, especially when coupled with the possibility of a variety of biases in scoring, some of which may be specific to a particular case but others of which may be assessor-based. Factor 1 scores, containing those items that are least relevant to risk assessment and most likely to influence decision-makers, appear to be particularly hard to score reliably (Edens et al., 2018).

Do unreliable scores have a place in psycho-legal contexts? If use of the PCL-R continues to grow, then investigations of practical methods for improving reliability are an urgent priority. Hare and others provide comprehensive training on how to use the PCL-R (e.g., Darkstone Research Group), and some efforts have been made in particular jurisdictions to provide post-workshop training or supervision. Hare (2003) expressed confidence that people could become competent in administration of the PCL-R with Darkstone, or organizational in-house training, and described research in support of reliability of scoring. However, evidence is mounting to suggest that it may be more difficult than expected to achieve adequate reliability, especially across the full range of people who are using it.

For example, Blais et al. (2017) investigated interrater reliability across items, facets, factors and total PCL-R scores in 280 people who completed Darkstone's PCL-R training and then scored 6 practice cases based on a packet of file information, 20 min of video interview and a full transcript of the video. A high level of variability was found for items and facets, with a particularly low ICC for the Affective facet (.51). But Factor and Total scores achieved good reliability (.65–.78), no systematic patterns of scoring bias were noted, and scores were more reliable for higher scoring cases.

These are encouraging results and more reassuring than a number of other studies reported earlier in the chapter, but Blais et al. (2017) also noted that some raters were consistently unreliable, leading them to recommend training changes and including follow-up supervision of assessments to criterion[3]. In practice, the court has no way of knowing the accuracy of a particular expert. Taken together, the findings on variable reliability suggest that the relevant professions should investigate or develop accreditation, quality assurance, and ongoing competency standards for those who use the PCL scales in their legal evaluation work.

On a different tack, the value of the PCL measures as risk assessment instruments is not exceptional. Their predictive accuracy compares relatively favorably with newer measures designed specifically for the purposes of risk assessment in assessing recidivism in the community. But the information provided by the use of a PCL is relatively limited. Good risk assessments include coverage of the applicable risk factors, their functional relevance, the level or type of risk identified, and consequent recommendations for management (Evans & Salekin, 2016). Newer instruments can address more of these components (e.g., the Level of Service scales with general recidivism; Olver et al., 2014; the Historical, Clinical, Risk Management-20 Version 2 (HCR-20 V2; Webster et al., 1997; V3 (Douglas et al., 2013). We are also beginning to see the development of "look-up" tables for some instruments that can be used to provide expected recidivism rates across the full range of scores for one or more fixed follow-up periods (Hanson et al., 2010; Hanson et al., 2012), including risk-change information (Mundt, 2015; Olver et al., 2018a, b). So far, the PCL scales are not among them.

Research into better ways to communicate risk information has been going on parallel to developments in ways of assessing risk, based on the recognition that assessors need to do the best they can to contribute to decision-makers accurately interpreting the risk information communicated to them (Evans & Salekin, 2016). Categorical approaches are still strongly favored, though not unanimously, and particularly not when they are not used to consistently refer to specific bands of outcomes (Scurich, 2017).

The publication of the Hanson et al. (2016) report on standardizing risk categories has stimulated a series of studies with a range of risk instruments (e.g., Hanson et al., 2017). Research into developing criterion-referenced measures, as Hanson et al. (2017) propose, requires an understanding of the distribution of scores through the population that is the basis for prediction. Then, that population is divided into categories based on uniform criteria, such as those suggested by Hanson et al. (Hanson et al., 2017; e.g., Coulter et al., 2019; Davies & Helmus, 2019; Moore & Grace, 2019; Olver et al., 2018a, b). Of course, the usefulness of this information is still limited if decision-makers themselves are only interested in dichotomously diagnosing dangerousness (Helmus, 2018). But all in all, there is an argument to be made that risk estimation and communication have been developing for some time well beyond either what the PCL scales can offer, or at least beyond what they are currently validated to do.

Another obvious ethical issue arises when the PCL scales are used for purposes in which they currently have no evidence base (e.g., risk of incestuous offending; Edens, 2001; malingered mental illness; DeMatteo & Edens, 2006). A group of concerned experts has recently drawn attention to the use of the PCL-R for predicting institutional violence. They reached the conclusion that in capital sentencing assessments, when attempting to predict serious violence in high security settings, the evidence suggests that use of the PCL-R cannot be justified, based on a lack of precision or accuracy (DeMatteo et al., 2020).

In the case of treatment amenability, the PCL scales also have little predictive validity. The evidence we have about treatment amenability in people with high PCL-psychopathy scores also suggests that we should be, where possible, encouraging courts and parole boards to take a less dichotomous view (i.e., treatable or not). For one thing, the data suggest (Polaschek, 2014) that people high on PCL-psychopathy are more difficult to treat, but not untreatable, and further, that we currently have no way of establishing ahead of time how effective treatment will be for a given individual (e.g., Olver et al., 2013). The PCL-R therefore appears to convey little useful information on this issue. But an assessment that includes the VRS or VRS:SO, in particular, can provide a considerable amount of information about current treatment amenability, and the targets for intervention, as well as generating risk assessment information that appears to be at least as accurate. A variety of other measures are also sensitive to change through repeated reassessment, and some also contain protective factors which is another useful addition, particularly when considering recommendations for management (Helmus, 2018). Progress appears to be faster in the sexual risk assessment field at present.

There are practical issues associated with the use of the PCL-scales. The PCL-psychopathy scales take considerable training to use well, can only be administered by highly qualified people (e.g., clinical psychologists), and are time consuming to score. In New Zealand, PCL-psychopathy assessments are used less than they were a decade ago, probably because of the combination of the expense involved in completing them and the relatively limited utility compared to other available options. One advantage of how PCL-Rs and PCL:SVs are completed by New Zealand's correctional psychologists is the use of an evidence recording sheet, in which the assessor documents the evidence used for each item to reach the score given. Such documentation can readily reveal sources of scoring disparity between assessors, including differences in evidence accessed, and systematic scoring biases. But the practice can lead the administration of the scale to take as long as 6–10 h, depending on the amount of file documentation available.

So then, when is the PCL-R the best measure to use? Except when its use is mandated, the decision to use the PCL-R or any other measure in a psychological assessment should be dependent on the purposes of the assessment as understood by the assessor, how well the chosen instrument can contribute to that purpose, and whether the results of the instrument can be presented in such a way as to clearly communicate with the audience (Monahan & Skeem, 2014). One reason for using a PCL-psychopathy measure may simply be the large number of studies that have used it. Another obvious purpose would be when there is a need to diagnose psychopathy, perhaps in conjunction with other personality disorders, in order to consider particular treatment options (e.g., Chakhssi et al., 2010; Kirkpatrick et al., 2010). Its more extensive use in the US, for assessments that elsewhere might use other scales may be due to a relative lack of US-validated risk assessment scales (Desmarais et al., 2016)—especially for assessing risk other than for sexual offending—compared to the large volume of risk assessment research on the PCL-R. As

US correctional systems turn their attention to the need to reduce incarceration numbers, assessment of progress and directions for management will become more important. Developing better validated risk instruments in the US through further research is an important priority (Desmarais et al., 2016).

21.13 Conclusions

Almost 40 years after the first PCL scale (the PCL-R) was published, PCL-psychopathy continues to have strong popularity as an important measure in psycholegal contexts. Emerging issues with reliability, predictive validity, lack of validation (in some applications, nations, and ethnicities) and calibration, the unremarkable predictive accuracy of the measures, and the potential for overinterpreting what a high PCL-psychopathy score actually means for the person being evaluated and their future behavior, together suggest that we should rely on it less. Research on how the PCL is scored in practice (e.g., how much information is used to make ratings, whether that information is drawn from across the person's life or mainly from their criminal justice files; whether disconfirming evidence is included when present), is needed to identify how to improve reliability. And new types of research are needed if it is to keep up with the information now being provided by other instruments that were designed first and foremost to be risk assessment measures.

Scoring a PCL-R is an expensive and inefficient choice for some settings, where a shorter, or more automated option may be available that gives equivalent information. The development of more locally validated static risk assessment tools is warranted, especially in the US. Finally, developments in risk assessment and treatment for high risk offenders, in identifying the functions of risk factors, targets for treatment, and long-term management options, also suggest that the PCL scales are not the optimal assessment measures for a significant proportion of evaluations where they may be currently used.

This chapter began by considering current definitions and controversies about what psychopathy is or is not. Agreeing on a definition of psychopathy is essential to determining its relevance to the criminal justice system. One of the most problematic aspects of the term "psychopathy" is the very real risk of divergent understandings between people, leading to divergent expectations and decisions. Viewing psychopathy as a multiply configurable syndrome rather than a well-bounded discrete entity is important to the criminal justice system for at least two reasons. First, it challenges potentially reductionistic thinking that psychopathy is synonymous with criminality and therefore may cause it. Instead, it promotes are more complex view of psychopathy that is more akin to other personality disorders, some of which also are linked to offending, but do not, on their own, cause it.

Second, it helps to remind us of the importance of keeping the measurement of psychopathy separate from the latent construct. Different measures reflect different operationalizations of the characteristics, providing a richer, sometimes more confusing, but more robust picture of psychopathy and its relevance. The inclusion of

Boldness or Fearless Dominance, and recognition of the role of negative emotionality in some apparently psychopathic people is important to this endeavor.

Finally, using the more rounded, diversely configurable understanding of psychopathy described in the opening of this chapter may help to balance out the current tendency to exaggerate the explanatory depth of labelling someone as psychopathic in the criminal justice system (given that the label is often derived from the very behavior it is apparently explaining). It may be an aid to recognizing that, while still important, psychopathy, like other mental disorders, may be of a little less relevance to the basic functions of the criminal justice system than might be imagined by lay people and naïve users of the PCL scales.

References

Andrews, D. A., & Bonta, J. (2010). Rehabilitating criminal justice policy and practice. *Psychology, Public Policy, and Law, 16*, 39–55.

Anthony, T. (2017, June 6). *FactCheck Q & A: Are indigenous Australians the most incarcerated people on Earth?*. Retrieved from https://theconversation.com/factcheck-qanda-are-indigenous-australians-the-most-incarcerated-people-on-earth-78528

Auty, K. M. (2019). The intergenerational transmission of psychopathy. In M. DeLisi (Ed.), *Routledge international handbook of psychopathy and crime* (pp. 136–153). Routledge.

Bakker, L., Riley, D., & O'Malley, J. (1999). *Risk of reconviction: Statistical models predicting four types of re-offending*. Retrieved from Wellington, NZ.

Bartak, A., Andrea, H., Spreeuwenberg, M. D., Ziegler, U. M., Dekker, J., Rossum, B. V., Hamers, E. F., Scholte, W., Aerts, J., Busschbach, J. J., Verheul, R., Stijnen, T., & Emmelkamp, P. M. (2011). Effectiveness of outpatient, day hospital, and inpatient psychotherapeutic treatment for patients with cluster B personality disorders. *Psychotherapy and Psychosomatics, 80*, 28–38. https://doi.org/10.1159/000321999

Bateman, A. W., Gunderson, J., & Mulder, R. T. (2015). Treatment of personality disorder. *The Lancet, 385*, 735–743.

Blais, J., Solodukhin, E., & Forth, A. E. (2014). A meta-analysis exploring the relationship between psychopathy and instrumental versus reactive violence. *Criminal Justice and Behavior, 41*, 797–821. https://doi.org/10.1177/0093854813519629

Blais, J., Forth, A. E., & Hare, R. D. (2017). Examining the interrater reliability of the Hare psychopathy checklist—Revised across a large sample of trained raters. *Psychological Assessment, 29*, 762–775. https://doi.org/10.1037/pas0000455

Boccaccini, M. T., Rufino, K. A., Jeon, H., & Murrie, D. C. (2017). Does the predictive validity of psychopathy ratings depend on the clinical experience of the raters. *International Journal of Forensic Mental Health, 16, 130–138.* https://doi.org/10.1080/14999013.2016.1266421.

Boccaccini, M. T., Turner, D. B., & Murrie, D. C. (2008). Do some evaluators report consistently higher or lower PCL-R scores than others: Findings from a statewide sample of Sexually Violent Predator evaluations. *Psychology, Public Policy, and Law, 14*, 262–283. https://doi.org/10.1037/a0014523

Bonta, J., & Andrews, D. A. (2016). *The psychology of criminal conduct* (6th ed.). Routledge.

Bonta, J., Blais, J., & Wilson, H. A. (2014). A theoretically informed meta-analysis of the risk for general and violent recidivism for mentally disordered offenders. *Aggression and Violent Behavior, 19*, 278–287. https://doi.org/10.1016/j.avb.2014.04.014

Boomen, M. (2018). Where New Zealand stands internationally: A comparison of offence profiles and recidivism rates. *Practice: The New Zealand Corrections Journal, 6*(1). Retrieved from https://www.corrections.govt.nz/resources/research_and_statistics/journal/volume_6_

issue_1_july_2018/where_new_zealand_stands_internationally_a_comparison_of_offence_profiles_and_recidivism_rates.html

Caldwell, M. F., & Van Rybroek, G. (2005). Reducing violence in serious juvenile offenders using intensive treatment. *International Journal of Law and Psychiatry, 28*, 622–636. https://doi.org/10.1016/j.ijlp.2004.07.001

Caldwell, M. F., & Van Rybroek, G. (2013). Effective treatment programs for violent adolescents: Programmatic challenges and promising features. *Aggression and Violent Behavior, 18*, 571–578. https://doi.org/10.1016/j.avb.2013.06.004

Caldwell, M. F., Skeem, J., Salekin, R., & Van Rybroek, G. (2006a). Treatment response of adolescent offenders with psychopathy features. *Criminal Justice and Behavior, 33*, 571–596.

Caldwell, M. F., Vitacco, M., & Van Rybroek, G. J. (2006b). Are violent delinquents worth treating? A cost-benefit analysis. *Journal of Research in Crime and Delinquency, 43*, 148–168.

Caldwell, M. F., McCormick, D. J., Umstead, D., & Van Rybroek, G. J. (2007). Evidence of treatment progress and therapeutic outcomes among adolescent offenders with psychopathy features. *Criminal Justice and Behavior, 34*, 573–587. https://doi.org/10.1177/0093854806297511

Camp, J., Skeem, J. L., Barchard, K., Lilienfeld, S., & Poythress, N. G. (2013). Psychopathic predators? Getting specific about the relation between psychopathy/antisociality and violence. *Journal of Consulting & Clinical Psychology, 81*, 467–480. https://doi.org/10.1037/a0031349

Chakhssi, F., de Ruiter, C., & Bernstein, D. (2010). Change during forensic treatment in psychopathic vs. nonpsychopathic offenders. *The Journal of Forensic Psychiatry and Psychology, 21*, 660–682.

Chauhan, P., Reppucci, N. D., & Burnett, M. (2007). Application and impact of the psychopathy label to juveniles. *International Journal of Forensic Mental Health, 6*, 3–14.

Cima, M., & Raine, A. (2009). Distinct characteristics of psychopathy relate to different sybtypes of aggression. *Personality and Individual Differences, 47*, 835–840. https://doi.org/10.1016/j.paid.2009.06.031

Cleckley, H. M. (1988). *The mask of sanity: An attempt to reinterpret the so-called psychopathic personality* (5th ed.). Mosby.

Coid, J., Yang, M., Ullrich, S., Roberts, A., & Hare, R. D. (2009). Prevalence and correlates of psychopathic traits in the household population of Great Britain. *International Journal of Law and Psychiatry, 32*, 65–73. https://doi.org/10.1016/j.ijlp.2009.01.002

Cooke, D. J. (1995). Psychopathic disturbance in the Scottish prison population: The cross-cultural generalisability of the Hare psychopathy checklist. *Psychology, Crime and Law, 2*, 101–118.

Cooke, D. J. (1998). Psychopathy across cultures. In D. J. Cooke, A. E. Forth, J. Newman, & R. D. Hare (Eds.), *Psychopathy: Theory, research, and implications for society* (pp. 13–45). Kluwer Academic Publishers.

Cooke, D. J., & Michie, C. (1999). Psychopathy across cultures: North America and Scotland compared. *Journal of Abnormal Psychology, 108*, 58–68.

Cooke, D. J., & Michie, C. (2001). Refining the construct of psychopathy: Towards a hierarchical model. *Psychological Assessment, 13*, 171–188.

Cooke, D. J., Kosson, D. S., & Michie, C. (2001). Psychopathy and ethnicity: Structural item and test generalizability of the Psychopathy Checklist-Revised (PCL-R) in Cauasian and African-American participants. *Psychological Assessment, 13*, 531–542.

Copestake, S., Gray, N. S., & Snowden, R. J. (2011). A comparison of a self-report measure of psychopathy with the Psychopathy Checklist-Revised in a UK sample of offenders. *The Journal of Forensic Psychiatry & Psychology, 22*, 169–182. https://doi.org/10.1080/14789949.2010.545134

Costa, P. T., & McCrae, R. R. (1992). *Revised NEO personality inventory (NEO PI-R) and NEO five-factor inventory (NEO-FFI) professional manual*. Psychological Assessment Resources.

Coulter, D., Lloyd, C. D., & Serin, R. (2019, May 31). *Combining static, stable, acute, and protective ratings into risk estimates within the standardized five-level framework*. Paper presented at the 4th North American Correctional and Criminal Justice Psychology Conference, Nova Scotia, Canada.

Craig, L. A., Dixon, L., & Gannon, T. A. (Eds.). (2013). *What works in offender rehabilitation: An evidence-based approach to assessment and treatment*. Wiley.

Crego, C., & Widiger, T. A. (2016). Cleckley's psychopaths: Revisited. *Journal of Abnormal Psychology, 125*, 75–87. https://doi.org/10.1037/abn0000130

Daly, T. E. (2017). *Why are psychopaths difficult to treat? Testing the two-component model for the treatment of PCL psychopaths*. Doctor of Philosophy Thesis, Victoria University of Wellington.

Daly, T. E., Fletcher, G. J. O., & Polaschek, D. L. L. (2017). *The relevance of PCL-psychopathy to in-treatment behaviour: An examination with high-risk violent male prisoners*. Article in preparation.

Davies, S., & Helmus, L. (2019, May 31). *The five-level risk and needs framework and violent recidivism: Applying the framework to the VRAG-R*. Paper presented at the 4th North American Correctional and Criminal Justice Psychology Conference, Nova Scotia, Canada.

DeLisi, M. (2016). *Psychopathy as unified theory of crime*. Palgrave Macmillan.

DeLisi, M. (2019). Psychopathy and crime are inextricably linked. In M. DeLisi (Ed.), *Routledge international handbook of psychopathy and crime* (pp. 3–12). Routledge.

DeMatteo, D., & Edens, J. F. (2006). The role and relevance of the Psychopathy Checklist-Revised in court: A case law survey of U.S. courts (1991–2004). *Psychology, Public Policy, and Law, 12*, 214–241. https://doi.org/10.1037/1076-8971.12.2.214

DeMatteo, D., Edens, J. F., & Hart, A. (2010). The use of measures of psychopathy in violence risk assessment. In R. K. Otto & K. S. Douglas (Eds.), *Handbook of violence risk assessment* (pp. 19–40). Routledge.

DeMatteo, D., Edens, J. F., Galloway, M., Cox, J., Smith, S. T., Koller, J. P., & Bersoff, B. (2014). Investigating the role of the Psychopathy Checklist-Revised in United States case law. *Psychology, Public Policy, and Law, 20*, 96–1067. https://doi.org/10.1037/a0035452

DeMatteo, D., Hodges, H., & Fairfax-Columbo, J. (2016). An examination of whether Psychopathy Checklist-Revised evidence satisfies the relevance/prejudice admissability standard. In B. H. Bornstein & M. K. Miller (Eds.), *Advances in psychology and law 2*. Springer.

DeMatteo, D., Murrie, D. C., Edens, J. F., & Lankford, C. (2019). Psychopathy in the courts. In M. DeLisi (Ed.), *Routledge international handbook of psychopathy and crime* (pp. 645–664). Routledge.

DeMatteo, D., Hart, S. D., Heilbrun, K., Boccaccini, M. T., Cunningham, M. D., Douglas, K. S., Dvoskin, J. A., Edens, J. F., Guy, L. S., Murrie, D. C., Otto, R. K., Packer, I. K., & Reidy, T. J. (2020). Statement of concerned experts on the use of the Hare Psychopathy Checklist—Revised in capital sentencing to assess risk for institutional violence. *Psychology, Public Policy, and Law, 26*(2), 133–144. https://doi.org/10.1037/law0000223

Desmarais, S. L., Johnson, K. L., & Singh, J. P. (2016). Performance of recidivism risk assessment instruments in U.S. correctional settings. *Psychological Services, 13*, 206–222. https://doi.org/10.1037/ser0000075

Douglas, K. S., Hart, S. D., Webster, C. D., & Belfrage, H. (2013). *HCR- 20 V3: Assessing risk for violence—User guide*. Mental Health, Law, and Policy Institute, Simon Fraser University.

Eckhouse, L., Lum, K., Conti-Cook, C., & Ciccolini, J. (2019). Layers of bias: A unified approach for understanding problems with risk assessment. *Criminal Justice and Behavior, 46*, 185–209. https://doi.org/10.1177/0093854818811379

Edens, J. F. (2001). Misuses of the Hare Psychopathy Checklist-Revised in court: Two case examples. *Journal of Interpersonal Violence, 16*, 1082–1093. https://doi.org/10.1177/088626001016010007

Edens, J. F., Cox, J., Smith, S. T., DeMatteo, D., & Sörman, K. (2015). How reliable are Psychopathy Checklist-Revised scores in Canadian criminal trials? A case law review. *Psychological Assessment, 27*, 447–456. https://doi.org/10.1037/pas0000048

Edens, J. F., Petrila, J., & Kelley, S. E. (2018). Legal and ethical issues in the assessment and treatment of psychopathy. In C. J. Patrick (Ed.), *Handbook of psychopathy* (2nd ed., pp. 732–751). Guiilford.

Evans, S. A., & Salekin, K. L. (2016). Violence risk communication: What do judges and forensic clinicians prefer and understand? *Journal of Threat Assessment and Management, 3*, 143–164. https://doi.org/10.1037/tam0000062

Fanti, K. A., Lordos, A., Sullivan, E. A., & Kosson, D. S. (2018). Cultural and ethnic variations in psychopathy. In C. J. Patrick (Ed.), *Handbook of psychopathy* (2nd ed., pp. 529–569). Guiilford.

Farrington, D. P. (2003). Developmental and life-course criminology: Key theoretical and empirical issues—The 2002 Sutherland Award address. *Criminology, 41*, 221–255.

Farrington, D. P. (2005). The importance of child and adolescent psychopathy. *Journal of Abnormal Child Psychology, 33*, 489–497.

Farrington, D. P. (2015). Prospective longitudinal research on the development of offending. *Australian and New Zealand Journal of Criminology, 48*, 314–335. https://doi.org/10.1177/0004865815590461

Farrington, D. P. (2018). Family background and psychopathy. In C. J. Patrick (Ed.), *Handbook of psychopathy* (2nd ed., pp. 354–379). Guilford.

Farrington, D. P., Ullrich, S., & Salekin, R. T. (2010). Environmental influences on child and adolescent psychopathy. In R. T. Salekin & D. R. Lynam (Eds.), *Handbook of child and adolescent psychopathy* (pp. 202–230). Guilford.

Forth, A. E., Kosson, D. S., & Hare, R. D. (2003). *Hare psychopathy checklist: Youth version*. Multi-Health Systems.

Fox, B. H., Jennings, W. G., & Farrington, D. P. (2015). Bringing psychopathy into developmental and life-course criminology theories and research. *Journal of Criminal Justice, 43*, 274–289. https://doi.org/10.1016/j.jcrimjus.2015.06.003

Gardner, B. O., Boccaccini, M. T., & Murrie, D. C. (2018). Which PCL-R scores best predict forensic clinicians' opinions of offender risk. *Criminal Justice and Behavior, 45*, 1404–1419. https://doi.org/10.1177/0093854818789974

Glazebrook, S. (2010). Risky business: Predicting recidivism. *Psychiatry, Psychology and Law, 17*, 88–120. https://doi.org/10.1080/13218710903040421

Gottfredson, D. M., & Hirschi, T. (1990). *A general theory of crime. Stanford University Press.*

Guy, L. S., Anthony, C., Edens, J. F., & Douglas, K. S. (2005). Does psychopathy predict institutional misconduct among adults? A meta-analytic investigation. *Journal of Consulting and Clinical Psychology, 73*, 1056–1064.

Guy, L. S., Kusaj, C., Packer, I. K., & Douglas, K. S. (2015). Influence of the HCR-20, LS/CMI, and PCL-R on decisions about parole suitability among lifers. *Law and Human Behavior, 39*, 232–243. https://doi.org/10.1037/lhb0000111

Haag, A. M., Boyes, A., Cheng, J., MacNeil, A., & Wirove, R. (2016). An introduction to the issues of cross-cultural assessment inspired by Ewert v. Canada. *Journal of Threat Assessment and Management, 3*, 65–75. https://doi.org/10.1037/tam0000067

Hanson, R. K., Helmus, L., & Thornton, D. (2010). Predicting recidivism amongst sexual offenders: A multi-site study of Static-2002. *Law and Human Behavior, 34*, 198–211. https://doi.org/10.1007/s10979-009-9180-1

Hanson, R. K., Babchishin, K. M., & Thornton, D. (2012). Quantifying the relative risk of sex offenders: Risk ratios for the Static-99R. *Sexual Abuse: A Journal of Research & Treatment, 25*, 482–515. https://doi.org/10.1177/1079063212469060

Hanson, R. K., Bourgon, G., McGrath, R. J., Kroner, D., D'Amora, D. A., Thomas, S. S., & Tavarez, L. P. (2016). *A five-level risk and needs system: Maximizing assessment results in corrections through the development of a common language*. Justice Center Council of State Governments.

Hanson, R. K., Babchishin, K. M., Helmus, L. M., Thornton, D., & Phenix, A. (2017). Communicating the results of criterion referenced prediction measures: Risk categories for the Static-99R and Static-2002R sexual offender risk assessment tools. *Psychological Assessment, 27*, 582–597. https://doi.org/10.1037/pas0000371

Hare, R. D. (1991). *The Hare psychopathy checklist-revised*. Multi-Health Systems.

Hare, R. D. (1996). Psychopathy and antisocial personality disorder: A case of diagnostic confusion. *Psychiatric Times, 8*(1). Retrieved from https://www.psychiatrictimes.com/antisocial-personality-disorder/psychopathy-and-antisocial-personality-disorder-case-diagnostic-confusion

Hare, R. D. (2003). *The Hare psychopathy checklist-revised technical manual* (2nd ed.). Multi-Health Systems.

Hare, R. D. (2016). Psychopathy, the PCL-R, and criminal justice: Some new findings and current issues. *Canadian Psychology, 57*, 21–34. https://doi.org/10.1037/cap0000041

Hart, S. D., Hare, R. D., & Forth, A. E. (1994). Psychopathy as a risk marker for violence: Development and validation of a screening version of the revised psychopathy checklist. In J. Monahan & H. J. Steadman (Eds.), *Violence and mental disorder: Developments in risk assessment* (pp. 81–98). University of Chicago.

Hawes, S. W., Boccaccini, M. T., & Murrie, D. C. (2013). Psychopathy and the combination of psychopathy and sexual deviance as predictors of sexual recidivism:Meta-analytic findings using the psychopathy checklist-revised. *Psychological Assessment, 25*, 233–243. https://doi.org/10.1037/a0030391

Hecht, L. K., Latzman, R. D., & Lilienfeld, S. O. (2018). The psychological treatment of psychopathy: Theory and research. In D. David, S. J. Lynn, & G. H. Montgomery (Eds.), *Evidence based psychotherapy: The state of the science and practice* (pp. 271–298). Wiley.

Helmus, L. M. (2018). Sex offender risk assessment: Where are we and where are we going? *Current Psychiatric Reports, 20*, 1–9. https://doi.org/10.1007/s11920-018-0909-8

Hemphill, J. F., Hare, R. D., & Wong, S. C. P. (1998). Psychopathy and recidivism: A review. *Legal and Criminological Psychology, 3*, 139–170.

Hicks, B. M., Clark, D. A., & Durbin, C. E. (2017). Person-centered approaches to the study of personality disorders. *Personality Disorders: Theory, Research, and Treatment, 8*, 288–297. https://doi.org/10.1037/per0000212

Hughes, M. A., Stout, J. C., & Dolan, M. C. (2013). Concurrent validity of the psychopathic personality inventory-revised and the psychopathy checklist: Screening version in an Australian offender sample. *Criminal Justice and Behavior, 40*, 802–813. https://doi.org/10.1177/0093854812475135

Hurducas, C. C., Singh, J. P., de Ruiter, C., & Petrila, J. (2014). Violence risk assessment tools: A systematic review of surveys. *International Journal of Forensic Mental Health, 13*, 181–192.

Jeandarme, I., Edens, J. F., Habets, P., Bruckers, L., Oei, K., & Bogaerts, S. (2017). PCL-R field validity in prison and hospital settings. *Law and Human Behavior, 41*, 29–43. https://doi.org/10.1037/lhb0000222

Kelley, S. E., Edens, J. F., Mowle, E. N., Peonson, B. N., & Rulseh, A. (2019). Dangerous, depraved, and death-worth: A meta-analysis of the correlates of perceived psychopathy in jury simulation studies. *Journal of Clinical Psychology, 75*, 627–643. https://doi.org/10.1002/jclp.22726

Kemp, E., & Baskin-Sommers, A. (2019). Using an experimental therapeutics approach to target psychopathy. In S. Dimidjian (Ed.), *Evidence-based practice in action: Bridging clinical science and intervention* (pp. 258–269). Guilford.

Kennealy, P. K., Skeem, J. L., Walters, G. D., & Camp, J. (2010). Do core interpersonal and affective traits of PCL-R psychopathy interact with antisocial behavior and disinhibition to predict violence? *Psychological Assessment, 22*, 569–580.

Kirkpatrick, J. T., Draycott, S., Freestone, M., Cooper, S., Twiselton, K., Watson, N., Evans, J., Hawes, V., Jones, L., Moore, C., Andrews, K., & Bd, T. (2010). A descriptive evaluation of patients and prisoners assessed for dangerous and severe personality disorder. *The Journal of Forensic Psychiatry and Psychology, 21*, 264–282. https://doi.org/10.1080/1478994093388978

Kroner, D. G., Mills, J. F., & Reddon, J. R. (2005). A coffee can, factor analysis, and prediction of antisocial behavior: The structure of criminal risk. *International Journal of Law and Psychiatry, 28*, 360–374.

Leistico, A., Salekin, R. T., DeCoster, J., & Rogers, R. (2008). A large-scale meta-analysis relating the Hare measures of psychopathy to antisocial conduct. *Law and Human Behavior, 32*, 28–45. https://doi.org/10.1007/s10979-007-9096-6

Lewis, K., Olver, M. E., & Wong, S. C. P. (2013). The violence risk scale: Predictive validity and linking treatment changes with recidivism in a sample of high risk and personality disordered offenders. *Assessment, 20*, 150–164. https://doi.org/10.1177/1073191112441242

Lilienfeld, S. O., & Widows, M. (2005). *Psychopathic personality inventory–revised professional manual*. PAR.

Lilienfeld, S. O., Patrick, C. J., Benning, S. D., Berg, J., Sellbom, M., & Edens, J. F. (2012). The role of fearless doiminance in psychopathy: Confusions, controversies, and clarifications. *Personality Disorders: Theory, Research, and Treatment, 3*, 327–340. https://doi.org/10.1037/a0026987

Lilienfeld, S. O., Smith, S. F., Sauvigné, K. C., Patrick, C. J., Drislane, L. E., Latzman, R. D., & Krueger, R. F. (2016). Is boldness relevant to psychopathic personality? Meta-analyitic relations with non-psychopathy checklist-based measures of psychopathy. *Psychological Assessment, 28*, 1172–1185. https://doi.org/10.1037/pas0000244

Lloyd, C. D., Clark, H. J., & Forth, A. E. (2010). Psychopathy, expert testimony, and indeterminate sentences: Exploring the relationship be- tween psychopathy checklist-revised testimony and trial outcome in Canada. *Legal and Criminological Psychology, 15*, 323–339. https://doi.org/10.1348/135532509X468432

Lynam, D. R., & Miller, J. D. (2019). Structural models of psychopathy. In M. DeLisi (Ed.), *Routledge international handbook of psychopathy and crime* (pp. 28–45). Routledge.

McGuire, J. (2002). Integrating findings from research reviews. In J. McGuire (Ed.), *Offender rehabilitation and treatment: Effective programmes and policies to reduce re-offending* (pp. 3–38). Wiley.

Miller, A. K., Rufino, K. A., Boccaccini, M. T., Jackson, R. L., & Murrie, D. C. (2011). On individual differences in person perception: Raters' personality traits relate to their psychopathy checklist—Revised scoring tendencies. *Assessment, 18*, 253–260. https://doi.org/10.1177/1073191111402460

Miller, C. S., Kimonis, E. R., Otto, R. K., Kline, S. M., & Wasserman, A. L. (2012). Reliability of risk assessment measures used in sexually violent predator proceedings. *Psychological Assessment, 24*, 944–953. https://doi.org/10.1037/a0028411

Moffitt, T. E. (1993). Adolescence-limited and life-course-persistent antisocial behavior: A developmental taxonomy. *Psychological Review, 100, 674–701.*

Moffitt, T. E., Caspi, A., Dickson, N., Silva, P. A., & Stanton, W. (1996). Childhood-onset versus adolescent-onset antisocial conduct in males: Natural history from age 3 to 18. *Development and Psychopathology, 8*, 399–424.

Moffitt, T. E., Caspi, A., Harrington, H., & Milne, B. J. (2002). Males on the life-course-persistent and adolescence-limited antisocial pathways: Follow-up at age 26 years. *Development and Psychopathology, 14*, 179–207.

Monahan, J., & Skeem, J. L. (2014). Risk redux: The resurgence of risk assessment in criminal sanctioning. *Federal Sentencing Reporter, 26*, 158–166. https://doi.org/10.1525/fsr.2014.26.3.158

Moore, L., & Grace, R. C. (2019, May 31). *CRMSO: Improving the communication of risk for sexual offenders in New Zealand*. Paper presented at the 4th North American Correctional and Criminal Justice Psychology Conference, Nova Scotia, Canada.

Mundt, J. C. (2015). *VRS-SO calculator*. Retrieved from http://www.psynergy.ca

Murrie, D. C., Boccaccini, M. T., Johnson, J. T., & Janke, C. (2008). Does interrater (dis)agreement on psychopathy checklist scores in sexually violent predator trials suggest partisan allegiance in forensic evaluations? *Law and Human Behavior, 32*, 352–362. https://doi.org/10.1007/s10979-007-9097-5

Murrie, D. C., Boccaccini, M. T., Turner, D., Meeks, M., Woods, C., & Tussey, C. (2009). Rater (dis)agreement on risk assess- ment measures in sexually violent predator proceedings: Evidence of adversarial allegiance in forensic evaluation? *Psychology, Public Policy, and Law, 15*, 19–53. https://doi.org/10.1037/a0014897

Murrie, D. C., Boccaccini, M. T., Guarnera, L. A., & Rufino, K. A. (2013). Are forensic experts biased by the side that retains them? *Psychological Science, 24*, 1889–1897. https://doi.org/10.1177/0956797613481812

Murrie, D. C., Cornell, D. G., & McCoy, W. K. (2005). Psychopathy, conduct disorder, and stigma: Does diagnostic labeling influence juvenile probation officer recommendations? *Law and Human Behavior, 29, 323–342.*

Neumann, C. S., & Hare, R. D. (2008). Psychopathic traits in a large community sample: Links to violence, alcohol use and intelligence. *Journal of Consulting & Clinical Psychology, 76*, 893–899. https://doi.org/10.1037/0022-006X.76.5.893

Odgers, C. L., Moffitt, T. E., Broadbent, J. M., Dickson, N., Hancox, R. J., Harrington, H., Poulton, R., Sears, M. R., Thomson, W. M., & Caspi, A. (2008). Female and male antisocial trajectories: From childhood origins to adult outcomes. *Development and Psychopathology, 20*, 673–716. https://doi.org/10.1017/S0954579408000333

Olver, M. (2019). Psychopathy and sex offender recidivism. In M. DeLisi (Ed.), *Routledge international handbook of psychopathy and crime* (pp. 598–609). Routledge.

Olver, M. E., & Wong, S. C. P. (2009). Therapeutic responses to psychopathic sexual offenders: Treatment attrition, therapeutic change, and long-term recidivism. *Journal of Consulting and Clinical Psychology, 77*, 328–336. https://doi.org/10.1037/a0015001

Olver, M. E., & Wong, S. C. P. (2013). Treatment programs for high risk sexual offenders: Program and offender characteristics, attrition, treatment change and recidivism. *Aggression and Violent Behavior, 18*, 579–591. https://doi.org/10.1016/j.avb.2013.06.002

Olver, M., & Wong, S. C. P. (2019). Psychopathy and risk assessment. In M. DeLisi (Ed.), *Routledge international handbook of psychopathy and crime* (pp. 665–683). Routledge.

Olver, M. E., Stockdale, K. C., & Wormith, J. S. (2009). Risk assessment with young offenders: A meta-analysis of three assessment measures. *Criminal Justice and Behavior, 36*, 329–353.

Olver, M. E., Lewis, K., & Wong, S. C. P. (2013). Risk reduction treatment of high risk psychopathic offenders: The relationship of psychopathy and treatment change to violent recidivism. *Personality Disorders: Theory, Research, and Treatment, 4*, 160–167. https://doi.org/10.1037/a0029769

Olver, M. E., Stockdale, K. C., & Wormith, J. S. (2014). Thirty years of research on the level of service scales: A meta-analytic examination of predictive accuracy and sources of variability. *Psychological Assessment, 26*, 156–176. https://doi.org/10.1037/a0035080

Olver, M. E., Mundt, J. C., Thornton, D., Beggs Christofferson, S. M., Kingston, D. A., Sowden, J. N., Nicholaichuk, T. P., Gordon, A., & Wong, S. (2018a). Using the violence risk scale-sexual offense version in sexual violence risk assessments: Updated risk categories and recidivism estimates from a multisite sample of treated sexual offenders. *Psychological Assessment, 30*, 941–955. https://doi.org/10.1037/pas0000538

Olver, M., Neumann, C. S., Sewell, L. A., Lewis, K., Hare, R. D., & Wong, S. C. P. (2018b). A comprehensive examination of the psychometric properties of the psychopathy checklist-revised in Canadian multi-site sample of indigenous and non-indigenous offenders. *Psychological Assessment, 30*, 779–792. https://doi.org/10.1037/pas0000533

Patrick, C. J. (2010). *Operationalising the triarchic conceptualisation of psychopathy: Description of brief scales for assessment of boldness, meanness and disinhibition*. Unpublished manual.

Patrick, C. J. (Ed.). (2018). *Handbook of psychopathy* (2nd ed.). Guilford.

Patrick, C. J., & Drislane, L. E. (2015). Triarchic model of psychopathy: Origins, operationalizations, and observed linkages with personality and general psychopathology. *Journal of Personality, 83*, 627–643. https://doi.org/10.1111/jopy.12119

Patrick, C. J., Fowles, D. C., & Krueger, R. F. (2009). Triarchic conceptualization of psychopathy: Developmental origins of disinhibition, boldness, and meanness. *Development and Psychopathology, 21*, 913–938. https://doi.org/10.1017/S0954579409000492

Patrick, C. J., Drislane, L. E., & Strickland, C. (2012). Conceptualizing psychpathy in triarchic terms: Implications for treatment. *International Journal of Forensic Mental Health, 11*, 253–266.

Polaschek, D. L. L. (2008). *Rimutaka violence prevention unit evaluation report V: Interim/progress report on prospective evaluation*. Unpublished report for the New Zealand Department of Corrections.

Polaschek, D. L. L. (2011). High-intensity rehabilitation for violent offenders in New Zealand: Reconviction outcomes for high- and medium-risk prisoners. *Journal of Interpersonal Violence, 26*, 664–682. https://doi.org/10.1177/0886260510365854

Polaschek, D. L. L. (2014). Adult criminals with psychopathy: Common beliefs about treatability and change have little empirical support. *Current Directions in Psychological Science, 23*, 296–301. https://doi.org/10.1177/0963721414535211

Polaschek, D. L. L. (2020). *Making the most of the risk-need-responsivity model.* Manuscript in preparation.

Polaschek, D. L. L., & Daly, T. (2013). Treatment and psychopathy in forensic settings. *Aggression and Violent Behavior, 18*, 592–603. https://doi.org/10.1016/j.avb.2013.06.003

Polaschek, D. L. L., & Skeem, J. L. (2018). Treatment of adults and juveniles with psychopathy. In C. J. Patrick (Ed.), *Handbook of psychopathy* (2nd ed., pp. 710–731). Guilford.

Polaschek, D. L. L., Wilson, N. J., Townsend, M., & Daly, L. (2005). Cognitive-behavioral rehabilitation for high-risk violent offenders: An outcome evaluation of the violence prevention unit. *Journal of Interpersonal Violence, 20*, 1611–1627.

Polaschek, D. L. L., Yesberg, J. A., Bell, R. K., Casey, A. R., & Dickson, S. R. (2016). Intensive psychological treatment of high-risk violent offenders: Outcomes and pre-release mechanisms. *Psychology, Crime & Law, 22*, 344–365. https://doi.org/10.1080/1068316X.2015.1109088

Poy, R., Segarra, P., Esteller, A., López, R., & Moltó, J. (2014). FFM description of the triarchic conceptualization of psychopathy in men and women. *Psychological Assessment, 26*, 69–76. https://doi.org/10.1037/a0034642

Poythress, N. G., Edens, J. F., Skeem, J. L., Lilienfeld, S. O., Douglas, K. S., Frick, P. J., Patrick, C. J., Epstein, M., & Wang, T. (2010a). Identifying subtypes among offenders with antisocial personality disorder: A cluster-analytic study. *Journal of Abnormal Psychology, 119*, 389–400.

Poythress, N. G., Lilienfeld, S. O., Skeem, J. L., Douglas, K. S., Edens, J. F., Epstein, M., & Patrick, C. J. (2010b). Using the PCL-R to help estimate the validity of two self-report measures of psychopathy with offenders. *Assessment, 17*, 206–219. https://doi.org/10.1177/1073191109351715

Prochaska, J. O., DiClemente, C. C., & Norcross, J. C. (1992). In search of how people change: Applications to addictive behaviors. *American Psychologist, 47*, 1102–1114.

Reidy, D. E., Kearns, M. C., & DeGue, S. (2013). Reducing psychopathic violence: A review of the treatment literature. *Aggression and Violent Behavior, 18*, 527–538. https://doi.org/10.1016/j.avb.2013.07.008

Rocket, J. L., Murrie, D. C., & Boccaccini, M. T. (2007). Diagnostic labeling in juvenile justice settings: Do psychopathy and conduct disorder findings influence clinicians? *Psychological Services, 4*, 107–122. https://doi.org/10.1037/1541-1559.4.2.107

Salekin, R. T. (2002). Psychopathy and therapeutic pessimism: Clinical lore or clinical reality? *Clinical Psychology Review, 22*, 79–112.

Salekin, R. T., Rogers, R., & Sewell, K. W. (1996). A review and meta-analysis of the psychopathy checklist and psychopathy checklist-revised: Predictive validity of dangerousness. *Clinical Psychology: Science and Practice, 3*, 203–215.

Salekin, R. T., Trobst, K. K., & Krioukova, M. (2001). Construct validity of psychopathy in a community sample. *Journal of Personality Disorders, 15*, 425–441.

Salekin, R. T., Worley, C., & Grimes, R. D. (2010). Treatment of psychopathy: A review and brief introduction to the mental model approach for psychopathy. *Behavioral Sciences & the Law, 28*, 235–266.

Scurich, N. (2017). The case against categorical risk estimates. *Behavioral Sciences & the Law, 36*, 554–564. https://doi.org/10.1002/bsl.2382

Sewell, L. A., & Olver, M. E. (2018). Psychopathy and treatment outcome: Results from a sexual violence reduction program. *Personality Disorders: Theory, Research, & Treatment, 10*, 59–69. https://doi.org/10.1037/per0000297

Shepherd, S. M. (2016). Violence risk instruments may be culturally unsafe for use with indigenous patients. *Australasian Psychiatry, 24*, 565–567. https://doi.org/10.1177/1039856216665287

Singh, J. P., Grann, M., & Fazel, S. (2011). A comparative study of violence risk assessment tools: A systematic review and metaregression analysis of 68 studies involving 25,980 participants. *Clinical Psychology Review, 31*, 499–513.

Sissons, M. K. A., & Polaschek, D. L. L. (2018). *Exploring personality and psychopathology profiles, criminal risk and recidivism in high risk, psychopathic prisoners.* Manuscript under revision.

Skeem, J. L., & Polaschek, D. L. L. (2020). High risk not hopeless: Correctional intervention with people at risk for violence. *Marquette Law Review, 103*(3), 1129–1148.

Skeem, J. L., Edens, J. F., Camp, J., & Colwell, L. H. (2004). Are there ethnic differences in levels of psychopathy?: A meta-analysis. *Law and Human Behavior, 28*, 505–527.

Skeem, J. L., Polaschek, D. L. L., Patrick, C. J., & Lilienfeld, S. O. (2011). Psychopathic personality: Bridging the gap between scientific evidence and public policy. *Psychological Science in the Public Interest, 12*, 95–162. https://doi.org/10.1177/1529100611426706

Stanley, J. H., Wygant, D. B., & Sellbom, M. (2013). Elaborating on the construct validity of the Triarchic psychopathy measure. *Journal of Personality Assessment, 95*, 343–350.

Sturup, J., Edens, J. F., Sörman, K., Karlberg, D., Fredriksson, B., & Kristiansson, M. (2014). Field reliability of the psychopathy checklist-revised among life sentenced prisoners in Sweden. *Law and Human Behavior, 38*, 315–332. https://doi.org/10.1037/lhb0000063

Sullivan, E. A., & Kosson, D. S. (2006). Ethnic and cultural variations in psychopathy. In C. J. Patrick (Ed.), *Handbook of psychopathy*. Guilford.

Tamatea, A. J. (2017). Culture is our business: Issues and challenges for forensic and correctional psychologists. *Australian Journal of Forensic Sciences, 49*, 564–578. https://doi.org/10.1080/00450618.2016.1237549

Thornton, D., & Blud, L. (2007). The influence of psychopathic traits on response to treatment. In H. Herve & J. C. Yuille (Eds.), *The psychopath: Theory, research, and practice* (pp. 505–539). Lawrence Erlbaum Associates.

Vermote, R., Lowyck, B., Luyten, P., Vertommen, H., Corveleyn, J., Verhaest, Y., Stroobants, R., Vandeneede, B., Vansteelandt, K., & Peuskens, J. (2010). Process and outcome in psychodynamic hospitalization-based treatment for patients with a personality disorder. *The Journal of Nervous and Mental Disease, 198*, 110–115. https://doi.org/10.1097/NMB.0b013e3181cc0d59

Viljoen, J. L., MacDougall, E. A. M., Gagnon, N. C., & Douglas, K. S. (2010). Psychopathy evidence in legal proceedings involving adolescent offenders. *Psychology, Public Policy and Law, 16*, 254–283. https://doi.org/10.1037/a0019649

Walsh, T. C. (1999). Psychopathic and non-psychopathic violence among alcoholic offenders. *International Journal of Offender and Comparative Criminology, 43*, 34–48.

Walters, G. D. (2003). Predicting institutional adjustment and recidivism with the psychopathy checklist factor scores: A meta-analysis. *Law and Human Behavior, 27*, 541–558.

Walters, G. D. (2004). The trouble with psychopathy as a general theory of crime. *International Journal of Offender Therapy and Comparative Criminology, 48*, 133–148.

Webster, C. D., Douglas, K. S., Eaves, D., & Hart, S. D. (1997). *HCR-20: Assessing risk for violence (version 2)*. Mental Health, Law, and Policy Institute, Simon Fraser University.

Wong, S. C. P. (2013). Treatment of psychopathy in correctional settings. In O. Thienhaus & M. Piasecki (Eds.), *Textbook on correctional psychiatry* (pp. 6–1–6–26). Civic Research Press.

Wong, S. C. P., & Gordon, A. (2006). The validity and reliability of the violence risk scale: A treatment-friendly violence risk assessment tool. *Psychology, Public Policy, and Law, 12*, 279–309. https://doi.org/10.1037/1076-8971.12.3.279

Wong, S. C. P., & Gordon, A. (2013). The violence reduction program: A treatment program for violence prone forensic clients. *Psychology, Crime & Law, 11*, 461–475. https://doi.org/10.1080/1068316X.2013.758981

Wong, S. C. P., & Gordon, A. (2016). *Violence risk scale*. CreateSpace Independent Publishing Platform.

Wong, S. C. P., & Hare, R. D. (2005). *Guidelines for a psychopathy treatment program*. Multi-Health Systems.

Wong, S. C. P., Olver, M. E., Nicholaichuk, T. P., & Gordon, A. E. (2003). *The violence risk scale—sexual offense version (VRS–SO)*. CreateSpace Independent Publishing Platform.

Wong, S. C. P., Gordon, A., Gu, D., Lewis, K., & Olver, M. E. (2012). The effectiveness of violence reduction treatment for psychopathic offenders: Empirical evidence and a treatment model. *International Journal of Forensic Mental Health, 11*, 336–349. https://doi.org/10.1080/14999013.2012.746760

Woodworth, M., & Porter, S. (2002). In cold blood: Characteristics of criminal homicides as a function of psychopathy. *Journal of Abnormal Psychology, 111*, 436–445. https://doi.org/10.1037//0021-843X.111.3.436

Yang, M., Wong, S. C. P., & Coid, J. W. (2010). The efficacy of violence prediction: A meta-analytic comparison of nine risk assessment tools. *Psychological Bulletin, 136*, 740–767.

Chapter 22
Public Health Considerations in Psychopathy

Dennis E. Reidy and Katherine W. Bogen

Abstract Public health is a discipline that aims to ensure health, safety, and well-being for the entire population. Psychopathy, a personality construct relevant to public health because of its link to injurious violence. However, there are other means by which psychopathy impedes the public health which have gone largely unaddressed. This is likely because psychopathy has primarily been viewed through a criminal justice lens. This singular focus has hindered efforts to develop prevention strategies for psychopathy and the adverse outcomes with which it is associated. In this chapter, we argue that adopting a public health framework for psychopathy will not only elucidate the full magnitude of its health impact, but also inspire innovation in the way we work to ameliorate said impact. We consider the importance of viewing and addressing psychopathy through a public health lens to facilitate the development of appropriate goals for its prevention, treatment, and management as both a means of preventing violent crime and promoting health.

Keywords Public health · Epidemiology · Prevention · Violence · Health

22.1 Introduction

Public health is a discipline that aims to ensure health, safety, and wellbeing for all individuals, communities, and societies. Psychopathy, a personality construct linked to a number of deleterious outcomes, constitutes a burden to all members of society. We have argued, as have others before us, that psychopathy is a pressing public health concern given its association with chronic and severe violence perpetrated by

D. E. Reidy (✉)
School of Public Health & Center for Research on Interpersonal Violence, Georgia State University, Atlanta, Georgia
e-mail: dreidy@gsu.edu

K. W. Bogen
Department of Psychology, University of Nebraska-Lincoln, Lincoln, Nebraska, USA

J. E. Vitale (ed.), *The Complexity of Psychopathy*, Dangerous Behavior in Clinical and Forensic Psychology, https://doi.org/10.1007/978-3-030-83156-1_22

those evincing such personality characteristics (Coid & Yang, 2011; Lynam, 1996; Reidy et al., 2015). Yet, while violence itself has been globally recognized as a public health problem (Krug et al., 2002a), the field of public health has generally neglected research, prevention efforts, or even discussion of psychopathy. This may be due, in part, to an erroneous assumption that the consequences of psychopathic persons' violence are relatively constrained to a minority of the population. Admittedly, psychopathic persons are a small fraction of the population; however, they are disproportionately responsible for rates of violence and subsequent population burden imposed by such behavior (Coid & Yang, 2011; Reidy et al., 2015). But, we argue that it is not violence alone through which psychopathy undermines health. Moreover, the adverse impact on health is magnified when considering how the consequences of psychopathic persons' behavior may diffuse across levels of the social ecology to impair the health and wellness of all members of society (Reidy et al., 2019a). Unfortunately, attention to how psychopathy impedes the public health through means other than violence is scarce.

Of course, given its well-established links to violence and crime, it is not surprising that psychopathy has primarily been viewed through a criminal justice lens. We suggest that this singular focus has hindered efforts to develop prevention strategies for psychopathy and the adverse outcomes with which it is associated. We suspect that adopting a public health framework for psychopathy will not only elucidate the full magnitude of its health impact, but also inspire innovation in the way we work to ameliorate said impact. In this chapter, we consider the importance of viewing and addressing psychopathy (especially among youth) through a public health lens to facilitate the development of appropriate goals for its prevention, treatment, and management as both a means of preventing crime and promoting health.

22.2 Overview of the Public Health Model

Public health, as a discipline, encompasses a wide variety of issues ranging from infectious and chronic diseases such as tuberculosis and diabetes to birth defects, injuries, mental health, and many more. A hallmark of the public health discipline is the application of a proactive approach to disease (and violence) focused on preventing it before it occurs- that is, primary prevention. Primary prevention is distinctive in its focus on attempting to forestall the *onset* of disease and injury which includes preventing the initiation of behaviors responsible for adverse health (e.g., violence, sexual risk behavior, substance use, nutritional habits, etc.). In this respect, primary prevention differs from secondary and tertiary prevention, which aim to reduce recurrence of disease and to ameliorate the short- and long-term consequences. While the fields of medical, behavioral, and mental health practice aim to diagnose and treat patients presenting with specific health problems (i.e., secondary and tertiary prevention), public health researchers and practitioners aim to study the distribution of such problems in the population, identify factors that increase the risk for or protect against the them, and implement programs, practices, and policies to prevent these harms from occurring in the first place (i.e., primary prevention). In reference to violence, the public health system works in tandem with the criminal justice system, which emphasizes the secondary and tertiary levels of prevention (Moore, 1995; Reidy et al., 2015).

Public health activities include broad actions such as vaccinating children and youth, educating the public on the harms related to certain behaviors (e.g., cigarette smoking), and implementing policies such as those that increase medical insurance coverage and inherently prevent negative health outcomes. A particularly crucial public health activity is the tracking and monitoring of health problems (i.e., surveillance) so their distribution within and burden upon the general public are well understood. Surveillance within the field of public health monitors the epidemiology of health problems, serves as an early warning system for impending public health emergencies, informs public health policy and strategies, and documents the impact of those strategies (WHO, 2014). Additionally, surveillance systems help to identify whether particular groups are at higher risk than others to experience negative health outcomes and why they may be at increased risk.

Understanding how health, including mental and behavioral health, manifests as a function of the larger population requires an understanding of the social determinants of health. These determinants drive and shape the health of individuals within a population. Specifically, health is influenced not only by genetic factors, but by the wider contexts into which people are born and develop. The latter encompass the social and physical makeup of their environment, including access to care, quality of education, workplace safety, ability to maintain income, availability of affordable housing, and quality of interpersonal relationships. These determinants of health allow researchers to explore and explain why certain populations are able to achieve and sustain greater health than others, as well as reasons why a given population may be at risk for both adverse health and criminal adjudication. For example, poverty, crime, and chronic health ailments tend to all congregate in certain populations (e.g., Haan et al., 1987; Nikulina et al., 2011; Piquero et al., 2007). Further, examination of the social determinants of health allows researchers, practitioners, policymakers, and community stakeholders to take effective action to alleviate health inequities by intervening to address the pertinent health determinants.

The social ecological model (Bronfenbrenner, 1977) has often been applied to trace the influence of the social determinants of health, and their compounding effects on various populations. This model addresses the relationship between a person and his or her changing environment, including not only immediate social settings, but larger social networks through which human beings learn, grow, and function. Bronfenbrenner's evaluation of social ecology allows public health researchers and practitioners to trace the determinants of health across social "levels," including *individual, relational, organizational, community,* and *societal*. In order to maximize effectiveness and impact, researchers designing interventions to improve public health are advised to consider how these efforts – for example, efforts to prevent violence, reduce the population-level burden of psychopathy, or improve community health outcomes – may utilize and impact multiple levels of the social ecology. However, public health interventions often focus on the outer levels of the social ecology, mobilizing actors with greater access to institutional resources and leaving potential avenues for targeted intervention, such as those focused on high-risk individuals, underexplored.

Fundamentally, public health focuses on achieving change at the population level to provide the greatest benefit to the maximum number of people (Dahlberg, 2007; Hemenway & Miller, 2013). The public health approach has often produced global prevention initiatives that are implemented at the community and societal levels (e.g., policies mandating seatbelts, media campaigns educating public about effects of tobacco, fluoridation of drinking water). Community level interventions of this nature have the potential to reach a much larger base of people. However, for those individuals most at risk, particularly for entrenched pathologies, prevention strategies may require an intervention with more significant intensity, dosage, or potency (Centers for Disease Control and Prevention [CDC], 2016; Reidy et al., 2013). Thus, prevention efforts must attend to risk factors across multiple levels of the social ecology, suggesting that individual-level factors remain an important component of prevention (e.g., CDC, 2016; Reidy et al., 2015). For this reason, identifying targeted prevention strategies for indicated persons most at risk is a critical component of a comprehensive public health approach to violence prevention and health promotion (CDC, 2016; Reidy et al., 2015), and may serve as a complement to interventions conducted at the outer levels of the social ecology.

This public health approach to prevention is a multistage process that includes (1) defining the problem, conducting surveillance and data collection; (2) identifying risk and protective factors; (3) developing and testing interventions; and (4) disseminating and implementing efficacious prevention interventions with continued measurement to evaluate effectiveness and cost-effectiveness (Mercy et al., 1993). While it may appear that these steps would occur in a linear order, they in fact are ongoing, and thus often operate in tandem: surveillance systems may be used to identify risk and protective factors or to evaluate the effectiveness of prevention strategies; pertinent risk and protective factors may moderate the efficacy of prevention strategies; dissemination and implementation of efficacious strategies to different populations may require translation based on unique risk and protective factors; and the development and evaluation of prevention interventions may involve identification and assessment of new risk and protective factors (Mercy et al., 1993).

22.3 Conceptual Definitions of Psychopathy

The conceptualization of psychopathy has varied and evolved significantly over the last century. Generally, it is agreed that the construct comprises a behaviorally deviant nature occurring in tandem with a cluster of interpersonally exploitative and emotionally calloused features (Patrick et al., 2009). Early conceptualizations portray violence as a defining characteristic of psychopathy (e.g., Kraepelin, 1915; McCord & McCord, 1964). Some theorists have suggested that the emotional deficits are a core etiology that give rise to manipulative, predatory, and violent behavior (Blair, 2013; McCord & McCord, 1964; Reidy et al., 2017). However, there has been spirited debate as to whether crime and violence are central features, or indeterminate consequences of psychopathy (e.g., Hare & Neumann, 2010; Skeem & Cooke, 2010a, b). In his seminal writings, *The Mask of Sanity,* Cleckley (1941, 1976) placed less emphasis on violence and crime than others before him. Though he described attributes of emotional detachment and socially deviant behavior (e.g., impulsive and irresponsible behavior), Cleckley highlighted the appearance of positive adjustment (e.g., good social skills, lack of dysregulated emotional expression) as a key attribute of the psychopath. Indeed, many of the clinical case examples he presented were of doctors, lawyers, businesspersons, etc. (Cleckley, 1941, 1976). Schneider (1958), much like Cleckley, believed psychopathy was prevalent among the general public regardless of criminality and even speculated that some psychopaths might make highly successful community leaders.

Arguably, the most researched and clinically utilized operationalization to date, Hare's Psychopathy Checklist-Revised (PCL-R; Hare, 1991, 2003) was developed based on the prototypical psychopath put forth by Cleckley (Hare, 1991; Skeem & Cooke, 2010a). Initial factor analytic studies of the PCL identified two moderately correlated factors (Hare, 1991; Harpur et al., 1989). The *Emotional Detachment* factor, commonly referred to as Factor 1, includes emotional and interpersonal features, such as affective shallowness, absence of empathy, lack of remorse, lack of shame, superficial charm, manipulative style, grandiosity, and lying. The *Social Deviance* factor, referred to as Factor 2, encompasses impulsivity, aggression, substance abuse, high sensation seeking, low socialization, proneness to boredom, irresponsibility, lack of concern or plans for the future, low motivation, and early life behavioral problems and delinquency. Hare (2003) later advanced a four-facet model in which the original Factor 1 was decomposed into the *Interpersonal* and *Affective* facets, and Factor 2 was split into the *Lifestyle* and Antisocial facets.

Although originally based on Cleckley's description, the family of PCL measures – which includes the Psychopathy Checklist: Screening Version (PCL:SV; Hart et al., 1995) and the Psychopathy Checklist: Youth Version (PCL:YV; Forth et al., 2003) – has evolved primarily to assess deviance while neglecting the "well-adjusted" and adaptive attributes described by Cleckley (Patrick et al., 2009; Skeem & Cooke, 2010a). In fact, Cleckley (1976) described the psychopath as unlikely to commit severe acts of violence and deviance. Yet, the PCL measures are generally predictive of some of the most extreme forms of violence (Reidy et al., 2011; Reidy et al., 2017). Despite these disparities between construct and measure, the Hare psychopath has become the most widely accepted model of psychopathy, likely due to the widespread adoption and implementation of the PCL measures in forensic populations. However, experts have raised valid concerns about conflating the construct of psychopathy with an operationalized measure of psychopathy. Skeem and Cooke (2010b) note an "almost routine confusion of the PCL-R's factor structure with the model of psychopathy itself" (p. 456) and have called for testing of alternative models of psychopathy.

In this vein, Patrick et al. (2009) have introduced the Triarchic model as an attempt to reconcile different historical conceptions of psychopathy and methods of assessing the construct. Patrick et al. (2012) have described this model as a "meta-conceptualization" that integrates previous conceptualizations and the findings across them rather than a novel conception. The Triarchic model orients psychopathy within three phenotypically distinct facets: (1) disinhibition, (2) boldness, and (3) meanness (Patrick et al., 2009). Disinhibition refers to general proneness toward impulse control problems and impaired affect regulation. Boldness encompasses social effectiveness, self-confidence, and stress resiliency. Meanness resembles the more criminal delinquent conceptions of psychopathy and encompasses shallow affect, deficient empathy, lack of close attachments, and exploitativeness (Patrick et al., 2009, 2012). Thus far, studies have demonstrated theoretically meaningful associations with related constructs offering initial support for this model. However, much of this associational research is based in survey methods and continued validation of the Triarchic model across other assessment domains (e.g., biological, behavioral, etc.) is necessary (Patrick & Drislane, 2015). Nevertheless, the Triarchic model of psychopathy offers promise to integrate differing conceptualizations and discrepant research findings generated over the past century (e.g., Drislane et al., 2014b).

Among youth, there are a number of different assessment inventories for psychopathic traits including the PCL:YV (Forth et al., 2003), the Antisocial Process Screening Device (Frick & Hare, 2001), the Inventory of Callous-Unemotional Traits (Frick, 2004), the Child Psychopathy Scale (Lynam, 1997), and the Youth Psychopathic Traits Inventory (Andershed et al., 2002). The varying content and factor structures of these disparate measures would seem to suggest a lack of congruity in conceptualization of youth psychopathy. However, evidence suggests that psychopathic characteristics in children and adolescents manifest similarly to those of adults (Blair, 2013; Frick & White, 2008; Lynam & Gudonis, 2005; Somma et al., 2016). In particular, the most widely referenced form of youth psychopathy, *Callous-Unemotional* (CU) traits, appear to mirror the core affective-interpersonal dysfunction of psychopathy seen in adults (Reidy et al., 2015). These CU traits are moderately associated with conduct disorder and delinquency; however, they can be reliably assessed (at an early age) and distinguished from these behavioral disorders (Loeber et al., 2009; Lynam & Gudonis, 2005; Reidy et al., 2015). Though the content and structure of extant youth psychopathy measures vary, they all tap the CU traits that are thought to be the core feature of psychopathy. Moreover, all of these measures are generally correlated moderately and have been shown to fit within the Triarchic model of psychopathy (Drislane et al., 2014a, b).

22.4 Burden of "Disease"

Traditional public health conceptions of disease burden have commonly focused on biomedical and economic burdens. In thinking about the biomedical burden of disease, the goal is to gauge the impact of disease on the body from onset to death or remission. This includes measures of the quality of life and premature loss of life in years. The economic burden focuses on the financial consequences of disease or disability for the individual, household, communities, healthcare systems, and society at large. These consequences include both direct (e.g., costs of treatment and care) and indirect costs (e.g., lost income due to illness-related absences from or complete inability to work, reduced productivity at work, and loss of tax revenue from premature death). Given the connection to violence, these measures of burden are particularly salient and straightforward means of quantifying disease burden for psychopathy. In 2017, there were nearly 20,000 deaths and 2.3 million injuries stemming from violence in the U. S. (Centers for Disease Control and Prevention [CDC], n.d.) and violence-related health care, law enforcement and judicial services, lost work days, and reduced productivity cost the U.S. economy trillions of dollars (Peterson et al., 2017; Peterson et al., 2018a, b). Youth and adults manifesting a high degree of psychopathic traits are responsible for a disproportionate amount of this violence (Coid & Yang, 2011; Reidy et al., 2015; Vaughn et al., 2014) and are therefore responsible for a disproportionate amount of adverse health and economic consequences.

For example, in the U.S., theorists contend that roughly 1% of noninstitutionalized men age 18 and over are psychopaths (Blair et al., 2005; Hare, 1996), but approximately 16% of incarcerated men in the U.S. meet the clinical criteria for psychopathy (Kiehl & Hoffman, 2011), indicating psychopathic individuals comprise a disproportionate number of male inmates in the U.S.. Kiehl and Hoffman (2011) estimate that this constitutes annual cost of $460 billion for the criminal justice system, alone. Further, while only 62% of male inmates in the U.S. are incarcerated for a violent offense (Cornell et al., 1996), it is estimated that 78% of psychopathic inmates are violent offenders (Hart et al., 1988; Kiehl & Hoffman, 2011). Coid and Yang (2011) reported that individuals with psychopathy had a prevalence rate of 0.7% in the general population of Great Britain, yet were responsible for approximately 18% of violent incidents over a 5 year period. Reidy et al. (2019b) collected data from an online sample of U.S. men. The authors found that psychopathy was even more strongly predictive of violent assaults among men with no arrest history compared to men who had been arrested. In this sample, relative to men scoring one standard deviation below the mean, men scoring one standard deviation above the mean on the affective facet of psychopathy reported a rate of assault with a weapon that was 1316% higher. The rate of violent assaults that caused injury was 720% higher. While base rates for such violence are low, and lower in the general population than forensic populations, the rarity of such events does not negate their burden. The average combined medical and work loss cost of a single violent assault injury treated in an emergency department is approximately US$7052, and this number jumps to nearly US$162,755 for assaults requiring hospitalization (CDC, n.d.). Moreover, each homicide imposes a burden of more than US$1.5 million in health care and lost wages (CDC, n.d.). Thus, these violent behaviors create a considerable burden for healthcare and criminal justice agencies, affecting community-level socioeconomic factors and potentially diverting resources away from other in-need groups. These findings suggest psychopathy, however rare, has a significant and disproportionate impact on population-levels of violence and consequently proffers a significant disease burden.

Pertinently, the biomedical and economic indices of disease burden have been criticized as being overly narrow and failing to account for pain and suffering and the indirect effects of disease on other members of the individual's social network (Thacker et al., 2006). Nor can this narrow view capture the ways in which disease burden may diffuse through society to affect the health of communities for current and future generations. Obviously, when considering the public health burden of psychopathy, it is necessary to consider the immediate risk for the direct victims of violence. But, it is not violence alone through which psychopathy influences the health of the population. As Robert Hare noted in his address to the Canadian Police Association, "Not all psychopaths are in prison. Some are in the boardroom" (Hare, 2002). Indeed, mean levels of psychopathic traits are higher among corporate samples than community samples (Babiak et al., 2010). High psychopathy individuals are seemingly prone to rise to positions of leadership and power in organizations (Babiak et al., 2010; Boddy, 2011; Boddy et al., 2010a; Howe et al., 2014) likely due to their ability charm, interpersonally manipulate others, cheat, and deceive others for personal gain.

As psychopathic individuals rise to positions of power and dominance within organizations, they have the opportunity not only to corrupt the culture of such environments, but to adversely affect the mental and physical health of its members (Boddy, 2014; Watson et al., 2017). Boddy et al. (2010b) found that under the leadership of corporate psychopaths, employees rated their company as less likely to do business in a way that demonstrates commitment to employees, their accomplishments as less likely to be recognized, and their work as less likely to be appreciated and rewarded. Boddy (2014) reported that the work environments under the leadership of corporate psychopaths were marked by significant hostility, interpersonal conflict, and bullying compared to work environments without psychopathic leaders. The tone and culture of the workplace that leaders establish can be critical because working in a hostile and/or stressful environment has a marked effect on the mental and physical health of its members (Fattori et al., 2015; Stansfeld & Candy, 2006; Theorell et al., 2015; Verkuil et al., 2015). In one study, victims of workplace harassment were more likely to report work-family balance conflict, sleep less than 6 h per night, smoke with greater frequency, report psychological distress, miss more days of work due to illness, have more days confined to bed because of illness, be obese, have a pain disorder, asthma, ulcers, diabetes, hypertension, and angina pectoris (Khubchandani & Price, 2015). Meta-analyses suggest that work stress is linked to an increased rate of recurrent coronary heart disease (Li et al., 2015) while employees who are bullied by supervisors are at risk of alcohol abuse, somatization, obesity, post-traumatic stress, depression, and suicide (Hansen et al., 2006; Luckhaupt et al., 2014; Martin & LaVan, 2010). Notably, Tokarev et al. (2017) reported that the association between leaders' psychopathy traits and employees' depression was mediated by workplace bullying. In fact, in multiples samples, ratings of supervisors' psychopathy traits have been linked to employees' ratings of their own adverse psychiatric health, work-family conflict, and job satisfaction (Boddy, 2014; Mathieu et al., 2014; Volmer et al., 2016).

The impact of corporate psychopaths can surpass the internal walls of their institutions to impact the broader population. In particular, the corruptive leadership of corporate psychopaths has the potential to influence the physical, mental, and financial well-being of persons, communities, and populations beyond the borders of their organization. For example, in a study of undergraduate business majors, Watson et al. (2017) had seniors complete self-report measures of psychopathy and their likelihood in engaging in unethical practices in 10 business scenarios. Among other unethical practices, psychopathic traits were positively associated with the likelihood of investing financially in violent reality television media, engaging in environmental pollution practices, and violating human rights for profit. Mounting evidence further suggests the presence of psychopathy traits predispose individuals to condoning and engaging in white collar and financial crimes such as deceptive accounting practices or insider-trading violations (Lingnau et al., 2017; Ragatz et al., 2012; Ray & Jones, 2011). In his sample of white collar workers drawn from business, professional, and managerial associations asked to rate supervisors on psychopathic traits, Boddy (2010) found the finance industry had the highest frequency of corporate psychopaths. Jeffrey Skilling (the former CEO of Enron), whose crimes included insider trading and financial statement fraud, demonstrated many of prototypical traits of the corporate psychopath (Fersch, 2006). Equally alarming is the potential of these corporate psychopaths to corrupt their institutions to such a degree that it can have a global impact. Some have gone as far as to suggest that the global financial crisis of 2008 was directly caused by corporate psychopaths (Boddy, 2011). Of course, this is potentially an extreme and overly simplistic interpretation that has not been empirically tested. But surely, individuals such as Bernie Madoff, Jeff Skilling, and others like them demonstrate a callousness and lack of empathy for their victims when they engage in their corporate deception. Importantly, the effect of these financial frauds is greater than just the loss of economic resources. After financial crises, rates of suicide increase significantly (Chang et al., 2013; Lopez Bernal et al., 2013; Stuckler et al., 2009).

22.5 Epidemiology

As the crux of public health, epidemiology is the scientific discipline concerned with the distribution (frequency, pattern) and determinants (causes, risk factors) of health-related states and events (e.g., health and diseases, morbidity, injury, disability, mortality) in specified populations (neighborhoods, schools, cities, states, countries, racial/ethnic, biological sex, age). The overarching objectives of this study are to describe, explain, and predict disease and health problems so that they may be prevented and/or controlled (Friis & Sellers, 2014).

Epidemiological research regarding the prevalence and patterns of psychopathy among affected populations is limited. As one might expect, psychopathy is most commonly studied in forensic and clinical settings. Clinical psychopathy (i.e., individuals manifesting psychopathic traits to a degree that would designate them diagnosed as a psychopath) is usually purported to manifest in about 0.5% - 2% of the general population and 15% - 25% of prison populations (Blair et al., 2005; Hare, 1996; Neumann & Hare, 2008). However, a number of studies with adults and youth have revealed that psychopathy is dimensional in nature (e.g., Coid & Yang, 2011; DeMatteo et al., 2006; Guay et al., 2007; Guay et al., 2018; Murrie et al., 2007). The dimensional nature substantiates the existence of psychopathy traits among all persons whether in the general or forensic population. Nevertheless, adequate population-based measurement of psychopathy is lacking, making it difficult to accurately assess rates of psychopathy and its impact on population health (Reidy et al., 2015).

We know of only one true rigorous epidemiological study. Coid and Yang (2011) utilized a stratified multi-stage cluster random sampling procedure to report on rates of psychopathy in the general population of Great Britain. The Postcode Address File (PAF) of Great Britain was used as the sampling frame for this study. The PAF is constructed by the Royal Mail as a list of all addresses, in England, Wales, and Scotland. In the first stage of sampling, 438 postal sectors were randomly selected as the primary sampling unit. Postal sectors were stratified by region and socioeconomic distribution. A postal sector contains an average of 2550 households. In the second stage of sampling, 36 mailing addresses were randomly selected from each postal sector yielding a 15,804 addresses. Interviewers then visited the 15,804 addresses to identify private households with at least one person aged 16 to 74 years. This resulted in the identification of 12,792 households eligible for interview. Within each of these eligible households, one person was randomly selected to take part in a two-phase survey. In the first phase of the survey, 8886 (69.5%) randomly selected adults agreed to participate and completed a computer-assisted interview that included a screen for personality disorders. In the second phase, 1036 subjects were selected on the basis of a screening process for psychosis and personality disorder; 638 (61.6%) agreed to participate and were interviewed by 7 psychologists trained in the in the use of the survey instruments (see Singleton et al., 2002 for more in depth description of the sampling methodology).

Psychopathy was assessed using the PCL:SV, a shortened 12-item rating scale based directly on the PCL-R. Notably, a full assessment of psychopathy using PCL measures involves conducting an in-depth clinical interview and a thorough review of collateral records and administrative data (e.g., criminal arrest history, institutional infractions, etc.). Given that these measures were designed to be used in forensic settings, a collateral records review is a reasonable and feasible expectation. However, such expectations are not possible with assessments in the general population given the lack of access to collateral files. Therefore PCL:SV assessments were based on clinical inferences obtained primarily from the interview (Coid & Yang, 2011). This is noteworthy because evidence suggests that scores from interview-only assessments are lower than from those that include adequate collateral information (Alterman et al., 1993). Therefore, these authors used cut-off scores of both 13 and 11 for probable and possible psychopathy. Normally, a score of 18 or greater is used as a cut-off score for probable psychopathy; and scores between 13 and 17 as an indication of possible psychopathy (Hart et al., 1995). Using these adjusted values, the authors reported prevalence rates of "probable psychopathy" to be 1.3% in men and 0% in women resulting in an overall prevalence rate of 0.7% in the general population. Using the more liberal cut score to diagnose "possible psychopathy," they found rates of 3.7% in men and 0.9% in women for an overall rate of 2.1%.

Among youth, some have suggested that prevalence rates of 3–5% for elevated callous-unemotional traits with or without conduct disorder (CD) among community and high-risk samples (Kimonis et al., 2015; McMahon et al., 2010). Perenc and Radochonski (2014) reported that 2.5% of a large community sample of Polish adolescents presented with elevated features of psychopathy. Considering the lifetime prevalence of CD in the general population is approximately 7–9% (Merikangas et al., 2010; Nock et al., 2006) and that approximately 10– 20% of youth in adjudicated populations with CD also manifest high levels of callous-unemotional traits in research samples (Christian et al., 1997; Vincent et al., 2003), it follows that a prevalence rate for CD with callous-unemotional traits is approximately 0.5–2% in the general population. These rates are generally consistent with rates of psychopathy reported for adults.

Evidence suggests psychopathy is less prevalent in women relative to men (Coid & Yang, 2011; Neumann & Hare, 2008; Wynn et al., 2012). Moreover, the pattern in which symptoms and associated behaviors manifest may be gender-specific. In one study, women in a large college sample scored higher than men on measures of egocentricity, carefree nonplanfulness (impulsivity), and blame externalization (Lee & Salekin, 2010). A large study of Swedish offenders found that high psychopathy women displayed significantly more lying behavior, deceitfulness, and lack of control relative to high psychopathy men (Strand & Belfrage, 2005). Conversely, high psychopathy men demonstrated more antisocial behavior compared to their female counterparts (Strand & Belfrage, 2005). Whereas these disparities are stark, robust research has yet to be conducted on the relationships between gendered socialization, such as ascription to strict gender norms, and psychopathic traits, though this may be a useful avenue for exploration.

Further exploring the impact of demography on psychopathy, studies have generally revealed small statistical differences. In their meta-analysis of offenders, Skeem et al. (2004) detected a significant difference for the affective facet and total score on the PCL-R wherein African-Americans scored higher, but these differences were statistically small (d = .10 & .11) suggesting a lack of meaningful difference. McCoy and Edens (2006) reported similar findings in their meta-analysis of youthful offenders. Though African-American youth scored higher than Caucasian youth on the total psychopathy score, the effect was again small (d = .20). In fact, these differences translate into approximately a 1-point difference on the 40 point scale of PCL measures (McCoy & Edens, 2006; Skeem et al., 2004). In a study of female offenders (Vitale et al., 2002), African-American women scored significantly higher than Caucasian women did on Factor 1 of the PCL-R, but the effect size was again small (d = .26).[1] A more recent large scale study of 1742 offenders from five U.S. states found that African-Americans relative to Caucasians scored higher on the affective, interpersonal, and antisocial facets of the PCL-R (Gatner et al., 2018). Again, the degree of these differences were statistically small though slightly larger than the previous studies (*d's* = .36–.37). Additionally, there were no differences on psychopathy scores for Hispanic offenders and any other population (Gatner et al., 2018). Sullivan et al. (2006) found no differences between Latino and Caucasian offenders, but found that African-Americans scored higher than Latinos on the total score and affective facet and higher than Caucasians on the interpersonal facet of the PCL-R (*d's* = .36–.44).[2]

At this point it is important to acknowledge that establishing prevalence estimates of psychopathy may be a double-edged sword. It is necessary for the purposes of determining the population burden that is attributable to psychopathy. But, obtaining prevalence rates requires classifying individuals into a binary classification (i.e. psychopathic vs. non-psychopathic, high callous-unemotional vs. not high) via cut scores on the continuum of psychopathic traits. This classification incorrectly assumes that psychopathy below the cutoff has no impact on behavior or other health related outcomes. For example, Coid and Yang (2011) reported that 18.7% of population violence of Great Britain was attributable to persons scoring 11 or higher on the PCL-SV. Therefore, eradicating psychopathy among those scoring at or above diagnostic levels would reduce population levels of violence by nearly 20%. However, this type of binary analysis inherently assumes that psychopathy at a score of 10 or below is unrelated to violent behavior. Yet, even at "subclinical" levels, psychopathy is related to violence (e.g., Reidy et al., 2011, 2019b). Developing effective treatment and prevention strategies for psychopathy and associated outcomes would also have an effect on the violence of these people scoring below the arbitrary diagnostic cut score. Thus, in reference to Coid and Yang's (2011) findings, preventing the adverse features of psychopathy would likely reduce population rates of violence by more than 20%.

Psychopathy is a dimensional construct in youth and adults (Guay et al., 2007, 2018; Murrie et al., 2007) which means all individuals demonstrate psychopathic traits to some degree (e.g., Lilienfeld, 1994; Patrick & Drislane, 2015; Reidy et al., 2011, 2019b). Furthermore, the correlates of such features are the same in community samples as they are in forensic samples (Lilienfeld, 1994; Vachon et al., 2012). Therefore, it is necessary to empirically determine what degree of psychopathic traits reflect pathology. To make this determination, good population-based epidemiological studies are necessary. It is necessary to go beyond the forensic and clinical focus of psychopathy to understand the true public health impacts of psychopathy. Whereas individuals with a high-level psychopathic traits may require secure care and custody, there are various "lower-level" or "high-functioning" psychopaths in

---

[1] Tests of mean differences and effects were not reported in the published article. We computed them based on presented descriptive data.

[2] Effects sizes were computed based on published descriptive data.

the community, including substance abusers, child and spouse abusers, and criminals with psychopathic traits below a diagnosable threshold (Coid & Yang, 2008). These individuals still have a significant impact on community health, not only through criminal behaviors that go undetected by the criminal justice system (Aharoni & Kiehl, 2013; Reidy et al., 2019b), but also through their impact on community norms and resources (Reidy et al., 2019a). Good epidemiological studies could identify critical ranges of psychopathy for risk, those populations most at risk, and focus areas for intervention, thereby decreasing population-level risk and improving health and safety standards for communities. The epidemiology of psychopathy has been hindered by a narrow disciplinary focus. By expanding the lens and incorporating a public health perspective, epidemiological research and ultimately the prevention of psychopathy (or its adverse consequences) will be advanced.

22.6 Etiology, Risk, & Protective Factors

An essential step in the public health model of prevention is the identification of risk and protective factors (Mercy et al., 1993). Data from twin studies, molecular genetics, and neuroimaging suggest the development and expression of psychopathy is, in part, the consequence of biology (Reidy et al., 2015; Viding & McCrory, 2018). Research across child, adolescent, and adult samples indicates psychopathic traits are moderately to strongly heritable and modestly influenced by environmental factors (Reidy et al., 2015; Viding & McCrory, 2018). Likewise, the *stability* of such traits over time is largely driven by genetic influence (Viding & McCrory, 2018). Twin studies further illustrate a strong genetic correlation between CU traits and antisocial behavior (including proactive aggression) whereas antisocial behavior absent of psychopathic traits is more strongly driven by environmental influences (Bezdjian et al., 2011; Taylor et al., 2003; Viding & McCrory, 2018). Psychopathic traits and behaviors are also associated with anomalies in a variety of brain regions including the amygdala, striatum, and prefrontal cortex (Blair, 2013; Reidy et al., 2015; Stratton et al., 2015; Viding & McCrory, 2018). These abnormalities appear to be highly similar across youth and adult samples and generally predict neurocognitive deficits in the affective responses to others' distress, decision-making, and reinforcement learning (e.g., Blair, 2013; Craig et al., 2009; Fairchild et al., 2011; Reidy et al., 2017; Viding & McCrory, 2018). Taken together, these lines of research suggest that genetic vulnerability influences the neurobiological profile and subsequent neurocognitive deficits associated with psychopathy, which in turn, bring about the adverse behavioral expressions (i.e., violence, substance use, crime, etc.) of psychopathy (Blair, 2013; Viding & McCrory, 2018).

However, as Blair (2013) notes, these neurocognitive dysfunctions alone will not establish the core features of psychopathy. A number of studies, both cross-sectional and longitudinal, have identified adverse family factors (e.g., high-conflict, harsh parenting, neglect, maternal psychopathology, mother attachment to child, etc.) as risk factors for psychopathy (Barker et al., 2011; Farrington, 2006; Lynam et al., 2008; Reidy et al., 2015). Likewise, substantial evidence indicates trauma exposure, abuse, and exposure to violence is positively associated with the degree of psychopathy traits in youth (Carlson et al., 2015; Howard et al., 2012; Kimonis et al., 2008, 2013, 2017; Krstic et al., 2016; Meffert et al., 2018). It is important to acknowledge that many of these risk factors may be confounded by genetic factors, including gene-environment correlations or interactions (Viding & McCrory, 2018). For example, using a longitudinal community sample of 4500+ twins, Viding et al. (2009) demonstrated that the association between harsh parenting and psychopathy traits reflected a shared genetic risk. Alternatively, some identified risk factors may be the consequence of parenting a callous-unemotional child (Hawes et al., 2011). Additionally, an individual's genetic predisposition influences the environments an individual seeks out and may modify the environment in which they exist (Jaffee & Price, 2007; Plomin et al., 1977). Therefore, it is possible that a genetic predisposition for psychopathic traits may create more hostile and conflict-filled interactions with parents, resulting in abuse by caregivers at greater intensity and frequency. Likewise, the tendency towards thrill-seeking and novelty associated with this genetic predisposition may lead these individuals to seek out dangerous situations that put them at risk for exposure to trauma. Thus, disentangling the true environmental etiological factors from genetic vulnerability for psychopathy is difficult.

It is widely believed that one's genome constrains their phenotypic expression, but it does not predetermine how they will turn out. In one study, Viding et al. (2009) reported that within MZ twin pairs, the twin receiving more negative parental discipline at 7 years had more conduct problems (but not more callous-unemotional traits) at 12 years. Thus, while the genetic vulnerability for psychopathy traits themselves was not impacted by parenting practices, the behavioral expression of those traits was altered. Additionally, adoption studies have shown that the level of antisocial behavior and fearlessness in the biological mother predicted early callous-unemotional features in toddlers who had been adopted; however, the use of positive reinforcement parenting practices by the adoptive mother buffered against the heritable risk for callous-unemotional features (Hyde et al., 2016; Waller et al., 2016). These findings are consistent with prior review of the treatment literature that indicated only interventions focused on positively reinforcing prosocial behavior were effective in preventing future violence by youth high in psychopathic traits (Reidy et al., 2013, 2015).

22.7 Community Response and Prevention

For the most part, community response and prevention efforts for psychopathy, and the burdens it imposes, are lacking. The current approach to mitigating the impact of psychopathy tends to be reactive rather than proactive, with society's primary response being incarceration. When treatment is implemented, it is most commonly forensic in nature, delivered to persons who have already been adjudicated (Reidy et al., 2013, 2015). However, incarceration is not a "cure" for psychopathy (or any social ailment) and it has no impact on those psychopathic individuals that manage to evade the criminal justice system. Nor does it address the burden posed by those in the general population manifesting sub-diagnostic levels of psychopathic traits. Moreover, it cannot abrogate the economic and health consequences that have already been rendered by such individuals. Thus, a shift toward community and population level strategies to *prevent* the sequelae of psychopathy *before they occur* is necessary. The public health model, in particular, focuses on the primary prevention of problematic behavior or illness before its onset (Mercy et al., 1993). In reference to psychopathy and its unfavorable outcomes, this means intervening early in life.

Increasing awareness of the health burden posed by psychopathy across the social ecology, and ultimately recognizing that psychopathy is a public health issue may stimulate work to develop primary prevention strategies. In fact, it is already known that juvenile antisocial behavior and delinquency is a health issue. The most severe and chronic delinquent offenders will go on to have the highest rates of illness, injury, hospitalization, disability, and premature death as adults (Piquero et al., 2007, 2011; Shepherd et al., 2009). Thus, youth with psychopathic traits, whose delinquent behavior tends to onset earlier and persist longer across the lifespan, reflect a public health burden not only through their impact on the health of others, but also based on their own adverse health outcomes. As such, researchers, practitioners, policy-makers etc. should be integrating a health vernacular into the discussion of psychopathy. There needs to be a shift in thinking pertaining to delinquency as a juvenile justice issue. Rather, viewing these behaviors through a public health lens may increase efficacy in motivating communities to engage in developing, implementing, and adequately funding an integrated set of individual-, family-, community-, and societal-level prevention strategies via a consortium of key agencies and stakeholders.

The transition between conceptualizing psychopathy as a criminal justice matter, as opposed to a public health matter, could be compared to the proliferation of public health efforts to address the opioid crisis. Whereas illegal drug use, such as use of opiates, has often been viewed and responded to as criminal behavior – taking a forensic perspective – significant efforts have been made to take a more public health oriented approach to opioid misuse and addiction, highlighting the prescribing, proliferation, and use of these drugs as a national public health crisis (Kolodny et al., 2015). The re-framing of opioid use away from a solely forensic lens and toward a public health perspective has included a re-imagining of national vocabulary surrounding drug use. The rise of opioid misuse has been characterized, not as a crisis of moral character, but as an "epidemic," co-opting health-oriented language in order to emphasize the public health risks and impacts of opioid use (Franklin et al., 2015; Volkow et al., 2014). In a related vein, the seemingly exponential rise of mass shootings in schools and public venues has contributed to the framing of gun violence as a public health issue by physicians, researchers, and subsequently (some) politicians (Cook, 2018; Hemenway & Miller, 2013; H.R. 1114, 2019).

Applying a similar framing to psychopathy could help inspire opportunities to prevent the associated harmful public-health sequelae.

To be clear, it is not our contention that the violent, criminal, or harmful behavior of individuals with psychopathy should be excused as an uncontrollable consequence of their "illness." Nor do we argue that these individuals should be immune from prosecution and incarceration if they do commit such violations of socially acceptable behavior. These are questions and debates beyond our competencies. Rather, we are suggesting a more holistic integration and utilization of both the public health and forensic systems to curb the population burden of psychopathy. For example, public health applies a "systems" approach that is broad and inclusive, engaging as many people and institutions as possible to build coalitions that reinforce one another (Hemenway & Miller, 2013). Recognizing that many of these youth begin as victims themselves either by witnessing violence or through direct victimization (Carlson et al., 2015; Howard et al., 2012; Kimonis et al., 2008, 2013, 2017; Krstic et al., 2016; Meffert et al., 2018), agencies such as child protective services, foster care, family courts, and youth detention centers among others, could partner together to develop coordinated community responses (e.g., Goldman et al., 2003) that provide multiple successive and overlapping opportunities for intervention that may prevent or mitigate the adverse behavioral expressions of psychopathy. A particular strength of the public health system is the ability to coordinate multi-disciplinary and multi-sectoral efforts, and its role in assuring the availability of services for victims (Krug et al., 2002b).

Of course, no single effort or strategy is sufficient. In their discussion of the public health model for violence prevention, Mercy et al. (1993) note that a coordinated and sustained effort at all levels of the social ecology is necessary to curb the spread of violence. The same is true for the health burdens imposed by psychopathy. From a public health approach, this involves changing social norms (Hemenway & Miller, 2013; Mercy et al., 1993), not just about how the problem of psychopathy is viewed, but norms surrounding contributory etiological factors. For example, given what is known about the exacerbating effect of harsh and physical parenting strategies on the phenotypic expression of psychopathic traits (e.g., Hyde et al., 2016; Viding et al., 2009; Waller et al., 2016), social norms campaigns to reduce the use of physical punishment (e.g., Durrant, 1996; Taylor et al., 2011) may be an important prevention strategy for psychopathy. At a complementary institutional level, a public health model might involve ensuring the widespread dissemination and adoption of empirically informed best practices for shaping prosocial behavior among youth by school administrators and staff. The evidence base on reinforcement learning and conditioning among youth with psychopathic traits (Reidy et al., 2017) suggests that this would involve advancing behavioral strategies that minimize a focus on punishing deviant behavior and emphasize explicitly rewarding prosocial behavior. This same strategy could be (and often is) implemented with parent training resources. These strategies have already demonstrated some efficacy with youth scoring high psychopathy traits (Reidy et al., 2013, 2017). In fact, effective responsive interventions such as Mendota Juvenile Treatment Center (MJTC: Caldwell,

2011; Caldwell et al. 2006a, b, 2007, 2012) could potentially be adapted and implemented as effective primary prevention strategies.

The main philosophical principles of the MJTC are the reduction of sanctions for negative behavior and the implementation of a type of token economy to positively reinforce prosocial behavior. In other treatment models, the use of punitive sanctions for violent and disruptive behavior often results in expulsion or temporary removal from treatment programs, which paradoxically reinforces the undesired behavior. At the MJTC, when increased security measures are required, a concomitant increase in individualized treatment contact occurs precluding negative reinforcement of disruptive behavior. The MJTC appears to shift reinforcement from negative behaviors to the desired prosocial behaviors: the program relies on a system of rapidly increasing incentives for positive interpersonal functioning, behavioral control, and participation in treatment (see Caldwell & Van Rybroek, 2005 for more details). The MJTC, which has demonstrated efficacy in preventing violent recidivism among severely violent psychopathic youth, would likely be even more efficacious if implemented sooner, before these youth have accumulated and started to become entrenched in delinquency. Such a prevention strategy could be adapted for implementation in schools with more recalcitrant youth that affect the learning and well-being of other students. Such a strategy may influence the school-to-prison pipeline (Heitzeg, 2009; Wald & Losen, 2003) thereby increasing educational attainment, employment opportunity and stability, and subsequent access to social determinants of health (Apel & Sweeten, 2010; CDC, 2013; Tanner et al., 1999).

Obviously, these examples are extremely rudimentary and not intended as the proposed solutions to psychopathy and its harmful effects. The goal is not to lay out what a public health prevention approach to psychopathy would look like in specificity here. At this stage, this cannot be known. However, shifting perspective from a primarily criminal justice orientation to an integrated public health perspective will likely offer new opportunities, methods, and resources to abate this societal issue.

22.8 Conclusions

The true nature and burden of psychopathy will remain unknown as long as we continue to address the issue as though it is solely a criminal justice problem. We propose that psychopathy is likewise a public health problem influencing the health and well-being of individuals across the social ecology. While the burdens and health consequences imposed by the many acts of violence committed by psychopathic individuals are self-evident, not all psychopathic individuals are violent. Yet, they may still adversely influence the health and well-being of others through their potential to corrupt social norms and values, especially if they are in positions of power or leadership. We believe viewing psychopathy through a public health lens will stimulate population based epidemiological studies that allow us to determine accurate prevalence rates of psychopathic traits in the general population and reveal the true magnitude of the impact of psychopathy on health in the general population. Furthermore, we suspect this will advance knowledge about potentially modifiable risk and protective factors; possibly elucidate those factors that have the most salience for altering the maladaptive phenotypic expression of psychopathy; and ultimately inform the development of prevention efforts and where we should target such efforts.

References

Aharoni, E., & Kiehl, K. A. (2013). Evading justice: Quantifying criminal success in incarcerated psychopathic offenders. *Criminal Justice and Behavior, 40*, 629–645.

Alterman, A. I., Cacciola, J. S., & Rutherford, M. J. (1993). Reliability of the revised psychopathy checklist in substance abuse patients. *Psychological Assessment, 5*, 442–448.

Andershed, H., Kerr, M., Stattin, H., & Levander, S. (2002). Psychopathic traits in non-referred youths: Initial test of a new assessment tool. In E. Blaauw, J. M. Philippa, K. C. M. P. Ferenschild, & B. van Lodensteijn (Eds.), *Psychopaths: Current international perspectives* (pp. 131–158). Elsevier.

Apel, R., & Sweeten, G. (2010). The impact of incarceration on employment during the transition to adulthood. *Social Problems, 57*, 448–479.

Babiak, P., Neumann, C. S., & Hare, R. D. (2010). Corporate psychopathy: Talking the walk. *Behavioral Sciences & the Law, 28*, 174–193.

Barker, E. D., Oliver, B. R., Viding, E., Salekin, R. T., & Maughan, B. (2011). The impact of prenatal maternal risk, fearless temperament and early parenting on adolescent callous-unemotional traits: A 14-year longitudinal investigation. *Journal of Child Psychology and Psychiatry, 52*, 878–888.

Bezdjian, S., Raine, A., Baker, L. A., & Lynam, D. R. (2011). Psychopathic personality in children: Genetic and environmental contributions. *Psychological Medicine, 41*, 589–600.

Blair, R. J. R. (2013). The neurobiology of psychopathic traits in youths. *Nature Reviews Neuroscience, 14*, 786–799.

Blair, J., Mitchell, D., & Blair, K. (2005). *The psychopath: Emotion and the brain*. Blackwell Publishing.

Boddy, C. R. (2010). Corporate psychopaths and organizational type. *Journal of Public Affairs, 10*, 300–312.

Boddy, C. R. (2011). The corporate psychopaths theory of the global financial crisis. *Journal of Business Ethics, 102*, 255–259.

Boddy, C. R. (2014). Corporate psychopaths, conflict, employee affective well-being and counterproductive work behavior. *Journal of Business Ethics, 121*, 107–121.

Boddy, C. R., Ladyshewsky, R., & Galvin, P. (2010a). Leaders without ethics in global business: Corporate psychopaths. *Journal of Public Affairs, 10*, 121–138.

Boddy, C. R., Ladyshewsky, R. K., & Galvin, P. (2010b). The influence of corporate psychopaths on corporate social responsibility and organizational commitment to employees. *Journal of Business Ethics, 97*, 1–19.

Bronfenbrenner, U. (1977). Toward an experimental ecology of human development. *American Psychologist, 32*, 513.

Caldwell, M. F. (2011). Treatment related changes in behavioral outcomes of psychopathy facets in adolescent offenders. *Law and Human Behavior, 35*, 275–287.

Caldwell, M. F., & Van Rybroek, G. J. (2005). Reducing violence in serious juvenile offenders using intensive treatment. *International Journal of Law & Psychiatry, 28*, 622–636.

Caldwell, M. F., Skeem, J. L., Salekin, R. L., & Van Rybroek, G. J. (2006a). Treatment response of adolescent offenders with psychopathy features: A two-year follow-up. *Criminal Justice and Behavior, 33*, 571–596.

Caldwell, M. F., Vitacco, M., & Van Rybroek, G. J. (2006b). Are violent delinquent worth treating? A cost-benefit analysis. *Journal of Research in Crime & Delinquency, 43*, 148–168.

Caldwell, M. F., McCormick, D. J., Umstead, D., & Van Rybroek, G. J. (2007). Evidence of treatment progress and therapeutic outcomes among adolescents with psychopathic features. *Criminal Justice and Behavior, 34*, 573–587.

Caldwell, M. F., McCormick, D. J., Wolfe, J., & Umstead, D. (2012). Treatment related changes in psychopathy features and behavior in adolescent offenders. *Criminal Justice and Behavior, 39*, 144–155.

Carlson, M., Oshri, A., & Kwon, J. (2015). Child maltreatment and risk behaviors: The roles of callous/unemotional traits and conscientiousness. *Child Abuse & Neglect, 50*, 234–243.

Centers for Disease Control & Prevention. (2016). *Preventing multiple forms of violence: A strategic vision for connecting the dots*. Division of Violence Prevention, National Center for Injury Prevention & Control, Centers for Disease Control & Prevention.

Centers for Disease Control and Prevention. (2013). CDC health disparities and inequalities report – United States, 2013. *Morbidity and Mortality Weekly Report, 62*(Suppl 3), 1–186.

Centers for Disease Control and Prevention. (n.d.). *Web-based injury statistics query and reporting system (WISQARS)*. Retrieved from http://www.cdc.gov/injury/wisqars

Chang, S. S., Stuckler, D., Yip, P., & Gunnell, D. (2013). Impact of 2008 global economic crisis on suicide: Time trend study in 54 countries. *BMJ, 347*, f5239.

Christian, R. E., Frick, P. J., Hill, N. L., Tyler, L., & Frazer, D. R. (1997). Psychopathy and conduct problems in children: Implications for subtyping children with conduct problems. *Journal of the American Academy of Child & Adolescent Psychiatry, 36*, 233–241.

Cleckley, H. (1941). *The mask of sanity: An attempt to reinterpret the so-called psychopath*. The C.V. Mosby Company.

Cleckley, H. (1976). *The mask of sanity* (5th ed.). Mosby.

Coid, J., & Yang, M. (2008). The distribution of psychopathy among a household population: Categorical or dimensional? *Social Psychiatry and Psychiatric Epidemiology, 43*, 773–781.

Coid, J., & Yang, M. (2011). The impact of psychopathy on violence among the household population of Great Britain. *Social Psychiatry and Psychiatric Epidemiology, 46*, 473–480.

Cook, P. J. (2018). Expanding the public health approach to gun violence prevention. *Annals of Internal Medicine, 169*, 723–724.

Cornell, D. G., Warren, J., Hawk, G., Stafford, E., Oram, G., & Pine, D. (1996). Psychopathy in instrumental and reactive violent offenders. *Journal of Consulting and Clinical Psychology, 64*, 783–790.

Craig, M. C., Catani, M., Deeley, Q., Latham, R., Daly, E., Kanaan, R., Picchioni, M., McGuire, P. K., Fahy, T., & Murphy, D. G. (2009). Altered connections on the road to psychopathy. *Molecular Psychiatry, 14*, 946–907.

Dahlberg, L. D. (2007). Public health and violence: Moving forward in a global perspective. In D. J. Flannery, A. T. Vazsonyi, & I. D. Waldman (Eds.), *The Cambridge handbook of violent behavior and aggression* (pp. 465–485). Cambridge University Press.

DeMatteo, D., Heilbrun, K., & Marczyk, G. (2006). An empirical investigation of psychopathy in a noninstitutionalized and noncriminal sample. *Behavioral Sciences & the Law, 24*, 133–146.

Drislane, L. E., Brislin, S., Kendler, K., Andershed, H., Larsson, H., & Patrick, C. J. (2014a). A triarchic model analysis of the youth psychopathic traits inventory. *Journal of Personality Disorders, 28*, 1–27.

Drislane, L. E., Patrick, C. J., & Arsal, G. (2014b). Clarifying the content coverage of differing psychopathy inventories through reference to the Triarchic psychopathy measure. *Psychological Assessment, 26*, 350–362.

Durrant, J. E. (1996). The Swedish ban on corporal punishment: Its history and effects. In D. Frehsee, W. Horn, & K. D. Bussmann (Eds.), *Family violence against children* (pp. 19–25). Walter de Gruyter and.

Fairchild, G., Passamonti, L., Hurford, G., Hagan, C. C., von dem Hagen, E. A., van Goozen, S. H., Goodyer, I. M., & Calder, A. J. (2011). Brain structure abnormalities in early-onset and adolescent-onset conduct disorder. *The American Journal of Psychiatry, 168*, 624–633.

Farrington, D. P. (2006). Family background and psychopathy. In C. J. Patrick (Ed.), *Handbook of psychopathy* (pp. 229–250). The Guilford Press.

Fattori, A., Neri, L., Aguglia, E., et al. (2015). Estimating the impact of workplace bullying: Humanistic and economic burden among workers with chronic medical conditions. *BioMed Research International*. https://doi.org/10.1155/2015/708908

Fersch, E. (2006). *Thinking about psychopaths and psychopathy*. iUniverse. Forth.

Forth, A. E., Kosson, D. S., & Hare, R. D. (2003). *The Hare PCL:YV*. Multi-Health Systems.

Franklin, G., Sabel, J., Jones, C. M., Mai, J., Baumgartner, C., Banta-Green, C. J., Nevin, D., & Tauben, D. J. (2015). A comprehensive approach to address the prescription opioid epidemic in Washington state: Milestones and lessons learned. *American Journal of Public Health, 105*, 463–469.

Frick, P. J. (2004). *Inventory of callous-unemotional traits*. Unpublished rating scale, University of New Orleans.

Frick, P. J., & Hare, R. (2001). *Antisocial process screening device*. Multi-Health Systems.

Frick, P. J., & White, S. F. (2008). Research review: The importance of callous-unemotional traits for developmental models of aggressive and antisocial behavior. *Journal of Child Psychology & Psychiatry, 49*, 359–375.

Friis, R. H., & Sellers, T. A. (2014). *Epidemiology for public health practice*. Jones & Bartlett Publishers.

Gatner, D. T., Blanchard, A. J., Douglas, K. S., Lilienfeld, S. O., & Edens, J. F. (2018). Psychopathy in a multiethnic world: Investigating multiple measures of psychopathy in Hispanic, African American, and Caucasian offenders. *Assessment, 25*, 206–221.

Goldman, J., Salus, M. K., Wolcott, D., & Kennedy, K. Y. (2003). *A coordinated response to child abuse and neglect: The foundation for practice*. US Department of Health and Human Services, Administration for Children and Families, Administration on Children, Youth and Families, Children's Bureau, Office on Child Abuse and Neglect.

Guay, J. P., Ruscio, J., Knight, R. A., & Hare, R. D. (2007). A taxometric analysis of the latent structure of psychopathy: Evidence for dimensionality. *Journal of Abnormal Psychology, 116*, 701–716.

Guay, J. P., Knight, R. A., Ruscio, J., & Hare, R. D. (2018). A taxometric investigation of psychopathy in women. *Psychiatry Research, 261*, 565–573.

Haan, M., Kaplan, G. A., & Camacho, T. (1987). Poverty and health prospective evidence from the alameda county study. *American Journal of Epidemiology, 125*, 989–998.

Hansen, Å. M., Hogh, A., Persson, R., Karlson, B., Garde, A. H., & Ørbaek, P. (2006). Bullying at work, health outcomes, and physiological stress response. *Journal of Psychosomatic Research, 60*, 63–72.

Hare, R. D. (1991). *The Hare psychopathy checklist—Revised manual*. Multi-Health Systems.

Hare, R. D. (1996). Psychopathy: A clinical construct whose time has come. *Criminal Justice and Behavior, 23*, 25–54.

Hare, R. D. (2002). *The predators among us*. Keynote address. Canadian Police Association Annual General Meeting, St. John's, Newfoundland and Labrador, August 27, 2002.

Hare, R. D. (2003). *The Hare psychopathy checklist—Revised (PCL–R) manual* (2nd ed.). Multi-Health Systems.

Hare, R., & Neumann, C. (2010). The role of antisociality in the psychopathy construct: Comment on Skeem and Cooke (2010). *Psychological Assessment, 22*, 446–454.

Harpur, T. J., Hare, R. D., & Hatskian, A. R. (1989). Two-factor conceptualization of psychopathy: Construct validity and assessment implications. *Psychological Assessment: A Journal of Consulting and Clinical Psychology, 56*, 741–747.

Hart, S. D., Kropp, P. R., & Hare, R. D. (1988). Performance of male psychopaths following conditional release from prison. *Journal of Consulting and Clinical Psychology, 56*, 227–232.

Hart, S. D., Cox, D. N., & Hare, R. D. (1995). *Manual for the psychopathy checklist: Screening version (PCL: SV)*. Multi-Health Systems.

Hawes, D. J., Dadds, M. R., Frost, A. D., & Hasking, P. A. (2011). Do childhood callous-unemotional traits drive change in parenting practices? *Journal of Clinical Child & Adolescent Psychology, 40*, 507–518.

Heitzeg, N. A. (2009). Education or incarceration: Zero tolerance policies and the school to prison pipeline. In *Forum on public policy online*. (Vol. 2009, No. 2). Oxford Round Table.

Hemenway, D., & Miller, M. (2013). Public health approach to the prevention of gun violence. *New England Journal of Medicine, 368*, 2033–2035.

H.R. 1114, 116th Congress. (2019). House Bill to require the Surgeon General of the Public Health Service to submit to Congress an annual report on the effects of gun violence on public health

Howard, A. L., Kimonis, E. R., Muñoz, L. C., & Frick, P. J. (2012). Violence exposure mediates the relation between callous-unemotional traits and offending patterns in adolescents. *Journal of Abnormal Child Psychology, 40*, 1237–1247.

Howe, J., Falkenbach, D., & Massey, C. (2014). The relationship among psychopathy, emotional intelligence, and professional success in finance. *International Journal of Forensic Mental Health, 13*, 337–347.

Hyde, L. W., Waller, R., Trentacosta, C. J., Shaw, D. S., Neiderhiser, J. M., Ganiban, J. M., Reiss, D., & Leve, L. D. (2016). Heritable and nonheritable pathways to early callous-unemotional behaviors. *American Journal of Psychiatry, 173*, 903–910.

Jaffee, S. R., & Price, T. S. (2007). Gene–environment correlations: A review of the evidence and implications for prevention of mental illness. *Molecular Psychiatry, 12*, 432–442.

Khubchandani, J., & Price, J. H. (2015). Workplace harassment and morbidity among US adults: Results from the National Health Interview Survey. *Journal of Community Health, 40*, 555–563.

Kiehl, K. A., & Hoffman, M. B. (2011). The criminal psychopath: History, neuroscience, treatment, and economics. *Jurimetrics, 51*, 355–397.

Kimonis, E. R., Frick, P. J., Munoz, L. C., & Aucoin, K. J. (2008). Callous-unemotional traits and the emotional processing of distress cues in detained boys: Testing the moderating role of aggression, exposure to community violence, and histories of abuse. *Development and Psychopathology, 20*, 569–589.

Kimonis, E. R., Fanti, K. A., Isoma, Z., & Donoghue, K. (2013). Maltreatment profiles among incarcerated boys with callous-unemotional traits. *Child Maltreatment, 18*, 108–121.

Kimonis, E. R., Fanti, K. A., Frick, P. J., Moffitt, T. E., Essau, C., Bijttebier, P., & Marsee, M. A. (2015). Using self-reported callous-unemotional traits to cross-nationally assess the DSM-5 "With limited prosocial emotions" specifier. *The Journal of Child Psychology & Psychiatry, 56*, 1249–1261.

Kimonis, E. R., Fanti, K. A., Goulter, N., & Hall, J. (2017). Affective startle potentiation differentiates primary and secondary variants of juvenile psychopathy. *Development and Psychopathology, 29*, 1149–1160.

Kolodny, A., Courtwright, D. T., Hwang, C. S., Kreiner, P., Eadie, J. L., Clark, T. W., & Alexander, G. C. (2015). The prescription opioid and heroin crisis: A public health approach to an epidemic of addiction. *Annual Review of Public Health, 36*, 559–574.

Kraepelin, E. (1915). *Psychiatrie. Lehrbuch fur Studeierende und Arzte* [Psychiatry. A Textbook for students and physicians] Band IV, (8th ed., Vol. 4). Barth.

Krstic, S., Knight, R. A., & Robertson, C. A. (2016). Developmental antecedents of the facets of psychopathy: The role of multiple abuse experiences. *Journal of Personality Disorders, 30*, 677–693.

Krug, E. G., Dahlberg, L. L., Mercy, J. A., Zwi, A. B., & Lozano, R. (Eds.). (2002a). *World report on violence and health*. World Health Organization.

Krug, E. G., Mercy, J. A., Dahlberg, L. L., & Zwi, A. B. (2002b). The world report on violence and health. *The Lancet, 360*(9339), 1083–1088.

Lee, Z., & Salekin, R. T. (2010). Psychopathy in a noninstitutional sample: Differences in primary and secondary subtypes. *Personality Disorders: Theory, Research, and Treatment, 1*, 153–169.

Li, J., Zhang, M., Loerbroks, A., Angerer, P., & Siegrist, J. (2015). Work stress and the risk of recurrent coronary heart disease events: A systematic review and meta-analysis. *International Journal of Occupational Medicine and Environmental Health, 28*, 8–19.

Lilienfeld, S. O. (1994). Conceptual problems in the assessment of psychopathy. *Clinical Psychology Review, 14*, 17–38.

Lingnau, V., Fuchs, F., & Dehne-Niemann, T. E. (2017). The influence of psychopathic traits on the acceptance of white-collar crime: Do corporate psychopaths cook the books and misuse the news? *Journal of Business Economics, 87*, 1193–1227.

Loeber, R., Burke, J. D., & Pardinin, D. A. (2009). Development and etiology of disruptive and delinquent behavior. *Annual Review of Clinical Psychology, 5*, 291–310.

Lopez Bernal, J. A., Gasparrini, A., Artundo, C. M., & McKee, M. (2013). The effect of the late 2000s financial crisis on suicides in Spain: An interrupted time-series analysis. *The European Journal of Public Health, 23*, 732–736.

Luckhaupt, S. E., Cohen, M. A., Li, J., & Calvert, G. M. (2014). Prevalence of obesity among US workers and associations with occupational factors. *American Journal of Preventive Medicine, 46*, 237–248.

Lynam, D. R. (1996). Early identification of chronic offenders: Who is the fledgling psychopath? *Psychological Bulletin, 120*, 209–234.

Lynam, D. R. (1997). Pursuing the psychopath: Capturing the fledgling psychopath in a nomological net. *Journal of Abnormal Psychology, 106*, 425–438.

Lynam, D. R., & Gudonis. (2005). The development of psychopathy. *Annual Review of Clinical Psychology, 1*, 381–407.

Lynam, D. R., Loeber, R., & Stouthamer-Loeber, M. (2008). The stability of psychopathy from adolescence into adulthood: The search for moderators. *Criminal Justice and Behavior, 35*, 228–243.

Martin, W., & LaVan, H. (2010). Workplace bullying: A review of litigated cases. *Employee Responsibilities and Rights Journal, 22*, 175–194.

Mathieu, C., Neumann, C. S., Hare, R. D., & Babiak, P. (2014). A dark side of leadership: Corporate psychopathy and its influence on employee well-being and job satisfaction. *Personality and Individual Differences, 59*, 83–88.

McCord, W., & McCord, J. (1964). *The psychopath: An essay on the criminal mind*. Van Nostrand.

McCoy, W. K., & Edens, J. F. (2006). Do black and white youths differ in levels of psychopathic traits? A meta-analysis of the psychopathy checklist measures. *Journal of Consulting and Clinical Psychology, 74*, 386–392.

McMahon, R. J., Witkiewitz, K., Kotler, J. S., & the Conduct Problems Prevention Research Group. (2010). Predictive validity of callous-unemotional traits measured in early adolescence with respect to multiple antisocial outcomes. *Journal of Abnormal Psychology, 119*, 752–763.

Meffert, H., Thornton, L. C., Tyler, P. M., Botkin, M. L., Erway, A. K., Kolli, V., Pope, K., White, S. F., & Blair, R. J. R. (2018). Moderation of prior exposure to trauma on the inverse relationship between callous-unemotional traits and amygdala responses to fearful expressions: An exploratory study. *Psychological Medicine, 48*, 2541–2549.

Mercy, J. A., Rosenberg, M. L., Powell, K. E., Broome, C. V., & Roper, W. L. (1993). Public health policy for preventing violence. *Health Affairs, 12*, 7–29.

Merikangas, K. R., He, J., Burstein, M., Swanson, S. A., Avenevoli, S., Cui, L., Benjet, C., Georgiades, K., & Swendsen, J. (2010). Lifetime prevalence of mental disorders in U.S. adolescents: Results from the National Comorbidity Survey Replication – Adolescent supplement. *Journal of the Academy of Child & Adolescent Psychiatry, 49*, 980–989.

Moore, M. H. (1995). Public health and criminal justice approaches to prevention. In M. T. Tonry & D. P. Farrington (Eds.), *Building a safer society: Strategic approaches to crime prevention*. University of Chicago Press.

Murrie, D. C., Marcus, D. K., Douglas, K. S., Lee, Z., Salekin, R. T., & Vincent, G. (2007). Youth with psychopathy features are not a discrete class: A taxometric analysis. *Journal of Child Psychology & Psychiatry, 48*, 714–723.

Neumann, C. S., & Hare, R. D. (2008). Psychopathic traits in a large community sample: Links to violence, alcohol use, and intelligence. *Journal of Consulting and Clinical Psychology, 76*, 893.

Nikulina, V., Widom, C. S., & Czaja, S. (2011). The role of childhood neglect and childhood poverty in predicting mental health, academic achievement and crime in adulthood. *American Journal of Community Psychology, 48*(3–4), 309–321.

Nock, M. K., Kazdin, A. E., Hiripi, E., & Kessler, R. C. (2006). Prevalence, correlates, and subtypes of DSM-IV Conduct Disorder in the national comoribidity survey replication. *Psychological Medicine, 36*, 699–710.

Patrick, C. J., & Drislane, L. E. (2015). Triarchic model of psychopathy: Origins, operationalizations, and observed linkages with personality and general psychopathology. *Journal of Personality, 83*, 627–643.

Patrick, C. J., Fowles, D. C., & Krueger, R. F. (2009). Triarchic conceptualization of psychopathy: Developmental origins of disinhibition, boldness, and meanness. *Development and Psychopathology, 21*, 913–938.

Patrick, C., Drislane, L. E., & Strickland, C. (2012). Conceptualizing psychopathy in triarchic terms: Implications for treatment. *International Journal of Forensic Mental Health, 11*, 253–266.

Perenc, L., & Radochonski, M. (2014). Psychopathic traits and reactive-proactive aggression in a large community sample of polish adolescents. *Child Psychiatry & Human Development, 45*, 464–471.

Peterson, C., DeGue, S., Florence, C., & Lokey, C. N. (2017). Lifetime economic burden of rape among US adults. *American Journal of Preventive Medicine, 52*, 691–701.

Peterson, C., Florence, C., & Klevens, J. (2018a). The economic burden of child maltreatment in the United States, 2015. *Child Abuse & Neglect, 86*, 178–183.

Peterson, C., Kearns, M. C., McIntosh, W. L., Estefan, L. F., Nicolaidis, C., McCollister, K. E., Gordon, A., & Florence, C. (2018b). Lifetime economic burden of intimate partner violence among US adults. *American Journal of Preventive Medicine, 55*, 433–444.

Piquero, A. R., Daigle, L. E., Gibson, C., Piquero, N. L., & Tibbetts, S. G. (2007). Research note: Are life-course-persistent offenders at risk for adverse health outcomes? *Journal of Research in Crime and Delinquency, 44*, 185–207.

Piquero, A. R., Shepherd, I., Shepherd, J. P., & Farrington, D. P. (2011). Impact of offending trajectories on health: Disability, hospitalisation and death in middle-aged men in the Cambridge study in delinquent development. *Criminal Behaviour and Mental Health, 21*, 189–201.

Plomin, R., DeFries, J. C., & Loehlin, J. C. (1977). Genotype-environment interaction and correlation in the analysis of human behavior. *Psychological Bulletin, 84*, 309–322.

Ragatz, L., Fremouw, W., & Baker, E. (2012). The psychological profile of white-collar offenders: Demographics, criminal thinking, psychopathic traits, and psychopathology. *Criminal Justice and Behavior, 39*, 978–997.

Ray, J. V., & Jones, S. (2011). Self-reported psychopathic traits and their relation to intentions to engage in environmental offending. *International Journal of Offender Therapy and Comparative Criminology, 55*, 370–391.

Reidy, D. E., Shelley-Tremblay, J. F., & Lilienfeld, S. O. (2011). Psychopathy, reactive aggression, and precarious proclamations: A review of behavioral, cognitive, and biological research. *Aggression and Violent Behavior, 16*, 512–524.

Reidy, D. E., Kearn, M. C., & DeGue, S. (2013). Reducing psychopathic violence: A review of the treatment literature. *Aggression and Violent Behavior, 18*, 527–538.

Reidy, D. E., Kearns, M. C., DeGue, S., Lilienfeld, S. O., Massetti, G., & Kiehl, K. A. (2015). Why psychopathy matters: Implications for public health and violence prevention. *Aggression and Violent Behavior, 24*, 214–225.

Reidy, D. E., Krusemark, E., Kosson, D. S., Kearns, M. C., Smith-Darden, J., & Kiehl, K. A. (2017). The development of severe and chronic violence among youth: The role of psychopathic traits and reward processing. *Child Psychiatry & Human Development, 48*, 967–982.

Reidy, D. E., Bogen, K. W., & Lilienfeld, S. O. (2019a). The impact of youth with psychopathic traits on public health: A social-ecological perspective. In M. G. Vaughn, C. P. Salas-Wright, & D. B. Jackson (Eds.), *The international handbook of delinquency & health*. Routledge.

Reidy, D. E., Lilienfeld, S. O., Berke, D. S., Gentile, B., & Zeichner, A. (2019b). Psychopathy traits and violent assault among men with and without history of arrest. *Journal of Interpersonal Violence, 12*, 2438–2457.

Schneider, K. (1958). *Psychopathic personalities* (9th ed.). Cassell.

Shepherd, J. P., Shepherd, I., Newcombe, R. G., & Farrington, D. (2009). Impact of antisocial lifestyle on health: Chronic disability and death by middle age. *Journal of Public Health, 31*, 506–511.

Singleton, N., Lee, A., & Meltzer, H. (2002). *Psychiatric morbidity among adults living in private households, 2000*: Technical Report.

Skeem, J. L., & Cooke, D. J. (2010a). Is criminal behavior a central component of psychopathy? Conceptual directions for resolving the debate. *Psychological Assessment, 22*, 433.

Skeem, J. L., & Cooke, D. J. (2010b). One measure does not a construct make: Directions toward reinvigorating psychopathy research–reply to Hare and Neumann (2010). *Psychological Assessment, 22*, 455.

Skeem, J. L., Edens, J. F., Camp, J., & Colwell, L. H. (2004). Are there ethnic differences in levels of psychopathy? A meta-analysis. *Law and Human Behavior, 28*, 505–527.

Somma, A., Borroni, S., Drislane, L. E., & Fossati, A. (2016). Assessing the triarchic model of psychopathy in adolescence: Reliability and validity of the Triarchic Psychopathy Measure (TriPM) in three samples of Italian community-dwelling adolescents. *Psychological Assessment, 28*, e36–e48.

Stansfeld, S., & Candy, B. (2006). Psychosocial work environment and mental health—A meta-analytic review. *Scandinavian Journal of Work, Environment & Health, 32*, 443–462.

Strand, S., & Belfrage, H. (2005). Gender differences in psychopathy in a Swedish offender sample. *Behavioral Sciences & the Law, 23*, 837–850.

Stratton, J., Kiehl, K. A., & Hanlon, R. E. (2015). The neurobiology of psychopathy. *Psychiatric Annals, 45*, 186–194.

Stuckler, D., Basu, S., Suhrcke, M., Coutts, A., & McKee, M. (2009). The public health effect of economic crises and alternative policy responses in Europe: An empirical analysis. *The Lancet, 374*(9686), 315–323.

Sullivan, E. A., Abramowitz, C. S., Lopez, M., & Kosson, D. S. (2006). Reliability and construct validity of the psychopathy checklist-revised for Latino, European American, and African American male inmates. *Psychological Assessment, 18*, 382–392.

Tanner, J., Davies, S., & O'Grady, B. (1999). Whatever happened to yesterday's rebels? Longitudinal effects of youth delinquency on education and employment. *Social Problems, 46*, 250–274.

Taylor, J., Loney, B. R., Bobadilla, L., Iacono, W. G., & McGue, M. (2003). Genetic and environmental influences on psychopathy trait dimensions in a community sample of male twins. *Journal of Abnormal Child Psychology, 31*, 633–645.

Taylor, C. A., Hamvas, L., Rice, J., Newman, D. L., & DeJong, W. (2011). Perceived social norms, expectations, and attitudes toward corporal punishment among an urban community sample of parents. *Journal of Urban Health, 88*, 254–269.

Thacker, S. B., Stroup, D. F., Carande-Kulis, V., Marks, J. S., Roy, K., & Gerberding, J. L. (2006). Measuring the public's health. *Public Health Reports, 121*, 14–22.

Theorell, T., Hammarström, A., Aronsson, G., Träskman Bendz, L., Grape, T., Hogstedt, C., Marteinsdottir, I., Skoog, I., & Hall, C. (2015). A systematic review including meta-analysis of work environment and depressive symptoms. *BMC Public Health, 15*, 738.

Tokarev, A., Phillips, A. R., Hughes, D. J., & Irwing, P. (2017). Leader dark traits, workplace bullying, and employee depression: Exploring mediation and the role of the dark core. *Journal of Abnormal Psychology, 126*, 911–920.

Vachon, D. D., Lynam, D. R., Loeber, R., & Stouthamer-Loeber, M. (2012). Generalizing the nomological network of psychopathy across populations differing on race and conviction status. *Journal of Abnormal Psychology, 121*, 263–269.

Vaughn, M. G., Salas-Wright, C. P., DeLisi, M., & Maynard, B. R. (2014). Violence and externalizing behavior among youth in the United States: Is there a severe 5%? *Youth Violence and Juvenile Justice, 12*, 3–21.

Verkuil, B., Atasayi, S., & Molendijk, M. L. (2015). Workplace bullying and mental health: A meta-analysis on cross-sectional and longitudinal data. *PLoS One, 10*(8), e0135225.

Viding, E., & McCrory, E. J. (2018). Understanding the development of psychopathy: Progress and challenges. *Psychological Medicine, 48*, 566–577.

Viding, E., Fontaine, N. M., Oliver, B. R., & Plomin, R. (2009). Negative parental discipline, conduct problems and callous–unemotional traits: Monozygotic twin differences study. *The British Journal of Psychiatry, 195*, 414–419.

Vincent, G. M., Vitacco, M. J., Grisso, T., & Corrado, R. R. (2003). Subtypes of adolescent offenders: Affective traits and antisocial behavior patterns. *Behavioral Sciences & the Law, 21*, 695–712.

Vitale, J. E., Smith, S. S., Brinkley, C. A., & Newman, J. P. (2002). The reliability and validity of the psychopathy checklist–revised in a sample of female offenders. *Criminal Justice and Behavior, 29*, 202–231.

Volkow, N. D., Frieden, T. R., Hyde, P. S., & Cha, S. S. (2014). Medication-assisted therapies—Tackling the opioid-overdose epidemic. *New England Journal of Medicine, 370*, 2063–2066.

Volmer, J., Koch, I. K., & Göritz, A. S. (2016). The bright and dark sides of leaders' dark triad traits: Effects on subordinates' career success and well-being. *Personality and Individual Differences, 101*, 413–418.

Wald, J., & Losen, D. J. (2003). Defining and redirecting a school-to-prison pipeline. *New Directions for Youth Development, 2003*, 9–15.

Waller, R., Trentacosta, C. J., Shaw, D. S., Neiderhiser, J. M., Ganiban, J. M., Reiss, D., Leve, L. D., & Hyde, L. W. (2016). Heritable temperament pathways to early callous–unemotional behaviour. *The British Journal of Psychiatry, 209*, 475–482.

Watson, G. W., Teaque, B. T., & Papamarcos, S. D. (2017). Functional psychopathy in morally relevant business decisions. *Ethics & Behavior, 27*, 458–485.

World Health Organization. Public health surveillance. *WHO*. N.p., n.d. Web. 31 July 2014. http://www.who.int/topics/public_health_surveillance/en/

Wynn, R., Høiseth, M. H., & Pettersen, G. (2012). Psychopathy in women: Theoretical and clinical perspectives. *International Journal of Women's Health, 4*, 257–263.

Index

J. E. Vitale (ed.), *The Complexity of Psychopathy*, Dangerous Behavior in Clinical and Forensic Psychology, https://doi.org/10.1007/978-3-030-83156-1

B

C

R